AF745298

Food and Cancer

Food and Cancer

Food and Cancer

Edited by

Sheetanshu Gupta
Department of Food Safety and Quality Assurance, College of Food Technology, Central Agricultural University (CAU), Imphal, Manipur, India

Sarfraj Ahmad Siddiqui
Department of Biochemistry,
King George's Medical University, U.P., India

Praneeth Juvvi
Department of Food Processing Technology, College of Food Technology, Central Agricultural University, Imphal, Manipur, India

Ng. Joykumar Singh
Department of Food Process Engineering, College of Food Technology, Central Agricultural University (CAU), Imphal, Manipur, India

Lokesh Kumar Mishra
Department of BPME, College of Agriculture,
Central Agricultural University (CAU), Imphal, Manipur, India

-EPH-
Elite Publishing House

CRC Press
Taylor & Francis Group
Boca Raton London New York

CRC Press is an imprint of the
Taylor & Francis Group, an **informa** business

First published 2027
by CRC Press
4 Park Square, Milton Park, Abingdon, Oxon, OX14 4RN

and by CRC Press
2385 NW Executive Center Drive, Suite 320, Boca Raton FL 33431

CRC Press is an imprint of Informa UK Limited

© 2026 2027 selection and editorial matter, Sheetanshu Gupta, Sarfraj Ahmad Siddiqui, Praneeth Juvvi, Ng. Joykumar Singh, Lokesh Kumar Mishra; individual chapters, the contributors

The right of Sheetanshu Gupta, Sarfraj Ahmad Siddiqui, Praneeth Juvvi, Ng. Joykumar Singh, Lokesh Kumar Mishra to be identified as the authors of the editorial material, and of the authors for their individual chapters, has been asserted in accordance with sections 77 and 78 of the Copyright, Designs and Patents Act 1988.

All rights reserved. No part of this book may be reprinted or reproduced or utilised in any form or by any electronic, mechanical, or other means, now known or hereafter invented, including photocopying and recording, or in any information storage or retrieval system, without permission in writing from the publishers.

For permission to photocopy or use material electronically from this work, access www.copyright.com or contact the Copyright Clearance Center, Inc. (CCC), 222 Rosewood Drive, Danvers, MA 01923, 978-750-8400. For works that are not available on CCC please contact mpkbookspermissions@tandf.co.uk

For Product Safety Concerns and Information please contact our EU representative GPSR@taylorandfrancis.com. Taylor & Francis Verlag GmbH, Kaufingerstraße 24, 80331 München, Germany.

Trademark notice: Product or corporate names may be trademarks or registered trademarks, and are used only for identification and explanation without intent to infringe.

Print edition not for sale in India

British Library Cataloguing-in-Publication Data
A catalogue record for this book is available from the British Library

ISBN: 9781041371649 (hbk)
ISBN: 9781041378808 (pbk)
ISBN: 9781042010387 (ebk)

DOI: 10.1201/9781042010387

Typeset in A Caslon Pro
by Elite Publishing House

-EPH-

Contents

Preface

Eating has served as ritual and solace deeply within human culture since the dawn of civilization, perhaps negotiating mortality silently and profoundly. Ancient healers instinctively grasped that consumed substances profoundly shaped health long before microbiology or molecular biology existed, often phrasing it crudely. Genuine scientific puzzles and fragmented data obscured this age-old connection as the complexities of the human body and its diseases became clearer, particularly in the enigmatic field of cancer pathology. Cancer casts a darkly ominous shadow across modern life eerily. Its presence pervades myriad existences, igniting deep within humans a fundamental yearning for comprehension and total eradication of painful suffering.

Food emerges as a focal point once again in this rather arduous quest. Intuitively, our food choices feel like a potent lever against this behemoth, largely fueling our very being with the necessary blocks and energy. Yet a vexing enigma remains very persistently, namely how formidable it actually proves in certain rather obscure contexts. Does it serve as shield or sword, or just some feeble crutch born of utter desperation and abject hopelessness? Popular press outlets veer wildly between outlandish pronouncements of miracle remedies and scornful doubt, leaving people bewildered amidst a deluge of contradictory counsel. The book The Food and Cancer endeavors earnestly through a complex, often strongly contradictory landscape with considerable trepidation and some treacherous uncharted territory. Not a tome of disparate dietary regimens nor a collection of folksy success stories gathered haphazardly over years. A mosaic woven from threads of rigorous research contributed by experts from diverse disciplines globally is presented with meticulous curation. Our aim is very much to debunk prevalent myths and illuminate the underlying mechanisms behind cancer development while presenting current evidence-based understanding very thoroughly. Journeying into this realm unfolds sporadically downwards in unpredictably meandering paths beneath surface expectations of linearity.

Enzymes frantically break down complex molecules with every single bite while nutrients get absorbed and transported through various bodily pathways. Against such a backdrop, cancer initiation and progression, a disease rooted deeply in cellular chaos, becomes a canvas painted subtly by dietary choices. Such strokes may foster cellular harmony or contribute inadvertently down a path of cancerous cellular transformation with chaotic consequences lurking beneath. Grasping such intricate relationships necessitates venturing fairly deep into the realms of molecular biology and epidemiology alongside clinical immunology practice. This edited volume serves quite effectively as a compass navigating readers through rather uncharted territory on that odyssey.

Certain dietary components and patterns offer protective benefits while others pose significant risks amidst complex dose-response relationships and considerable individual variability. Cutting-edge research on carcinogenesis is explored in this book, focusing on the gut microbiome's mediating role in dietary effects very thoroughly. It probes the complex interplay between diet and immune system rather deeply, and epigenetic tweaks caused by food intake are also examined thoroughly alongside the latest clinical trial results guiding dietary advice for cancer sufferers.

Conversation around food and cancer has been grossly dichotomized for far too long, veering wildly between reductionist platitudes and generalized wishy-washy guidance. Food and Cancer endeavors rather quietly to bridge such a gap. A diverse audience will find it useful, including seasoned researchers seeking a broad overview of recent developments and postgraduate students embarking on discovery journeys. Editors must curate a vast array of expertise very carefully, ensuring scientific rigor and clarity while judiciously including impactful research findings often. We have endeavored vehemently to present a narrative bursting with sheer scientific savvy yet still riveting and mind-bending, inviting readers ponder deeply the evidence marshalled in support of the ongoing pursuit of knowledge.

Each chapter stands as a testament to the dedication of authors who painstakingly summarized vast bodies of literature and distilled years of research into concise arguments. Contributions from them sit squarely at the heart of this hefty volume, offering quite a fascinating glimpse into oncology's nutritional frontiers nowadays. Science being an evolving tapestry by its very nature, this book hardly constitutes a final word on the subject matter. Novel findings surface rapidly nowadays, refining existing frameworks and drastically altering the perception of reality every single day. Food and Cancer embodies a crucial juncture in human understanding, presented with hopes of sparking savvy choices and fostering research effectively worldwide against cancer.

Editors

About the Editors

Dr. Sheetanshu Gupta is currently working as an Assistant Professor (Plant Biochemistry) at the College of Food Technology, Central Agriculture University, Imphal, Manipur. Earlier, he was Examiner of Patents and Design (Gazetted A Officer) in the Ministry of Commerce at the IPO office in Delhi. He was an alumnus of G.B. Pant University of Agriculture & Technology, Pantnagar, Uttarakhand, India, from the last 13 years. Dr Gupta completed his PhD (Biochemistry) in 2011 from G.B. Pant University of Agriculture & Technology, Pantnagar, Uttarakhand, India. He cleared ICAR ARS NET (Plant Biochemistry and Plant Physiology) and CSIR NET. Dr. Gupta gained valuable experience in the areas of environmental problems, aeroponics and hydroponics, and protein biochemistry. His work showcased his expertise in applying innovative farming techniques and exploring novel approaches to plant protection. Dr. Gupta researched on tissue culture hydroponics and mushroom farming, contributing to the advancement of these fields. Dr. Gupta's academic qualifications, research experience, and expertise in biochemistry and biotechnology make him a valuable asset in the field. With his passion for teaching and research, dedication to innovative farming techniques, and student advocacy, Dr. Gupta continues to contribute significantly to the advancement of agricultural and biochemical sciences with more than 35 published books, more than 250 chapters, and nearly 23 Research/ Review papers.

Dr. Sarfraj Ahmad Siddiqui is a Young Scientist in ICMR DHR at the Department of Biochemistry, King George's Medical University, U.P., India. He has completed his M, Sc. in Biotechnology from Allahabad University and Ph.D degrees in Biotechnology with specialization in Animal biology, Neurobiology from Babasaheb Bhimrao Ambedkar University, Lucknow, India in 2018. Dr. Sarfraj served as a Postdoctoral fellow at University of Lucknow for 3 years between 2019-2022, followed by a Young Scientist at KGMU. Dr. Sarfraj has 8 book chapters, 12 Research papers, and 2 awards to his credit. He has presented papers in over 15 conferences/seminars/workshops, etc., both with national and international importance. He is also a recipient of several national and international awards.

Dr. Praneeth Juvvi is currently working as an Assistant Professor (Food Processing Technology) at the College of Food Technology, Central Agricultural University (CAU), Imphal, Manipur. He holds a Ph.D. in Food Technology from CSIR-Central Food Technological Research Institute (CFTRI), Mysuru, an M.Tech. in Food Engineering and Technology from SLIET, Punjab, and a B.Tech. in Food Science from ANGRAU, Bapatla, Andhra Pradesh. He has qualified for the ICAR-ASRB-NET (2014) in Food Technology and cleared the GATE examination in Engineering Sciences twice, with All India Rank 163rd in 2009 and 295th in 2011. Dr. Praneeth has over five years of research experience at CFTRI, where he contributed to the design and development of innovative food processing equipment, process optimization for healthy snack production, and quality analysis using advanced instrumentation. He has authored multiple peer-reviewed research articles, holds a patent, and has received several best poster awards at national and international conferences. His academic and research efforts continue to advance innovation and capacity-building in the field of food technology.

Dr. Ng. Joykumar Singh obtained his B Tech Agricultural Engineering degree from Dharward Agricultural University (UAS) Karnataka, in 1994, M Tech Agricultural Processand Food Engineering from University of Agricultural University (UAS), Bangalore (1996) and PhD in Process and Food Engineering from GBPUAT, Pantnagar (2009 in-service). Dr. Joykumar started his career as teaching faculty in the Agricultural Engineering Division, College of Agriculture, Central Agricultural University, Imphal, since 2001 till date.

Dr. Joykumar has been actively involved in teaching, research and extension for the last 20 years. He has been granted 5 patents till date. He has many external aided research projects funded by DST, DBT, Ministry of Science and Technology, Govt. of India. He is also heading the AICRP on Post-harvest Engineering and Technology, CAU, Imphal, as Principal Investigator. He has more than 25 publications (including 20 research papers in reputed National & International journals, and proceedings of seminar/workshops/book chaptersand many bulletins in the field of Post-harvest Technology). His broad research areas are design and development of small/medium food processing machines which are eco-friendly and drudgery-free, value addition of fruits and vegetables. He was involved in development of various value-added products from the locally available and underutilized fruits. He has also received the 'Distinguished award in the field of Agricultural Engineering, Best Centre performance Award of AICRP-PHET, and best paper presentation awards in National Seminars.

Dr Lokesh Kumar Mishra obtained his Post-Graduate and Doctorate degree in Biochemistry from Narendra Deva University of Agriculture and Technology, Faizabad, Uttar Pradesh. The dissertation work of the author focused on the impact of fertilizers on the nutritional components of the cereal crops, mainly wheat. He started his academic career as Assistant Professor in Biochemistry at ND University, Faizabad. He later served as Assistant Professor at VBS Purvanchal University, Jaunpur, UP. Presently, he is working as Professor (Biochemistry) at Central Agricultural University, Imphal, Manipur. He is involved in teaching Biochemistry for the last fourteen years. The author has also handled research projects funded by different agencies of the Government of India. The focus of these projects is metabolic profiling of the indigenous food products of North East India and the development of new products utilizing the biodiversity of the NE India. He has authored several research papers and review articles in International and National Journals of repute and is associated with many national and international Societies in the field of Plant Biochemistry. The Author worked as DBT Overseas Visiting Associate at Department of Plant Sciences North Dakota State University, Fargo, United States. The focus of the research at North Dakota State University was the exploration of phenolic-linked antioxidant activities of food systems for health promotion and combating metabolic syndromes like type-2 diabetes and hypertension. In recognition of his work in the field of medicinal plants and agricultural research and development, he has been awarded a fellowship for the year 2019 by the International Society of Noni Science, Chennai.

Chapter 1

Dietary Intervention and Oncogenesis: Foundational Principles

Sarfraj Ahmad Siddiqui[1], Sheetanshu Gupta[2], Praneeth Juvvi[3], and Lokesh Kumar Mishra[4*]

[1]Department of Biochemistry, King George's Medical University, U.P., India
[2]Department of Food Safety and Quality Assurance, College of Food Technology, Central Agricultural University (CAU), Imphal, Manipur, India
[3]Department of Food Processing Technology, College of Food Technology-Central Agricultural University, Imphal, Manipur, India
[4]Department of BPME, College of Agriculture, Central Agricultural University (CAU), Imphal, Manipur, India

Abstract

Dietary factors influence oncogenesis significantly, with mounting evidence suggesting interventions can alter cancer risk substantially in recent years. The Foundational This provide a comprehensive exploration of the underlying mechanisms through which diet influences cancer development and prevention thoroughly. Cellular metabolism unravels rather slowly as fats and micronutrients mingle with signalling pathways amidst inflamed genetic instability and quirky protein structures. Gut microbiome's role gets explored thoroughly, highlighting its considerable impact on cancer risk and potential as a target for novel dietary strategies. Emerging data on dietary patterns such as plant-based diets and Mediterranean diets, along with calorie restriction, are reviewed alongside their effects on oncogenesis in preclinical studies and clinical trials. Effective dietary strategies for cancer prevention and therapy are formulated considering genetic predispositions, microbiome composition, and various lifestyle factors very carefully nowadays.

Keywords: Dietary Intervention, Oncogenesis, Cancer Prevention, Tumour Microenvironment, Nutrient-Sensitive Pathways, Chemoprevention

1. Introduction

Scientific inquiry has extensively scrutinized human health impacts stemming from varied dietary patterns over long periods, rather thoroughly nowadays. Cancer development remains deeply entangled with dietary factors in modern times and poses significant challenges to healthcare systems globally nowadays. Research

DOI: 10.1201/9781042010387-1

into dietary intervention influencing oncogenesis has emerged as a vital field drawing heavily on nutrition science and molecular biology insights lately. Uncovering strategies for cancer prevention and management hinges on grasping how dietary factors mesh with various genetic and lifestyle variables. The diet and cancer connection involves myriad intricate mechanisms directly and indirectly through various bodily processes and external factors simultaneously (Nagy et al, 2023; Pal et al, 2012).

Oncogenesis unfolds via multiple convoluted steps entailing subtle alterations at genetic and epigenetic levels and metabolic pathways, resulting in abnormal cells proliferating uncontrollably. Diet impacts various stages of this process very significantly, from initiation of genetic mutations and the promotion of tumour metastasis, rather quickly. Certain foods and nutrients trigger cancer risk via inflammation and oxidative stress, while others potentially reduce risk or halt malignant cell progression entirely. Nutritional modulation underlies a key foundational principle linking diet and oncogenesis fundamentally within complex biological systems. Nutrients like vitamins and phytochemicals heavily influence cellular processes in very complex ways that can either vigorously support or significantly hinder cancer development (Koya and Ibrahim, 2024; Dakal et al, 2020).

Dietary antioxidants counteract oxidative stress that contributes rather heavily to DNA damage and carcinogenesis, while specific fatty acids regulate cell membrane integrity, somewhat crucially for tumour progression. Diets heavy in processed food and saturated fats foster an environment ripe for chronic disease, including cancer development, quite readily nowadays. Duality highlights a critical need for balanced evidence-based dietary intervention remarkably. Growing recognition of gut microbiome as a vital component in cancer biology has recently opened fresh avenues for assiduous research endeavors nowadays (Reuter et al, 2010; Jiang et al, 2021). Gut microbiota plays a significant role in maintaining immune function deeply inside the human body, modulating inflammation and influencing various metabolic pathways erratically. Gut microbiome disruptions caused by an imbalanced diet or factors like antibiotics and chronic stress have been associated with various cancer forms recently. Evidence abounds suggesting dietary tweaks ranging from gorging on fibrous veggies and whole grains or ditching junk food altogether can recalibrate gut bacteria very significantly, thereby lowering the odds of getting cancer. Inflammation plays a crucial role in comprehending links between dietary habits and cancer development. Diet plays a critical role in modulating inflammatory processes while chronic low-grade inflammation drives cancer quite relentlessly nowadays (Randeni et al, 2024; Wu and Wu, 2012).

Diets heavy with pro-inflammatory foods like red meat and sugary drinks can crank up inflammatory pathways and spur tumourigenesis rapidly. Anti-inflammatory diets typically comprising copious fruits, vegetables, whole grains, and healthy fats may counteract such deleterious effects and foster cancer prevention. Obesity serves as a key risk factor for various cancers like breast cancer, pancreatic cancer and colorectal cancer, tied closely to metabolic state. Precision nutrition emerges as a crucial concept underlying dietary intervention strategies in cancer prevention and its treatment effectively nowadays. This approach acknowledges impact of diet on oncogenesis varies greatly depending on individual genetic predispositions and existing health issues or cancer subtypes (Yu et al, 2024; Scheiber and Mank, 2023).

Personalized dietary strategies become remarkably effective when nutritional interventions are cleverly tailored according to genetic profiles and molecular characteristics of patients. Advances in nutritional genomics alongside personalized oncology medicine hold promise for a more cohesive cancer care strategy with dietary interventions deeply embedded in treatment regimens (Singar et al, 2024). Evidence increasingly suggests that dietary interventions play crucial roles in cancer management and treatment alongside prevention-focused research endeavors. Cancer patients frequently undergo drastic weight loss and muscle wasting alongside severe nutritional deficiencies that adversely impact various treatment outcomes significantly. Dietary changes might somewhat effectively alleviate the nasty side effects of chemo very significantly, and boost overall well-being remarkably. Emerging studies explore the potential of ketogenic diets or caloric restriction in cancer progression and improving responses quite significantly to conventional therapies (Mittelman SD, 2020). The principles of dietary intervention and oncogenesis necessitate acknowledgement of rapidly evolving nuances within this fairly complex field nowadays. Substantial progress has been made, but challenges are still very deeply entrenched in translating basic research into actual clinical practice. Human metabolism's intricate nature and cancer's heterogeneous manifestations, alongside dietary interplay with various lifestyle factors, render the formulation of universal guidelines rather arduous. This chapter provides a foundation for grasping molecular and cellular mechanisms whereby diet affects cancer development, alongside emerging clinical applications holding promise.

2. Oncogenesis: Mechanisms and Molecular Pathways

Oncogenesis involves normal cells morphing into cancerous ones through a convoluted multi-step process driven by genetic and epigenetic factors alongside environmental influences. Tumour cells bypass normal regulatory mechanisms of growth, survival and differentiation quite readily, leading to proliferative chaos and very much uncontrolled metastatic spread. Mechanisms underlying oncogenesis are ridiculously complex, involving gnarly signalling pathways, genomic mutations, epigenetic changes and interactions within the tumour microenvironment, quite dynamically. Oncogenesis is driven by complex molecular pathways that facilitate the acquisition of malignancy hallmarks in cancer cells through various deeply rooted biological processes (Pedraza-Fariña LG, 2006; Cheng and O'Neill, 2009).

2.1. Genetic Mutations and the Hallmarks of Cancer

Oncogenesis unfolds as normal cells mutate into cancerous entities via a tortuous multistage pathway fueled by genetic aberrations and stochastic epigenetic perturbations. Tumour cells quite readily eschew normal regulatory mechanisms of growth and survival leading to proliferative chaos and wildly uncontrolled metastatic spread. Gnarly signaling pathways and genomic mutations intricately interact within tumour microenvironment fostering oncogenesis extremely dynamically through multiple epigenetic changes. Malignancy hallmarks are acquired in cancer cells via deeply rooted biological processes driven by intricate molecular pathways fostering oncogenesis robustly (Sorscher et al, 2009; Pedraza-Fariña LG, 2006).

2.2. Oncogenes and Tumour Suppressors

Oncogenesis occurs quite haphazardly at the molecular level driven by dysregulation of oncogenes and tumour suppressor genes, rather rapidly. Mutated forms of normal genes called proto-oncogenes get overexpressed, driving cell growth excessively in rather abnormal and quite frantic manners. Activation of an oncogene results from various point mutations or gross amplifications, and sometimes chromosomal translocations occur simultaneously. Noteworthy instances of oncogenes are MYC and HER2 whereas some archetypes comprise RAS and EGFR in various cancerous tissues obviously. Genes like these frequently encode proteins deeply embedded in cell signalling cascades regulating cell proliferation, differentiation and survival mechanisms simultaneously. Mutated, they push cells into frenzied unregulated proliferation, thereby significantly contributing to oncogenesis (Dakal et al, 2024; Stojchevski et al, 2025). Tumour suppressor genes act as brakes on cell proliferation very aggressively and survival mechanisms get thwarted somewhat effectively. Mutated or inactivated genes lose regulatory functions leading very much to unchecked growth and survival of cells rather haphazardly. Tumour suppressor genes like TP53 and BRCA2 are deeply embedded in processes including cell cycle regulation and DNA repair mechanisms. Loss of p53 function often dubbed genome guardian results in inability to repair damaged DNA or kickstart apoptosis allowing cells with shaky genomic integrity to thrive (Abreu et al, 2015; Joyce et al, 2023).

2.3. Signaling Pathways in Oncogenesis

Changes occur very frequently in numerous crucial signaling pathways during oncogenesis unfolding rapidly in fairly complex biological processes. Various cellular processes like growth survival differentiation and metabolism are governed by these pathways somewhat irregularly. Key pathways driving oncogenesis encompass PI3K/AKT/mTOR pathway which promotes cellular survival metabolism and growth in various cancers very frequently. Mutations or amplification of genes like PIK3CA AKT and mTOR encoding pathway components lead to downstream signaling activation enhancing cell survival.

RAS/RAF/MEK/ERK Pathway: The RAS family of small GTPases, including KRAS, NRAS, and HRAS, are often mutated in various cancers. RAS/RAF/MEK/ERK pathway involves KRAS NRAS and HRAS small GTPases frequently mutated in diverse cancer types very obviously. Mutations trigger RAS-RAF-MEK-ERK signaling cascade involved in cell proliferation differentiation and survival very vigorously (Song et al, 2022).

Wnt/β-catenin Pathway: The Wnt signaling pathway regulates cell fate determination, proliferation, and stem cell renewal. RAS mutations occur frequently in pancreatic cancers and colon malignancies and sometimes in lung tumours too apparently. Wnt signaling pathway intricately governs cell fate determination and proliferation alongside stem cell renewal via β-catenin mediation extremely effectively (He and Gan, 2023).

TGF-β Signaling: Transforming Growth Factor-beta (TGF-β) plays a dual role in cancer. Wnt ligands bind Frizzled receptors triggering accumulation of β-catenin in cytoplasm which subsequently translocates into nucleus initiating gene expression there. Aberrant Wnt pathway activation manifests frequently in cancers notably colorectal malignancies harbouring APC gene mutations that severely disrupt β-catenin regulation (Song et al, 2022).

Notch Signalling: The Notch pathway regulates cell fate decisions, and its dysregulation has been implicated in various cancers. Transforming Growth Factor-beta plays a rather complex dual role in cancer progression and sometimes surprisingly in tumour suppression mechanisms.

2.4. Genomic Instability and Mutagenesis

Genomic instability manifests aberrantly in cancer cells, resulting from defects in machinery maintaining genomic integrity largely beneath cellular surface. Failure of the DNA damage response fuels genomic instability rampantly in cancer cells, largely due to unrepaired DNA lesions accumulating rapidly. Genetic mutations in ATM BRCA1 and MRE11 disrupt DNA damage response pathways fostering accumulation of chromosomal aberrations that drive oncogenic processes rapidly. Defects in DNA repair mechanisms such as mismatch repair or base excision repair, can lead rather quickly to accumulation of mutations driving cancer. Genomic instability in tumours fosters rapid evolution of cancer cells fairly quickly acquiring mutations that confer growth advantages and evade immune surveillance (Yoshioka et al, 2021; Bartek J., 2011).

2.5. Tumour Microenvironment and Oncogenesis

The tumour microenvironment (TME) is a dynamic and complex environment composed of various cell types, extracellular matrix components, and signaling molecules that interact with the tumour cells. TME plays crucial roles in tumour progression and metastasis and often fuels angiogenesis quite vigorously and immune evasion too. Tumour cells often manipulate the TME to create a favorable environment for their survival and proliferation. Tumours get oxygen and nutrients via angiogenesis and employ sneaky immune evasion mechanisms that help them dodge detection by immune system cells. Stroma comprising fibroblasts macrophages and endothelial cells often furtively secretes various growth factors and cytokines promoting proliferation and invasion of cancer cells (Anderson and Simon, 2020; Biray et al, 2024).

2.6. Metastasis: The Final Stage of Oncogenesis

Cancer cells spread haphazardly to distant organs in a critically important process that significantly worsens patient prognosis very drastically. Molecular mechanisms underlying metastasis intricately involve numerous steps including invasion into surrounding tissue and intravasation into bloodstream quite rapidly. Molecular players crucial in metastasis encompass E-cadherin regulating cell adhesion and matrix metalloproteinases degrading extracellular matrix facilitating tumour cell invasion vigorously. Oncogenesis involves myriad genetic mutations and signaling pathways disrupted in tumour microenvironments with very complex interactions occurring rapidly therein (Martin et al, 2013). Cancer cells hijack normal bodily functions rather haphazardly and spread quickly through tissues far away from original sites. Grasping such underlying mechanisms thoroughly is crucial for devising novel treatments that target peculiar molecular pathways and thwart cancer hallmarks effectively. Our grasp of oncogenesis's molecular underpinnings deepens remarkably and fosters designing super effective personalized cancer treatments quite rapidly nowadays (Cooper GM, 2000).

3. The Role of Nutrition in Cancer Development and Progression

Cancer persists as a top cause of morbidity globally and remains a significant factor in mortality rates worldwide nowadays. Genetics influences cancer susceptibility significantly but a increasing amount of research implies nutrition and dietary factors pivotally drive cancer initiation and progression. Estimates indicate dietary factors heavily influence almost 30-40% of all cancer cases underscoring a crucial link between nutrition and cancer. Diet impacts cancer in myriad ways with both salubrious and pernicious effects on cellular processes like DNA mending and cell division rapidly. Nutrition plays a strongly complex role in cancer development and progression with diet influencing myriad stages of cancer biology (Anand et al, 2008).

3.1. Nutrition and Carcinogenesis: Initiation and Promotion

Malignant cells emerge through a intricate multi-step process fuelled by genetic mutations and drastic alterations in surrounding tissue. Process breaks down quite haphazardly into three main stages namely initiation promotion and then surprisingly progression occurs afterwards effectively. Cells undergo genetic mutations very frequently during initiation phase often triggered by exposure to weird carcinogenic substances that damage DNA directly. Mutations spawned by environmental stressors like tobacco radiation or specific dietary components kickstart cancer development fairly quickly sometimes. Certain dietary constituents can function as both potent carcinogens and anticarcinogenic agents simultaneously in human bodies under various circumstances (Koya and Ibrahim, 2025).

Foods loaded with processed meats saturated fats and refined sugars ramp up cancer risk by fostering inflammation and oxidative stress deeply. Nitrosamines lurking in processed meats like bacon or sausages are known carcinogens capable of triggering mutations in DNA leading cancer. Heterocyclic amines and polycyclic aromatic hydrocarbons formed during grilling or frying meat have been linked to increased risk of various cancers. Certain bioactive compounds found in plant-based foods conversely thwart cancer initiation by neutralizing carcinogens or promoting cellular DNA repair mechanisms vigorously. Fruits and vegetables contain flavonoids and carotenoids that exhibit strong antioxidant properties helping scavenge free radicals and protect DNA from oxidative damage (Santarelli et al, 2008).

Cruciferous veggies like broccoli and kale contain glucosinolates which are thought to detoxify carcinogens and inhibit enzyme activity facilitating carcinogenesis heavily. Promotion phase begins subsequently after initiation occurs. Cells with prior mutations proliferate rapidly often due to actions of growth factors or changes in surrounding tissue very quickly nowadays. Obesity, increasingly prevalent in modern societies stands out as a significant dietary risk factor promoting various types of cancer effectively nowadays (Esteve M., 2020). Excess adiposity fuels chronic low-grade inflammation and ramps up insulin levels while boosting estrogen production which can promote cancer. Increased insulin-like growth factor signaling observed in obese individuals can enhance cell growth vigorously and proliferation occurs rapidly meanwhile adipokines released by fat cells alter immune responses favouring tumour progression (Kim DS, Scherer et al, 2021).

3.2. Nutritional Factors in Tumour Progression and Metastasis

Tumours evolve and acquire more genetic alterations and interact with surrounding tissue enabling uncontrollable growth and spreading into other body parts via metastasis. Nutrition plays a crucially important role in cancer progression at this stage, influencing tumour cell behavior and ability to colonize distant tissues quite significantly. Omega-6 fatty acids lurking in corn oil and sunflower oil can badly exacerbate inflammation, driving tumour progression very quickly. Omega-3 fatty acids found in fatty fish and walnuts have profoundly anti-inflammatory effects and may curtail cancer spread by altering tumour behavior drastically. Emerging evidence suggests lipid metabolism plays a crucial role in tumour growth and metastasis, particularly in breast, colon and prostate cancer (Martin et al, 2013).

Tumours develop their own blood supply very quickly and metastasize through angiogenesis a critical aspect of cancer progression. Extensive studies have been done on dietary compounds regulating angiogenesis deeply. Phytonutrients like curcumin found in turmeric and catechins abundant in green tea have been shown quite effectively to inhibit vascular endothelial growth factor. Compounds effectively thwart formation of new vasculature thereby stunting tumour growth and subsequent metastasis in various bodily tissues quite rapidly. Microorganisms residing in human gut have surfaced as key instigators in cancer progression fairly recently alongside other obscure health factors (Lugano et al, 2020). Dysbiosis or gut microbiota imbalance has been linked rather tenuously to elevated risk of several cancers, including very aggressive colorectal cancer. Diets rich in fibre and fermented foods heavily promote a healthy gut microbiome which can modulate immune responses rather effectively and reduce nasty inflammation. A diet replete with processed food and saccharine delights fosters the growth of pro-inflammatory bacteria thereby contributing significantly to tumour progression.

3.3. Nutrition and Immune Modulation in Cancer

Cancers evolve sneaky mechanisms quite rapidly to evade detection by a person's immune system which plays a crucial role in eliminating tumour cells. Diet profoundly impacts cancer immune surveillance either encourage immune system's ability to sniff out and annihilate tumour cells or crippling it allowing tumours to flourish vigorously. Vitamin D and zinc profoundly modify immune function and may thwart cancer development by encourage immune responses quite effectively. Vitamin D has been shown to exhibit profoundly anti-inflammatory properties and regulate expression of genes involved heavily in cell apoptosis and growth (Kim and Cho, 2022). Antioxidants present abundantly in various fruits and veggies can help maintain redox balance in certain immune cells thereby greatly enhancing their ability quite remarkably to recognize tumour cells and respond accordingly. Dietary patterns rich in saturated fats and refined carbs can induce immune suppression fostering growth of tumour cells quite readily and create pro-inflammatory environments. Diets ridiculously high in sugar spur production of advanced glycation end products which sabotage immune cell function and foster chronic inflammation very badly (Rahaman et al, 2020).

3.4. Dietary Interventions for Cancer Prevention and Therapy

Growing interest in nutritional interventions stems largely from understanding nutrition's role in cancer development and its potential to thwart cancer progression and recurrence. Caloric restriction and intermittent fasting show considerable promise in preclinical research and some early stage clinical trials by markedly slowing the growth of tumours and improving the efficacy of chemotherapy and radiation therapy. Plant-based diets rich in fruits, vegetables, whole grains and legumes garner growing recognition nowadays for cancer-protective properties. These diets furnish a trove of bioactive compounds and antioxidants that synergistically quell inflammation and abet DNA repair in immune system support (Mercier et al, 2022).

Mediterranean diets rich in healthy fats from olive oil, nuts and fatty fish have been linked with reduced risks of various cancers, particularly digestive system malignancies. Nutrition therapy plays an essential role in cancer treatment on the clinical side everywhere nowadays. Dietitians and nutritionists collaborate with oncologists ensuring cancer patients maintain peak nutrition during treatment addressing side effects like dysgeusia and nausea, preventing weight loss and muscle wasting cachexia often seen in advanced cancer stages. Nutrition plays a pivotal role in cancer development and progression through various mechanisms including modulation of cellular signaling and immune function rather quietly (Mentella et al, 2019). Some dietary factors may heighten cancer risk while others confer protection, potentially thwarting carcinogenesis or retarding tumour growth significantly over time. Research will progressively reveal links between diet metabolism and cancer biology and the role of nutrition in cancer prevention becomes increasingly vital (Donaldson MS, 2004). Promoting healthier dietary patterns at the population level and integrating nutritional interventions into cancer care offers a promising strategy for improving public health outcomes significantly.

4. Key Nutrients and Their Impact on Tumourigenesis

Nutrition plays a crucial albeit often overlooked role in tumourigenesis, profoundly influencing initiation and metastatic spread of various cancer types. Evidence increasingly suggests key nutrients such as carbohydrates, proteins and fats or vitamins minerals, and phytochemicals can either spur or thwart cancer development, depending on type quantity and consumption context. Specific dietary components profoundly affect molecular pathways involved in cell proliferation DNA repair, inflammation and immune function during tumourigenesis. A balanced diet replete with protective nutrients can mitigate cancer risk yet certain dietary imbalances may foster the development of various malignancies (Haskins et al, 2020).

4.1. Antioxidant Vitamins and Their Role in Tumourigenesis

Vitamins A, C and E are widely known for their antioxidant properties, which help neutralize free radicals very effectively and reduce oxidative stress a factor in initiation of various cancers. Oxidative stress stems from an imbalance between the generation of reactive oxygen species and bodily ability to detoxify reactive radicals, ultimately cancer.

Vitamin A (Retinoids): Vitamin A and its active metabolites, including retinoic acid, play an essential role in regulating cell growth, differentiation, and apoptosis. Vitamin A and its active metabolites, including retinoic acid, play an essential role in regulating cell growth, differentiation and apoptosis. Retinoic acid modulates gene expression crucially in cellular differentiation, preventing unbridled cell proliferation fairly effectively under normal conditions (Zasada and Budzisz, 2019).

Vitamin C: Vitamin C (ascorbic acid) is a potent antioxidant that scavenges free radicals and protects cells from oxidative damage. Vitamin A deficiency boosts risk of cervical and lung cancers while supplementation curbs breast and prostate cancer development by fostering tumour cell differentiation and inhibiting metastasis quite effectively. Vitamin C or ascorbic acid powerfully scavenges free radicals thereby protecting cells from oxidative damage with considerable efficacy. It plays a crucial role in DNA repair and synthesizing collagen very effectively for maintaining healthy immune function basically (Kaźmierczak-Barańska et al, 2020).

Vitamin E: Vitamin E, particularly in its form of alpha-tocopherol, protects cellular membranes from oxidative damage and plays a role in regulating gene expression involved in cell growth and immune function. High doses of vitamin C possibly exhibit anticancer properties particularly when administered alongside other therapeutic regimens or interventions quite effectively. Cytotoxic effects of chemotherapy get a considerable boost from it especially in breast cancer and pancreatic cancer cells becoming super sensitive (Rizvi et al, 2014).

4.2. Minerals and Tumourigenesis

Minerals like selenium and zinc play crucial roles in various bodily functions including DNA repair and cellular metabolism quite effectively. Their influence on cancer development manifests diversely some acting as antioxidants while others potentially exacerbate oxidative damage or spark inflammation upon excessive consumption.

Selenium: Selenium is an essential trace mineral with antioxidant properties that protect cells from oxidative damage. Selenium possesses antioxidant properties that shield cells from oxidative stress and damage remarkably well under various physiological conditions. Selenium is a crucial constituent of enzyme glutathione peroxidase that neutralizes reactive oxygen species very effectively inside cells. Selenium potentially reduces risk of prostate lung and colorectal cancers through regulating cell apoptosis and inhibiting angiogenesis quite effectively (Tinggi U, 2008).

Zinc: Zinc plays an essential role in DNA repair, cell proliferation, and immune function. Supplementation with selenium has shown some promise in various clinical trials although effects vary wildly depending on baseline selenium status and form consumed. Zinc plays an essential role in DNA repair cell proliferation and immune function. It plays a crucial role in function of numerous enzymes and transcription factors and deficiency has been tenuously linked to increased DNA damage and cancer (Yildiz et al, 2019).

Iron: Iron is critical for cellular metabolism and oxygen transport, but its role in cancer is more controversial. Zinc supplementation exhibits profoundly protective effects against various cancers, including oesophageal cancer, prostate cancer, and oral cancer quite remarkably. Excessive zinc intake potentially messes with copper absorption, leading to wonky immune function and ramping up cancer risk very significantly. Iron plays a crucial role in cellular metabolism and oxygen transport, but its involvement in cancer development remains rather contentious nowadays. Iron plays a role in generating ROS during oxidative metabolism, which can badly damage DNA and heighten mutagenesis risk substantially (Guo et al, 2021).

4.3. Fatty Acids and Tumourigenesis

Fats play a critical role in cancer development, particularly with regard to their composition and delicate balance. Consumption of certain fatty acids significantly affects inflammation and tumour progression, with cell membrane integrity hanging precariously in the balance.

Omega-3 Fatty Acids: Omega-3 fatty acids (e.g., eicosapentaenoic acid (EPA) and docosahexaenoic acid (DHA)), predominantly found in fatty fish and flaxseeds, have well-documented anti-inflammatory effects. Omega-3 fatty acids like eicosapentaenoic acid and docosahexaenoic acid are found mostly in fatty fish and also in flaxseeds, having potent anti-inflammatory effects. Several cancer types, including breast, prostate and colon cancer, exhibit suppressed angiogenesis and inhibited cell proliferation alongside promoted apoptosis by these fats (Swanson et al, 2012).

Omega-6 Fatty Acids: While essential for health, omega-6 fatty acids (e.g., linoleic acid) found in vegetable oils may contribute to chronic inflammation when consumed in excess relative to omega-3s. Omega-3 fatty acids radically alter the activity of key signalling pathways like PI3K/AKT and NF-κB, both deeply implicated in tumourigenesis regulation. Omega-6 fatty acids like linoleic acid, found plentifully in various vegetable oils, may spur chronic inflammation when eaten excessively relative to omega-3s (Patterson et al, 2012).

Saturated Fat: Diets high in saturated fat (found in red meat, butter, and processed foods) have long been associated with an increased risk of several cancers, including colon and breast cancer. Chronic inflammation drives cancer progression markedly in tissues such as breast tissue and colon. High omega-6 intake correlates very strongly with elevated pro-inflammatory prostaglandins that can ramp up tumourigenesis by fostering cell proliferation quite vigorously and suppressing apoptosis rather markedly (Sivasubramanian et al, 2023).

4.4. Fibre and Its Protective Role in Tumourigenesis

Dietary fibre found predominantly in fruits and whole grains has been shown to protect against several cancer types, particularly colorectal cancer. Fermentation of fibre in the colon produces short-chain fatty acids like butyrate having anti-inflammatory effects and exhibit strikingly potent anticancer properties. Butyrate induces apoptosis fairly readily in cancerous cells and inhibits certain histone deacetylases very effectively, enhancing immune surveillance mechanisms. Fibre also helps to regulate insulin and glucose metabolism, both of which are involved in cancer development. Fibre helps regulate insulin and glucose metabolism, intricately involved in cancer development processes very deeply within bodily functions (Celiberto et al, 2023).

4.5. Phytochemicals and Their Anticancer Potential

Phytochemicals contain bioactive properties that modulate various molecular pathways involved heavily in cancerous tumour development within plant-based organisms naturally. Compounds like flavonoids and carotenoids have shown anticancer properties in various preclinical studies and some clinical trials remarkably. Flavonoids, found in fruits, vegetables, and tea, have antioxidant and anti-inflammatory properties that can inhibit tumour cell proliferation, induce apoptosis, and modulate signalling pathways like NF-κB and MAPK (Rudzińska et al, 2023).

Carotenoids like beta-carotene, lycopene, and lutein found in colourful fruits and vegetables have demonstrated anticancer effects through their antioxidant activity and ability to modulate gene expression involved in cell growth and differentiation. Glucosinolates, present in cruciferous vegetables such as broccoli, kale, and Brussels sprouts, have been shown to activate detoxification enzymes and inhibit carcinogen activation, thereby reducing cancer risk (Ağagündüz et asl, 2022). Flavonoids present in fruits, vegetables, and tea have antioxidant properties that inhibit tumour cell proliferation and induce apoptosis quite effectively. Beta-carotene, lycopene and lutein in brightly hued produce exhibit anticancer properties via antioxidant action and modulation of gene expression affecting cellular growth. Glucosinolates found in cruciferous veggies like broccoli and kale have been shown to rev up detox enzymes and somewhat inhibit carcinogen activation, thereby lowering cancer risk. Key nutrients play both directly and very indirectly in tumourigenesis, influencing various cancer biology aspects including DNA repair, cell proliferation, immune function and inflammation heavily (Pyo et al, 2024).

5. Dietary Patterns and Their Influence on Cancer Risk

The diet and cancer connection appears complex and deeply multifactorial, with growing evidence suggesting dietary patterns rather than isolated nutrients significantly impact cancer initiation and progression. Certain dietary habits and food patterns can ramp up the risk of developing specific cancers, while others mitigate it significantly in various populations. Significant shifts towards grasping how certain dietary patterns influence cancer risk have occurred, with considerable emphasis on the type and variety of foods consumed. Various dietary patterns linked to cancer risk are scrutinised here, and their impact on cellular pathways, inflammation and immune function is explored deeply (Nagy et al, 2023).

5.1. Western Diet and Cancer Risk

Western diet typified by hefty consumption of red and processed meats, saturated fats and sugary refined foods correlates strongly with elevated cancer risk, including colorectal, breast, prostate and pancreatic cancers. Energy-dense foods are characteristically abundant in this dietary pattern, thereby significantly contributing to obesity, a major risk factor for cancer. Obesity fosters insulin resistance remarkably and boosts levels of insulin-like growth factor IGF-1 significantly, promoting chronic inflammation that spawns cancer development environments.

Red and Processed Meats: High consumption of red meat (beef, pork, lamb) and processed meats (bacon, sausages, hot dogs) has been linked to an increased risk of colorectal cancer and possibly stomach and pancreatic cancers. High consumption of red meats like beef and lamb and processed fare such as sausages has been linked quite strongly to colorectal cancer (Jain S, 2022).

High-Sugar, Low-Fibre Diets: Diets rich in refined sugars, such as those found in soft drinks, pastries, and snacks, can increase the risk of cancer by contributing to obesity, insulin resistance, and chronic low-grade inflammation. Carcinogenic effects arise from compounds like heterocyclic amines and polycyclic aromatic hydrocarbons formed when meat is cooked really hot by grilling or frying. Diets rich in refined sugars found in soft drinks pastries and snacks can fuel cancer risk by exacerbating obesity and chronic inflammation heavily (Clemente-Suárez et al, 2022).

5.2. Mediterranean Diet and Cancer Protection

The Mediterranean diet, rich in fruits, vegetables whole grains, nuts, seeds, olive oil and fish, has been linked consistently to reduced cancer risk. This dietary pattern highlights antioxidant-rich foods and anti-inflammatory compounds that work very synergistically, protecting against cancer at various levels.

Olive Oil and Omega-3 Fatty Acids: Olive oil, a hallmark of the Mediterranean diet, is rich in monounsaturated fats and polyphenols like oleocanthal, which have anti-inflammatory and antioxidant properties. Olive oil, rich in monounsaturated fats and polyphenols like oleocanthal, has potent anti-inflammatory properties and significant antioxidant effects. Olive oil reduces oxidative stress quite significantly, and inflammation plays a huge role in cancer initiation and tumour progression (Infante et al, 2023).

Fruits, Vegetables, and Fibre: The Mediterranean diet is rich in fruits and vegetables, which provide fibre, vitamins, minerals, and phytochemicals. Mediterranean diet abounds with omega-3 fatty acids found abundantly in fish like salmon and sardines, which thwart tumour-feeding angiogenesis and dial down inflammatory cytokines. Mediterranean diet comprises heaps of fruits and veggies bursting with vitamins, minerals, phytochemicals and loads of fibre naturally (Tosti et al, 2018).

Wine and Phytochemicals: Moderate consumption of red wine, a common component of the Mediterranean diet, provides resveratrol, a polyphenolic compound that has demonstrated anticancer properties by inhibiting cancer cell proliferation, inducing apoptosis, and suppressing angiogenesis. Flavonoids and carotenoids, alongside polyphenols, exhibit potent antioxidant properties protecting against DNA damage and cellular mutations rather effectively (Divella et al, 2020).

5.3. Plant-Based Diets and Cancer Prevention

Plant-based diets, including vegetarian and vegan diets, have gained attention for their potential to prevent and manage cancer. These diets focus on whole plant foods, including fruits, vegetables, legumes, whole grains, nuts, and seeds, while eliminating or minimising animal products. Evidence suggests that plant-based diets may reduce cancer risk by providing a rich array of fibre, antioxidants, phytochemicals, and anti-inflammatory fats.

Phytochemicals and Fibre: One of the primary protective mechanisms of plant-based diets lies in their phytochemical content, which includes compounds like flavonoids, saponins, terpenes, and glucosinolates, each of which has been shown to protect against cancer through their antioxidant, anti-inflammatory, and immune-modulating properties (Kumar et al, 2023).

Phytochemicals and Fibre: One of the primary protective mechanisms of plant-based diets lies in their phytochemical content, which includes compounds like flavonoids, saponins, terpenes, and glucosinolates, each of which has been shown to protect against cancer through their antioxidant, anti-inflammatory, and immune-modulating properties. Tumour suppressor genes get regulated by these compounds, which induce apoptosis and inhibit carcinogen activation thereby contributing to cancer prevention (Kumar et al, 2023).

Reduced Animal Protein Intake: Plant-based diets are typically low in animal protein, which has been associated with an increased risk of certain cancers, especially colorectal cancer. Additionally, the high fibre content in plant-based diets promotes gut health, regulates insulin metabolism, and reduces the production of pro-inflammatory compounds that can contribute to cancer development (Sieri et al, 2020).

Soy and Isoflavones: A notable aspect of plant-based diets is the inclusion of soy products, such as tofu, tempeh, and soy milk, which are rich in phytoestrogens, particularly isoflavones like genistein. Plant-based diets tend to be low in animal protein which correlates with heightened risk of certain malignancies, especially colorectal cancer (Messina M, 2016).

5.4. Low-Carbohydrate Diets and Cancer Risk

Ongoing research investigates the role of carbohydrates in cancer risk, suggesting low-carb diets rich in whole foods may lower the incidence of breast and pancreatic cancers.

Insulin and IGF-1: Diets that are low in refined sugars and carbohydrates help regulate insulin and IGF-1 levels, both of which are known to promote cancer cell growth and inhibit apoptosis. Diets low in refined sugars help regulate insulin and IGF-1 levels, which promote cancer cell growth and inhibit apoptosis somewhat naturally (Klement and Fink, 2016).

Ketogenic Diet: The ketogenic diet, which is extremely low in carbohydrates and high in fats, has gained attention for its potential therapeutic effects in cancer treatment. Low-carbohydrate diets may help diminish circulating levels of certain growth factors, thus potentially mitigating risk of various cancers somewhat. The ketogenic diet, extremely low in carbs and ridiculously high in fats, has gained considerable attention for potential therapeutic effects in treating cancer (Masood et al, 2025).

5.5. Global Diets and Cancer Risk

Diets differ wildly across cultures, and some global dietary patterns have been shown recently to confer significant protection against various cancers. Traditional Japanese diets rich in fish, soy products, and veggies have been linked very strongly with significantly lower rates of various cancers. Traditional Asian diets rich in rice, legumes, vegetables and green tea have been associated with significantly reduced incidence of oesophageal and liver cancers. Dietary patterns play a crucial albeit often underappreciated role in determining overall risk of developing various forms of cancer (Gabriel et al, 2018).

Diets rich in fruits and whole grains with healthy fats are protective against cancer and may reduce the risk of several common malignancies. Western-style diets rich in unhealthy fats, sugars and animal products can conversely promote tumourigenesis through insulin resistance and heightened oxidative stress. Our comprehension of dietary patterns linked closely with cancer evolves rapidly, offering valuable fodder for crafting potent preventive measures and novel therapeutic regimens (Gabriel et al, 2018).

6. Bioactive Compounds

Naturally occurring substances exerting beneficial effects on human health are abundantly present in fruits and vegetables and various whole grains. Compounds capable of modulating myriad biological pathways make them pivotal in the prevention and management of maladies like cancer quite effectively. Growing research highlights the role of bioactive compounds heavily influencing cancer pathways like cell proliferation, apoptosis and metastasis in various bodily processes. Their effects are mediated via activation of specific enzymes and receptors involved heavily in various physiological processes fairly frequently (Lobo et al, 2010). Polyphenols and flavonoids, alongside carotenoids, glucosinolates and terpenes, are scrutinised here for profoundly impacting cancer-related molecular pathways quite extensively nowadays. Compounds exhibit antioxidant, anti-inflammatory and antitumour properties and have potential for modulating epigenetic changes, making them rather attractive cancer chemoprevention candidates.

6.1. Polyphenols and Their Role in Cancer Modulation

Polyphenols constitute a vast array of phytochemicals abundant in fruits and vegetables and also found in tea, coffee, and red wine. Flavonoids, stilbenes, phenolic acids and lignans are fairly well-known polyphenols. Various cellular processes, including oxidative stress and cell cycle regulation, are influenced by these compounds, which have demonstrated anticancer properties effectively.

Flavonoids

Flavonoids rank among highly studied polyphenolic compounds owing largely to potent antioxidant and profoundly anti-inflammatory effects. Quercetin and catechins, found mostly in tea, and anthocyanins prevalent in various berries, are common flavonoids alongside apigenin present in parsley. Flavonoids exert anticancer effects through multiple mechanisms, including inhibition of cell proliferation by regulating key cell cycle regulators like cyclins. Quercetin can hinder cell cycle progression rather effectively by modulating cyclin-dependent kinases essential for cell division (Panche et al, 2016).

Induction of apoptosis: Many flavonoids promote programmed cell death (apoptosis) by activating caspases and modulating the Bcl-2 family of proteins. Flavonoids induce apoptosis vigorously by activating caspases and modulating Bcl-2 family proteins deeply in cells under certain conditions, apparently (Abotaleb et al, 2018).

Inhibition of angiogenesis: Flavonoids also interfere with angiogenesis (the formation of new blood vessels), which is crucial for tumour growth and metastasis. Apigenin triggers apoptosis in breast cancer cells by downregulating anti-apoptotic proteins and boosts the expression of pro-apoptotic proteins remarkably well (Wei and Zhang, 2024).

Other Polyphenols

Resveratrol, a stilbene polyphenol found in red wine and grapes, has demonstrated anti-cancer effects by modulating tumour suppressor genes and growth factor signalling pathways like PI3K/Akt and MAPK, which regulate cell survival and proliferation. Resveratrol, a stilbene polyphenol present in red wine and various grapes has shown anti-cancer properties by modulating certain tumour suppressor genes and growth factor signaling pathways.

Curcumin, the active compound in turmeric, is another polyphenol with significant anticancer activity. NF-κB pathway gets inhibited quite heavily, exhibiting profoundly anti-inflammatory effects often upregulated mercilessly in most cancerous cells.

6.2. Carotenoids

Carotenoids comprise a vibrant assortment of phytochemicals, including β-carotene, lycopene, lutein and zeaxanthin, typically inhabiting brightly hued fruits and various vegetables. Carotenoids possess antioxidant properties mainly by neutralising reactive oxygen species and free radicals that severely damage DNA, thereby facilitating carcinogenesis.

Lycopene

Lycopene, a carotenoid pigment responsible for red colouration in tomatoes, has garnered considerable attention recently owing largely to its anticancer properties. Lycopene significantly inhibits tumour growth and induces apoptosis in various cancer types, including prostate cancer cells quite effectively nowadays. It achieves this by modulating AKT/mTOR signalling pathway involved heavily in cell growth, survival, and various metabolic processes downstream. Lycopene inhibits angiogenesis and invasion by downregulating various pro-angiogenic factors, including VEGF, quite effectively in various cellular contexts (Imran et al, 2020).

β-Carotene and Lutein

β-carotene, a precursor to vitamin A, has been shown to modulate immune function and enhance the activity of natural killer (NK) cells, which are crucial for detecting and eliminating cancer cells. β-carotene, a precursor to vitamin A, has been shown quite effectively to modulate immune function and boost the activity of natural killer cells crucial for detecting cancer cells. Lutein, found in spinach and kale, has protective effects against lung cancer and breast cancer by reducing oxidative stress and preventing DNA damage. It inhibits pro-inflammatory cytokines fairly effectively and suppresses cell proliferation vigorously in various cellular contexts apparently (Ashfaq et al, 2000).

6.3. Glucosinolates

Sulfur-containing compounds called glucosinolates occur very frequently in cruciferous veggies such as broccoli and kale, and sometimes Brussels sprouts. Myrosinase hydrolyses these compounds rather quickly, producing isothiocyanates like sulforaphane, which possess documented anticancer properties in various medical studies.

Sulforaphane

Sulforaphane induces apoptosis and inhibits tumour cell proliferation by activating the Nrf2 pathway, which regulates the expression of various antioxidant and detoxification enzymes. Activation enhances bodily ability quite rapidly to detoxify various carcinogens and protects against oxidative damage very effectively, meanwhile. Sulforaphane inhibits angiogenesis by downregulating VEGF and impairs epithelial-to-mesenchymal transition, a process intricately involved in metastasis (Su et al, 2018).

Indole-3-Carbinol (I3C)

Indole-3-carbinol, present in cruciferous veggies, modulates estrogen metabolism and has been shown to reduce the risk of cancers related to hormones like breast cancer. I3C exerts effects by influencing cytochrome P450 enzymes involved in estrogen metabolism and other hormone regulation very deeply inside cells (Centofanti et al, 2023).

6.4. Terpenes and Their Impact on Cancer Pathways

Terpenes comprise a vast array of bioactive compounds present in essential oils and aromatic flora like turmeric or oregano naturally. D-Limonene and β-caryophyllene exhibit notable anticancer properties, having been extensively studied as terpenes in various research endeavours. D-limonene, found in citrus fruits, has been shown rather effectively to induce apoptosis and reduce significant inflammation, inhibiting tumour growth. It acts on multiple signalling pathways, including AKT/mTOR and MAPK pathways, to inhibit cell proliferation vigorously and angiogenesis quite effectively. D-limonene promotes immune surveillance rather vigorously by activating natural killer cells and T lymphocytes very effectively in the body (Yu et al, 2018). Terpene found in the essential oil of cloves and oregano has been shown recently to reduce inflammation drastically by binding the CB2 cannabinoid receptor. β-caryophyllene's anti-inflammatory effects are significant in reducing cancer risk by modulating the NF-κB pathway.

6.5. Bioactive Compounds as Potential Cancer Modulators

Bioactive compounds spearhead chemoprevention research owing largely to their ability to target multiple facets of cancer biology like oxidative stress and cell proliferation. Bioactive compounds from fruits and veggies modulate cancer pathways very effectively and reduce the risk of carcinogenesis significantly in various bodily systems. Growing evidence supports the potential of bioactive compounds quite vigorously in the prevention of various cancer types and possibly as adjunctive therapy too. Incorporating a variety of bioactive-rich foods into the diet may help reduce cancer risk and improve outcomes for patients with certain molecular pathways involved heavily in tumourigenesis. Further clinical trials are desperately needed now to confirm optimal dosing, bioavailability and therapeutic applications of such compounds in preventing cancer effectively (Yuan et al, 2022).

7. Molecular Targets of Dietary Interventions in Cancer Prevention

Cancer manifests as a heterogeneous disease fraught with markedly dysregulated cellular activity, including unbridled proliferation and evasion of apoptotic mechanisms. Molecular oncology and nutrition science evidence has highlighted the potential for dietary interventions modulating key targets involved in cancer initiation and metastasis, but rather slowly. Bioactive compounds lurking in dietary components sway molecular pathways energetically, providing an opportunity for chemoprevention using natural substances, preventing cancer entirely. Molecular targets underlying cancer prevention via dietary interventions are examined with particular focus on oncogenic signalling pathways and gene expression modulation occurring therein. Dietary compounds influence hallmarks of cancer such as cell cycle regulation, apoptosis and oxidative stress through various intricate mechanisms very effectively (Maleki et, 2023).

7.1. Cell Cycle Regulation and Dietary Interventions

A series of events unfolds fairly rapidly, leading to cell division and replication within eukaryotic cells under normal conditions. Tumour cells frequently subvert normal checkpoints controlling cellular proliferation and division, resulting in dysregulation of the cycle being a cancer hallmark. Cyclins and cyclin-dependent kinases, along with tumour suppressor genes like p53 and retinoblastoma protein, govern cell cycle progression irregularly. Several dietary compounds heavily influence cell cycle progression by modulating the activity of molecules, thus halting the proliferation of cancer cells (Abreu Velez and Howard, 2015).

Polyphenols and Cell Cycle Regulation

Polyphenolic compounds like epigallocatechin gallate in green tea and resveratrol found in grapes interfere with cell cycle progression at several key points. EGCG inhibits CDK2 activity, thereby inducing G1 phase arrest in cancer cells, which prevents entry into the S-phase of the cell cycle. Curcumin induces cell cycle arrest rather effectively by downregulating cyclin D1 gene expression and upregulating p21 a cyclin-dependent kinase inhibitor very significantly (Alam et al, 2024).

Retinoids

Retinoids derived from vitamin A specifically retinoic acid are famously known for regulating cell cycle progression by modulating the expression of cyclin-dependent kinase inhibitors like p21 and p27 quite effectively. Compounds modulate retinoic acid receptors, which regulate transcription of genes controlling G1/S transition fairly precisely through various molecular pathways. Retinoids show promise in preventing various cancers, particularly in epithelial tissues by inducing arrest of the cell cycle and promoting cellular differentiation fast (Chen and Ross, 2004).

7.2. Apoptosis Modulation through Dietary Interventions

Apoptosis or programmed cell death serves as a crucial defence mechanism against cancer in various organisms. Cancer cells frequently accrue myriad mutations enabling evasion of apoptosis, thereby facilitating uncontrolled survival within affected tissue. Bioactive compounds found in the diet can restore apoptotic mechanisms normally disrupted in cancer cells, offering a pathway for prevention. Quercetin and apigenin promote apoptosis vigorously in cancer cell lines by activating caspases and modulating the expression of pro-apoptotic proteins. Apigenin, for instance, can trigger mitochondrial-mediated apoptosis in breast cancer cells and prostate cancer cells by activating caspase-3 and caspase-9 (Choi and Kim, 2009). Curcumin induces apoptosis through activation of caspases, particularly caspase-8 and the mitochondrial pathway in turmeric remarkably. Curcumin downregulates anti-apoptotic proteins like BCL-2 and boosts expression of pro-apoptotic molecules such as BAX, promoting mitochondrial dysfunction quite effectively (Wang et al, 2009).

7.3. Modulation of Angiogenesis by Dietary Compounds

Tumour growth and metastasis rely heavily on angiogenesis, a vital process involving the formation of new blood vessels quite rapidly. Tumours need a blood supply for delivering nutrients and oxygen by upregulating pro-angiogenic factors such as vascular endothelial growth factor or VEGF. Certain dietary compounds can thwart angiogenesis rather effectively by messing with VEGF signalling or blocking activation of key pro-angiogenic transcription factors. Quercetin and epigallocatechin gallate EGCG exhibit anti-angiogenic effects by markedly suppressing VEGF-induced proliferation and migration of endothelial cells. EGCG has been found for instance, to downregulate the expression of VEGF in tumour cells and inhibit PI3K/AKT signalling pathway essential for angiogenesis. Genistein, found in soy, suppresses angiogenesis heavily by inhibiting the HIF-1α pathway, a transcription factor promoting VEGF expression under hypoxic conditions, very effectively (Zhu et al, 2011). Curcumin has been studied very extensively owing largely to its ostensibly potent anti-angiogenic properties in various cellular contexts. It works by inhibiting the activation of NF-κB, a transcription factor regulating the expression of various pro-angiogenic molecules, including VEGF, in a downstream. Curcumin also blocks the activity of the MAPK pathway involved heavily in cell survival mechanisms and angiogenesis processes, quite significantly. Curcumin hampers tumour growth potential drastically by limiting angiogenesis through various mechanisms reducing their ability to develop a blood supply substantially (Sharifi-Rad et al, 2020).

7.4. Inflammation and Its Impact on Cancer: Dietary Modulation

Cancer progression and metastasis are significantly fueled by chronic inflammation remarkably deep within bodily tissues over long periods of time. Tumour cells exploit inflammatory pathways creating a microenvironment that supports progression and fosters immune evasion rather stealthily. NF-B and pro-inflammatory cytokines play quite an integral role in tumourigenesis alongside COX-2 rather mysteriously in various contexts. Omega-3 polyunsaturated fatty acids particularly EPA and DHA from fish oil have shown considerable promise in various inflammatory pathways recently. Omega-3s suppress production of pro-inflammatory cytokines such as TNF-α and IL-6 which significantly contribute rather markedly to tumour growth and metastasis. Fatty acids modulate NF-B signaling thereby markedly reducing expression of pro-inflammatory mediators and COX-2 quite effectively downstream. Omega-3s help reduce chronic inflammation often found in tumour microenvironments by heavily dampening inflammation quite effectively over time (Calder PC, 2013). Curcumin inhibits NF-B pathway very effectively and it plays a central role in regulating inflammation within various cancer cells. Curcumin reduces production of pro-inflammatory cytokines and enzymes like COX-2 and iNOS by suppressing NF-B activation associated with tumour progression. Curcumin becomes an alluring dietary intervention targeting inflammatory microenvironment supporting cancer growth vigorously inside human bodies naturally everyday (Peng et al, 2021).

7.5. Antioxidants and DNA Damage Repair

Oxidative stress caused by wildly fluctuating reactive oxygen species and bodily antioxidant defenses plays a fiendishly pivotal role in cancer initiation quite rapidly. ROS induces genetic damage very frequently leading to mutations that spur tumourigenesis rather haphazardly in some cases and with alarming rapidity. Dietary antioxidants restore balance by neutralizing ROS and enhancing mechanisms that repair DNA very effectively. Vitamin C or ascorbic acid enhances activity of DNA repair enzymes thereby facilitating repair of oxidative DNA damage quite effectively. Studies imply vitamin C ramps up expression of genes tied deeply into base excision repair fixing oxidative DNA damage quite efficiently. It acts as cofactor for enzymes involved heavily in collagen synthesis and reduces metastasis of cancer quite effectively meanwhile maintaining tissue integrity (Konopacka M, 2004). Selenium found in food like Brazil nuts enhances DNA repair capacity of cells by activating proteins and reducing accumulation of mutations quite effectively. Selenium's antioxidant properties shield cells from oxidative stress thereby preventing mutations that can conceivably lead to cancerous growth very quickly (Tinggi U, 2008).

7.6. Epigenetic Modulation by Dietary Compounds

Epigenetic changes like DNA methylation and histone modification play a crucial role in cancer initiation quite rapidly through various mechanisms. Dietary compounds influence these processes either by reactivating silenced tumour suppressor genes or inhibiting expression of certain oncogenes quite effectively. Epigallocatechin gallate a polyphenol in green tea has been shown to modulate DNA methylation patterns reactivating silenced tumour suppressor genes in various cancer cells effectively. EGCG profoundly modifies histone acetylation thereby rendering it a mighty epigenetic regulator within cancer prevention contexts quite effectively nowadays (Nandakumar et al, 2011).

7.7. Curcumin and Epigenetic Regulation

Curcumin affects histone deacetylases very significantly and inhibits expression of certain genes by removing acetyl groups from histones quite effectively. Curcumin influences gene expression quite profoundly by modulating HDAC activity and restores function of tumour suppressor genes effectively. Dietary interventions targeting molecular pathways in cancer prevention represent a promising strategy for reducing cancer risk and encourage treatment regimens effectively. Bioactive compounds in fruits and spices influence tumour biology at molecular level by modulating cell cycle regulation and apoptosis heavily. Molecular targets identified provide valuable insight into how diet can play a preventive role slowly in various cancer cases naturally. Understanding nutrition's interaction with molecular cancer pathways enables development of super personalized dietary regimens alongside existing cancer prevention methods and therapies (Verza et al, 2020).

8. Future Directions: Integrating Diet with Cancer Therapy and Prevention

Cancer remains a behemoth challenge in modern medicine with substantial efforts geared towards finding innovative treatments and devising novel prevention strategies. Conventional therapies like surgery and chemotherapy improve survival rates for many cancers but often bring substantial side effects. Dietary interventions have gained traction rapidly as complementary cancer treatment approaches alongside conventional methods for prevention lately. Scientists are rapidly uncovering links between specific nutrients and cancer progression while intense research focuses on how bioactive compounds modulate body's biological pathways. Future directions in cancer therapy integrate diet with personalized nutrition and targeted dietary strategies alongside microbiome research potentially transforming cancer care landscape utterly (Anand et al, 2020).

Better understanding how nutrition complements existing treatments and enhances therapy effectiveness potentially prevents cancer onset altogether in various high-risk populations. Precision medicine evolves rapidly and growing recognition exists that tailored dietary recommendations based on genetic and lifestyle factors play a role in cancer treatment. Cancer manifests variably owing largely to genetic predispositions and myriad environmental stressors that modulate disease susceptibility and responsiveness to treatment regimens. Personalized nutrition endeavors quite deliberately for highly specific differences providing a fairly individualized approach in cancer care lately (Narimatsu H, Yaguchi, 2022).

Recent advances in genomics and epigenomics have opened fresh avenues for deciphering diet's influence on gene expression and cancer initiation processes deeply. Researchers are beginning to pinpoint genetic variants influencing response to certain nutrients or dietary patterns by analyzing a patient's genetic makeup quite thoroughly. Variations in genes related to folate metabolism and detoxification pathways may impact an individual's ability to metabolize certain compounds very effectively or defend against oxidative stress relevant in cancer prevention. Dietary factors like methyl donors found in folate-rich food can heavily influence DNA methylation patterns that play a crucial role in regulating gene expression . Greater insight into such mechanisms potentially guides modified nutrition strategies targeting cancer-linked epigenetic alterations deeply within cells (Tiffon C, 2018).

Metabolic profiling plays a crucial role alongside genetic factors in shaping personalized nutrition strategies effectively nowadays. Tumours undergo radical metabolic rewiring often dubbed Warburg effect relying heavily on glycolysis for energy production even when oxygen abounds freely. Reprogramming presents opportunity for dietary strategies modulating various metabolic pathways and hindering growth of tumours rapidly inside human body. Certain low-carb diets or interventions inducing ketosis greatly affect cancer cell metabolism by slashing glucose availability thus stifling tumour growth markedly. Personalized nutrition might consider factors such as insulin sensitivity gut microbiome makeup or capacity for nutrient absorption tailoring diets for optimal metabolic health and better cancer treatment outcomes (Burns and Manda, 2017). Diet plays a crucial role alongside conventional cancer therapies potentially enhancing their effectiveness greatly in various complex ways sometimes. Growing interest lies in dietary tactics that sensitize tumours chemotherapy and mitigate treatment toxicity thereby improving patient outcomes somewhat effectively. Certain dietary components surprisingly influence chemoresistance a significant hurdle in cancer treatment and potentially modulate chemotherapy sensitivity greatly nowadays. Tumours often develop chemotherapy resistance by drastically altering metabolism and supercharging drug efflux via pumps such as P-glycoprotein and boosting DNA repair mechanisms suddenly. Curcumin and resveratrol sensitize tumour cells remarkably by inhibiting pathways of drug resistance and modulating gene expression extensively. Radiation therapy supplemented with specific dietary regimens can significantly alter treatment outcomes in patients undergoing oncological interventions (Mittelman SD, 2020).

Diet has potential quite remarkably to amplify effectiveness of radiation therapy. Antioxidants have been shown to mitigate radiation-induced toxicity remarkably in healthy tissues thereby enhancing therapeutic index of radiation noticeably. Antioxidants role in radiation therapy remains contentious with some research indicating they may shield cancer cells from radiation-induced harm . Future research must figure out how best balance antioxidant intake during radiation therapy protecting normal cells while ramping up effects on tumour cells. Cancer therapies such as chemotherapy and radiation pose considerable toxicity problems and managing them remains a particularly daunting task.

Cancer patients often suffer terribly from nasty side effects like nausea, fatigue and weight loss which hampers treatment adherence so badly. Specific nutritional adjustments and carefully planned dietary regimens may somewhat alleviate such adverse reactions fairly effectively sometimes. Omega-3 fatty acids present in fish oil and flavonoid-rich foods such as fruits and veggies possess anti-inflammatory properties that mitigate treatment-induced inflammation. Probiotics and prebiotics potentially help maintain gut health during harsh chemotherapy treatments, preventing diarrhoea and nasty gut dysbiosis very often. Gut microbiome sprawls wildly with trillions of microbes inhabiting the gastrointestinal tract and plays a crucial role in modulating inflammation quietly (Milliron et al, 2022).

Recent research has shown gut microbiome profoundly influences cancer development and impacts treatment response with various therapy-related side effects severely. Dietary tweaks influencing gut microbiota might drastically revamp cancer prognoses significantly amidst emerging research on oncology nutrition frontiers. Gut microbiome composition profoundly influences immune response to tumours and impacts efficacy of immunotherapy substantially in various cancer scenarios. High-fibre diets rich in prebiotics have been linked to a more diverse microbiome which may enhance immune surveillance and diminish chronic inflammation significantly. Fermented foods like yogurt and kimchi harbour beneficial probiotics which modulate gut microbiome very effectively under certain conditions. Probiotics may enhance immunotherapy via gut-associated lymphoid tissue enhancement and activation of T cells and natural killer cells simultaneously maybe. Polyphenols present in foods like blueberries green tea and grapes can positively influence microbiome by promoting growth of beneficial bacteria and reducing abundance of pathogenic microbes. Cancer therapy's efficacy can be enhanceed by grasping microbiome intricacies thereby unlocking novel dietary regimens that augment immunotherapy chemotherapy and radiotherapy outcomes remarkably. Certain dietary compounds can modulate gut microbiome and thereby enhance the efficacy of immune checkpoint inhibitors by promoting proliferation of various immune cells deeply within tumour microenvironment (Mazziotta et al, 2023).

Dietary fibre supports production of short-chain fatty acids by gut bacteria known to possess anti-cancer properties and improves immune function significantly. Public health initiatives will ostensibly play a crucial role in translating increasing knowledge about diet and cancer into prevention strategies nationwide. Nutritional education and community-based interventions will be crucial in promoting adoption of healthy dietary habits that can mitigate cancer risk significantly. Global nutrition policies must assimilate rigorously researched guidelines on cancer prevention focusing on diets heavy in veggies and whole grains. Integration of dietary interventions into cancer therapy and prevention remains a rapidly evolving field full of promise somewhat surprisingly nowadays. Moving forward personalized nutrition microbiome modulation and synergistic effects of diet and therapy hold immense potential for revolutionizing cancer care utterly. Future research must intricately unravel molecular underpinnings of dietary influence on cancer and devise modified strategies for optimizing clinical outcomes effectively. Diet may play a central role increasingly in preventing cancer and enhancing therapy so survivorship outcomes improve remarkably over time.

9. Conclusion

A new era of integrative oncology has been ushered in by mounting evidence linking dietary factors with cancer prevention therapy and survivorship. Nutrition plays a crucial role nowadays in cancer care no longer just a secondary aspect but a key player in prevention and therapeutic outcomes. Dietary interventions can potentially modify tumour microenvironment deeply inside bodily tissues and enhance immune responses quite significantly for chemoprevention. Integration of diet with conventional cancer treatment holds immense promise particularly in realms of personalized nutrition and increasing microbiome research lately. Personalized approaches might enhance treatment efficacy remarkably by dovetailing nutritional regimens with individual patients genetic and metabolic peculiarities quite effectively.

Growing recognition of gut microbiome's role in cancer development presents a new frontier for dietary modulation suggesting interventions could be tailored. Robust clinical trials and longitudinal studies are desperately needed now as cancer biology research progresses rapidly through increasingly sophisticated methods. Existing evidence remains mostly inconclusive owing largely to cancer heterogeneity and need for more rigorous protocols surrounding dietary factors. A multidisciplinary approach involving biotechnologists and epidemiologists will be essential in translating latest research findings into very actionable guidelines quickly. Public health initiatives play a crucial role in fostering adoption of cancer-preventive diets remarkably across various populations nationwide every year.

Evidence-based nutrition-driven cancer prevention measures must be incorporated rapidly into global health strategies benefiting broader populations considerably worldwide now. Policy reforms and nutritional guidelines should promote diets rich in whole grains and fibre while reducing intake of sugars and red meats implicated in cancer risk. Integrating dietary interventions into cancer therapy and prevention is a garrulous strategy essentially promising for oncology's gloomily shrouded future maybe slowly.

Dietary compounds modulate molecular targets heavily involved in cancer initiation and progression thereby opening up fresh avenues for innovative therapeutic interventions. Research will likely uncover new ways diet impacts cancer prompting a surge in modified treatments pairing food changes with standard therapies. Integrating diet with cancer care remains somewhat nascent still but a bright future beckons practitioners fairly obviously now. Ongoing research and cross-disciplinary collaboration very much ensures nutrition as medicine will be realized ultimately improving cancer prevention strategies greatly for individuals affected.

References

Abotaleb M, Samuel SM, Varghese E, Varghese S, Kubatka P, Liskova A, Büsselberg D. Flavonoids in Cancer and Apoptosis. Cancers (Basel). 2018 Dec 28;11(1):28. doi: 10.3390/cancers11010028. PMID: 30597838; PMCID: PMC6357032.

Abreu Velez AM, Howard MS. Tumour-suppressor Genes, Cell Cycle Regulatory Checkpoints, and the Skin. N Am J Med Sci. 2015 May;7(5):176-88. doi: 10.4103/1947-2714.157476. PMID: 26110128; PMCID: PMC4462812.

Ağagündüz D, Şahin TÖ, Yılmaz B, Ekenci KD, Duyar Özer Ş, Capasso R. Cruciferous Vegetables and Their Bioactive Metabolites: from Prevention to Novel Therapies of Colorectal Cancer. Evid Based Complement Alternat Med. 2022 Apr 11;2022:1534083. doi: 10.1155/2022/1534083. PMID: 35449807; PMCID: PMC9017484.

Alam M, Gulzar M, Akhtar MS, Rashid S, Zulfareen, Tanuja, Shamsi A, Hassan MI. Epigallocatechin-3-gallate therapeutic potential in human diseases: molecular mechanisms and clinical studies. Mol Biomed. 2024 Dec 27;5(1):73. doi: 10.1186/s43556-024-00240-9. PMID: 39725830; PMCID: PMC11671467.

Anand P, Kunnumakkara AB, Sundaram C, Harikumar KB, Tharakan ST, Lai OS, Sung B, Aggarwal BB. Cancer is a preventable disease that requires major lifestyle changes. Pharm Res. 2008 Sep;25(9):2097-116. doi: 10.1007/s11095-008-9661-9. Epub 2008 Jul 15. Erratum in: Pharm Res. 2008 Sep;25(9):2200. Kunnumakara, Ajaikumar B [corrected to Kunnumakkara, Ajaikumar B]. PMID: 18626751; PMCID: PMC2515569.

Anand U, Dey A, Chandel AKS, Sanyal R, Mishra A, Pandey DK, De Falco V, Upadhyay A, Kandimalla R, Chaudhary A, Dhanjal JK, Dewanjee S, Vallamkondu J, Pérez de la Lastra JM. Cancer chemotherapy and beyond: Current status, drug candidates, associated risks and progress in targeted therapeutics. Genes Dis. 2022 Mar 18;10(4):1367-1401. doi: 10.1016/j.gendis.2022.02.007. Erratum in: Genes Dis. 2024 Jan 20;11(4):101211. doi: 10.1016/j.gendis.2024.101211. PMID: 37397557; PMCID: PMC10310991.

Anderson NM, Simon MC. The tumour microenvironment. Curr Biol. 2020 Aug 17;30(16):R921-R925. doi: 10.1016/j.cub.2020.06.081. PMID: 32810447; PMCID: PMC8194051.

Ashfaq MK, Zuberi HS, Anwar Waqar M. Vitamin E and beta-carotene affect natural killer cell function. Int J Food Sci Nutr. 2000;51 Suppl:S13-20. PMID: 11271852.

Bartek J. DNA damage response, genetic instability and cancer: from mechanistic insights to personalized treatment. Mol Oncol. 2011 Aug;5(4):303-7. doi: 10.1016/j.molonc.2011.07.006. Epub 2011 Jul 22. PMID: 21843977; PMCID: PMC5528317.

Biray Avci C, Goker Bagca B, Nikanfar M, Takanlou LS, Takanlou MS, Nourazarian A. Tumour microenvironment and cancer metastasis: molecular mechanisms and therapeutic implications. Front Pharmacol. 2024 Nov 12;15:1442888. doi: 10.3389/fphar.2024.1442888. PMID: 39600368; PMCID: PMC11588459.

Burns JS, Manda G. Metabolic Pathways of the Warburg Effect in Health and Disease: Perspectives of Choice, Chain or Chance. Int J Mol Sci. 2017 Dec 19;18(12):2755. doi: 10.3390/ijms18122755. PMID: 29257069; PMCID: PMC5751354.

Calder PC. Omega-3 polyunsaturated fatty acids and inflammatory processes: nutrition or pharmacology? Br J Clin Pharmacol. 2013 Mar;75(3):645-62. doi: 10.1111/j.1365-2125.2012.04374.x. PMID: 22765297; PMCID: PMC3575932.

Celiberto F, Aloisio A, Girardi B, Pricci M, Iannone A, Russo F, Riezzo G, D'Attoma B, Ierardi E, Losurdo G, Di Leo A. Fibres and Colorectal Cancer: Clinical and Molecular Evidence. Int J Mol Sci. 2023 Aug 31;24(17):13501. doi: 10.3390/ijms241713501. PMID: 37686308; PMCID: PMC10488173.

Centofanti F, Buono A, Verboni M, Tomino C, Lucarini S, Duranti A, Pandolfi PP, Novelli G. Synthetic Methodologies and Therapeutic Potential of Indole-3-Carbinol (I3C) and Its Derivatives. Pharmaceuticals (Basel). 2023 Feb 5;16(2):240. doi: 10.3390/ph16020240. PMID: 37259386; PMCID: PMC9960368.

Chen Q, Ross AC. Retinoic acid regulates cell cycle progression and cell differentiation in human monocytic THP-1 cells. Exp Cell Res. 2004 Jul 1;297(1):68-81. doi: 10.1016/j.yexcr.2004.02.017. PMID: 15194426; PMCID: PMC3843129.

Cheng X, O'Neill HC. Oncogenesis and cancer stem cells: current opinions and future directions. J Cell Mol Med. 2009 Nov-Dec;13(11-12):4377-84. doi: 10.1111/j.1582-4934.2008.00664.x. Epub 2009 Jan 16. PMID: 19175465; PMCID: PMC4515053.

Choi EJ, Kim GH. Apigenin Induces Apoptosis through a Mitochondria/Caspase-Pathway in Human Breast Cancer MDA-MB-453 Cells. J Clin Biochem Nutr. 2009 May;44(3):260-5. doi: 10.3164/jcbn.08-230. Epub 2009 Apr 25. PMID: 19430615; PMCID: PMC2675027.

Clemente-Suárez VJ, Mielgo-Ayuso J, Martín-Rodríguez A, Ramos-Campo DJ, Redondo-Flórez L, Tornero-Aguilera JF. The Burden of Carbohydrates in Health and Disease. Nutrients. 2022 Sep 15;14(18):3809. doi: 10.3390/nu14183809. PMID: 36145184; PMCID: PMC9505863.

Cooper GM. The Cell: A Molecular Approach. 2nd edition. Sunderland (MA): Sinauer Associates; 2000. The Development and Causes of Cancer. Available from: https://www.ncbi.nlm.nih.gov/books/NBK9963/

Dakal TC, Dhabhai B, Pant A, Moar K, Chaudhary K, Yadav V, Ranga V, Sharma NK, Kumar A, Maurya PK, Maciaczyk J, Schmidt-Wolf IGH, Sharma A. Oncogenes and tumour suppressor genes: functions and roles in cancers. MedComm (2020). 2024 May 31;5(6):e582. doi: 10.1002/mco2.582. PMID: 38827026; PMCID: PMC11141506.

Divella R, Daniele A, Savino E, Paradiso A. Anticancer Effects of Nutraceuticals in the Mediterranean Diet: An Epigenetic Diet Model. Cancer Genomics Proteomics. 2020 Jul-Aug;17(4):335-350. doi: 10.21873/cgp.20193. PMID: 32576579; PMCID: PMC7367609.

Donaldson MS. Nutrition and cancer: a review of the evidence for an anti-cancer diet. Nutr J. 2004 Oct 20;3:19. doi: 10.1186/1475-2891-3-19. PMID: 15496224; PMCID: PMC526387.

Esteve M. Mechanisms Underlying Biological Effects of Cruciferous Glucosinolate-Derived Isothiocyanates/Indoles: A Focus on Metabolic Syndrome. Front Nutr. 2020 Sep 2;7:111. doi: 10.3389/fnut.2020.00111. PMID: 32984393; PMCID: PMC7492599.

Gabriel AS, Ninomiya K, Uneyama H. The Role of the Japanese Traditional Diet in Healthy and Sustainable Dietary Patterns around the World. Nutrients. 2018 Feb 3;10(2):173. doi: 10.3390/nu10020173. PMID: 29401650; PMCID: PMC5852749.

Guo Q, Li L, Hou S, Yuan Z, Li C, Zhang W, Zheng L, Li X. The Role of Iron in Cancer Progression. Front Oncol. 2021 Nov 10;11:778492. doi: 10.3389/fonc.2021.778492. PMID: 34858857; PMCID: PMC8631356.

Haskins CP, Champ CE, Miller R, Vyfhuis MAL. Nutrition in Cancer: Evidence and Equality. Adv Radiat Oncol. 2020 May 24;5(5):817-823. doi: 10.1016/j.adro.2020.05.008. PMID: 33083643; PMCID: PMC7557144.

He K, Gan WJ. Wnt/β-Catenin Signaling Pathway in the Development and Progression of Colorectal Cancer. Cancer Manag Res. 2023 May 23;15:435-448. doi: 10.2147/CMAR.S411168. PMID: 37250384; PMCID: PMC10224676.

Imran M, Ghorat F, Ul-Haq I, Ur-Rehman H, Aslam F, Heydari M, Shariati MA, Okuskhanova E, Yessimbekov Z, Thiruvengadam M, Hashempur MH, Rebezov M. Lycopene as a Natural Antioxidant Used to Prevent Human Health Disorders. Antioxidants (Basel). 2020 Aug 4;9(8):706. doi: 10.3390/antiox9080706. PMID: 32759751; PMCID: PMC7464847.

Infante R, Infante M, Pastore D, Pacifici F, Chiereghin F, Malatesta G, Donadel G, Tesauro M, Della-Morte D. An Appraisal of the Oleocanthal-Rich Extra Virgin Olive Oil (EVOO) and Its Potential Anticancer and Neuroprotective Properties. Int J Mol Sci. 2023 Dec 10;24(24):17323. doi: 10.3390/ijms242417323. PMID: 38139152; PMCID: PMC10744258.

Jain S. Processed meat and its relationship with cancer: Literature review. IP Journal of Nutrition, Metabolism and Health Science. 2022;5(2):38–43.

Jiang S, Liu H, Li C. Dietary Regulation of Oxidative Stress in Chronic Metabolic Diseases. Foods. 2021 Aug 11;10(8):1854. doi: 10.3390/foods10081854. PMID: 34441631; PMCID: PMC8391153.

Joyce C, Rayi A, Kasi A. Tumour-Suppressor Genes. [Updated 2023 Aug 28]. In: StatPearls [Internet]. Treasure Island (FL): StatPearls Publishing; 2025 Jan-. Available from: https://www.ncbi.nlm.nih.gov/books/NBK532243/

Kaźmierczak-Barańska J, Boguszewska K, Adamus-Grabicka A, Karwowski BT. Two Faces of Vitamin C-Antioxidative and Pro-Oxidative Agent. Nutrients. 2020 May 21;12(5):1501. doi: 10.3390/nu12051501. PMID: 32455696; PMCID: PMC7285147.

Kim DS, Scherer PE. Obesity, Diabetes, and Increased Cancer Progression. Diabetes Metab J. 2021 Nov;45(6):799-812. doi: 10.4093/dmj.2021.0077. Epub 2021 Nov 22. PMID: 34847640; PMCID: PMC8640143.

Kim SK, Cho SW. The Evasion Mechanisms of Cancer Immunity and Drug Intervention in the Tumour Microenvironment. Front Pharmacol. 2022 May 24;13:868695. doi: 10.3389/fphar.2022.868695. PMID: 35685630; PMCID: PMC9171538.

Klement RJ, Fink MK. Dietary and pharmacological modification of the insulin/IGF-1 system: exploiting the full repertoire against cancer. Oncogenesis. 2016 Feb 15;5(2):e193. doi: 10.1038/oncsis.2016.2. PMID: 26878387; PMCID: PMC5154349.

Konopacka M. Role of vitamin C in oxidative DNA damage]. Postepy Hig Med Dosw (Online). 2004;58:343-8. Polish. PMID: 15459552.

Koya AI, Ibrahim SA. Carcinogenesis. [Updated 2024 Oct 2]. In: StatPearls [Internet]. Treasure Island (FL): StatPearls Publishing; 2025 Jan-. Available from: https://www.ncbi.nlm.nih.gov/books/NBK604463/

Kumar A, P N, Kumar M, Jose A, Tomer V, Oz E, Proestos C, Zeng M, Elobeid T, K S, Oz F. Major Phytochemicals: Recent Advances in Health Benefits and Extraction Method. Molecules. 2023 Jan 16;28(2):887. doi: 10.3390/molecules28020887. PMID: 36677944; PMCID: PMC9862941.

Lobo V, Patil A, Phatak A, Chandra N. Free radicals, antioxidants and functional foods: Impact on human health. Pharmacogn Rev. 2010 Jul;4(8):118-26. doi: 10.4103/0973-7847.70902. PMID: 22228951; PMCID: PMC3249911.

Lugano R, Ramachandran M, Dimberg A. Tumour angiogenesis: causes, consequences, challenges and opportunities. Cell Mol Life Sci. 2020 May;77(9):1745-1770. doi: 10.1007/s00018-019-03351-7. Epub 2019 Nov 6. PMID: 31690961; PMCID: PMC7190605.

Maleki EH, Bahrami AR, Matin MM. Cancer cell cycle heterogeneity as a critical determinant of therapeutic resistance. Genes Dis. 2023 Jan 14;11(1):189-204. doi: 10.1016/j.gendis.2022.11.025. PMID: 37588236; PMCID: PMC10425754.

Martin TA, Ye L, Sanders AJ, et al. Cancer Invasion and Metastasis: Molecular and Cellular Perspective. In: Madame Curie Bioscience Database [Internet]. Austin (TX): Landes Bioscience; 2000-2013. Available from: https://www.ncbi.nlm.nih.gov/books/NBK164700/

Masood W, Annamaraju P, Khan Suheb MZ, et al. Ketogenic Diet. [Updated 2023 Jun 16]. In: StatPearls [Internet]. Treasure Island (FL): StatPearls Publishing; 2025 Jan-. Available from: https://www.ncbi.nlm.nih.gov/books/NBK499830/

Mazziotta C, Tognon M, Martini F, Torreggiani E, Rotondo JC. Probiotics Mechanism of Action on Immune Cells and Beneficial Effects on Human Health. Cells. 2023 Jan 2;12(1):184. doi: 10.3390/cells12010184. PMID: 36611977; PMCID: PMC9818925.

Mentella MC, Scaldaferri F, Ricci C, Gasbarrini A, Miggiano GAD. Cancer and Mediterranean Diet: A Review. Nutrients. 2019 Sep 2;11(9):2059. doi: 10.3390/nu11092059. PMID: 31480794; PMCID: PMC6770822.

Mercier BD, Tizpa E, Philip EJ, Feng Q, Huang Z, Thomas RM, Pal SK, Dorff TB, Li YR. Dietary Interventions in Cancer Treatment and Response: A Comprehensive Review. Cancers (Basel). 2022 Oct 20;14(20):5149. doi: 10.3390/cancers14205149. PMID: 36291933; PMCID: PMC9600754.

Messina M. Soy and Health Update: Evaluation of the Clinical and Epidemiologic Literature. Nutrients. 2016 Nov 24;8(12):754. doi: 10.3390/nu8120754. PMID: 27886135; PMCID: PMC5188409.

Milliron BJ, Packel L, Dychtwald D, Klobodu C, Pontiggia L, Ogbogu O, Barksdale B, Deutsch J. When Eating Becomes Torturous: Understanding Nutrition-Related Cancer Treatment Side Effects among Individuals with Cancer and Their Caregivers. Nutrients. 2022 Jan 14;14(2):356. doi: 10.3390/nu14020356. PMID: 35057538; PMCID: PMC8781744.

Mittelman SD. The Role of Diet in Cancer Prevention and Chemotherapy Efficacy. Annu Rev Nutr. 2020 Sep 23;40:273-297. doi: 10.1146/annurev-nutr-013120-041149. Epub 2020 Jun 16. PMID: 32543948; PMCID: PMC8546934.

Nagy S, Petrosky SN, Demory Beckler M, Kesselman MM. The Impact of Modern Dietary Practices on Cancer Risk and Progression: A Systematic Review. Cureus. 2023 Oct 7;15(10):e46639. doi: 10.7759/cureus.46639. PMID: 37937022; PMCID: PMC10627144.

Nandakumar V, Vaid M, Katiyar SK. (-)-Epigallocatechin-3-gallate reactivates silenced tumour suppressor genes, Cip1/p21 and p16INK4a, by reducing DNA methylation and increasing histones acetylation in human skin cancer cells. Carcinogenesis. 2011 Apr;32(4):537-44. doi: 10.1093/carcin/bgq285. Epub 2011 Jan 5. PMID: 21209038; PMCID: PMC3066414.

Narimatsu H, Yaguchi YT. The Role of Diet and Nutrition in Cancer: Prevention, Treatment, and Survival. Nutrients. 2022 Aug 14;14(16):3329. doi: 10.3390/nu14163329. PMID: 36014835; PMCID: PMC9414571.

Pal D, Banerjee S, Ghosh AK. Dietary-induced cancer prevention: An expanding research arena of emerging diet related to healthcare system. J Adv Pharm Technol Res. 2012 Jan;3(1):16-24. doi: 10.4103/2231-4040.93561. PMID: 22470889; PMCID: PMC3312721.

Panche AN, Diwan AD, Chandra SR. Flavonoids: an overview. J Nutr Sci. 2016 Dec 29;5:e47. doi: 10.1017/jns.2016.41. Erratum in: J Nutr Sci. 2025 Jan 29;14:e11. doi: 10.1017/jns.2024.73. PMID: 28620474; PMCID: PMC5465813.

Patterson E, Wall R, Fitzgerald GF, Ross RP, Stanton C. Health implications of high dietary omega-6 polyunsaturated Fatty acids. J Nutr Metab. 2012;2012:539426. doi: 10.1155/2012/539426. Epub 2012 Apr 5. PMID: 22570770; PMCID: PMC3335257.

Pedraza-Fariña LG. Mechanisms of oncogenic cooperation in cancer initiation and metastasis. Yale J Biol Med. 2006 Dec;79(3-4):95-103. PMID: 17940619; PMCID: PMC1994802.

Peng Y, Ao M, Dong B, Jiang Y, Yu L, Chen Z, Hu C, Xu R. Anti-Inflammatory Effects of Curcumin in the Inflammatory Diseases: Status, Limitations and Countermeasures. Drug Des Devel Ther. 2021 Nov 2;15:4503-4525. doi: 10.2147/DDDT.S327378. PMID: 34754179; PMCID: PMC8572027.

Pyo Y, Kwon KH, Jung YJ. Anticancer Potential of Flavonoids: Their Role in Cancer Prevention and Health Benefits. Foods. 2024 Jul 17;13(14):2253. doi: 10.3390/foods13142253. PMID: 39063337; PMCID: PMC11276387.

Rahaman MM, Hossain R, Herrera-Bravo J, Islam MT, Atolani O, Adeyemi OS, Owolodun OA, Kambizi L, Daştan SD, Calina D, Sharifi-Rad J. Natural antioxidants from some fruits, seeds, foods, natural products, and associated health benefits: An update. Food Sci Nutr. 2023 Jan 13;11(4):1657-1670. doi: 10.1002/fsn3.3217. PMID: 37051367; PMCID: PMC10084981.

Randeni N, Bordiga M, Xu B. A Comprehensive Review of the Triangular Relationship among Diet-Gut Microbiota-Inflammation. Int J Mol Sci. 2024 Aug 29;25(17):9366. doi: 10.3390/ijms25179366. PMID: 39273314; PMCID: PMC11394685.

Reuter S, Gupta SC, Chaturvedi MM, Aggarwal BB. Oxidative stress, inflammation, and cancer: how are they linked? Free Radic Biol Med. 2010 Dec 1;49(11):1603-16. doi: 10.1016/j.freeradbiomed.2010.09.006. Epub 2010 Sep 16. PMID: 20840865; PMCID: PMC2990475.

Rizvi S, Raza ST, Ahmed F, Ahmad A, Abbas S, Mahdi F. The role of vitamin e in human health and some diseases. Sultan Qaboos Univ Med J. 2014 May;14(2):e157-65. Epub 2014 Apr 7. PMID: 24790736; PMCID: PMC3997530.

Rudzińska A, Juchaniuk P, Oberda J, Wiśniewska J, Wojdan W, Szklener K, Mańdziuk S. Phytochemicals in Cancer Treatment and Cancer Prevention-Review on Epidemiological Data and Clinical Trials. Nutrients. 2023 Apr 14;15(8):1896. doi: 10.3390/nu15081896. PMID: 37111115; PMCID: PMC10144429.

Santarelli RL, Pierre F, Corpet DE. Processed meat and colorectal cancer: a review of epidemiologic and experimental evidence. Nutr Cancer. 2008;60(2):131-44. doi: 10.1080/01635580701684872. PMID: 18444144; PMCID: PMC2661797.

Scheiber A, Mank V. Anti-Inflammatory Diets. [Updated 2023 Oct 28]. In: StatPearls [Internet]. Treasure Island (FL): StatPearls Publishing; 2025 Jan-. Available from: https://www.ncbi.nlm.nih.gov/books/NBK597377/

Sharifi-Rad J, Rayess YE, Rizk AA, Sadaka C, Zgheib R, Zam W, Sestito S, Rapposelli S, Neffe-Skocińska K, Zielińska D, Salehi B, Setzer WN, Dosoky NS, Taheri Y, El Beyrouthy M, Martorell M, Ostrander EA, Suleria HAR, Cho WC, Maroyi A, Martins N. Turmeric and Its Major Compound Curcumin on Health: Bioactive Effects and Safety Profiles for Food, Pharmaceutical, Biotechnological and Medicinal Applications. Front Pharmacol. 2020 Sep 15;11:01021. doi: 10.3389/fphar.2020.01021. PMID: 33041781; PMCID: PMC7522354.

Sieri S, Agnoli C, Pala V, Grioni S, Palli D, Bendinelli B, Macciotta A, Ricceri F, Panico S, De Magistris MS, Tumino R, Fontana L, Krogh V. Dietary Intakes of Animal and Plant Proteins and Risk of Colorectal Cancer: The EPIC-Italy Cohort. Cancers (Basel). 2022 Jun 13;14(12):2917. doi: 10.3390/cancers14122917. PMID: 35740583; PMCID: PMC9221300.

Singar S, Nagpal R, Arjmandi BH, Akhavan NS. Personalized Nutrition: Tailoring Dietary Recommendations through Genetic Insights. Nutrients. 2024 Aug 13;16(16):2673. doi: 10.3390/nu16162673. PMID: 39203810; PMCID: PMC11357412.

Sivasubramanian BP, Dave M, Panchal V, Saifa-Bonsu J, Konka S, Noei F, Nagaraj S, Terpari U, Savani P, Vekaria PH, Samala Venkata V, Manjani L. Comprehensive Review of Red Meat Consumption and the Risk of Cancer. Cureus. 2023 Sep 15;15(9):e45324. doi: 10.7759/cureus.45324. PMID: 37849565; PMCID: PMC10577092.

Song Y, Bi Z, Liu Y, Qin F, Wei Y, Wei X. Targeting RAS-RAF-MEK-ERK signaling pathway in human cancer: Current status in clinical trials. Genes Dis. 2022 May 20;10(1):76-88. doi: 10.1016/j.gendis.2022.05.006. PMID: 37013062; PMCID: PMC10066287.

Sorscher SM, Hill A, Sorscher EJ. Evolutionary maintenance of oncogenesis. J Cancer Res Clin Oncol. 2009 Jan;135(1):159-62. doi: 10.1007/s00432-008-0426-y. Epub 2008 May 30. PMID: 18512072; PMCID: PMC12160312.

Stojchevski R, Sutanto EA, Sutanto R, Hadzi-Petrushev N, Mladenov M, Singh SR, Sinha JK, Ghosh S, Yarlagadda B, Singh KK, Verma P, Sengupta S, Bhaskar R, Avtanski D. Translational Advances in Oncogene and Tumour-Suppressor Gene Research. Cancers (Basel). 2025 Mar 17;17(6):1008. doi: 10.3390/cancers17061008. PMID: 40149342; PMCID: PMC11940485.

Su X, Jiang X, Meng L, Dong X, Shen Y, Xin Y. Anticancer Activity of Sulforaphane: The Epigenetic Mechanisms and the Nrf2 Signaling Pathway. Oxid Med Cell Longev. 2018 Jun 6;2018:5438179. doi: 10.1155/2018/5438179. PMID: 29977456; PMCID: PMC6011061.

Swanson D, Block R, Mousa SA. Omega-3 fatty acids EPA and DHA: health benefits throughout life. Adv Nutr. 2012 Jan;3(1):1-7. doi: 10.3945/an.111.000893. Epub 2012 Jan 5. PMID: 22332096; PMCID: PMC3262608.

Tiffon C. The Impact of Nutrition and Environmental Epigenetics on Human Health and Disease. Int J Mol Sci. 2018 Nov 1;19(11):3425. doi: 10.3390/ijms19113425. PMID: 30388784; PMCID: PMC6275017.

Tinggi U. Selenium: its role as antioxidant in human health. Environ Health Prev Med. 2008 Mar;13(2):102-8. doi: 10.1007/s12199-007-0019-4. Epub 2008 Feb 28. PMID: 19568888; PMCID: PMC2698273.

Tosti V, Bertozzi B, Fontana L. Health Benefits of the Mediterranean Diet: Metabolic and Molecular Mechanisms. J Gerontol A Biol Sci Med Sci. 2018 Mar 2;73(3):318-326. doi: 10.1093/gerona/glx227. PMID: 29244059; PMCID: PMC7190876.

Verza FA, Das U, Fachin AL, Dimmock JR, Marins M. Roles of Histone Deacetylases and Inhibitors in Anticancer Therapy. Cancers (Basel). 2020 Jun 23;12(6):1664. doi: 10.3390/cancers12061664. PMID: 32585896; PMCID: PMC7352721.

Wang JB, Qi LL, Zheng SD, Wu TX. Curcumin induces apoptosis through the mitochondria-mediated apoptotic pathway in HT-29 cells. J Zhejiang Univ Sci B. 2009 Feb;10(2):93-102. doi: 10.1631/jzus.B0820238. PMID: 19235267; PMCID: PMC2644749.

Wei Q, Zhang YH. Flavonoids with Anti-Angiogenesis Function in Cancer. Molecules. 2024 Mar 31;29(7):1570. doi: 10.3390/molecules29071570. PMID: 38611849; PMCID: PMC11013936.

Wu HJ, Wu E. The role of gut microbiota in immune homeostasis and autoimmunity. Gut Microbes. 2012 Jan-Feb;3(1):4-14. doi: 10.4161/gmic.19320. Epub 2012 Jan 1. PMID: 22356853; PMCID: PMC3337124.

Yildiz A, Kaya Y, Tanriverdi O. Effect of the Interaction Between Selenium and Zinc on DNA Repair in Association With Cancer Prevention. J Cancer Prev. 2019 Sep;24(3):146-154. doi: 10.15430/JCP.2019.24.3.146. Epub 2019 Sep 30. PMID: 31624720; PMCID: PMC6786808.

Yoshioka KI, Kusumoto-Matsuo R, Matsuno Y, Ishiai M. Genomic Instability and Cancer Risk Associated with Erroneous DNA Repair. Int J Mol Sci. 2021 Nov 12;22(22):12254. doi: 10.3390/ijms222212254. PMID: 34830134; PMCID: PMC8625880.

Yu X, Lin H, Wang Y, Lv W, Zhang S, Qian Y, Deng X, Feng N, Yu H, Qian B. d-limonene exhibits antitumour activity by inducing autophagy and apoptosis in lung cancer. Onco Targets Ther. 2018 Apr 4;11:1833-1847. doi: 10.2147/OTT.S155716. PMID: 29670359; PMCID: PMC5894671.

Yu X, Pu H, Voss M. Overview of anti-inflammatory diets and their promising effects on non-communicable diseases. Br J Nutr. 2024 Oct 14;132(7):898-918. doi: 10.1017/S0007114524001405. Epub 2024 Oct 16. PMID: 39411832; PMCID: PMC11576095.

Yuan M, Zhang G, Bai W, Han X, Li C, Bian S. The Role of Bioactive Compounds in Natural Products Extracted from Plants in Cancer Treatment and Their Mechanisms Related to Anticancer Effects. Oxid Med Cell Longev. 2022 Feb 15;2022:1429869. doi: 10.1155/2022/1429869. PMID: 35211240; PMCID: PMC8863487.

Zasada M, Budzisz E. Retinoids: active molecules influencing skin structure formation in cosmetic and dermatological treatments. Postepy Dermatol Alergol. 2019 Aug;36(4):392-397. doi: 10.5114/ada.2019.87443. Epub 2019 Aug 30. PMID: 31616211; PMCID: PMC6791161.

Zhu BH, Chen HY, Zhan WH, Wang CY, Cai SR, Wang Z, Zhang CH, He YL. (-)-Epigallocatechin-3-gallate inhibits VEGF expression induced by IL-6 via Stat3 in gastric cancer. World J Gastroenterol. 2011 May 14;17(18):2315-25. doi: 10.3748/wjg.v17.i18.2315. PMID: 21633597; PMCID: PMC3098399.

Chapter 2

Epidemiological Insights: Dietary Patterns and Cancer Incidence

Sheetanshu Gupta[1], Ng. Joykumar Singh[2], Sarfraj Ahmad Siddiqui[3], and Praneeth Juvvi[4*]

[1]Department of Food Safety and Quality Assurance, College of Food Technology, Central Agricultural University (CAU), Imphal, Manipur, India

[2]Department of Food Process Engineering, College of Food Technology, Central Agricultural University (CAU), Imphal, Manipur, India

[3]Department of Biochemistry, King George's Medical University, U.P., India

[4]Department of Food Processing Technology, College of Food Technology, Central Agricultural University, Imphal, Manipur, India

Abstract

The relationship between dietary patterns and cancer incidence is a critical area of investigation in epidemiology, with substantial implications for public health strategies and cancer prevention. Dietary patterns significantly influence cancer incidence, sparking intense investigation in epidemiology with huge implications for public health and prevention strategies. Cancer incidence varies greatly across different populations influenced heavily by eating habits, such as the Western diet and plant-based diets. Epidemiological research yields key findings that underscore the protective effects of fruits and antioxidants against various cancer types, while red meat and processed foods promote cancer. Chapter discussions encompass confounding factors like socioeconomic status and genetic predisposition, which may significantly amplify or obscure dietary cancer associations. It delves into increasing trends in precision nutrition, highlighting how modified dietary advice stemming from genetic metabolic profiling might yield cancer prevention strategies that are more efficacious. Cancer rates are highlighted through cross-cultural and cross-temporal analyses in this chapter, focusing on dietary shifts across various nations.

Keywords: Dietary Patterns, Cancer Epidemiology, Cancer, Nutritional Epidemiology, Preventive Nutrition

1. Introduction

Epidemiology plays a pivotal role in grasping complex relationships between lifestyle factors, including dietary habits and the incidence of various cancers. Cancer represents a gargantuan public health quandary

DOI: 10.1201/9781042010387-2

worldwide, prompting extensive research into the prevention of this frequently fatal disease. Diet has emerged as a crucial modifiable factor influencing the development and progression of various cancer types amidst genetic predispositions and environmental exposures. Cancer epidemiology revolves around studying dietary patterns at population level and their links with the incidence of various cancers quite intensely nowadays. Diet comprises diverse foods, nutrients and eating habits interacting intricately with personal biology, genetic predispositions and surrounding environmental conditions in convoluted manners. Examining the impact of dietary patterns on cancer risk necessitates a rather comprehensive approach, going far beyond the study of individual nutrients or specific foods (Sharman et al, 2024).

Epidemiological research increasingly focuses on pinpointing weird dietary patterns, namely peculiar combos of food and nutrients ingested over quite some time, possibly linked with heightened cancer risk. Identifying patterns across diverse cancer types and populations requires deciphering their underlying biological mechanisms and assessing their significance quite thoroughly. Diet and cancer linkage appears multifaceted and heavily context-dependent, often under various influences simultaneously outside simple causal pathways. Dietary patterns deemed protective in one population may not have same effect in another, owing partly to genetic variations and differing lifestyles elsewhere. Dietary influence on cancer risk demands nuanced understanding grounded deeply in cultural practices of specific populations and their socio-economic status (Chu et al, 2025).

Global variability in dietary habits and cancer rates underscores the necessity for cross-cultural investigations unraveling complexities of this oft-misunderstood relationship quite thoroughly. Several overarching trends linking dietary habits with cancer risk have been identified upon examining various dietary patterns very thoroughly nowadays. Western diet typified by substantial consumption of red and processed meats, refined grains, sugars and fats correlates strongly with elevated cancer incidence rates particularly colorectal, breast and prostate cancers. Plant-based diets rich in fruits and whole grains have been found to be protective against many forms of cancer quite effectively, it seems (Ennouri et al, 2024). Dietary epidemiology requires distinguishing association from causation very carefully amidst often murky evidence and confounding variables. Many studies found links between certain dietary habits and risk of cancer but approaching these findings with caution is utterly essential. Epidemiological studies frequently encounter numerous challenges mainly due to confounding factors and biases that heavily influence cancer incidence rates. Robust conclusions about relationship between certain dietary patterns and cancer risk have emerged gradually from diverse studies including many cohort studies (Nagy et al, 2023).

Accurate assessment of diet remains a crucial and key challenge within dietary epidemiology quite often nowadays apparently. Traditional methods like food frequency questionnaires and 24-hour dietary recalls rely heavily on self-reporting and often yield inaccurate results especially when estimating portion sizes or figuring out cooking methods and frequency of eating specific foods. Dietary patterns fluctuate somewhat over time making it rather tough to quantify lifetime exposure to specific nutrients or certain food items. Advancements in dietary assessment methodologies including use of biomarkers and digital tracking tools are improving accuracy of dietary data gradually nowadays.

Macronutrients and micronutrients play a crucial role sometimes in prevention and occasionally in promotion of various cancer forms naturally. Epidemiological research suggests specific nutrients may either enhance or thwart cancer development via their role in various cellular processes like DNA repair and apoptosis. Certain types of dietary fat found in red meat and processed foods have been implicated in promoting inflammation and altering metabolic pathways, favouring cancer cell survival. On the other hand, antioxidants like vitamins C and E, and compounds found in cruciferous vegetables, berries, and other plant foods, have shown protective effects against oxidative DNA damage and tumourigenesis. In addition to individual nutrients, dietary patterns that emphasise whole food consumption, high dietary fibre, and polyphenol-rich foods have been found to have cancer-protective effects (Fagbohun et al, 2023). Fibre reduces colorectal cancer risk noticeably through effects on gut microbiota and regulation of intestinal transit, alongside reduction of carcinogenic bile acids. Polyphenols found in tea fruits and veggies have demonstrated anti-inflammatory, antioxidant, and anticarcinogenic properties in numerous preclinical studies and some clinical trials. Globally a drastic shift toward urbanisation and adoption of westernised diets has precipitated a stark rise in lifestyle-associated cancers nationwide. In developing countries, rapid urbanization has resulted in a rise in cancer cases that were traditionally less prevalent, often due to the adoption of Western dietary patterns. These transitions also come with challenges related to food security, socioeconomic disparities, and the prevalence of obesity, which is now recognized as a significant risk factor for several cancers (Celiberto et al, 2023). Profound implications arise from shifting dietary patterns globally not just for individual health but also public health policies and cancer prevention strategies.

2. The Link between Diet and Cancer

Cancer persists as a paramount global health scourge with mortality rates swelling public health coffers to the breaking point worldwide nowadays. Diet plays a significant role in the prevention and development of various cancers, with genetic factors and environmental exposures contributing heavily too. Epidemiological studies examining patterns and effects of health conditions in specific populations have yielded fascinating insights into dietary patterns and cancer risk factors. Diet plays a complex, multifaceted role in cancer development, involving interplay between specific nutrients, food components and overall eating patterns erratically. Understanding carcinogenesis requires a broad approach incorporating individual food constituents like antioxidants and omega-3 fatty acids, and whole dietary patterns. Major studies furnish evidence linking diet and cancer via complex biological mechanisms that inform public health policy on cancer prevention strategies effectively (Britten and Tosi, 2024).

2.1. The Role of Diet in Cancer Etiology:

Dietary patterns emerge as a significant modifiable risk factor for cancer in numerous epidemiological studies conducted over several decades quite rigorously. Unhealthy diets replete with red meats, saturated fats and refined sugars are associated with elevated cancer risk, including colorectal and pancreatic cancers. Diets teeming with fruits and veggies and whole grains and fibre and plant-based fats have been remarkably associated with lowered cancer risk remarkably.

Western Diet and Cancer Risk

High consumption of red meat and processed foods alongside refined sugars in Western diets correlates strongly with elevated cancer risk generally. Epidemiological evidence suggests folks gobbling Western-style food are rather more likely to develop certain cancers especially breast and prostate cancers. Western diet's meagre fibre and sky-high saturated fat levels ostensibly foster inflammation and insulin resistance, thereby fuelling oxidative stress that spurs tumourigenesis. A large cohort study published in The Lancet indicated that individuals with high consumption of red meat had a significantly increased risk of colorectal cancer. Formation of carcinogenic compounds like heterocyclic amines and polycyclic aromatic hydrocarbons happens during the cooking process very frequently, and heme iron in red meat wreaks havoc on the gastrointestinal tract terribly (Qian et al, 2020).

Mediterranean Diet and Cancer Prevention

Mediterranean diet emphasising consumption of fruits, vegetables, whole grains, olive oil and moderate amounts of fish or poultry, has been consistently linked with reduced cancer risk. Research indicates people eating Mediterranean-style diets often exhibit significantly lower rates of various cancers, including breast cancer and lung cancer. Antioxidant-rich foods in this dietary pattern, including polyphenols from olive oil and flavonoids from various fruits and vegetables, may reduce oxidative stress. High omega-3 fatty acid content in fish and olive oil possibly modulates inflammatory pathways and enhances immune function, further reducing cancer risk somewhat (Widmer et al, 2015).

Plant-Based Diets and Cancer Protection

Epidemiological literature abundantly documents a markedly reduced cancer risk associated with largely plant-based dietary regimens. Vegetarian and vegan diets have been associated with reduced cancer rates, especially colorectal cancer and other digestive system malignancies, more frequently. Diets high in fibre play a crucial role in promoting gut health and regular bowel movements quite effectively every day. Fibre reduces the formation of carcinogenic compounds in the colon and helps maintain a healthy gut microbiome, thereby lowering overall cancer risk significantly. Plant-based diets tend to be markedly lower in saturated fats and red meat, which notoriously foster inflammation and oxidative stress linked with cancer development (Orlich et al, 2015).

2.2. Mechanisms: How Diet Influences Cancer Development

Mechanisms underlying cancer development via dietary influences are multifaceted, involving genetic predispositions and various environmental stressors simultaneously. Several well-established pathways are purportedly underlying links between diet and cancer.

Inflammation and Oxidative Stress

Oxidative stress and chronic inflammation fuel cancer development deeply within tissues. Diets rich in saturated fats and red meat can foster low-grade systemic inflammation implicated in the initiation of various cancers quite mysteriously. Fruits, vegetables and whole grains found in the Mediterranean diet have profoundly anti-inflammatory effects and are rich in antioxidants, counteracting oxidative stress (Saha et al, 2017).

Insulin Resistance and Obesity

Obesity and insulin resistance stem from dietary patterns strongly linked with heightened risk of various cancers, including breast cancer and pancreatic cancer. Consuming loads of refined carbs and sugary stuff alongside saturated fats often results in weight gain and heightened adiposity disrupting insulin signaling normally. Elevated insulin levels and insulin-like growth factors spur tumour cell proliferation and squash apoptosis thereby fueling cancer progression quite rapidly (Seiler et al, 2018).

DNA Repair and Epigenetic Changes

Compounds found in cruciferous veggies like broccoli and Brussels sprouts, turmeric and green tea can heavily influence DNA repair and epigenetic regulation mechanisms. Sulforaphane, found in cruciferous veggies, has been shown to enhance DNA repair mechanisms via modulation of Nrf2 pathway under oxidative stress conditions. Certain dietary patterns may induce epigenetic changes like DNA methylation or histone modification that influence gene expression, thereby lowering cancer risk (Mitra et al, 2022).

2.3. Public Health Implications and Future Directions

A critical need exists for incorporating dietary recommendations into cancer prevention strategies, given compelling evidence linking diet with heightened cancer risk. Healthy eating habits can be fostered by initiatives emphasising whole grains and veggies over processed food and sugary treats very effectively nowadays. Policymakers and healthcare professionals must collaboratively ensure culturally relevant dietary guidelines reach disparate populations effectively nationwide every single year. Future research oughta keep probing molecular mechanisms whereby diet impacts cancer and scrutinize personalized nutrition's role in cancer prevention very deeply (Donaldson MS, 2004).

Nutrigenomics and nutritional epigenetics hold potential to thoroughly revolutionise cancer prevention therapy by studying individual genetic variations and their influence on bodily response. Further studies conducted over lengthy periods are needed to assess the long-term impacts of dietary changes on the incidence of cancer recurrence and survival rates. Developing comprehensive cancer prevention strategies will be crucial alongside integrating diet with other aspects like physical activity and medical treatments, somewhat effectively. Epidemiological evidence unequivocally supports a significant role of diet in cancer prevention and development, quite markedly nowadays (Nicastro et al, 2012). Diets comprising largely processed foods, red meats, and unhealthy fats drastically heighten cancer risk, while those rich in fruits and whole grains confer protection. Deciphering the molecular underpinnings behind such correlations will be vital in crafting modified nutritional regimens that mitigate oncogenic hazards and enhance therapeutic efficacy remarkably. Integrating nutrition into cancer prevention and therapy holds great promise for reducing global cancer burden and vastly improving public health outcomes eventually.

3. Exploring Global Dietary Trends and Their Impact on Cancer Rates

Nearly 10 million cancer-related deaths occurred worldwide in 2020, alongside an estimated 19.3 million new cases of cancer globally. Dietary habits have garnered considerable attention lately for their potential impact on cancer development and progression variably over several years. Global cancer burden stems largely from dietary patterns that are sometimes protective and often risk-enhancing according to various epidemiological findings. Devising effective strategies to mitigate cancer incidence and enhance survival outcomes requires grasping global dietary trends and their correlation with cancer rates. Dietary trends worldwide are rapidly influencing cancer rates rapidly shedding light on the complex interplay between lifestyle factors and the prevalence of specific cancer types (Sung et al, 2021).

3.1. Global Dietary Patterns: A Snapshot of Changing Trends

Global diets now morph rapidly, driven by urban sprawl globalization forces and shifts in cultural mores across disparate regions. Westernised diets high in processed foods, red meats, sugars and refined grains are supplanting traditional eating habits based on whole foods locally sourced. Dietary shifts in low and middle-income nations are frequently characterised by abandoning plant-based diets for more meat, dairy and fast food options.

The Western Diet

Western diet typified by copious processed foods sugar-sweetened beverages, red meat, fried food and saturated fats offers minimal fruits and fibre. This diet has become quite prevalent in nations like the United States and Canada and many European countries and is linked strongly with higher rates of cancer, especially colon and breast cancer (Clemente-Suárez et al, 2023).

The Mediterranean Diet

The Mediterranean diet, rich in fruits, vegetables, whole grains, olive oil, fish and nuts, has long been associated with significantly lower cancer risk. Countries surrounding Mediterranean, including Italy and Greece, traditionally follow this dietary pattern, and evidence suggests it contributes to a lower incidence of cancers like breast and colorectal cancer. Mediterranean diet emphasizes anti-inflammatory antioxidant heart-healthy fats like omega-3 fatty acids which may modulate cancer-related pathways involved in oxidative stress heavily (Mentella et al, 2019).

Plant-Based Diets in Asia and Africa

Diets in many African countries have been rooted deeply in plant based traditions with emphasis on legumes, whole grains, rice and various vegetables. Diets like these are often very low in stuff from animals and extremely high in fibre and various phytonutrients and antioxidants. China and India boast rich histories of herbivorous dietary habits featuring copious amounts of soy, tofu rice and vegetables very frequently. Many parts of Sub-Saharan Africa predominantly follow diets revolving around starchy tubers, leafy greens and beans with minimal intake of red meat. Cancer rates in some regions are generally lower compared to Western countries, surprisingly. Colorectal cancer rates are significantly lower in Asia and Africa compared to most Western nations, obviously nowadays. Cancer rates have started rising sharply in these regions amidst rapid urbanization and westernization particularly for breast, prostate and liver cancers. Higher consumption of processed foods and sugary edibles often correlates with rising cancer cases in these areas amidst sedentary lifestyles (Oniang'o et al, 2025).

3.2. The Influence of Dietary Fat and Protein on Cancer Rates

A major factor driving the association between dietary patterns and cancer risk is the intake of **dietary fat** and **protein**, both of which vary considerably between regions.

Animal Fats and Processed Meats

Diets rich in saturated fats, typically sourced from animal products and processed meats like bacon and sausages, increase cancer risk significantly. Incidence of such cancers appears markedly higher in regions with diets heavy in processed and red meat products like those found in the United States and parts of Europe. Processed meats harbour carcinogenic properties ostensibly stemming from the presence of nitrates and nitrites or heterocyclic amines produced during high-temperature cooking, damaging DNA. Countries emphasising diets rich in plant-based fats from sources like olive oil, Mediterranean diets, avocados and nuts have lower cancer incidence rates, probably owing largely to anti-inflammatory and antioxidant properties inherent in such fats (Aykan NF, 2015).

Protein and Cancer Risk

Protein consumption's link with cancer risk appears decidedly more multifaceted nowadays. Red meat and processed meats harbouring animal protein have ostensibly been tied rather strongly to elevated cancer risk in prior discussions. Plant-based proteins like legumes and whole grains apparently offer protective effects and haven't been found to pose similar risks whatsoever. Protein type consumed heavily influences cancer risk modulation, alongside quantity and frequency of intake, very significantly over time. A diet replete with soy protein correlates very strongly with diminished breast cancer risk in certain Asian demographic groups, apparently (Sivasubramanian et al, 2023).

3.3. Dietary Carbohydrates, Sugars, and Cancer Rates

Refined carbs and copious amounts of added sugars intrinsic in Western dietary patterns have been tenuously linked to heightened oncological risks. High glycemic diets foster insulin resistance and obesity, which are risk factors for various cancers, including pancreatic, liver and breast cancer. Rising cancer rates, especially hormone-related ones like breast cancer, correlate with increasing prevalence of diabetes and obesity, mostly in developed nations. Nations like China, undergoing frenetic economic expansion and rampant urbanization have witnessed obesity rates and type 2 diabetes swell precipitously, fueling a surge in cancer cases. Cancer rates are projected to keep rising rapidly as regional diets increasingly shift toward fast foods and sugar-sweetened beverages elsewhere nowadays (Jiao et al, 2009).

3.4. Impact of Alcohol Consumption on Global Cancer Rates

Cancer risk increases substantially with boozy habits, being yet another crucial dietary consideration often linked heavily to oncogenic tendencies. IARC classified alcohol as a Group 1 carcinogen, linking it rather ominously mostly to liver cancer oral cancer and oesophagal cancer alongside breast cancer. Alcohol consumption differs markedly across various regions, with per capita rates being extremely high in certain European countries like France and Russia. Many Asian and African nations report relatively low levels of alcohol consumption, although rates surge rapidly in increasing urban populations nowadays. Higher alcohol consumption poses a considerable threat, particularly when coupled with smoking or obesity, thereby heightening cancer risk substantially (Rumgay et al, 2021).

3.5. Dietary Trends and Cancer Prevention: A Public Health Approach

Integrating dietary strategies into public health initiatives might prove remarkably effective for thwarting cancer onset in diverse populations worldwide very effectively. Governments worldwide ought to staunchly advocate for drastic dietary changes emphasizing vastly increased consumption of fruits and various whole grains rapidly.

- » Reduction in processed meats, red meat, and sugary foods.
- » Promotion of healthy fats, such as those found in olive oil, avocados, and omega-3-rich fish.
- » Promotion of physical activity and maintenance of a healthy weight.

Cut back drastically on sugary foods and processed meats alongside red meat for a healthier diet, apparently. Promotion of healthy fats occurs through consumption of foods like omega-3-rich fish, avocados and olive oil naturally. Fostering regular exercise habits and upkeep of a relatively healthy bodily mass is crucial nowadays, apparently. Public health initiatives should educate populations in nations experiencing dietary shifts about the perils of consuming copious animal fats and refined sugars. Global dietary trends correlate intricately with cancer rates, highlighting the importance of nutrition in prevention and cancer control efforts worldwide. Widespread adoption of Western diets rich in processed foods and saturated fats has been linked with higher cancer rates, mostly in affluent nations (Enkhmaa et al, 2018).

4. Nutrient Consumption and Cancer Risk

Modern nutritional epidemiology concentrates heavily on deciphering links between cancer risk and nutrient consumption patterns nowadays. Scientists are frantically trying to figure out how certain foods and nutrients inside them influence cancer risk worldwide very slowly. Mounting evidence suggests proteins, fats and carbohydrates alongside vitamins, minerals and trace elements play crucial roles in initiating cancer and its metastasis. The influence of nutrient consumption on cancer risk gets complicated by various genetic and environmental factors and different types of cancer. Extensive research into cancer risk and nutrient consumption highlights key nutrients that potentially exacerbate or mitigate oncogenic processes fairly significantly. Nutrients exert effects through various obscure mechanisms, and emerging trends in nutritional cancer research will be highlighted alongside implications for public health (Nagy et al, 2023).

4.1. The Role of Macronutrients in Cancer Risk

Dietary Fats and Cancer

Consumption of dietary fats sparks heated debate quite frequently around cancer risk factors and various associated health problems. Unsaturated fats found in nuts and plant-based oils may play a role differently than saturated fats in meat and dairy products.

» **Saturated fats:** Numerous studies have shown a positive correlation between high consumption of saturated fats and increased cancer risk, particularly in breast, colon, and prostate cancers. Numerous studies show that high consumption of saturated fats correlates with increased risk of breast, colon, and prostate cancers fairly strongly nowadays. High-fat diets possibly foster cancer development through the induction of chronic inflammation and drastically altered cell signalling pathways in various tissues (Mei et al, 2024).

» **Monounsaturated and polyunsaturated fats:** On the other hand, the Mediterranean diet, which is high in monounsaturated fats (particularly olive oil) and omega-3 fatty acids (found in fatty fish), has been associated with a reduced risk of several cancers, including breast, colorectal, and endometrial cancer. Consumption of copious red and processed meats frequently high in saturated fats has been tenuously linked to colorectal cancer owing to the formation of carcinogenic compounds during searing hot cooking (Caprara et al, 2021).

Dietary Carbohydrates and Cancer Risk

Refined sugars and high-glycemic index foods have been studied extensively for a role in cancer risk alongside other carbohydrates very thoroughly.

» **Refined carbohydrates:** Diets high in sugary foods, soft drinks, and refined grains can lead to hyperinsulinemia and insulin resistance, conditions known to promote the development of obesity, type 2 diabetes, and ultimately, cancer. Diets rich in sugary foods and refined grains can lead to hyperinsulinemia and insulin resistance fueling development of obesity and type 2 diabetes, and ultimately cancer. Elevated insulin levels and quirky insulin-like growth factors spur cancer cells' proliferation wildly and squash apoptosis very effectively (Clemente-Suárez et al, 2022).

» **Fibre and complex carbohydrates:** Conversely, fibre-rich diets, especially those high in whole grains, fruits, and vegetables, have been associated with reduced cancer risk. High intake of refined carbs correlates very strongly with heightened risk of various cancers namely pancreatic, liver and breast cancer. Conversely, diets rich in fibre especially whole grains fruits and veggies, have been associated with significantly reduced risk of various cancers apparently (Makarem et al, 2016).

Protein and Cancer Risk

Protein consumption correlates with cancer risk in complex ways with animal-based proteins frequently linked to elevated risk and plant-based proteins seemingly offering protection.

» **Animal-based proteins:** High consumption of red and processed meats (e.g., beef, pork, sausages) has been strongly linked to an increased risk of colorectal cancer, primarily due to the presence of carcinogenic compounds such as heterocyclic amines and polycyclic aromatic hydrocarbons, which form when meat is cooked at high temperatures. High consumption of red meats like beef and processed stuff such as sausages strongly correlates with elevated colorectal cancer risk owing largely to the presence of nasty chemicals formed when cooked at scorching temperatures. Heme iron present in red meat apparently promotes intestinal inflammation and DNA damage quite extensively in colon cells, contributing heavily to carcinogenesis (Santarelli et al, 2008).

» **Plant-based proteins:** In contrast, diets rich in plant-based proteins, such as those found in legumes, tofu, lentils, and nuts, have not been associated with the same cancer risks. Processed meats contain high levels of nitrates and nitrites, which can morph into nitrosamines, a notoriously nasty class of carcinogens. Diets rich in plant-based proteins found in legumes, tofu, lentils, and nuts have not been associated with the same cancer risks, apparently.

4.2. The Role of Micronutrients in Cancer Prevention

Micronutrients like vitamins and minerals play crucial roles in various cellular processes that either thwart or spur cancerous growth quite significantly. Deficiencies in some micronutrients heighten cancer risk quite substantially, while adequate intake of other specific nutrients may offer considerable protection.

Antioxidant Vitamins: Vitamins C, E, and A

Vitamin C: Vitamin C is a potent antioxidant that can scavenge reactive oxygen species (ROS) and prevent oxidative DNA damage, a key factor in cancer initiation. Vitamin C proves potent antioxidant properties by scavenging reactive oxygen species and thwarting oxidative DNA damage quite effectively in cancer initiation processes. Adequate consumption of vitamin C from various fruits and veggies possibly correlates with reduced oesophagal cancer risk and lower incidence of stomach malignancies (Pawlowska et al, 2019).

Vitamin E: Like vitamin C, vitamin E is another powerful antioxidant that may help protect against lipid peroxidation and cellular damage. Large clinical trials have failed miserably to confirm the benefits of high-dose vitamin C supplementation in cancer prevention, suggesting dietary sources beat supplements hands down (Traber and Stevens, 2011).

Vitamin A and beta-carotene: The provitamin A compound beta-carotene, found in carrots, sweet potatoes, and dark leafy greens, is essential for immune function and skin health. Vitamin E is a robust antioxidant rivalling vitamin C, potentially safeguarding against lipid peroxidation and some forms of cellular damage quite effectively. High dietary intake of vitamin E possibly mitigates risk of prostate and lung cancers but mixed findings necessitate further rigorous investigation (Grune et al, 2010).

Vitamin D and Cancer Risk

Vitamin D has gained increasing attention in cancer research due to its potential role in immune modulation and cell differentiation. Epidemiological studies suggest that individuals with low vitamin D levels may be at higher risk for several types of cancer, including breast, colon, prostate, and ovarian cancers. Vitamin D receptor appears quite ubiquitously in cancer cells and vitamin D possibly helps regulate growth and cellular apoptosis rather slowly. Further research into optimal levels for cancer prevention in various populations is sorely needed despite promising results from supplementation trials (Vuolo et al, 2012).

Minerals: Selenium and Zinc

Selenium: Selenium is a trace mineral with antioxidant properties that has been linked to a reduced risk of several cancers, including prostate and lung cancer. Selenium a trace mineral boasting antioxidant properties has been associated with lower risk of various cancers including prostate cancer and lung malignancies. Brazil nuts fish and whole grains rich in selenium possibly inhibit proliferation of cancer cells and foster repair of DNA quite effectively (Jiang et al, 2023).

Zinc: Zinc plays a role in DNA synthesis, immune function, and cell division, and deficiencies have been linked to increased cancer risk. Selenium supplementation's protective effects remain somewhat inconclusive with certain studies indicating little tangible benefit overall nonetheless (Jiang et al, 2023).

4.3. The Impact of Diet on Cancer Prevention:

Evidence linking nutrient consumption cancer risk underscores importance of dietary interventions for prevention of various cancers naturally. Whole foods and balanced diets rich in veggies and lean proteins could play a significant role globally in reducing cancer rates markedly. Dietary education should heavily stress cutting back on processed meats and refined carbs alongside excessive booze consumption which fuels cancer risk. Cancer risk gets influenced heavily by dietary patterns and genetics and lifestyle factors in a multifaceted manner through nutrient consumption. Certain nutrients like saturated fats and red meats are linked to increased cancer risk, while others, such as fibre and omega-3 fatty acids, may help protect against it. Public health strategies should focus on promoting a balanced diet rich in nutrients alongside lifestyle tweaks that entail regular physical exertion and weight control. Crucial research into mechanisms whereby specific nutrients influence cancer development significantly aids the development of targeted nutritional interventions in oncology therapy (Donaldson MS, 2004).

5. The Role of Dietary Patterns in Cancer Prevention and Development

Diet exerts influence quite profoundly on the development of various chronic ailments, and cancer stands out as the most researched outcome. Epidemiological research has consistently revealed that dietary habits significantly impact cancer risk and progression in various, surprisingly subtle yet profound ways. Dietary patterns involve a convoluted dance of numerous foodstuffs and groups consumed by individuals, unlike the impact of singular nutrients on health. These patterns sway myriad biological pathways implicated in carcinogenesis and tumour progression alongside inflammation, oxidative stress, and aberrant immune function (Nagy et al, 2023). Various dietary patterns contribute significantly towards cancer prevention or development, with some traditional diets being notably different from modern trends. Specific food groups will be scrutinised alongside their interactions within dietary habits and their potential bearing on cancer risk propensity. We will scrutinise mounting evidence on dietary interventions potentially alleviating cancer burden worldwide with significant implications for global health initiatives (Nagy et al, 2023).

5.1. Traditional Diets and Cancer Prevention

Many populations globally stuck fairly rigidly to old-school eating habits rich in veggies and relatively bereft of processed food. Dietary patterns fluctuating wildly across geographical areas correlate with markedly lower cancer incidence and significantly enhanced overall well-being. Diets rich in fruits and whole grains typically come from varied healthy sources like nuts, olive oil, and fish.

The Mediterranean Diet

The Mediterranean diet is a thoroughly examined traditional eating pattern that has been linked to do with lowering the risk of cancer in general, among those populations who follow it. The countries that lie along the shores of the Mediterranean Sea have, from time immemorial, been consuming a diet that is not only rich in olive oil, whole grains, fruits, veggies, fish, and legumes but also low in red meat. Several studies indicate that the Mediterranean diet gives a very strong shield from all kinds of cancers, such as breast cancer, lung cancer, and most importantly, colorectal cancer. The anti-cancer properties of the Mediterranean diet may point to the presence of omega-3 fatty acids in fish and olive oil, which are the main components of the diet and are very effective in the case of inflammation (Mentella et al, 2019). High intake of antioxidants from fruits and vegetables, which protect cells from oxidative DNA damage, is a key step in cancer initiation. The presence of polyphenols from olive oil and wine has been shown to induce apoptosis in cancer cells and inhibit tumour growth. A low intake of saturated fats and red meat, which are the main culprits of higher risks of cancers like colon cancer (Mentella et al, 2019).

Plant-Based Diets

Populations across parts of Asia and Africa traditionally eat diets heavily centred around rice, legumes, veggies fruits and tofu basically. Diets rich in fibre and phytonutrients contain vitamins and minerals but have low amounts of processed foods and animal proteins. The Asian diet typically correlates with significantly lower incidence of colorectal cancer and breast cancer, alongside prostate cancer, quite remarkably. High fibre content fosters gut health and regular bowel movements, reducing risk of colorectal cancer while abundance of phytonutrients from soy products like isoflavones may protect against hormone-related cancers such as breast cancer vigorously. Traditional African diets emphasizing whole grains and veggies are linked to remarkably lower cancer rates very much everywhere. Diets rich in fibre and various micronutrients have profoundly protective effects against certain cancers notably esophageal and colon cancer quite remarkably (Oniang'o et al, 2025).

5.2. Modern Dietary Patterns and Cancer Risk

Modern Westernized diets feature copious processed foods refined sugars saturated fats and animal proteins alongside rather low fruit vegetable and whole grain consumption. Rising cancer rates are often associated with adoption of this diet globally particularly in countries with high incomes fairly recently.

The Western Diet and Cancer

There is an increased risk of cancer including breast, colon, and pancreatic cancer, due to the western diet. Processed red and meat products are consumed greatly which contain nitrosamines that are carcinogenic and cooked, and which during colon digestion, oxidative stress and damage is very. Diets rich in red meats also contain heme iron and processed rich foods, which increases the risk of cancer in the body. Increased consumption of carbohydrates and refined sugar, foods such as fast food and sugar-sweetened beverages are associated with obesity and insulin resistance, which increases the risk of breast, pancreatic, and liver cancer. Decreased consumption of phytonutrients and plant food which increases the risk of cancer, also lowers fibre and vitamin intake. Moreover, processed foods also lead to higher insulin resistance (Sivasubramanian et al, 2023).

Dietary Fat and Cancer Risk

Consumption of saturated fats and trans fats often lurking in fast food and processed nosh has been tied up with elevated cancer risk notably prostate cancer. Fats fuel chronic inflammation extremely and insulin resistance occurs partly because of hormonal regulation changes thereby heightening risk of cancer significantly. Replacement of saturated fats with monounsaturated fats like olive oil and omega-3 fatty acids found abundantly in fish and flaxseeds has been linked quite strongly to lower cancer risk owing largely to anti-inflammatory and antioxidant properties (He et al, 2025).

5.3. The Protective Role of Specific Dietary Patterns

Research indicates dietary habits rather than isolated nutrients may offer quite a comprehensive method for preventing cancer effectively nowadays. Multiple biological pathways involved in cancer initiation and progression are purportedly influenced by certain dietary habits including inflammation and hormone regulation.

The Anti-Cancer Potential of Fibre-Rich Diets

Dietary fibre plays surprisingly a crucial role in prevention of various kinds of cancer very effectively. People who eat lots of fibre from fruits vegetables whole grains and legumes tend to have relatively low rates of various cancers especially colorectal cancer. Fibre fosters regularity in bowel movements and reduces transit time through intestines very quickly and may act prebiotically supporting growth of beneficial bacteria. Fibre gets metabolized into short-chain fatty acids in colon which exhibit anti-cancer properties by inhibiting inflammation and tumourigenesis quite effectively (Hu et al, 2023).

Plant-Based Diets and Cancer Prevention

Diets rich in veggies fruits and whole grains are linked very strongly with a markedly lower risk of getting cancer. Diets rich in nutrients provide abundance of antioxidants polyphenols flavonoids and phytochemicals that help neutralize free radicals and prevent DNA damage crucially in cancer initiation. Plant-based diets tend to be markedly lower in saturated fats and refined sugars which notoriously promote inflammation and subsequent cancer progression rapidly (Rahaman et al, 2023).

5.4. The Role of Alcohol and Processed Foods in Cancer Development

Alcohol and processed foods emerge as significant dietary risk factors for cancer development quite frequently in various medical research studies. Alcohol consumption poses a markedly heightened risk for various malignancies, including oral cancer oesophagal cancer and liver cancer quite frequently. Alcohol ramps up levels of acetaldehyde, a notorious carcinogen and messes with immune function, thereby spurring cancer cell proliferation rapidly. Consumption of processed foods, especially highly processed meats like sausages and bacon, has been very consistently linked to heightened risk of colorectal cancer. Nitrates, nitrites and heterocyclic amines produced during processing and cooking meats are recognised carcinogens frequently found in highly processed foods nowadays (Ratna and Mandrekar, 2017). An increasing trove of data highlights the significance of eating habits in cancer prophylaxis and tumourigenesis across various populations worldwide. Mediterranean and Asian diets rich in whole foods and antioxidants show promise in reducing cancer risk through emphasis on healthy fats. Modern Western dietary patterns high in processed foods and refined sugars are strongly linked with heightened risk of various cancers. Public health initiatives should heavily promote whole food-based diets rich in fruits and fibre while severely limiting consumption of processed foods and alcohol. We can significantly slash the worldwide cancer burden by adopting more protective dietary habits very quickly and fairly easily nowadays. Future research oughta deeply probe complex links between dietary habits and cancer, focusing on personalised nutrition factoring in genetic predispositions and sundry lifestyle variables (Mentella et al, 2019).

6. Environmental and Genetic Factors in Diet-Cancer Interactions

The diet and cancer connection proves intricate largely because numerous genetic and environmental factors interplay with foods consumed daily. Diet plays a crucial role in cancer risk modulation, yet myriad other factors contribute significantly to overall disease susceptibility. Cancer development is driven by a complex mix of factors such as genetic predispositions and exposures from highly polluted environments. Grasping interactions between these elements and dietary habits yields valuable insights into cancer initiation mechanisms and progression under various treatment regimens.

6.1. Genetic Factors in Cancer Risk and Diet Response

Genetics play a fundamental role in cancer risk, influencing how the body metabolizes certain nutrients quite rapidly and responds erratically to dietary components. Gene mutations and polymorphisms variably modulate bodily ability quite significantly to metabolise foods absorb vital nutrients, or detoxify potentially carcinogenic substances. Genetic variability manifests differently in individuals, and same diet can have profoundly disparate effects on cancer risk somewhat unpredictably.

Genetic Variability and Nutrient Metabolism

Certain genetic variations may affect how efficiently the body processes nutrients, which can influence cancer risk. Folate metabolism involves a B-vitamin found in leafy greens and legumes and citrus fruits critical for DNA synthesis very much everywhere. People having certain genetic variations in MTHFR gene involved deeply in metabolizing folate may struggle converting it into an active usable form. Such individuals might be at elevated risk for malignancies like colorectal cancer owing largely to suboptimal DNA repair mechanisms and heightened genomic instability. Vitamin D metabolism entails essential processes for immune function maintenance and cell differentiation which significantly enhance cancer prevention mechanisms naturally (Duthie SJ, 2011).

Variants of VDR gene namely vitamin D receptor may alter body's response to vitamin D affecting its cancer prevention ability quite significantly. Individuals harbouring specific VDR gene variants may face elevated cancer risk notably breast prostate or colon cancer especially with inadequate vitamin D consumption or meager sun exposure. GST enzymes crucially facilitate detoxification of various carcinogens quite effectively. Genetic polymorphisms within GST genes can ostensibly hinder one's capacity quite severely to metabolize carcinogens stemming from various environmental exposures or dietary sources. Individuals sporting GSTM1-null genotype resulting in absence of GSTM1 enzymes face heightened lung cancer risk upon smoking or getting exposed to environmental toxins because they inefficiently detoxify carcinogenic compounds (Duthie SJ, 2011).

Gene-Diet Interactions in Cancer Prevention

Genetic factors heavily influence bodily responses to certain dietary components having profoundly protective effects beyond mere nutrient metabolism occasionally. Cruciferous veggies like broccoli and cauliflower contain sulforaphane which activates detoxifying enzymes providing antioxidant protection quite effectively in human bodies. Individuals harbouring peculiar genetic polymorphisms within Nrf2 pathway that governs bodily antioxidant defenses may not reap full benefits from such protective compounds. Omega-3 fatty acids found mainly in fish and some plant oils exhibit markedly anti-inflammatory and anticancer properties rather remarkably. Genetic variations within fatty acid desaturase gene cluster heavily influence individual ability to derive cancer-protective benefits from plant-based omega-3 sources effectively (Ağagündüz et al, 2022).

6.2. Environmental Exposures and Diet-Cancer Interactions

Genetic factors predispose individuals to cancer risk and environmental exposures sometimes trigger or markedly accelerate cancer development rapidly over time. These exposures intricately interact with bodily metabolic processes and handling of dietary components occurs in profoundly varied ways naturally. Lifestyle factors like boozing heavily and being a couch potato alongside environmental toxins can radically alter diet's impact on cancer risk.

Environmental Pollutants and Diet

Environmental pollutants like pesticides and heavy metals alongside air pollution have been linked with heightened cancer risk particularly when paired with some dietary habits. Pesticides are linked very strongly with elevated cancer risk in agriculture particularly for non-Hodgkin lymphoma and brain cancer among farmers . Diets heavy in organic produce grown sans synthetic pesticides may significantly help mitigate risk somewhat effectively over time naturally. Research shows pesticide exposure coupled with meager antioxidant intake can markedly exacerbate oxidative stress DNA damage and cancer initiation quite severely. Arsenic and cadmium found in tainted food or soil are very potent carcinogens lurking ominously in contaminated water supplies everywhere (Alengebawy et al, 2021).

Diets rich in seafood particularly shellfish can sometimes be a significant source of arsenic in its methylated form naturally occurring abundantly. People with meager consumption of antioxidant-rich edibles or fibre-dense food may face an elevated cancer risk notably skin lung and bladder malignancies. Long-term exposure to air pollutants such as particulate matter and benzene has been tenuously linked to development of lung cancer recently. Pollutants mingling with dietary factors like super fatty foods or fibreless food exacerbate inflammation and cellular mutations thereby upsurging cancer risk quite drastically (Alengebawy et al, 2021).

Lifestyle Factors and Diet Interactions

Smoking and obesity severely impact cancer risk interacting with diet in myriad obscure ways alongside physical activity and alcohol consumption patterns. Cigarette smoke contains carcinogens that heighten risk of various cancers notably lung cancer very significantly under certain conditions obviously. Diets high in fruits vegetables and fibre provide protection against carcinogenic effects of smoking by reducing oxidative stress quite significantly through various pathways. Smokers with meager antioxidant consumption often face heightened cancer risk from synergistic DNA damage courtesy of fags and woeful eating habits (Land et al, 2014).

Excessive booze intake links heavily to various cancers including breast liver and esophageal cancer and alcohol stands as notoriously toxic carcinogen. Diets rich in folate and antioxidants may offer protection against alcohol-induced carcinogenesis but boozing excessively often spawns deficiencies in vitamin A and B vitamins. Obesity driven by diets high in calories but low in nutrients contributes significantly to chronic inflammation and insulin resistance thereby increasing risk of cancers like breast colon and endometrial cancer. Fast food availability and sedentary behaviour largely exacerbate such risks under various environmental conditions very significantly nowadays. Diets rich in fibre whole grains, and veggies may help reduce cancer risk related to obesity fairly significantly nowadays (Land et al, 2014).

6.3. Gene-Environment-Diet Interactions and Personalised Nutrition

Genetic factors intricately intertwined with dietary habits and environmental exposures underscore a pressing need for modified nutrition strategies in cancer prevention. People aren't equally susceptible to cancer, and dietary advice should factor in individual genetic makeup and lifestyle factors alongside environmental influences. Ideally personalized nutrition involves tailored dietary interventions factoring in genetic susceptibilities towards nutrient metabolism alongside various environmental exposures very intricately. Individuals harbouring particular genetic polymorphisms in folate metabolic pathways may reap benefits from supranormal folate consumption, reducing colorectal cancer risk somewhat effectively (Elsamanoudy et al, 2016).

People with genetic predispositions benefiting from diets rather low in refined carbs and very high in healthy fats or fibre may reduce insulin-related cancer risks. Dietary factors and genetic susceptibility intertwine intricately with environmental exposures, central to grasping cancer's complex initiation and prevention mechanisms somewhat nebulously. Genetics lays a shaky foundation for individual risk, and environmental factors significantly influence cancer outcomes, alongside dietary habits, remarkably. Growing research on gene-environment diet interactions underscores the importance of tailored nutrition, factoring in genetic predispositions and varied lifestyle choices simultaneously nowadays. We can gain deeper insight into cancer's complex, multifaceted nature and devise innovative prevention strategies quite effectively by weighing various factors (Elsamanoudy et al, 2016).

7. Epidemiological Studies

Cancer manifests through a complex interplay of genetic predispositions and various external factors, including lifestyle choices and environmental exposures. Identifying modifiable risk factors is crucial for understanding cancer etiology and diet remains a significantly influential factor in this regard. Epidemiological studies over many years back up claims that cancer risk intertwines deeply with dietary habits and patterns of food consumption. Studies have been pivotal in unveiling how specific foods, nutrients, and overall dietary patterns drastically affect the development of various cancers naturally (Parsa N, 2012).

Diet and cancer have a convoluted relationship with numerous variables intersecting in perplexing ways not easily deciphered. Epidemiological research plays a crucial role in uncovering links between food consumption and cancer risk, highlighting both strengths and inherent methodological limitations. Epidemiological approaches have unearthed various dietary risk factors and protective foods influencing susceptibility to cancer in somewhat obscure dietary patterns. Researchers studying complex multifactorial relationships face numerous challenges, and future research directions could yield clearer insights into diet and cancer risk (Parsa N, 2012).

7.1. Epidemiological Study Designs in Cancer Research

Epidemiological studies play a crucial role in exploring associations between various dietary factors and diverse cancer outcomes fairly extensively nowadays. Cohort studies and case-control studies are two primary study designs used very frequently in cancer epidemiology, yielding crucial insights into diet-cancer relationships.

Cohort Studies

Researchers track sizable populations over prolonged periods, gathering data on dietary habits and various extraneous lifestyle factors simultaneously. Participants get grouped by diet type, such as high-fat versus low-fat or maybe something entirely different. Low-fat diets pit starkly against ridiculously high-fibre regimens. Participants eating low-fibre diets are tracked over time, and the incidence of cancer gets observed very frequently afterwards. Prospective studies follow participants forward in time thereby establishing temporal relationships between diet and various forms of cancer quite effectively (Mozaffarian et al, 2011).

Decades-long scrutiny of sizable cohorts comprising women and men yielded profound insights into links between dietary fat and cancer risk factors namely breast and colorectal cancer. Cohort studies possess considerable strength in establishing causal links between various dietary factors and development of cancer effectively. These studies are notoriously expensive and ridiculously time-consuming requiring fairly large sample sizes for statistically significant results. Dietary data tends to be self-reported rather haphazardly leading to potential biases like gross underreporting of junk food consumption or grossly overreporting health-conscious eating habits (Mozaffarian et al, 2011).

Case-Control Studies

Researchers compare cancer patients and healthy counterparts looking retrospectively for disparate dietary patterns and various other potentially confounding risk factors. Case-control studies typically gaze backward in time to gather data retrospectively unlike cohort studies which mostly proceed forward in some manner. Studies of this nature tend to be relatively quick and cheap but very prone to bias such as recall bias whereby participants having cancer possibly overemphasize or misremember dietary habits. Case-control studies have been very instrumental in identifying potential risk factors for cancer linked somewhat vaguely to dietary habits. Numerous case-control studies demonstrate high consumption of red meat and processed meats correlates with increased risk of colorectal cancer somewhat surprisingly. Case-control studies suggest fruit and vegetable consumption may sizably reduce risk of various cancers including lung cancer and oral cancers very significantly (Nemati et al, 2012).

7.2. Dietary Risk Factors Identified Through Epidemiological Studies

Research in epidemiology highlights various dietary components strongly associated with heightened cancer risk or conversely remarkable protective effects. Certain trends have emerged offering quite compelling evidence for a role of diet in cancer prevention and progression rather sporadically.

Red and Processed Meats

Red meat and processed meats like bacon and sausages are notoriously linked with heightened risk of cancer especially colorectal cancer in epidemiological research findings. High consumption of red meat correlates with elevated colorectal cancer risk probably owing largely to nitrosamines and heterocyclic amines formed during cooking. Processed meats have been classified carcinogenic (Group 1) by World Health Organization and red meat probably carcinogenic (Group 2A) to humans (Santarelli et al, 2008).

Fruits and Vegetables

A diet teeming with fruits and veggies has consistently been linked with lowered risk of various cancer types including lung mouth and stomach cancers. Protective effects are largely attributed to antioxidants fibre and phytochemicals present abundantly in various whole plant-based foods naturally. Carotenoids found in vibrant orange and yellow fruits and veggies like carrots and sweet potatoes have been tied rather strongly to reduced cancer risk especially in lungs (Donaldson MS, 2004).

Alcohol Consumption

Epidemiological studies provide conclusive evidence that drinking alcohol boosts risk of various cancers including liver and esophageal cancers quite significantly. Cancer risk escalates precipitously alongside copious alcohol intake and heavy drinking gets tied up with heightened oncological hazards rather ominously. Ethanol can be metabolized into acetaldehyde a carcinogenic compound damaging DNA inside cells fairly quickly under certain conditions. Alcohol can impair absorption of folate quite significantly and this micronutrient plays a critical role in DNA repair mechanisms somewhat effectively (Rumgay et al, 2021).

Fibre Intake

Dietary fibre found in fruits and whole grains has been shown quite effectively to protect against colorectal cancer development. Fibre supposedly fosters regular bowel movements thus reducing time potentially carcinogenic substances spend in contact with colon lining. Fibre helps produce short-chain fatty acids with anti-inflammatory and anti-cancer properties quite rapidly inside human gut mostly (Kunzmann et al, 2015).

Omega-3 Fatty Acids

Evidence mounts that omega-3 fatty acids present in oily fish such as salmon mackerel and herring exert profoundly protective anticancer effects. Fats like these have been shown quite effectively to reduce inflammation which plays a pivotal role in progression of various cancers. Epidemiological studies have tenuously linked copious omega-3 intake with remarkably reduced cancer risks namely breast prostate and colorectal malignancies (Freitas et al, 2019).

7.3. The Complexity of Diet-Cancer Relationships

Epidemiological studies yield valuable yet perplexing insights into diet-cancer relationships and several challenges persist in data interpretation somewhat problematically.

Confounding Factors

Numerous factors intricately affect diet and cancer risk making causality quite difficult to establish with utmost certainty. People who chow down on plenty fruits and veggies often exhibit other salubrious habits like exercising regularly and eschewing cigarettes. Factors like these can really muddy relationship between diet and cancer making the effects of specific foods or nutrients super hard to discern (Key et al, 2020).

The Role of Genetics

Genetic factors largely influence individual responses drastically to various dietary habits under certain conditions with obvious profound effects. Genetic polymorphisms influence bodily metabolism of certain nutrients and some folks may be extremely susceptible to cancers related to diet because of genetic predispositions. Individuals possessing specific MTHFR gene variants may face elevated colorectal cancer risk with suboptimal folate consumption. Cancer epidemiology necessitates consideration of both environmental influences and genetic predispositions very thoroughly nowadays in research circles (Kiani et al, 2022).

The Complexity of Dietary Patterns

Dietary patterns are inherently complex involving interaction of various foods and myriad nutrients in deeply intricate ways. Overall dietary patterns tend to have a much greater impact on cancer risk than specific foods eaten in isolation typically do. A Mediterranean diet rich in fruits and veggies may slash cancer risk through a medley of dietary factors rather than one lone nutrient (Dominguez et al, 2021).

Future Directions in Diet-Cancer Epidemiology

Emerging research areas are gaining traction slowly as understanding deepens between diet and cancer. Advances in genomics are allowing researchers to explore individual genetic profiles influencing dietary responses quite intricately and cancer risk varies accordingly. Personalized dietary advice stemming from genetic profiles might result in fairly effective strategies for preventing various forms of cancer very successfully. Future cohort studies following individuals over protracted periods will ostensibly elucidate long-term effects of diverse dietary regimens on oncogenesis and survivability (Nicastro et al, 2012).

Randomized controlled trials intervening in individual diets and tracking cancer outcomes might furnish stronger evidence of causal relationships. Epidemiological studies have unearthed links between diet and cancer risk by identifying risk factors and protective foods quite effectively nowadays. Significant strides have been made recently but complexity of diet-cancer relationships necessitates further investigation very urgently nowadays for cancer prevention. Integration of genetic factors and longitudinal studies alongside personalized nutrition approaches will be crucial in advancing understanding of diet's role in cancer significantly (Nicastro et al, 2012).

8. Addressing Dietary Interventions in Cancer Prevention:

Numerous epidemiological studies underscore potential of specific foods and nutrients in reducing cancer risk through dietary interventions long recognized as pivotal. Evidence amassed over several decades demonstrates diet plays a crucial quasi causal role in cancer prevention and pathological progression simultaneously. Epidemiological perspective offers a singular lens for grasping intricate interplay between dietary habits environment and heightened cancer risk factors. Researchers have identified various modifiable dietary factors promoting or inhibiting cancer development through analysis of large populations and long-term dietary habits.

Epidemiological studies investigating dietary interventions in cancer prevention yield fascinating findings that we will explore thoroughly in this section. Dietary patterns and specific nutrients have shown promise in reducing cancer risk alongside various challenges associated with dietary interventions. Implications of these findings for public health strategies and future research in nutritional oncology will be deliberated quite thoroughly afterwards .

8.1. Epidemiological Evidence on Dietary Interventions in Cancer Prevention

Epidemiological studies via cohort studies and meta-analyses have consistently underscored effectiveness of dietary interventions in reducing incidence of various cancers. Dietary tweaks influence cancer risk profoundly over time shedding light on potential mechanisms linking food intake roughly to carcinogenic processes.

Dietary Patterns for Cancer Prevention

Overall dietary patterns play a significant role in reducing cancer risk rather than individual foods or specific nutrients being solely responsible. Dietary patterns consider interactions among various foods eaten within specific contexts emphasizing importance of holistic approaches nutritionally speaking very broadly.

- » **Mediterranean Diet:** The Mediterranean diet, which is rich in fruits, vegetables, whole grains, legumes, nuts, and olive oil, has been consistently associated with a lower risk of several cancers, including colorectal, breast, and prostate cancer. Mediterranean diet rich in fruits vegetables whole grains legumes nuts and olive oil has been consistently linked with lower risk of several cancers (Mentella et al, 2019).
- » **Plant-based Diets:** The plant-based diet, which focuses on the consumption of plant-derived foods while minimizing animal products, has shown promising results in reducing the incidence of cancer, particularly in relation to colon and lung cancers. This diet's anti-inflammatory properties largely attributed to high monounsaturated fat content and antioxidants are thought to mitigate cancer risk somewhat by reducing oxidative stress and encourage DNA repair (Mentella et al, 2019).
- » **Western Diet:** In contrast, the Western diet, which is characterized by high intake of processed foods, red meat, refined sugars, and saturated fats, has been associated with an increased risk of developing various types of cancer, particularly colorectal, pancreatic, and breast cancers. Plant-based diets yield promising results in cancer reduction especially regarding colon and lung cancers by mainly consuming plant-derived foods (Mentella et al, 2019).

Specific Nutrients and Cancer Risk

Epidemiological studies have identified specific nutrients that can either ramp up or mitigate cancer risk through various dietary patterns. Nutrients typically exert influence via various cellular signaling pathways and immune modulation or antioxidant protection with effects varying wildly across genetic backgrounds.

» **Folate:** Folate, a water-soluble B-vitamin, plays a crucial role in DNA synthesis, repair, and methylation, processes that are vital for maintaining genome stability. Folate a water-soluble B-vitamin plays a crucial role in DNA synthesis repair and methylation vital for genome stability maintenance . Epidemiological evidence suggests adequate folate intake may help prevent colorectal cancer by supporting various DNA-related processes somewhat effectively. Folate plays a dicey role somewhat because high-dose supplementation has been tenuously linked to heightened prostate cancer risk in certain dodgy studies (Crider et al, 2012).

» **Vitamin D:** Vitamin D is well-known for its role in maintaining bone health, but accumulating evidence also suggests that it has anticancer properties. Dietary folate from sources like leafy greens and fortified grains apparently provides very optimal protection against certain health issues naturally. Vitamin D plays a crucial role in maintaining bone health but emerging evidence sporadically suggests some very potent anticancer properties too. Low levels of vitamin D correlate with heightened risk of various cancers including breast prostate and colorectal malignancies quite frequently (Laird et al, 2010).

» **Omega-3 Fatty Acids:** Omega-3 fatty acids, found in fatty fish and certain plant oils, are known for their anti-inflammatory and anti-cancer properties. Vitamin D regulates several crucial cellular functions including apoptosis and cell differentiation thereby helping prevent cancerous transformations somewhat effectively. Optimal cancer prevention requires consuming vitamin D-rich foods such as fatty fish and egg yolks or getting adequate sunlight exposure daily (Gutiérrez et al, 2019).

» **Antioxidants:** Antioxidants, including vitamins C and E, flavonoids, and polyphenols, found in fruits and vegetables, help combat oxidative stress by neutralizing free radicals that can cause DNA damage and promote cancer. Omega-3 fatty acids found in fatty fish and certain plant oils are known for their highly touted anti-inflammatory properties remarkably. Higher intake of omega-3s especially EPA and DHA has been linked with reduced risk of various cancers including breast cancer and colorectal cancer (Pruteanu et al, 2023).

8.2. Challenges and Limitations of Dietary Interventions in Cancer Prevention

Epidemiological studies offer valuable insights into relationships between diet and cancer but have plenty of glaring methodological shortcomings inherently. Multiple factors confound efforts quite seriously to discern efficacy of various dietary regimens in preventing cancer occurrence effectively nowadays.

Methodological Challenges

Diet complexity makes isolating effects of specific nutrients or certain foods on cancer risk extremely challenging very much always nowadays. Numerous factors like caloric intake and genetic predispositions heavily influence cancer outcomes alongside exercise and alcohol consumption in varied dietary patterns. Self-reported dietary data suffers from recall bias and misreporting thereby potentially grossly distorting findings in a rather significant way. Socio-economic status and smoking habits alongside physical activity must be factored into epidemiological research to avoid skewing results substantially.

Long-Term vs. Short-Term Effects

Cancer develops over a protracted timeframe and impact of dietary habits on cancer risk becomes glaringly apparent decades after interventions start. Some cohort studies yield lengthy insights but many investigations get bogged down in fairly short observation periods rather quickly. Assessing full effects of dietary interventions on cancer prevention proves arduous owing largely to inherent complexities surrounding such evaluations.

Variability in Individual Response

People metabolize nutrients differently and react uniquely to various dietary elements while being exposed somewhat variably to environmental carcinogens. Polymorphisms in genes related to folate metabolism or vitamin D receptor genes influence cancer risk by interacting with various dietary factors somewhat differently. Personalized dietary interventions tailored rather intricately to an individual's unique genetic makeup may prove remarkably more effective than broad generalized recommendations.

External Environmental Factors

Pollution and toxins interfere with effects of dietary interventions while lifestyle factors like smoking and boozing play a role too. Exposure to carcinogens from various environmental sources can severely undermine even a fairly well balanced nutrient rich diet occasionally.

8.3. Future Directions in Dietary Cancer Prevention

Growing evidence from epidemiological studies offers direction for public health interventions and cancer prevention strategies through advances in personalized nutrition somewhat effectively nowadays. Advances in nutrigenomics and precision nutrition will enable fairly tailored dietary recommendations accounting quirky individual genetic profiles and health history messily. Genetic variants influence diet-cancer interactions and personalized dietary interventions might be developed slowly with surprising optimism for cancer prevention.

» **Interventional Trials:** Randomized controlled trials (RCTs) that test specific dietary interventions in populations at risk for cancer are needed to establish definitive cause-and-effect relationships. Randomized controlled trials testing specific dietary interventions in cancer-prone populations are crucial for establishing definitive cause-and-effect relationships between diet and cancer development effectively.

» **Dietary Guidelines:** As the evidence base grows, updated dietary guidelines that emphasize cancer prevention should be developed. RCTs help ascertain optimal nutrient amounts such as omega-3 fatty acids or vitamin D required for preventing cancer effectively nowadays. Updated dietary guidelines emphasizing cancer prevention should be developed as evidence mounts steadily over time. Guidelines must be somewhat adaptable for different demographics with varying cultural proclivities and unequal access to nutritional sustenance and local carcinogenic hazards. Epidemiological studies yield invaluable insights into diet's role in cancer prevention identifying both protective dietary facets and risk-associated factors simultaneously. Dietary patterns emphasizing whole grains and healthy fats show considerable promise for cancer prevention yet no universal approach exists (Donaldson MS, 2004).

9. Conclusion

Growing epidemiological evidence profoundly underscores impact of various dietary patterns on cancer incidence rates across diverse global populations. Overall dietary patterns reflecting complexity and synergy of human diet offer robust insights into cancer risk prevention quite effectively now. Cohort and case-control studies have shown that plant-based diets rich in nutrients like those found in Mediterranean patterns lower cancer incidence markedly. Diets rich in fruits and whole grains alongside legumes and healthy fats often feature minimal red meat and refined sugars. Beneficial influences on gut microbiota and hormonal balance are thought to arise from anti-inflammatory properties and antioxidant effects simultaneously.

Diets heavy in saturated fats and added sugars have been tied partly to heightened carcinogenesis risk due to chronic inflammation and insulin resistance. Such dietary habits often coexist with other modifiable risk factors like obesity and smoking, compounding cancer risk heavily in vulnerable demographics. Challenges stubbornly remain despite valuable insights gleaned from epidemiological research. Difficulties arise in accurately measuring dietary intake and accounting for confounding variables and complex genetic interactions within various environments. Longitudinal studies quite remarkably continue refining our understanding of how dietary behaviours influence cancer risk across diverse populations over considerable time spans.

Integrating epidemiological findings into public health strategies has become utterly imperative as cancer incidence rises rapidly worldwide. Policymakers, healthcare providers, and researchers must collaborate fairly intensely, translating scientific evidence into rather practical dietary guidelines and somewhat innovative community-based interventions. Advancements in technology and nutritional science, such as digital dietary tracking and microbiome profiling,, offer fresh tools supporting dietary change at the individual level now. Evidence pointing clearly towards a crucial role for diet in thwarting cancer development is overwhelming very much across the board. Epidemiological insights guide dietary recommendations quite effectively and represent a somewhat powerful strategy for reducing global cancer burden.

References

Ağagündüz D, Şahin TÖ, Yılmaz B, Ekenci KD, Duyar Özer Ş, Capasso R. Cruciferous Vegetables and Their Bioactive Metabolites: from Prevention to Novel Therapies of Colorectal Cancer. Evid Based Complement Alternat Med. 2022 Apr 11;2022:1534083. doi: 10.1155/2022/1534083. PMID: 35449807; PMCID: PMC9017484.

Alengebawy A, Abdelkhalek ST, Qureshi SR, Wang MQ. Heavy Metals and Pesticides Toxicity in Agricultural Soil and Plants: Ecological Risks and Human Health Implications. Toxics. 2021 Feb 25;9(3):42. doi: 10.3390/toxics9030042. PMID: 33668829; PMCID: PMC7996329.

Aykan NF. Red Meat and Colorectal Cancer. Oncol Rev. 2015 Dec 28;9(1):288. doi: 10.4081/oncol.2015.288. PMID: 26779313; PMCID: PMC4698595.

Britten O, Tosi S. The role of diet in cancer: the potential of shaping public policy and clinical outcomes in the UK. Genes Nutr. 2024 Aug 3;19(1):15. doi: 10.1186/s12263-024-00750-9. PMID: 39097687; PMCID: PMC11298086.

Caprara G. Mediterranean-Type Dietary Pattern and Physical Activity: The Winning Combination to Counteract the Rising Burden of Non-Communicable Diseases (NCDs). Nutrients. 2021 Jan 28;13(2):429. doi: 10.3390/nu13020429. PMID: 33525638; PMCID: PMC7910909.

Celiberto F, Aloisio A, Girardi B, Pricci M, Iannone A, Russo F, Riezzo G, D'Attoma B, Ierardi E, Losurdo G, Di Leo A. Fibres and Colorectal Cancer: Clinical and Molecular Evidence. Int J Mol Sci. 2023 Aug 31;24(17):13501. doi: 10.3390/ijms241713501. PMID: 37686308; PMCID: PMC10488173.

Chu AH, Lin K, Croker H, Kefyalew S, Becerra-Tomás N, Dossus L, González-Gil EM, Ahmadi N, Park Y, Krebs J, Weijenberg MP, Baskin ML, Copson E, Lewis SJ, Seidell JC, Chowdhury R, Hill L, Chan DS, Lee DH, Giovannucci EL. Dietary patterns and colorectal cancer risk: Global Cancer Update Programme (CUP Global) systematic literature review. Am J Clin Nutr. 2025 May;121(5):999-1016. doi: 10.1016/j.ajcnut.2025.02.021. Epub 2025 Feb 25. PMID: 40010692; PMCID: PMC12107496.

Clemente-Suárez VJ, Beltrán-Velasco AI, Redondo-Flórez L, Martín-Rodríguez A, Tornero-Aguilera JF. Global Impacts of Western Diet and Its Effects on Metabolism and Health: A Narrative Review. Nutrients. 2023 Jun 14;15(12):2749. doi: 10.3390/nu15122749. PMID: 37375654; PMCID: PMC10302286.

Clemente-Suárez VJ, Mielgo-Ayuso J, Martín-Rodríguez A, Ramos-Campo DJ, Redondo-Flórez L, Tornero-Aguilera JF. The Burden of Carbohydrates in Health and Disease. Nutrients. 2022 Sep 15;14(18):3809. doi: 10.3390/nu14183809. PMID: 36145184; PMCID: PMC9505863.

Crider KS, Yang TP, Berry RJ, Bailey LB. Folate and DNA methylation: a review of molecular mechanisms and the evidence for folate's role. Adv Nutr. 2012 Jan;3(1):21-38. doi: 10.3945/an.111.000992. Epub 2012 Jan 5. PMID: 22332098; PMCID: PMC3262611.

Dominguez LJ, Di Bella G, Veronese N, Barbagallo M. Impact of Mediterranean Diet on Chronic Non-Communicable Diseases and Longevity. Nutrients. 2021 Jun 12;13(6):2028. doi: 10.3390/nu13062028. PMID: 34204683; PMCID: PMC8231595.

Donaldson MS. Nutrition and cancer: a review of the evidence for an anti-cancer diet. Nutr J. 2004 Oct 20;3:19. Doi: 10.1186/1475-2891-3-19. PMID: 15496224; PMCID: PMC526387.

Duthie SJ. Folate and cancer: how DNA damage, repair and methylation impact colon carcinogenesis. J Inherit Metab Dis. 2011 Feb;34(1):101-9. doi: 10.1007/s10545-010-9128-0. Epub 2010 Jun 11. PMID: 20544289.

Elsamanoudy AZ, Mohamed Neamat-Allah MA, Hisham Mohammad FA, Hassanien M, Nada HA. The role of nutrition-related genes and nutrigenetics in understanding the pathogenesis of cancer. J Microsc Ultrastruct. 2016 Jul-Sep;4(3):115-122. doi: 10.1016/j.jmau.2016.02.002. Epub 2016 Mar 8. PMID: 30023217; PMCID: PMC6014201.

Enkhmaa B, Surampudi P, Anuurad E, et al. Lifestyle Changes: Effect of Diet, Exercise, Functional Food, and Obesity Treatment on Lipids and Lipoproteins. [Updated 2018 Sep 11]. In: Feingold KR, Ahmed SF, Anawalt B, et al., editors. Endotext [Internet]. South Dartmouth (MA): MDText.com, Inc.; 2000-. Available from: https://www.ncbi.nlm.nih.gov/books/NBK326737/

Ennouri S, Daoud N, Berrazegua Y, El Benna H, Korbi S, Rachdi H, Mejri N, Labidi S, Boussen H. VARIATIONS IN DIETARY HABITS DURING CANCER TREATMENT: RESULTS OF A CROSS-SECTIONAL SURVEY. Acta Clin Croat. 2024 Apr;63(1):80-88. doi: 10.20471/acc.2024.63.01.10. PMID: 39959318; PMCID: PMC11827403.

Fagbohun OF, Gillies CR, Murphy KPJ, Rupasinghe HPV. Role of Antioxidant Vitamins and Other Micronutrients on Regulations of Specific Genes and Signaling Pathways in the Prevention and Treatment of Cancer. Int J Mol Sci. 2023 Mar 23;24(7):6092. doi: 10.3390/ijms24076092. PMID: 37047063; PMCID: PMC10093825.

Freitas RDS, Campos MM. Protective Effects of Omega-3 Fatty Acids in Cancer-Related Complications. Nutrients. 2019 Apr 26;11(5):945. doi: 10.3390/nu11050945. PMID: 31035457; PMCID: PMC6566772.

Grune T, Lietz G, Palou A, Ross AC, Stahl W, Tang G, Thurnham D, Yin SA, Biesalski HK. Beta-carotene is an important vitamin A source for humans. J Nutr. 2010 Dec;140(12):2268S-2285S. doi: 10.3945/jn.109.119024. Epub 2010 Oct 27. PMID: 20980645; PMCID: PMC3139236.

Gutiérrez S, Svahn SL, Johansson ME. Effects of Omega-3 Fatty Acids on Immune Cells. Int J Mol Sci. 2019 Oct 11;20(20):5028. doi: 10.3390/ijms20205028. PMID: 31614433; PMCID: PMC6834330.

He JW, Huang ZX, Su YF, Mo YQ. Dietary saturated fatty acids and prostate cancer: insights into NF-κB pathway and lipid metabolism mechanisms. Discov Oncol. 2025 Jun 20;16(1):1166. doi: 10.1007/s12672-025-03005-0. PMID: 40542303; PMCID: PMC12181547.

Hu J, Wang J, Li Y, Xue K, Kan J. Use of Dietary Fibres in Reducing the Risk of Several Cancer Types: An Umbrella Review. Nutrients. 2023 May 30;15(11):2545. doi: 10.3390/nu15112545. PMID: 37299507; PMCID: PMC10255454.

Jiang J, Chen B, Tang B, Wei Q. Selenium in Prostate Cancer: Prevention, Progression, and Treatment. Pharmaceuticals (Basel). 2023 Sep 5;16(9):1250. doi: 10.3390/ph16091250. PMID: 37765058; PMCID: PMC10536940.

Jiao L, Flood A, Subar AF, Hollenbeck AR, Schatzkin A, Stolzenberg-Solomon R. Glycemic index, carbohydrates, glycemic load, and the risk of pancreatic cancer in a prospective cohort study. Cancer Epidemiol Biomarkers Prev. 2009 Apr;18(4):1144-51. doi: 10.1158/1055-9965.EPI-08-1135. Epub 2009 Mar 31. PMID: 19336549; PMCID: PMC2687095.

Key TJ, Bradbury KE, Perez-Cornago A, Sinha R, Tsilidis KK, Tsugane S. Diet, nutrition, and cancer risk: what do we know and what is the way forward? BMJ. 2020 Mar 5;368:m511. doi: 10.1136/bmj.m511. Erratum in: BMJ. 2020 Mar 11;368:m996. doi: 10.1136/bmj.m996. PMID: 32139373; PMCID: PMC7190379.

Kiani AK, Bonetti G, Donato K, Kaftalli J, Herbst KL, Stuppia L, Fioretti F, Nodari S, Perrone M, Chiurazzi P, Bellinato F, Gisondi P, Bertelli M. Polymorphisms, diet and nutrigenomics. J Prev Med Hyg. 2022 Oct 17;63(2 Suppl 3):E125-E141. doi: 10.15167/2421-4248/jpmh2022.63.2S3.2754. PMID: 36479483; PMCID: PMC9710387.

Kunzmann AT, Coleman HG, Huang WY, Kitahara CM, Cantwell MM, Berndt SI. Dietary fibre intake and risk of colorectal cancer and incident and recurrent adenoma in the Prostate, Lung, Colorectal, and Ovarian Cancer Screening Trial. Am J Clin Nutr. 2015 Oct;102(4):881-90. doi: 10.3945/ajcn.115.113282. Epub 2015 Aug 12. PMID: 26269366; PMCID: PMC4588743.

Laird E, Ward M, McSorley E, Strain JJ, Wallace J. Vitamin D and bone health: potential mechanisms. Nutrients. 2010 Jul;2(7):693-724. doi: 10.3390/nu2070693. Epub 2010 Jul 5. PMID: 22254049; PMCID: PMC3257679.

Land SR, Liu Q, Wickerham DL, Costantino JP, Ganz PA. Cigarette smoking, physical activity, and alcohol consumption as predictors of cancer incidence among women at high risk of breast cancer in the NSABP P-1 trial. Cancer Epidemiol Biomarkers Prev. 2014 May;23(5):823-32. doi: 10.1158/1055-9965.EPI-13-1105-T. Epub 2014 Feb 25. PMID: 24569437; PMCID: PMC4011972.

Makarem N, Nicholson JM, Bandera EV, McKeown NM, Parekh N. Consumption of whole grains and cereal fibre in relation to cancer risk: a systematic review of longitudinal studies. Nutr Rev. 2016 Jun;74(6):353-73. doi: 10.1093/nutrit/nuw003. Epub 2016 May 5. PMID: 27257283; PMCID: PMC4892300.

Mei J, Qian M, Hou Y, Liang M, Chen Y, Wang C, Zhang J. Association of saturated fatty acids with cancer risk: a systematic review and meta-analysis. Lipids Health Dis. 2024 Jan 30;23(1):32. doi: 10.1186/s12944-024-02025-z. PMID: 38291432; PMCID: PMC10826095.

Mentella MC, Scaldaferri F, Ricci C, Gasbarrini A, Miggiano GAD. Cancer and Mediterranean Diet: A Review. Nutrients. 2019 Sep 2;11(9):2059. doi: 10.3390/nu11092059. PMID: 31480794; PMCID: PMC6770822.

Mitra S, Emran TB, Chandran D, Zidan BMRM, Das R, Mamada SS, Masyita A, Salampe M, Nainu F, Khandaker MU, Idris AM, Simal-Gandara J. Cruciferous vegetables as a treasure of functional foods bioactive compounds: Targeting p53 family in gastrointestinal tract and associated cancers. Front Nutr. 2022 Aug 4;9:951935. doi: 10.3389/fnut.2022.951935. PMID: 35990357; PMCID: PMC9386315.

Mozaffarian D, Hao T, Rimm EB, Willett WC, Hu FB. Changes in diet and lifestyle and long-term weight gain in women and men. N Engl J Med. 2011 Jun 23;364(25):2392-404. doi: 10.1056/NEJMoa1014296. PMID: 21696306; PMCID: PMC3151731.

Nagy S, Petrosky SN, Demory Beckler M, Kesselman MM. The Impact of Modern Dietary Practices on Cancer Risk and Progression: A Systematic Review. Cureus. 2023 Oct 7;15(10):e46639. doi: 10.7759/cureus.46639. PMID: 37937022; PMCID: PMC10627144.

Nemati A, Mahdavi R, Naghizadeh Baghi A. Case-control study of dietary pattern and other risk factors for gastric cancer. Health Promot Perspect. 2012 Jul 1;2(1):20-7. Doi: 10.5681/hpp.2012.003. PMID: 24688914; PMCID: PMC3963657.

Nicastro HL, Trujillo EB, Milner JA. Nutrigenomics and Cancer Prevention. Curr Nutr Rep. 2012 Mar 1;1(1):37-43. doi: 10.1007/s13668-011-0007-6. PMID: 24910810; PMCID: PMC4047824.

Oniang'o R, Maingi Z, Jaika S, Konyole S. Africa's contribution to global sustainable and healthy diets: a scoping review. Front Nutr. 2025 May 2;12:1519248. doi: 10.3389/fnut.2025.1519248. PMID: 40386220; PMCID: PMC12083016.

Orlich MJ, Singh PN, Sabaté J, Fan J, Sveen L, Bennett H, Knutsen SF, Beeson WL, Jaceldo-Siegl K, Butler TL, Herring RP, Fraser GE. Vegetarian dietary patterns and the risk of colorectal cancers. JAMA Intern Med. 2015 May;175(5):767-76. doi: 10.1001/jamainternmed.2015.59. PMID: 25751512; PMCID: PMC4420687.

Parsa N. Environmental factors inducing human cancers. Iran J Public Health. 2012;41(11):1-9. Epub 2012 Nov 1. PMID: 23304670; PMCID: PMC3521879.

Pawlowska E, Szczepanska J, Blasiak J. Pro- and Antioxidant Effects of Vitamin C in Cancer in Correspondence to Its Dietary and Pharmacological Concentrations. Oxid Med Cell Longev. 2019 Dec 24;2019:7286737. Doi: 10.1155/2019/7286737. PMID: 31934267; PMCID: PMC6942884.

Pruteanu LL, Bailey DS, Grădinaru AC, Jäntschi L. The Biochemistry and Effectiveness of Antioxidants in Food, Fruits, and Marine Algae. Antioxidants (Basel). 2023 Apr 2;12(4):860. doi: 10.3390/antiox12040860. PMID: 37107235; PMCID: PMC10135154.

Qian F, Riddle MC, Wylie-Rosett J, Hu FB. Red and Processed Meats and Health Risks: How Strong Is the Evidence? Diabetes Care. 2020 Feb;43(2):265-271. doi: 10.2337/dci19-0063. PMID: 31959642; PMCID: PMC6971786.

Rahaman MM, Hossain R, Herrera-Bravo J, Islam MT, Atolani O, Adeyemi OS, Owolodun OA, Kambizi L, Daştan SD, Calina D, Sharifi-Rad J. Natural antioxidants from some fruits, seeds, foods, natural products, and associated health benefits: An update. Food Sci Nutr. 2023 Jan 13;11(4):1657-1670. doi: 10.1002/fsn3.3217. PMID: 37051367; PMCID: PMC10084981.

Ratna A, Mandrekar P. Alcohol and Cancer: Mechanisms and Therapies. Biomolecules. 2017 Aug 14;7(3):61. doi: 10.3390/biom7030061. PMID: 28805741; PMCID: PMC5618242.

Rumgay H, Murphy N, Ferrari P, Soerjomataram I. Alcohol and Cancer: Epidemiology and Biological Mechanisms. Nutrients. 2021 Sep 11;13(9):3173. doi: 10.3390/nu13093173. PMID: 34579050; PMCID: PMC8470184.

Saha SK, Lee SB, Won J, Choi HY, Kim K, Yang GM, Dayem AA, Cho SG. Correlation between Oxidative Stress, Nutrition, and Cancer Initiation. Int J Mol Sci. 2017 Jul 17;18(7):1544. doi: 10.3390/ijms18071544. PMID: 28714931; PMCID: PMC5536032.

Santarelli RL, Pierre F, Corpet DE. Processed meat and colorectal cancer: a review of epidemiologic and experimental evidence. Nutr Cancer. 2008;60(2):131-44. doi: 10.1080/01635580701684872. PMID: 18444144; PMCID: PMC2661797.

Seiler A, Chen MA, Brown RL, Fagundes CP. Obesity, Dietary Factors, Nutrition, and Breast Cancer Risk. Curr Breast Cancer Rep. 2018 Mar;10(1):14-27. doi: 10.1007/s12609-018-0264-0. Epub 2018 Jan 19. PMID: 30662586; PMCID: PMC6335046.

Sharman R, Harris Z, Ernst B, Mussallem D, Larsen A, Gowin K. Lifestyle Factors and Cancer: A Narrative Review. Mayo Clin Proc Innov Qual Outcomes. 2024 Mar 4;8(2):166-183. doi: 10.1016/j.mayocpiqo.2024.01.004. PMID: 38468817; PMCID: PMC10925935.

Sivasubramanian BP, Dave M, Panchal V, Saifa-Bonsu J, Konka S, Noei F, Nagaraj S, Terpari U, Savani P, Vekaria PH, Samala Venkata V, Manjani L. Comprehensive Review of Red Meat Consumption and the Risk of Cancer. Cureus. 2023 Sep 15;15(9):e45324. doi: 10.7759/cureus.45324. PMID: 37849565; PMCID: PMC10577092.

Sung H, Ferlay J, Siegel RL, Laversanne M, Soerjomataram I, Jemal A, Bray F. Global Cancer Statistics 2020: GLOBOCAN Estimates of Incidence and Mortality Worldwide for 36 Cancers in 185 Countries. CA Cancer J Clin. 2021 May;71(3):209-249. doi: 10.3322/caac.21660. Epub 2021 Feb 4. PMID: 33538338.

Traber MG, Stevens JF. Vitamins C and E: beneficial effects from a mechanistic perspective. Free Radic Biol Med. 2011 Sep 1;51(5):1000-13. doi: 10.1016/j.freeradbiomed.2011.05.017. Epub 2011 May 25. PMID: 21664268; PMCID: PMC3156342.

Vuolo L, Di Somma C, Faggiano A, Colao A. Vitamin D and cancer. Front Endocrinol (Lausanne). 2012 Apr 23;3:58. Doi: 10.3389/fendo.2012.00058. PMID: 22649423; PMCID: PMC3355893.

Widmer RJ, Flammer AJ, Lerman LO, Lerman A. The Mediterranean diet, its components, and cardiovascular disease. Am J Med. 2015 Mar;128(3):229-38. doi: 10.1016/j.amjmed.2014.10.014. Epub 2014 Oct 15. PMID: 25447615; PMCID: PMC4339461.

Chapter 3

Molecular Dialogues: Nutritional Modulators of Cellular Homeostasis

Praneeth Juvvi[1], Sheetanshu Gupta[2*], Lokesh Kumar Mishra[3], and Sarfraj Ahmad Siddiqui[4]

[1]Department of Food Processing Technology, College of Food Technology-Central Agricultural University, Imphal, Manipur, India
[2]Department of Food Safety and Quality Assurance, College of Food Technology, Central Agricultural University (CAU), Imphal, Manipur, India
[3]Department of BPME, College of Agriculture, Central Agricultural University (CAU), Imphal, Manipur, India
[4]Department of Biochemistry, King George's Medical University, U.P., India

Abstract

Cellular homeostasis remains vital for sustaining normal cell function and thwarting pathological conditions like cancer or metabolic disorders very frequently nowadays. Nutritional modulators profoundly sway cellular homeostasis via complex molecular crosstalk, drastically affecting overall function and balance quite unpredictably. Vitamins and polyphenols deeply interact with cellular pathways that regulate homeostasis through autophagy and stress responses involving oxidative damage. Major cellular regulators such as mTOR and AMPK engage in molecular crosstalk with dietary signals, orchestrating survival, growth, differentiation, and apoptosis very intricately. Profound dietary influence significantly affects cellular pathways and homeostasis, often reinforcing health or precipitating disease development via diverse nutrient consumption patterns. Nutrients weirdly modulate epigenetic changes, influencing gene expression, significantly impacting health outcomes over prolonged periods, drastically, sometimes very badly. The gut microbiome serves as an intermediary between diet and cellular health, underscoring its heavy involvement in nutrient metabolism and immune modulation very effectively. Cutting-edge technologies like metabolomics and recent findings are harnessed effectively, providing a fairly comprehensive view of nutrition's modulatory role.

Keywords: Cellular Homeostasis, Nutritional Signalling, Metabolic Pathways, Autophagy, Oxidative Stress, Cellular Adaptation

DOI: 10.1201/9781042010387-3

1. Introduction

Nutrition profoundly influences human physiology by intricately linking diet and cellular health in a delicate balancing act of maintaining homeostasis. Stable internal conditions within cells and tissues are crucial for survival, ensuring bodily responses to external environmental changes happen effectively. Dysfunctional metabolic processes, inflammation, and oxidative stress can lead to the onset of cancer and various cardiovascular conditions suddenly. Nutrition plays a pivotal role in regulating various cellular processes, maintaining balance through bioactive components, making it essential for molecular biology and disease prevention. Cellular homeostasis is maintained through an intricate network of signalling pathways and metabolic processes responding quietly to intrinsic and extrinsic cues (Libretti and Puckett, 2025).

Genetic factors are often seen as a blueprint for cellular functions, but external factors like environmental toxins significantly influence gene expression. Emerging research highlights nutrients acting as modulators, fine-tuning molecular pathways that regulate various cellular functions deeply within cells. Nutrients ranging from proteins and fats to vitamins and minerals interact heavily with cellular machinery, influencing metabolic processes and gene expression significantly. Certain dietary components act as signalling molecules influencing key metabolic pathways crucial for maintaining cellular function very effectively. Pathways like AMP-activated protein kinase and mechanistic target of rapamycin regulate energy balance and cell growth amidst oxidative stress responses (Tiffon C, 2018).

Glucose and various bioactive compounds found in plant foods can modulate cell survival and apoptosis by activating or inhibiting certain pathways. Glucose, a primary energy source for most cells, exists as one most well-studied nutrients in the context of cellular homeostasis, evidently. Dysregulated glucose metabolism seen in conditions like obesity and type 2 diabetes disrupts cellular homeostasis, leading to insulin resistance, chronic inflammation and increased risk of diseases like cancer. Polyphenols found in fruits and tea, alongside fibre and unsaturated fats, have been shown to mitigate metabolic disruptions by modulating glucose metabolism quite effectively and reducing oxidative stress. Glucose availability in the body is tightly controlled by insulin and glucagon, and sundry hormones that regulate energy homeostasis are influenced heavily by dietary intake (Vaughn and Deshmukh, 2008).

mTOR pathway plays a crucial role in cellular homeostasis, regulating cell growth, metabolism and protein synthesis amidst varied nutrient availability and stress signals. Overactivation of mTOR has been heavily implicated in various nasty diseases, including cancer and weird neurodegenerative disorders. Amino acids, especially leucine and insulin, activate the mTOR pathway heavily, while caloric restriction or plant-based diets inhibit it, promoting longevity. Modulating mTOR via dietary regimens unveils promising therapeutic avenues aimed squarely at rejuvenating cellular homeostasis and thwarting maladies spawned by unruly cell proliferation. Inflammation plays a crucial role in maintaining cellular homeostasis, particularly in contexts fraught with chronic disease and turmoil (Saxton and Sabatini, 2017).

Dysregulated nutrient intake precipitates chronic low-grade inflammation, resulting in copious production of inflammatory cytokines and rampant oxidative stress. Disruption occurs, thereby precipitating aberrant cellular signalling and heightening the risk of various diseases such as cancer, cardiovascular malady or autoimmune disorder. Nutritional components like omega-3 fatty acids from fish oils and polyphenols can help counteract inflammation deeply within cellular processes. Omega-3 fatty acids influence the NF-kB pathway, a critical mediator of inflammation often overactive in various chronic diseases, very frequently nowadays (Reuter et al, 2010).

Recent research has brought attention sharply upwards towards the roles of epigenetics in cellular homeostasis alongside well-known nutrients. Epigenetic tweaks like DNA methylation or histone modification play a crucial role in gene expression regulation, very much sans DNA sequence alteration. Nutritional factors profoundly impact epigenetic mechanisms, thereby altering the function of cells greatly in various subtle yet significant ways. Certain nutrients like folate and vitamin B12 have been shown to influence DNA methylation patterns, thereby potentially affecting the expression of genes related to stress response. Molecular dialogue between diet and gene expression represents an increasing frontier in grasping how nutrition drastically reshapes cellular health mechanisms (Handy et al, 2011). Cells degrade damaged components via autophagy, a vital process playing a critical role in maintaining homeostasis within cells remarkably well under stressful conditions. Certain polyphenols and vitamins, alongside intermittent fasting and caloric restriction, modulate autophagy, enhancing the removal of damaged organelles and proteins very effectively. Cellular integrity and function are maintained, thereby thwarting the buildup of damage that can precipitate cancer and sundry other maladies quite rapidly. Various signalling pathways intricately mediate the diet's influence on autophagy, involving AMPK and mTOR pathways, amidst complex molecular mechanisms, rather elaborately. Molecular dialogues between nutrition and cellular homeostasis will be explored here, focusing on how diet components heavily modulate key pathways (Ortega et al, 2024).

2. Nutrient Sensing and Cellular Communication Pathways

The human body relies heavily on myriad complex signals and various cellular pathways for regulating energy balance, growth, repair and overall survival mechanisms. Crucial regulatory mechanisms maintain cellular homeostasis remarkably well amidst environmental flux and react swiftly to various metabolic cues. Cells detect changes in nutrient availability very intricately and respond accordingly, playing a rather crucial role in sustaining such vital processes. Disruptions in nutrient-sensing pathways increasingly play a key role in oncogenesis, whereby normal cells morph into decidedly cancerous ones quite rapidly. Cellular behaviour and cancer development are influenced by various nutrient-sensing pathways and mechanisms involved in cellular communication quite intricately. Major nutrient-sensing pathways such as the insulin/IGF-1 axis and mTOR signalling alongside the AMPK pathway, SIRT1, and hypoxia-inducible factors will be examined in depth now. Elucidating such pathways yields profound insight into how nutritional tweaks and dietary regimens influence cancer onset and malignant progression rapidly (Liu et al, 2025).

2.1. The Role of Cellular Pathways

The body has evolved remarkably sensitive mechanisms very quickly to detect various nutrients and thereby regulate myriad cellular functions fairly precisely. Cells adapt swiftly under varying nutrient availability conditions, and biosynthesis proceeds vigorously only when sufficient energy resources exist. Cells slow down growth and division drastically under low nutrient levels, while nutrient-rich conditions vigorously promote cell cycle progression and anabolic processes. Cancer cells often hijack nutrient-sensing systems, enabling rather uncontrolled growth and survival in very nutrient-poor environments almost always.

2.1.1. Insulin/IGF-1 Signaling Pathway

Insulin and insulin-like growth factor 1 signaling constitutes a crucial pathway for sensing nutrients remarkably well in various organisms. Insulin and IGF-1 play crucial roles in regulating cell survival quite intricately alongside growth and metabolism simultaneously. Insulin gets released very quickly after eating food, especially carbs, whereas IGF-1 plays a major role in cell proliferation and growth. Insulin signalling activates the insulin receptor, which triggers a cascade of downstream signalling events through the PI3K-AKT-mTOR pathway. Insulin signalling activates the insulin receptor, which triggers a cascade of downstream signalling events through the PI3K-AKT-mTOR pathway quite rapidly (Cheng et al, 20025).

Cell survival and protein synthesis heavily rely on this crucial pathway for regulating various aspects of cellular metabolism quite effectively. Similarly, IGF-1 signalling plays a significant role in cancer by promoting cell cycle progression and inhibiting apoptosis. Elevated insulin levels often manifest in cancer and drive tumour cell growth by persistently activating AKT and mTOR signalling pathways. IGF-1 signalling plays a significant role in cancer progression by heavily promoting cell cycle and vigorously inhibiting cellular apoptosis mechanisms (Simpson et al, 2017).

2.1.2. mTOR Pathway: The Central Hub of Nutrient Sensing

The major player in nutrient sensing and cell growth mTOR pathway, operates quite intricately within cells under various physiological conditions. mTOR integrates signals from growth factors and nutrients like glucose, lipids, and energy levels quite extensively. The mTOR pathway operates via two distinct complexes, mTORC1 and mTORC2, which regulate various cellular processes somewhat differently under diverse conditions (Jewell and Guan, 2013).

mTORC1 is particularly sensitive to nutrient availability, like amino acids, glucose, and insulin and regulates protein synthesis, heavily influencing cell growth and overall metabolism. mTORC1 stimulates translation of key proteins like ribosomal protein S6 and eukaryotic initiation factor 4E when nutrients abound and promotes cell growth and division vigorously. mTORC1 often goes haywire in cancer, promoting the relentless growth of tumour cells and survival under harsh conditions, normally inducing stress or cell death. mTORC2, on the other hand, is involved in cell survival and metabolism (Jewell and Guan, 2013). mTORC2 plays a role in cell survival very deeply and is tied closely with metabolism, on the other hand. The AKT signalling pathway gets heavily regulated by it, and cancer cell survival implicates this pathway very deeply in resistance to apoptosis. mTORC2 gets activated very frequently in diverse cancer types and fosters stubborn resistance of cancer cells against chemotherapy and many other therapies (Jewell and Guan, 2013). mTOR has become a tantalising target for novel anti-cancer therapies owing largely to its pivotal role in cancer cell metabolic processes.

2.1.3 AMPK Pathway

AMP-activated protein kinase, aka AMPK frequently dubbed the body's energy sensor quite ostensibly in most physiological contexts. AMPK gets activated under energy stress conditions like super low nutrient availability or intense exercise and hypoxia, and it conserves energy by ramping up catabolic processes such as fat oxidation while inhibiting anabolic ones like synthesising protein and lipid quite effectively. When cellular energy levels are low (e.g., low glucose or ATP), AMPK is activated and initiates a cascade of reactions that lead to the inhibition of mTORC1 and the activation of autophagy, a process that allows cells to degrade and recycle their own components to provide energy. In cancer, AMPK is frequently deregulated. Cells starved of glucose or ATP trigger activation of AMPK, which kicks off reactions inhibiting mTORC1 and sparking autophagy to recycle cellular components. Cancer often exhibits frequent deregulation of AMPK (Hardie DG, 2011).

2.1.4 SIRT1: The Nutrient-Sensing Deacetylase

SIRT1, a member of the sirtuin family proteins, plays a crucial role in regulating cellular metabolism in response to various nutrients very dynamically. Sirtuins deacetylate proteins that are intricately involved in metabolism and also in DNA repair or gene expression using NAD+. SIRT1 has been heavily implicated in the regulation of cellular stress responses and cancer development, alongside ageing in particular contexts. SIRT1 activity is modulated by caloric restriction, which has been shown to extend lifespan and reduce cancer incidence in multiple organisms. SIRT1 activity gets modulated somewhat by caloric restriction, which has been shown to extend lifespan rather significantly in multiple organisms. SIRT1 activates pathways promoting DNA repair and cell survival under nutrient scarcity, which can help shield cells from genetic damage leading to cancer. In many cancers, the expression and activity of SIRT1 are altered. Abundant nutrient levels may downregulate SIRT1 activity, thereby contributing heavily to tumourigenesis under certain physiological conditions quite rapidly. Expression and activity of SIRT1 are significantly altered in many types of cancer (Cantó and Auwerx, 2012).

2.1.5 Hypoxia-Inducible Factors (HIFs)

Transcription factors known as hypoxia-inducible factors regulate cellular response to low oxygen levels very effectively under various physiological conditions. Tumour cells frequently outstrip their blood supply, leading to hypoxic regions deep within the tumour mass under varying physiological conditions. HIFs get activated and crank up a metabolic shift heavily favouring anaerobic glycolysis or the Warburg effect, providing energy even without oxygen. HIF-1α, the most studied of the HIF family, activates the expression of genes involved in angiogenesis, metabolic reprogramming, and cell survival. HIF-1α activates the expression of genes heavily involved in angiogenesis and metabolic reprogramming quite profoundly alongside cell survival mechanisms. Cancer cells thrive remarkably well in hypoxic environments by ramping up glucose uptake significantly and supercharging glycolytic pathways. Targeting HIF signalling is an emerging therapeutic strategy, particularly in solid tumours where hypoxia is prevalent. HIFs facilitate tumour immune evasion by downregulating the activity of immune cells within the tumour microenvironment very effectively and quietly (Ziello and Jovin, 2007).

2.2. Integration of Nutrient-Sensing Pathways in Cancer

Nutrient-sensing pathways described above operate not in isolation but rather amidst complex cellular interactions normally. They form a complex network of signals deeply intertwined, regulating growth, survival and cellular metabolic processes fairly intricately. Insulin and IGF-1 signaling activates mTOR very readily, while AMPK activation inhibits mTORC1, thereby creating a delicate balance between anabolic processes and catabolism. SIRT1 intricately interacts with diverse pathways like AMPK and mTOR pathways under nutrient stress, maintaining cellular integrity very effectively. Cancer cells frequently hijack nutrient-sensing pathways, promoting unchecked proliferation and encouraging metabolic resilience against considerable stress. Pharmacological agents or gene therapy may interrupt nutrient-sensing mechanisms driving tumourigenesis, offering novel cancer therapy approaches quite effectively nowadays (Efeyan et al, 2015).

2.3. Implications for Cancer Prevention and Treatment

Nutrient sensing plays a crucial role in cancer development, thereby providing valuable insight into potentially efficacious therapeutic interventions and preventive strategies. Caloric restriction and intermittent fasting, alongside other dietary tweaks, can directly mess with nutrient-sensing pathways in very significant ways. Caloric restriction has been shown markedly reduce insulin/IGF-1 signalling and activate AMPK, leading rather slowly to reduced tumour growth in various animal models. Intermittent fasting can activate autophagy and SIRT1, improving cellular resilience to DNA damage and oxidative stress (Brandhorst and Longo, 2016).

Pharmacological agents, such as mTOR inhibitors, AMPK activators, and SIRT1 modulators, are being explored as potential cancer therapies to disrupt the metabolic pathways that sustain tumour growth. Intermittent fasting activates autophagy and SIRT1, very significantly improving cellular resilience against DNA damage under oxidative stress. Pharmacological agents like mTOR inhibitors and SIRT1 modulators are being explored as potential cancer therapies disrupting metabolic pathways sustaining tumour growth vigorously (Brandhorst and Longo, 2016).

3. The Role of Metabolic Signals in Homeostasis Regulation

Fundamental quite obviously essential to the health of all living organisms. It represents the body's ability to maintain remarkably stable internal conditions despite fluctuating external environments. It encompasses various physiological processes such as temperature regulation, fluid balance, and pH regulation, and crucially, maintenance of energy balance occurs. Molecular cues reflecting bodily energy status intricately orchestrate adaptive responses necessary for survival, growth, and repair deeply within this complex regulatory network. Signals play crucial roles in regulating various cellular processes like energy production and growth, alongside repair and nutrient storage mechanisms.

Metabolic signals play a crucial role in homeostasis regulation, particularly when maintaining glucose levels and lipid balance, intricately linked with protein turnover vital for optimal cellular functioning. Pathological conditions emerge from disruptions in intricate signal balances, resulting in metabolic disorders like obesity, type 2 diabetes, or cancer slowly. Key metabolic signals and various complex pathways intricately regulate homeostasis within bodily systems, rather quietly and effectively, every day. We will discuss deeply into bodily mechanisms sensing nutrient availability and energy requirements, transmitting such info governing vital metabolic functions. Disruptions in metabolic signalling contribute substantially to diseases, whereas therapeutic interventions targeting specific pathways offer novel strategies for prevention and treatment.

3.1. Key Metabolic Signals in Homeostasis Regulation

Regulation of energy homeostasis relies heavily on myriad molecular cues responding rapidly to shifting nutrient availability and fluctuating energy demands. Cells and organs communicate with each other via signals that coordinate myriad metabolic processes fairly intricately inside bodily systems.

3.1.1 Insulin and Glucagon: The Primary Hormones of Energy Regulation

The insulin and glucagon axis plays a crucial role in regulating blood glucose levels, deeply intertwined with overall energy homeostasis mechanisms. The pancreas secretes both insulin and glucagon in response to wildly fluctuating blood sugar levels, thus maintaining homeostasis of glucose somewhat. Insulin is released from pancreatic beta cells in response to elevated blood glucose levels, typically following a meal. Pancreatic beta cells release insulin in response to skyrocketing glucose levels, typically after eating a meal or sometimes even just snacking heavily. It signals cells throughout bodily systems, especially in liver muscles and adipose tissue, to uptake glucose and store it as glycogen or turn it into fat (Röder et al, 2016).

Glucagon, on the other hand, is released from pancreatic alpha cells when blood glucose levels are low, such as between meals or during fasting. Insulin vigorously promotes protein synthesis and quashes lipolytic processes and glycogen breakdown, thereby ensuring efficient energy storage when nutrients abound plentifully. Glucagon is released from pancreatic alpha cells when blood glucose levels drop drastically between meals or during prolonged periods of fasting. The liver gets signalled to break down glycogen into glucose and release it into the bloodstream, restoring normal blood glucose levels rapidly (Röder et al, 2016).

3.1.2 AMP-Activated Protein Kinase (AMPK):

AMP-activated protein kinase AMPK serves as a crucial sensor of cellular energy status within cells. AMPK helps cells adapt rather quickly to rather dire energy shortages signalled by a surge in AMP levels, indicating low energy availability. AMPK gets activated under gruelling conditions like severe nutrient deprivation or intense exercise and extremely low cellular ATP levels. AMPK activation leads to the promotion of catabolic processes, such as fatty acid oxidation and glucose uptake, and inhibits anabolic processes like lipogenesis and protein synthesis. AMPK activation spurs catabolic processes like fatty acid oxidation and glucose uptake while stifling anabolic ones, namely lipogenesis and protein synthesis heavily (Hardie DG, 2011). In addition to its role in cellular energy metabolism, AMPK has been shown to regulate key processes such as autophagy (the degradation of damaged cellular components) and mitochondrial biogenesis. Maximising energy production and conserving energy resources restores cellular energy balance very effectively under normal physiological conditions anyway. AMPK regulates crucial processes like autophagy, involving the degradation of damaged cell components and mitochondrial biogenesis, deeply within cellular energy metabolism (Hardie DG, 2011).

3.1.3 mTOR (Mechanistic Target of Rapamycin): The Growth Pathway

mTOR or mechanistic target of rapamycin intricately regulates cell growth and metabolism by integrating signals largely from nutrients and growth factors.mTOR manifests in two disparate complexes, namely mTORC1 and mTORC2, with distinct roles within various cellular processes, obviously. mTORC1 is particularly responsive to nutrient availability, such as amino acids, glucose, and lipids, as well as insulin and other growth factors. mTORC1 responds keenly to the availability of nutrients like glucose and lipids, as well as insulin and various other growth factors, normally. mTORC1 vigorously promotes protein synthesis and lipogenesis under ridiculously nutrient-rich conditions and facilitates cell cycle progression very quickly (Kennedy et al, 2016).

However, when nutrients are scarce or energy levels are low, mTORC1 activity is inhibited, leading to a shift toward catabolic processes, including autophagy (cellular recycling). Cellular growth and anabolism are facilitated by these processes, allowing the body to respond somewhat rapidly to abundant nutrient supply. mTORC2, while less understood, plays a role in cell survival and metabolic regulation by influencing AKT signalling, which controls cell proliferation and glucose metabolism. When nutrients are scarce or energy levels dwindle, mTORC1 activity gets inhibited, leading to catabolic processes such as autophagy, a cellular recycling mechanism. Such a drastic shift proves crucial under stress or during periods of extreme nutrient deprivation for maintaining cellular homeostasis effectively (Kennedy et al, 2016).

3.1.4 Sirtuins: Metabolic Regulators of Longevity

Sirtuins are a family of NAD+-dependent deacetylases regulating key cellular processes such as metabolism and DNA repair intricately within cells slowly. SIRT1 has emerged as a central player in the regulation of metabolic homeostasis, quite remarkably, within various studied contexts nowadays. SIRT1 is activated under conditions of caloric restriction or nutrient deprivation, where it promotes fat oxidation, mitochondrial function, and DNA repair. SIRT1 gets activated under caloric restriction or severe nutrient deprivation, where it vigorously promotes fat oxidation and enhances mitochondrial function.In addition to its role in metabolism, SIRT1 also influences processes such as autophagy and inflammation, which are critical for cellular survival and maintenance. SIRT1 maintains cellular integrity rather effectively under tremendous stress by activating various pathways that significantly enhance oxidative metabolism. SIRT1 heavily influences various processes, including autophagy and inflammation, which are crucial for cellular survival mechanisms under extremely stressful conditions (Mei et al, 2016).

3.1.5 Hypoxia-Inducible Factors (HIFs): Adapting to Low Oxygen Environments

Transcription factors known as hypoxia-inducible factors regulate responses of cells to low oxygen levels in a rather complex manner. These factors play a crucial role in tweaking cellular metabolism very rapidly under oxygen deprivation, mostly in tumour tissues or during fairly intense exercise. Under hypoxic conditions, HIF-1α is stabilised and activates a suite of genes involved in anaerobic metabolism (the Warburg effect), vascularisation (via angiogenesis), and cell survival. HIF-1α gets stabilised very quickly under hypoxic conditions and very much kicks off a slew of genes dealing with anaerobic metabolism via some gnarly vascularisation and cell survival mechanisms. HIFs also contribute to the metabolic reprogramming of cancer cells, enabling them to survive and proliferate in environments with limited nutrients and oxygen. Cells thrive quite vigorously in environments severely depleted of oxygen by drastically shifting metabolic processes toward glycolysis for generating energy (Dengler et al, 2014).

3.2. Integration of Metabolic Signals in Homeostasis

Metabolic signals don't operate in isolation and instead function intricately within complex physiological networks, ensuring homeostasis very effectively. Insulin and glucagon function antagonistically, regulating glucose metabolism; meanwhile, AMPK acts as an energy gauge, ensuring bodily adaptation during low-energy conditions. mTOR integrates signals from nutrients and growth factors to control cellular growth and repair, while also responding to changes in energy status. Sirtuins and HIFs contribute to cellular stress response and longevity, helping the body cope with both energy scarcity and environmental stress (Kahn et al, 2025).

mTOR integrates signals from various nutrients and growth factors, controlling cellular growth and repair amidst fluctuations in energy status. Sirtuins and HIFs enhance cellular stress response and longevity, helping the body cope with energy dearth and harsh environmental conditions quite effectively. These pathways interact with each other extensively in a highly coordinated fashion rather intricately (Kahn et al, 2025).

3.3. Implications for Disease and Therapeutic Strategies

Several diseases, including type 2 diabetes and cancer, are associated with disruptions in metabolic signalling pathways very frequently nowadays. Mutations or overactivation of pathways like mTOR and HIFs egregiously promote uncontrolled cell growth and metabolic reprogramming in cancerous tissues. Therapeutic strategies targeting metabolic signals like AMPK activators or SIRT1 modulators hold great potential in treating cancer and various metabolic diseases effectively. Lifestyle interventions like severe caloric restriction or periodic fasting may greatly help restore metabolic equilibrium and significantly reduce the risk of disease. Metabolic signals orchestrate bodily responses quite intricately amidst fluctuating nutrient availability and wildly shifting energy needs. Researchers develop novel therapeutic approaches by grasping intricate networks of metabolic pathways linked heavily to various diseases caused by dysregulation. Modulating specific pathways through targeted interventions unlocks new potential in prevention and treatment, improving overall health outcomes significantly (Yang et al, 2017).

4. Molecular Mechanisms

Gene expression governs cellular functions intricately by determining how cells grow rapidly and divide in response to various environmental cues. Regulation of gene expression plays a crucial role in the development and homeostasis of organisms across various species. Recent research has revealed that dietary nutrients such as vitamins and amino acids play a significant role in modulating gene expression, thus influencing cellular metabolism and disease development. Interaction between various nutrients and gene expression unfolds dynamically through multiple obscure molecular mechanisms beneath cellular surfaces. Epigenetic modifications and transcriptional regulation, alongside post-transcriptional regulation and protein synthesis, are encompassed by these mechanisms rather irregularly. Specific nutrients serve as regulatory signals influencing gene expression and interactions between these signals can drastically impact various physiological processes, including cancer metabolism (Bervoets I, Charlier et al, 2019).

4.1. Nutrients and Epigenetic Regulation of Gene Expression

Epigenetics entails modifications in gene expression unfolding without alterations to the underlying DNA sequence, very mysteriously, nowadays. Epigenetic mechanisms encompass DNA methylation and histone modification alongside the regulation of non-coding RNAs heavily. Nutrients can influence epigenetic marks, thereby playing a crucial role in regulating genes deeply inside cells.

4.1.1 DNA Methylation

Addition of a methyl group occurs at the carbon-5 position of cytosine residues in CpG islands within gene promoters epigenetically. Gene expression gets repressed typically by this modification, which prevents transcription factors and other regulatory proteins from binding DNA. Specific nutrients significantly influence DNA methylation patterns quite profoundly under certain conditions. Folate, a water-soluble B vitamin, serves as a crucial source of methyl groups utilised extensively in DNA methylation processes. Folate deficiency has been tenuously linked to aberrant DNA methylation, which may precipitously contribute development of cancer and various other maladies (Handy et al, 2011).

Methionine, an amino acid, and B-vitamins like B12 play a role in the methylation cycle, influencing gene silencing or activation mainly in cancer and ageing contexts. In cancer, hypermethylation of tumour suppressor genes often leads to their silencing, contributing to uncontrolled cell growth. Hypermethylation of tumour suppressor genes frequently precipitates their silencing in cancer, fostering rather uncontrolled cell proliferation. Hypomethylation, conversely, results in activation of certain oncogenes rather quietly underneath cellular surfaces (Handy et al, 2011).

4.1.2 Histone Modification and Acetylation

Gene expression regulation involves essential roles played by histone modifications such as phosphorylation and methylation, alongside acetylation, very frequently. Histone acetylation generally correlates with gene activation because it loosens histone grip on DNA, thereby facilitating access for transcriptional machinery. Butyrate, a short-chain fatty acid produced by fermenting dietary fibre in the gut, powerfully inhibits HDAC histone deacetylase activity, apparently. Butyrate inhibits HDACs, thereby enhancing histone acetylation very significantly, and it promotes gene expression related to cell differentiation or apoptosis (Lee et al, 2020).

Polyunsaturated fatty acids (PUFAs), particularly omega-3 fatty acids, also influence histone acetylation and have been shown to affect the expression of genes involved in inflammation and immune response. Polyunsaturated fatty acids, particularly omega-3 fatty acids, influence histone acetylation and affect the expression of genes involved in inflammation very significantly (Lee et al, 2020).

4.1.3 MicroRNAs and Nutrient Regulation

MicroRNAs post-transcriptionally regulate gene expression by binding messenger RNAs and inhibiting translation or catapulting them towards degradation pathways suddenly. Recent studies show dietary components like polyphenols and omega-3 fatty acids modulate the expression of specific miRNAs, influencing gene expression significantly. Curcumin, a bioactive compound extracted rather haphazardly from turmeric, has been shown to regulate the expression of miR-21 in various tumour cells vigorously. Omega-3 fatty acids influence miRNAs regulating inflammation and metabolism, suggesting a role in disease prevention via gene expression regulation post-transcriptionally (O'Brien et al, 2018).

4.2. Transcriptional Regulation by Nutrients

Proteins known as transcription factors bind specifically to certain DNA sequences, thereby regulating gene transcription quite intricately. Nutrients modulate the activity of transcription factors, influencing the expression of myriad genes involved deeply in growth metabolism and various disease processes.

4.2.1 The Role of Transcription Factors in Nutrient Sensing

Peroxisome proliferator-activated receptors and Liver X receptors respond rather vigorously to various fatty acids and lipids as key transcription factors. Receptors tweak gene expression intricately linked with metabolic fat processes and inflammation, alongside maintenance of cholesterol levels under sundry physiological states. Omega-3 fatty acids activate PPARγ protein, regulating the expression of genes involved deeply in lipid metabolism and implicated heavily in inflammation. Retinoic acid, an active form of vitamin A, binds to retinoic acid receptors RARs and regulates a different set of genes involved deeply in cell differentiation. Vitamin D acts through its receptor VDR, regulating genes influencing bone health and modulating immune function deeply within bodily tissues. Retinoic acid binds very tightly to retinoic acid receptors and heavily regulates a multitude of genes involved in cellular differentiation mechanisms, preventing cancer (Kersten S., 2008).

4.2.2 The Role of the mTOR Pathway in Nutrient Sensing

mTOR orchestrates an intricate ballet of protein synthesis, cell growth, and autophagy as a central hub sensing sundry nutrients rather effectively downstream. Cues from nutrients like amino acids, glucose, and lipids are synthesised by mTOR, coordinating gene expression tied up with cellular hypertrophy very intricately across vast swaths. Abundant nutrients activate mTOR, which in turn switches on transcription factors such as HIF-1 and SREBP, promoting anabolic processes very vigorously, it seems. In contrast, nutrient scarcity or stress activates AMPK, which inhibits mTOR activity and induces autophagy, the process by which cells degrade and recycle damaged proteins and organelles. Nutrient scarcity activates AMPK, which inhibits mTOR activity, inducing autophagy, a catabolic process whereby cells degrade damaged proteins and organelles quite thoroughly (Jewell and Guan, 2013).

4.3. Nutrient Regulation and Disease Implications

Gene expression regulated by nutrients has profoundly significant implications for human health and the onset of various debilitating diseases. Nutrients sway gene expression in ways that directly impact the development and progression of diseases like cancer and cardiovascular disease rather quietly.

4.3.1 Nutrients and Cancer Prevention

Cancer cells often exhibit freaky metabolic anomalies and unusual gene signatures, facilitating rampant proliferation deeply inside compromised tissue. Vitamin D and omega-3 fatty acids, alongside polyphenols, very effectively modulate gene expression and foster suppression of tumour growth extensively. Sulforaphane, present very abundantly in cruciferous veggies such as broccoli, modulates epigenetic pathways and activates various genes involved in detoxification. Omega-3 fatty acids exhibit potent anti-inflammatory effects, downregulating pro-inflammatory cytokines and inhibiting the activity of transcription factor NF-kB linked with tumourigenesis.

4.3.2 Nutrient Regulation in Metabolic Disease

Metabolic maladies like obesity and type 2 diabetes frequently manifest aberrant nutrient sensing alongside anomalous gene expression profiles, rather mysteriously simultaneously. Omega-3 fatty acids, fibre, and polyphenols regulate pathways of gene expression involved in insulin sensitivity and inflammation, rather quietly influencing the progression of various nasty diseases significantly. Incorporating such nutrients into one's diet significantly enhances metabolic health and slashes the risk of nasty diseases like cardiovascular issues. Nutrients act as potent regulators of gene expression, deeply influencing cellular growth, metabolism and various bodily functions in myriad obscure ways. Genes involved in thwarting disease, particularly some cancers and metabolic disorders, can be tweaked via post-transcriptional regulation and epigenetic mark modulation by dietary factors. Molecular machinery governing gene expression interacts with nutrients, unlocking modified dietary interventions and novel preventive nutrition pathways very effectively nowadays (Lam et al, 2025).

5. Interplay of Diet and Cell Function: A Molecular Perspective

Molecular foundation of life gets dictated by an intricate dance between the genetic blueprint and the cellular apparatus under the influence of sundry external factors. Diet profoundly influences energy availability among external factors and significantly alters cellular structure and overall bodily homeostasis. Bio-signals from ingested nutrients profoundly influence gene expression and modulate various metabolic pathways, regulating cellular functions simultaneously quite deeply. Epigenetic mods and nutrient-sensing mechanisms inside cells interact heavily with diet at the molecular level, mediating cell function dynamically. Dietary components intricately modulate cellular homeostasis and disease progression via molecular mechanisms that involve crucial signalling pathways operating rather quietly underneath. Grasping interactions impacting health and disease states like obesity emerges from new opportunities for modified interventions down various unconventional paths.

5.1. Nutrient-Sensing Pathways and Cellular Regulation

Cells detect nutrients with decent precision and react with remarkable intricacy underlying much overall cellular function and complex dietary interplay. Cells adapt rapidly via intricate molecular cascades that sense fluctuations in nutrient availability, thereby supporting homeostasis and fostering precarious energy equilibrium. Key signalling pathways activated in response to the absence or presence of nutrients have been identified as central regulators of various cellular processes.

5.1.1 AMP-Activated Protein Kinase (AMPK)

AMPK a central energy-sensing enzyme, plays a crucial role in regulating cellular energy homeostasis within cells rather effectively. A surge in the AMP-to-ATP ratio during fasting exercise or caloric restriction strongly indicates energy insufficiency and very clearly activates AMPK. AMPK swiftly triggers myriad adaptations upon activation, thereby restoring energy balance by firing up catabolic processes and inhibiting anabolic ones like lipogenesis. Promotion of autophagy, a process in which damaged cellular components are degraded and recycled to maintain cellular integrity (Hardie DG, 2011). Damaged cellular components get degraded and recycled via autophagy, thus maintaining cellular integrity very effectively under normal conditions. Blocking anabolic processes like lipogenesis and protein synthesis conserves energy rather effectively under certain taxing physiological circumstances.

5.1.2 mTOR Pathway

mTOR pathway intricately integrates signals from nutrients alongside growth factors and cellular energy status in a rather complex manner. The mTOR pathway manifests in two distinct complexes, mTORC1 and mTORC2, playing somewhat different roles. The presence of nutrients, especially amino acids, activates mTORC1, which in turn promotes protein synthesis, cellular growth and anabolism very robustly. Presence of nutrients, especially certain amino acids, vigorously activate mTORC1, which boosts protein synthesis, cellular growth and anabolic processes (Sengupta et al, 2010).

mTORC2 regulates cell survival and insulin signalling while being involved in actin cytoskeleton organisation somewhat mysteriously.mTORC2 assumes a crucial albeit somewhat enigmatic role partly through reorganisation of actin cytoskeleton and modulation of insulin signalling pathways inside cells. It heavily regulates lipogenesis and ribosome biogenesis in response to nutrients within cellular environments. Dysregulation of the mTOR pathway has been heavily implicated in various nasty metabolic diseases and some aggressive forms of cancer. Aggressive forms of cancer and nasty metabolic diseases have been very heavily linked to dysregulation (Sengupta et al, 2010).

5.1.3 Sirtuins and Nutrient Regulation

Sirtuins are a family of NAD+-dependent deacetylases intricately regulating various crucial cellular processes like metabolism, DNA repair, and ageing remarkably slowly. SIRT1 responds vigorously under caloric restriction or prolonged fasting in various cellular contexts to cellular stress signals and nutrient availability. Sirtuins somewhat haphazardly mediate cellular responses by deacetylating proteins, thereby significantly altering activity or surprisingly stability with various cellular components. SIRT1 promotes fatty acid oxidation and mitochondrial biogenesis and cell survival during periods of extreme nutrient scarcity. SIRT1 vigorously promotes fatty acid oxidation and mitochondrial biogenesis during nutrient deficiency periods and remarkably enhances cell survival (Gibril et al, 2024). Resveratrol, a polyphenolic compound found in grapes, is known to activate SIRT1, and its anti-ageing and anti-cancer effects are attributed somewhat nebulously to modulation of sirtuin activity. It maintains genomic stability rather mysteriously by activating DNA repair pathways and regulating telomere function with very high effectiveness.

5.2. Dietary Components and Cellular Metabolism

Dietary nutrients like proteins, fats, and carbs directly influence cellular metabolism profoundly under varying physiological conditions, obviously. Nutrients act as fundamental building blocks for various cellular structures and energy sources, fueling diverse metabolic processes, simultaneously serving as signalling molecules, regulating gene expression.

5.2.1 Amino Acids and Protein Metabolism

Amino acids play crucial roles, surprisingly beneath cellular surfaces, regulating vital metabolic pathways silently. The mTORC1 pathway gets activated very quickly when amino acids abound, stimulating protein synthesis quite vigorously and spurring cell growth rapidly. Glutamine and some other amino acids frequently reprogram metabolism deep inside cancer cells with very unusual regularity. Glutamine metabolism ramps up energetically in various cancers, fueling tumourigenesis very effectively in rapidly proliferating cells with high energy demands. Scientists nowadays investigate nutrient-based interventions targeting peculiar metabolic routes for possibly treating cancer effectively with various applications (Bar-Peled and Sabatini, 2014).

5.2.2 Fatty Acids and Lipid Metabolism

Crucial lipids, including saturated fats and cholesterol, maintain cellular structure effectively within lipid bilayer membranes. Fatty acids serve obscurely as signalling molecules regulating cellular metabolism and play a crucial structural role within cells. Fatty fish and flaxseeds are rich sources of omega-3 polyunsaturated fatty acids, harbouring profoundly anti-inflammatory properties that deeply regulate gene expression involved in lipid metabolism. Saturated fats, in contrast, promote insulin resistance and contribute heavily to inflammatory pathways, potentially leading to metabolic diseases like obesity and type 2 diabetes when consumed excessively. Gorging on copious amounts of saturated fats fuels inflammatory pathways very significantly and promotes nasty metabolic maladies like obesity or type 2 diabetes, rather alarmingly (Yoon et al, 2021).

5.2.3 Carbohydrates and Glucose Metabolism

Glucose acts as the primary energy source for most cells owing largely to its ready availability inside various bodily fluids under normal conditions. Glucagon plays a crucial role alongside insulin in regulating glucose metabolism vigorously by inhibiting glucose uptake somewhat in various tissues. Glucagon energetically stimulates the release of glucose during prolonged fasting or under conditions of extreme nutrient scarcity. Glucose metabolism undergoes radical alteration quite frequently, supporting rapid proliferation of tumour cells in cancer, a phenomenon now dubbed the Warburg effect. Cancer cells frequently rely quite heavily on glycolysis rather than oxidative phosphorylation for producing energy, even with abundant available oxygen. Ketogenic diets drastically alter glucose metabolism and are being probed for stifling tumour growth and boosting overall metabolic wellbeing significantly nowadays (Nakrani et al, 2025).

5.3. Nutritional Interventions and Disease Prevention

Diet profoundly influences cellular function at the molecular level, with far-reaching implications for preventing and treating various diseases effectively nowadays. Specific dietary tweaks potentially mitigate the risk of maladies such as cancer, neurodegenerative disorders and cardiovascular disease by targeting molecular pathways involved in inflammation.

5.3.1 Cancer Prevention and Nutritional Modulation

Polyphenols and vitamins exert antioxidant effects very slowly by modifying epigenetic pathways, which may hinder cancer progression somewhat effectively. Curcumin, present in turmeric, and green tea catechins found in various berries, modulate pathways critical quite effectively related to cell survival and apoptosis quite effectively.

5.3.2 Metabolic Disease Prevention

Modifying nutrient intake rather effectively regulates insulin sensitivity and lipid metabolism, holds considerable promise for the prevention of obesity and type 2 diabetes. Diets rich in fibre and omega-3 fatty acids tend to regulate blood sugar levels somewhat vigorously, supporting heart health and reducing inflammation deeply. Diet intersects cellular function through nutrient-sensing pathways and epigenetic tweaks amidst a maelstrom of concurrent metabolic machinations unfolding rapidly. Dietary components influence gene expression and cellular metabolism via various molecular mechanisms, enabling the formulation of effective preventive measures and therapeutic interventions against cancer and metabolic disorders. Research into molecular underpinnings of diet and disease has positioned nutritional genomics quite dramatically to utterly revamp health management practices (Azadbakht et al, 2011).

6. Molecular Responses to Nutrient Imbalance: Implications for Health

Nutrient imbalance catastrophically disrupts delicate molecular processes underpinning human health, owing largely to deficiency or glaringly wonky ratios of essential nutrients. Body systems intricately maintain homeostasis and adjust rapidly to fluctuations in nutrient availability fairly deep beneath the surface level quite quickly. Molecular responses get triggered by fluctuations beyond certain thresholds, disrupting metabolic pathways and severely boosting susceptibility to diseases like cancer or cardiovascular problems. Intricate pathways sensing nutrients quietly influence cellular stress responses and regulate metabolic homeostasis at the heart of such disruptions, somewhat mysteriously. Disruption of cellular function by molecular mechanisms underlying nutrient imbalances occurs significantly in disease states caused by deficiency or excess. Understanding various molecular responses accurately underpins the development of effective prevention strategies and treatment for diet-related health conditions (Kiani et al, 2022).

6.1. Nutrient Imbalance and Cellular Stress Responses

Coping with nutrient imbalances relies heavily on bodily detection of fluctuations in nutrient levels and swift responses accordingly under various physiological conditions. Cells have evolved rather sophisticated mechanisms for sensing fluctuations in various nutrients and activating specific signalling pathways that maintain homeostasis. Prolonged extreme imbalances can trigger responses that disrupt normal cellular function very badly and lead, rather quickly, to pathological changes.

6.1.1 Cellular Stress and Metabolic Reprogramming

Cells face brutal nutrient dearth during fasting or severe caloric restriction and subsequently spark various stress response pathways like AMPK and autophagy very rapidly. Pathways preserve energy and promote cell survival by ramping up production very effectively under stress and fixing damaged cellular bits rapidly. AMPK gets activated during low energy states with a high AMP to ATP ratio and plays a central role in regulating cellular metabolism vigorously by promoting catabolic processes like fatty acid oxidation and inhibiting anabolic processes such as protein synthesis or lipogenesis effectively. Autophagy is another key response that allows cells to degrade and recycle damaged organelles, proteins, and other macromolecules, thereby conserving energy and maintaining cellular integrity. Cells degrade damaged organelles and proteins through autophagy, thereby conserving energy and maintaining the integrity of cellular structures remarkably well.

6.1.2 The Role of Inflammation in Nutrient Imbalance

Excess nutrients frequently spark insidious inflammation, which fuels many diseases related to diet significantly from behind the scenes. Obesity correlates with excess adipose tissue accumulation, releasing pro-inflammatory cytokines such as TNF-α and IL-6 fairly often in various bodily regions. Inflammatory signals trigger a plethora of downstream molecular events that disrupt normal cellular function, rapidly fostering insulin resistance and tumourigenesis simultaneously. Grossly inadequate intake of certain vitamins or minerals can significantly impair immune response and foster susceptibility to various nasty opportunistic infections lurking everywhere. Molecular pathways mediating inflammation, like NF-κB and NLRP3 inflammasome, become dysregulated in both cases, fostering persistent inflammation, which exacerbates disease progression rapidly (Kawai et al, 2021).

6.2. Nutrient Deficiency and Molecular Impacts

Nutrient deficiency can significantly impair cellular homeostasis and disrupt normal metabolic pathways while altering gene expression radically overnight. Essential nutrients like vitamins and minerals, amino acids, and fatty acids act as cofactors for enzymatic reactions, structural cell components and signalling molecules regulating gene expression. Cellular dysfunction arises from a deficiency in certain nutrients and contributes massively to various obscure health problems.

6.2.1 Vitamin and Mineral Deficiencies

Gross nutrient imbalance occurs frequently in developing regions worldwide, mostly due to deficiencies of some extremely common micronutrient forms. Lack of vitamins such as Vitamin A or B-vitamins, and minerals like iron, zinc and magnesium can have fairly profound molecular repercussions ultimately. Vitamin D deficiency severely impairs immune system function and drastically reduces calcium absorption, increasing the risk of osteoporosis and various cardiovascular diseases. Vitamin D deficiency grossly hampers immune system function and severely curtails calcium absorption, ratcheting up the risk of osteoporosis or cardiovascular disease substantially. Iron deficiency precipitates anemia which impairs the oxygen-carrying capacity of red blood cells, disrupting cellular processes reliant on iron-dependent enzymes vital for DNA synthesis. Molecular actions of vitamin D transpire remarkably via the VDR receptor modulating gene expression related to calcium homeostasis and influencing cell proliferation greatly (Kaur et al, 2025).

6.2.2 Protein Deficiency and Amino Acid Imbalance

Proteins comprising diverse amino acids play vital roles everywhere in cellular operations under varying environmental conditions. Amino acid imbalance or protein deficiency severely disrupts cellular signalling and protein synthesis, affecting overall metabolic balance terribly in the body. Leucine is a crucial BCAA that activates the mTOR pathway, regulating cell growth and the synthesis of protein. Leucine plays a pivotal role in activating the mTOR pathway, which governs protein synthesis and spurs cell growth surprisingly fast in cells. Glutamine becomes vital during stress or disease states, especially in cancer cells that rely heavily on it for metabolic reprogramming. Leucine deficiency or scarcity of other crucial amino acids stifles mTOR activity, thereby significantly hindering cellular growth and crippling regeneration of tissue. Glutamine assumes paramount importance during stress states or disease, especially in cancer cells heavily reliant on it for metabolic flux reconfiguration (Ling et al, 2023).

6.3. Nutrient Excess and Molecular Pathology

Excessive intake of specific nutrients can trigger pernicious molecular reactions, and subsequently, metabolic chaos and various diseases unfold quite rapidly. Consuming too many macronutrients, such as carbs and lipids, or certain micronutrients, overloads cellular systems very quickly, contributing significantly to pathology.

6.3.1 Excess Carbohydrates and Insulin Resistance

Consuming refined sugars and simple carbs triggers elevated blood glucose levels, prompting a superfluous insulin release. Chronic high-insulin states typically culminate in insulin resistance underlying type 2 diabetes fairly typically over an extended period of time. Insulin resistance kicks in somewhat nebulously when insulin receptor and downstream signalling pathways like the PI3K/Akt pathway get blunted, impairing glucose uptake into cells really badly. Excessive carb intake fosters fat accumulation predominantly in visceral stores, spurring the release of pro-inflammatory cytokines that exacerbate insulin resistance quite severely (DiNicolantonio and O'Keefe, 2022).

6.3.2 Fat Excess and Lipotoxicity

Consuming excessive saturated and trans fats can trigger lipotoxicity, a state where fat accumulates rapidly inside non-adipose tissues such as the liver, disrupting cellular function badly. Lipotoxicity activates stress pathways such as endoplasmic reticulum stress, riling up inflammatory responses and spawning insulin resistance quite rapidly. Fatty liver disease, NAFLD, stems from excessive fat buildup in the liver and subsequently increases the risk of cirrhosis, liver cancer and cardiovascular issues.

6.3.3 Overactivation of the mTOR Pathway in Obesity and Cancer

Overconsumption of calories, particularly proteins and certain amino acids, results in overactivation of the mTOR pathway linked with rapid cellular proliferation. Overactivation of mTOR heavily promotes tumour development and contributes significantly, amidst obesity, to inflammation and various metabolic derangements often seen in cancer. Molecular pathways governing metabolism undergo significant disruptions as diet interacts intricately with cellular function in a profoundly complex manner. Nutrient deficiencies severely impair gene expression and damage essential cellular functions while weakening various immune responses significantly. Nutrients in excess, conversely, foster stress at the cellular level and metabolic dysregulation, promoting diseases like cancer and obesity very quietly alongside diabetes. Nutrient imbalances trigger molecular responses that present fertile ground for crafting modified interventions remarkably extending human lifespan and preventing maladies related to diet (Saxton and Sabatini, 2017).

7. Nutritional Stress and Cellular Adaptation Mechanisms

Profoundly debilitating effects on overall cellular health stem rather quietly from nutritional stress occasioned by copious excess or severe deficiency. Cells, tissues, and organs regularly confront vagaries in nutrient supply, and adaptability significantly determines the overall resilience of metabolic health. Nutritional stress often erupts suddenly from gross dietary imbalances or festers slowly through protracted fasting and severe malnutrition, sparking myriad cellular adaptations. Disease development and tissue damage may ensue very rapidly when adaptive mechanisms falter or become utterly overwhelmed, precipitating cellular dysfunction. Cells surprisingly thrive under extremely stressful conditions at the molecular level, with myriad complex and rather unorthodox tactics employed quite effectively.

Alterations transpire rapidly in diverse metabolic processes, whilst gene expression undergoes very frequent changes and stress-response pathways get activated meanwhile. Rapidly adapting cells under severe nutritional stress yield crucial insight into mechanisms underlying prevention efforts and novel disease-fighting therapeutic strategies. Nutrient imbalance triggers various cellular processes that mediate stress responses and regulate survival metabolism alongside genomic stability under harsh conditions.

7.1. Cellular Sensing of Nutritional Stress

Cells have highly specialised systems for sensing fluctuations in the availability of nutrients very quickly under various conditions. Molecular sensors and pathways intricately involved in such sensing systems finely tune cellular responses according to available resources. Cells maintain metabolic equilibrium via nutrient sensing and react suitably to nutrient level fluctuations, ensuring optimised cellular function for health survival.

7.1.1 AMP-Activated Protein Kinase (AMPK)

AMP-activated protein kinase or AMPK acts as the primary sensor of cellular energy status virtually everywhere within cells, basically. Under low nutrient availability, AMPK activation occurs with severely depleted glucose and oxygen, causing a surge in the AMP-to-ATP ratio. AMPK swiftly triggers multiple responses upon activation, conserving energy and encouraging survival mechanisms effectively in stressed cellular environments. Catabolic processes get activated somewhat vigorously, involving fatty acid oxidation and glucose uptake from blood with considerable energy liberation. Anabolic processes like lipogenesis and protein synthesis are inhibited very strongly to conserve energy (Hardie DG, 2011). Promotion of autophagy, which enables cells to break down and recycle damaged organelles, proteins, and other cellular debris to maintain energy homeostasis and prevent further damage. Promotion of autophagy enables cells to break down damaged organelles and recycle proteins and other cellular detritus, thereby maintaining homeostasis.

7.1.2 mTOR Pathway

The mechanistic target of rapamycin pathway crucially influences cellular responses heavily reliant on nutrient availability. mTOR intricately weaves together cues from insulin, glucose, oxygen, and amino acids, regulating growth, protein synthesis, and metabolic processes deeply within cells. Nutrient excess or deficit surprisingly affects mTOR activity very significantly under various physiological conditions, altering cellular function drastically.mTORC1 drives cell growth rapidly in ridiculously nutrient-rich conditions and stimulates protein synthesis vigorously. Cells shift towards catabolic processes, including autophagy, under nutrient deprivation or severe caloric restriction, suppressing mTORC1 activity. Cells drastically shift towards catabolic processes like autophagy under severe nutrient deprivation, suppressing mTORC1 activity fairly significantly. mTOR mediates crucial responses under nutrient stress, maintaining cellular homeostasis remarkably well (Wang et al, 2022).

7.1.3 Sirtuins: Nutrient-Sensitive Epigenetic Regulators

Sirtuins are NAD+-dependent deacetylases intricately regulating metabolism and modulating ageing processes very effectively under diverse stressful conditions. Sirtuins detect cellular energy and nutrient availability very effectively, influencing gene expression and metabolic reprogramming, and facilitating DNA repair remarkably well. SIRT1 reacts energetically by promoting catabolic processes such as fatty acid oxidation inside mitochondria and stifling numerous anabolic pathways during energy shortage. Sirtuins mediate stress adaptation partly by regulating cellular pathways controlling DNA damage repair mechanisms and cell survival or inflammatory responses. Activity of transcription factors such as p53 and NF-κB gets heavily modified, and they play crucial roles in various stress response regulations. Resveratrol, present in red wine and NAD+ precursors spur sirtuin activation, rendering them plausible targets for potentially therapeutic age-related disease interventions (Houtkooper et al, 2012).

7.2. Molecular Adaptations to Nutrient Stress

Cells undergo drastic molecular shifts, coping with nutritional stress and activating signalling pathways that enable metabolic reprogramming and cell survival mechanisms suddenly. Cells maintain metabolic balance and integrity remarkably well under challenging conditions, owing largely to adaptations essential for survival during extreme fluctuations in nutrient availability.

7.2.1 Autophagy:

Damaged organelles, proteins, and lipids get degraded very quickly via autophagy, a vital process triggered by severe nutrient stress, apparently. Autophagy gets ramped up rapidly under nutrient scarcity, furnishing cells with vital energy by degrading damaged junk inside cellular spaces quite quickly. Energy homeostasis is maintained rather effectively, and grossly misfolded proteins, along with badly damaged mitochondria, are removed with considerable efficacy. AMPK and mTOR, alongside SIRT1, integrate signals regarding nutrient availability, determining whether the cell activates autophagic processes rapidly under various conditions (He et al, 2018).

Under certain conditions, AMPK activation vigorously inhibits mTORC1 during periods of nutrient deprivation like fasting, thus somewhat promoting autophagy. Autophagy kicks in as a vital response mechanism enabling cells to function remarkably well under extremely dire circumstances with severely limited resources. Elevated nutrient availability precipitates autophagy inhibition as cells favour brisk growth and rambunctious anabolic processes over humdrum catabolism rather sluggishly. Obesity fuels the progression of metabolic diseases and cancer by causing chronic autophagy inhibition that leads to the accumulation of cellular damage (He et al, 2018).

7.2.2 Nutrient-Induced Epigenetic Reprogramming

Nutrient imbalances trigger epigenetic changes that subtly affect gene expression deeply inside cells, altering cellular function markedly with passing time. Folate, alongside various vitamins and fatty acids, modulates DNA methylation and histone modifications, yielding long-term changes in gene expression. Epigenetic modifications drastically alter stress responses in cells, thereby significantly contributing to the progression of various complex diseases. Epigenetic regulation of genes involved in inflammation gets drastically altered by excessive caloric intake, leading rapidly to obesity issues. Caloric restriction triggers beneficial epigenetic alterations fostering DNA repair and stress resistance, thereby potentially retarding ageing processes and significantly extending lifespan (Tiffon C, 2018).

7.2.3 The Role of Inflammation in Nutrient Stress

Excessive nutrient intake triggers inflammatory pathways rooted deeply in metabolic processes and chronic diseases that manifest slowly over long periods. High-fat diets induce adipose tissue dysfunction and release of pro-inflammatory cytokines such as TNF-α and IL-6 via chronic overnutrition pathways. Cytokines trigger key signalling pathways such as NF-κB and JAK/STAT, fueling systemic inflammation that rapidly exacerbates insulin resistance and cancer progression. Severe protein deficiency triggers inflammation rapidly by activating stress-related pathways like NF-κB under conditions of nutrient deprivation remarkably quickly. Inflammation can severely impair immune response, fostering cellular stress, which makes cellular recovery really tough under acute nutrient deficiency (Duan et al, 2018).

7.3. Implications of Nutritional Stress for Health and Disease

Cells respond quite vigorously to nutritional stress, maintaining homeostasis and staving off disease in a fundamentally crucial manner naturally. Nutritional stress turns chronic or excessive, and adaptive mechanisms falter, leading to cellular dysfunction, tissue damage and onset of disease.

7.3.1 Obesity and Metabolic Syndrome

Refined carbohydrates alongside excessive calories and saturated fats precipitate metabolic syndrome and obesity quite alarmingly in many unsuspecting individuals nowadays. Chronic inflammation heightens the risk for cardiovascular diseases, cancer, and diabetes significantly, alongside insulin resistance and severely dysfunctional endothelium. Developing therapeutic interventions that modulate metabolic pathways crucially reduces the burden of chronic diseases by targeting nutrient-induced inflammatory responses effectively these days.

7.3.2 Cancer and Nutritional Stress

Nutritional stress plays a pivotal albeit oft-overlooked role, remarkably enough, in cancer progression under diverse and sundry complex circumstances. High-fat diets fuel tumour growth vigorously by enhancing insulin resistance and promoting chronic inflammation and angiogenesis substantially in various bodily tissues. Vitamin and mineral shortages severely impair DNA repair, thereby heightening genomic instability, which plays a crucial role in cancer formation processes. Nutritional stress triggers diverse cellular responses at the molecular level, enabling cells cope with scarcity or excessive nutrient availability quite effectively. Activation of AMPK alongside autophagy and epigenetic reprogramming plays quite a crucial role in cellular health maintenance. Under certain circumstances, these mechanisms can rather quickly foment the development of chronic diseases like obesity, cancer or diabetes. Scientists concoct innovative tactics somewhat futuristically by grasping cellular reactions under nutritional duress, offering prospects of vastly improved health results (Ruban et al, 2025).

8. Dietary Modulation of Cell Signalling in Homeostasis Maintenance

Cellular homeostasis maintenance entails keeping internal conditions remarkably stable, and a balanced state underpins the proper functioning of cells, tissues and organs quite fundamentally. Cells react haphazardly under varying internal or external stimuli, modifying function fairly dynamically in response to bodily needs quite frequently nowadays. Diet modulates cellular signalling pathways, heavily influencing metabolic processes and sometimes drastically altering immune response in various physiological contexts. Dietary components drastically alter nutrient availability, thereby influencing key signalling pathways crucial for rapid cellular growth or survival, ultimately impacting overall long-term health badly (Libretti and Puckett, 2025).

Cell signalling pathways like insulin signaling mTOR, and NF-κB play crucial roles, basically through myriad mechanisms within cellular environments. Cells remarkably adjust metabolic functions and gene expression according to nutritional state, with pathways responding largely to various environmental factors. Cellular dysfunction and disease arise haphazardly from aberrant signalling pathways triggered by nutrient imbalance stemming from deficiency or gross surfeit. Dietary components intricately modulate crucial signalling pathways for homeostasis, and judiciously manipulating them can rather effectively stave off the onset of disease (Libretti and Puckett, 2025).

8.1. Nutrient Sensing and Signalling Pathways

Cells constantly assess nutrient availability via specialised sensors that tweak functions based on the presence of metabolites like glucose, lipids, and oxygen. Nutrient sensors assimilate various environmental cues and toggle certain pathways on or off, maintaining metabolic homeostasis, rather precariously, meanwhile.

8.1.1 The Role of mTOR in Nutrient Sensing

The mTOR pathway stands out exceptionally well as a rather well-known nutrient-sensing pathway in cellular physiology, on the whole. Signals from amino acids, glucose, lipids and insulin integrate to regulate cell growth, proliferation, protein synthesis and overall metabolic processes vigorously. mTOR very vigorously promotes anabolism under conditions of nutrient excess, supporting growth and division with the synthesis of proteins and lipids. Nutrient scarcity, conversely, slows mTOR activity down significantly and cellular resources are retained effectively, thereby conserving anabolic processes. Amino acids, especially leucine, potently activate mTORC1, stimulating protein synthesis and fostering cell growth very rapidly (Liu and Sabatini, 2020).

Insulin and glucose also promote mTOR activation, enhancing cellular growth and energy storage, particularly in tissues like muscle, fat, and liver. Caloric restriction or nutrient deprivation, on the other hand, leads to AMPK activation, which inhibits mTOR and switches the cell to a more energy-conserving state, promoting processes like autophagy and fatty acid oxidation. Insulin and glucose fuel mTOR activation, thereby encouraging cellular growth and storing energy mostly in muscle, fat and liver tissue quite vigorously (Liu and Sabatini, 2020).

8.1.2 AMPK as a Key Sensor of Energy Balance

AMPK serves as a vital energy sensor under diverse physiological states, helping cells manage wildly fluctuating energy levels quite effectively. AMPK gets activated rapidly under low energy status, marked by a heightened AMP/ATP ratio, and subsequently promotes catabolic processes like fatty acid oxidation. Caloric restriction and exercise activate AMPK, leading to improved metabolic efficiency and heightened insulin sensitivity under certain conditions, obviously. Polyphenols such as resveratrol (found in red wine) and compounds in green tea have been shown to activate AMPK, linking dietary bioactive compounds to enhanced metabolic control and health (Herzig and Shaw, 2018).

Resveratrol, found in red wine and certain green tea compounds, apparently activates AMPK, thereby linking bioactive dietary compounds to enhanced longevity and metabolic control. Caloric restriction and exercise remarkably activate AMPK, leading to improved metabolic efficiency with heightened insulin sensitivity quite effectively.

8.2. Dietary Modulation of Inflammation and Immune Signalling

Chronic inflammation manifests ubiquitously across various maladies, including cardiovascular disease, type 2 diabetes, obesity, and some forms of cancer. Dietary intake heavily influences the balance between pro-inflammatory signals and anti-inflammatory ones, particularly via consumption of certain fatty acids and phytochemicals. Dietary components intricately modulate immune cell signalling and inflammatory pathways, ensuring inflammation gets regulated according to bodily needs rather precisely.

8.2.1 NF-κB Signalling Pathway

NF-κB regulates the expression of genes involved in cell survival and orchestrates immune responses with intense inflammatory processes unfolding rapidly. Oxidative stress, cytokines, and infection induce activation of NF-κB among various stress signals linked with numerous chronic diseases very frequently. Dietary components in red meat and processed food spur NF-κB activation robustly, fueling chronic inflammation very significantly (Liu et al, 2018). Omega-3 fatty acids sourced from fish, flaxseeds, and walnuts, alongside polyphenols found in fruits, veggies, and tea, quell NF-κB activation, effectively mitigating systemic inflammation and encouraging immune function. Omega-3 fatty acids present in fish, flaxseeds and walnuts seem to thwart NF-κB activation, thereby mitigating inflammation very effectively and encouraging immune health (Liu et al, 2018).

8.2.2 Dietary Fibre and Gut Microbiota

Gut microbiota modulates immune response fairly vigorously within bodily systems, amidst inflammation, playing a rather pivotal role. Dietary fibre plays a crucial role in gut health, obviously largely through interaction with microbiota in myriad convoluted manners. Fermentable fibres found in various fruits and veggies get broken down very quickly by gut bacteria, producing short-chain fatty acids like butyrate. Butyrate and other SCFAs stifle activation of NF-κB and foster differentiation of Tregs, which help maintain immune tolerance and blunt excessively inflammatory responses. A high-fibre diet enhances gut microbiome health very thoroughly, providing various systemic benefits that counteract inflammation across most bodily systems (Wu and Wu, 2012).

8.3. Dietary Bioactive Compounds and Cell Signalling

Many bioactive compounds lurking in plant-based food potentially tweak crucial cell signalling pathways that keep homeostasis more or less intact. Phytochemicals such as flavonoids and terpenoids influence various signalling pathways heavily involved in processes like apoptosis and oxidative stress.

8.3.1 Polyphenols and Cellular Signalling

Polyphenols such as flavonoids and stilbenes are potent modulators of cell signalling pathways, with quercetin and resveratrol being exemplary compounds naturally. AMPK activation happens with these compounds and improves insulin sensitivity substantially while promoting fat oxidation, apparently, and inhibiting mTOR slows cell growth. Modulate NF-κB, reducing inflammation and protecting against chronic diseases such as cardiovascular disease and neurodegeneration (Mutha et al, 2021).

Modulate NF-κB, thereby somewhat downregulating inflammatory responses and safeguarding against a myriad of chronic diseases like cardiovascular maladies or neurodegeneration occurring simultaneously. Suppressing mTOR activity markedly curtails cell growth and proliferation, benefiting cancer prevention efforts greatly in diverse cellular environments (Mutha et al, 2021).

8.3.2 Curcumin and Apoptotic Pathways

Curcumin, another bioactive compound in turmeric, profoundly affects complex cell signalling pathways these days with remarkably notable effects, obviously. Curcumin quite effectively inhibits the NF-κB pathway, thereby markedly reducing inflammation in various cellular contexts, and modulates cell cycle regulators, promoting arrest in cancer cells. Induce apoptosis (programmed cell death) through the activation of pro-apoptotic signalling pathways (Sharifi-Rad et al, 2020).

Pro-apoptotic signalling pathways get activated, thereby inducing apoptosis or programmed cell death very rapidly inside cells. Cell cycle regulators undergo modulation, thereby very effectively fostering arrest in cancer cells with considerable efficacy under certain conditions. Pro-apoptotic signalling pathways get activated under certain conditions, triggering programmed cell death rapidly inside affected cells. Curcumin exhibits multifaceted effects, thereby possibly possessing considerable therapeutic potential in cancer and various other chronic ailments. Diet governs cellular signalling pathways entwined with homeostasis and bodily well-being remarkably through various physiological processes deeply inside the human body (Sharifi-Rad et al, 2020).

9. Conclusion

Intricate interplay of nutrition with cellular homeostasis represents a rather compelling frontier in fairly obscure areas of biomedical science these days. Nutrients now act as molecular messengers, influencing cellular pathways, deeply regulating growth and orchestrating repair or cell death mechanisms. Bioactive compounds sourced from food intricately modulate complex signalling pathways, maintaining physiological homeostasis or precipitating disease progression when dysregulated, thereby underpinning the molecular nutrition paradigm. Micronutrients and phytochemicals, alongside macronutrients such as fatty acids and amino acids, intricately interact with various cellular signalling pathways (Gomes and Blenis, 2015). Metabolic regulation occurs in various forms alongside redox balance, epigenetic modifications, inflammatory cascades and apoptosis under somewhat enigmatic circumstances. Dietary components can influence health at the molecular level, thereby promoting cellular stability or triggering adaptive stress responses quite effectively. Crucial implications emerge largely from this new understanding, which bears significantly on cancer prevention and informs novel therapeutic strategies. Malignant cells frequently subvert compromised cellular equilibrium, thereby fueling rampant proliferation and obstinate survival under gruelling environmental stress very quickly. Targeted nutritional regimens might somewhat restore equilibrium by reinforcing defensive mechanisms within normal cells or rendering cancer cells vulnerable to therapy (Wu et al, 2023).

Sulforaphane, curcumin, and omega-3 fatty acids demonstrate an ability to modulate key regulators like NF-κB or Nrf2, yielding novel therapeutic possibilities downstream. Molecular dialogues between diet and cellular function must be grasped deeply now as precision medicine gradually supplants conventional treatments entirely. Modified nutritional regimens informed by such knowledge quietly augment medicinal treatments and foster robust long-term wellbeing underneath pharmacological regimens rather effectively (Houghton et al, 2016). Translating insights into clinical practice demands a lot more research downstream with systems biology tools fairly comprehensively integrated, very often. Nutrition plays a crucial albeit oft-overlooked role in cell signalling and regulation rather than merely lurking as some nebulous background factor in human health or disease states. Nutritional modulators deeply impact cellular homeostasis, thus unlocking new paths for disease prevention and modified therapeutic strategies effectively.

References

Aykan NF. Red Meat and Colorectal Cancer. Oncol Rev. 2015 Dec 28;9(1):288. doi: 10.4081/oncol.2015.288. PMID: 26779313; PMCID: PMC4698595.

Azadbakht L, Rouhani MH, Surkan PJ. Omega-3 fatty acids, insulin resistance and type 2 diabetes. J Res Med Sci. 2011 Oct;16(10):1259-60. PMID: 22973318; PMCID: PMC3430014.

Bar-Peled L, Sabatini DM. Regulation of mTORC1 by amino acids. Trends Cell Biol. 2014 Jul;24(7):400-6. doi: 10.1016/j.tcb.2014.03.003. Epub 2014 Mar 31. PMID: 24698685; PMCID: PMC4074565.

Bervoets I, Charlier D. Diversity, versatility and complexity of bacterial gene regulation mechanisms: opportunities and drawbacks for applications in synthetic biology. FEMS Microbiol Rev. 2019 May 1;43(3):304-339. doi: 10.1093/femsre/fuz001. PMID: 30721976; PMCID: PMC6524683.

Brandhorst S, Longo VD. Fasting and Caloric Restriction in Cancer Prevention and Treatment. Recent Results Cancer Res. 2016;207:241-66. doi: 10.1007/978-3-319-42118-6_12. PMID: 27557543; PMCID: PMC7476366.

Britten O, Tosi S. The role of diet in cancer: the potential of shaping public policy and clinical outcomes in the UK. Genes Nutr. 2024 Aug 3;19(1):15. doi: 10.1186/s12263-024-00750-9. PMID: 39097687; PMCID: PMC11298086.

Cantó C, Auwerx J. Targeting sirtuin 1 to improve metabolism: all you need is NAD(+)? Pharmacol Rev. 2012 Jan;64(1):166-87. doi: 10.1124/pr.110.003905. Epub 2011 Nov 21. PMID: 22106091; PMCID: PMC3616312.

Caprara G. Mediterranean-Type Dietary Pattern and Physical Activity: The Winning Combination to Counteract the Rising Burden of Non-Communicable Diseases (NCDs). Nutrients. 2021 Jan 28;13(2):429. doi: 10.3390/nu13020429. PMID: 33525638; PMCID: PMC7910909.

Celiberto F, Aloisio A, Girardi B, Pricci M, Iannone A, Russo F, Riezzo G, D'Attoma B, Ierardi E, Losurdo G, Di Leo A. Fibres and Colorectal Cancer: Clinical and Molecular Evidence. Int J Mol Sci. 2023 Aug 31;24(17):13501. doi: 10.3390/ijms241713501. PMID: 37686308; PMCID: PMC10488173.

Cheng CL, Gao TQ, Wang Z, Li DD. Role of insulin/insulin-like growth factor 1 signalling pathway in longevity. World J Gastroenterol. 2005 Apr 7;11(13):1891-5. doi: 10.3748/wjg.v11.i13.1891. PMID: 15800976; PMCID: PMC4305707.

Chu AH, Lin K, Croker H, Kefyalew S, Becerra-Tomás N, Dossus L, González-Gil EM, Ahmadi N, Park Y, Krebs J, Weijenberg MP, Baskin ML, Copson E, Lewis SJ, Seidell JC, Chowdhury R, Hill L, Chan DS, Lee DH, Giovannucci EL. Dietary patterns and colorectal cancer risk: Global Cancer Update Programme (CUP Global) systematic literature review. Am J Clin Nutr. 2025 May;121(5):999-1016. doi: 10.1016/j.ajcnut.2025.02.021. Epub 2025 Feb 25. PMID: 40010692; PMCID: PMC12107496.

Clemente-Suárez VJ, Beltrán-Velasco AI, Redondo-Flórez L, Martín-Rodríguez A, Tornero-Aguilera JF. Global Impacts of Western Diet and Its Effects on Metabolism and Health: A Narrative Review. Nutrients. 2023 Jun 14;15(12):2749. doi: 10.3390/nu15122749. PMID: 37375654; PMCID: PMC10302286.

Clemente-Suárez VJ, Mielgo-Ayuso J, Martín-Rodríguez A, Ramos-Campo DJ, Redondo-Flórez L, Tornero-Aguilera JF. The Burden of Carbohydrates in Health and Disease. Nutrients. 2022 Sep 15;14(18):3809. doi: 10.3390/nu14183809. PMID: 36145184; PMCID: PMC9505863.

Dengler VL, Galbraith M, Espinosa JM. Transcriptional regulation by hypoxia-inducible factors. Crit Rev Biochem Mol Biol. 2014 Jan-Feb;49(1):1-15. doi: 10.3109/10409238.2013.838205. Epub 2013 Oct 7. PMID: 24099156; PMCID: PMC4342852.

DiNicolantonio JJ, O'Keefe JH. Added Sugars Drive Insulin Resistance, Hyperinsulinemia, Hypertension, Type 2 Diabetes and Coronary Heart Disease. Mo Med. 2022 Nov-Dec;119(6):519-523. PMID: 36588634; PMCID: PMC9762218.

Donaldson MS. Nutrition and cancer: a review of the evidence for an anti-cancer diet. Nutr J. 2004 Oct 20;3:19. Doi: 10.1186/1475-2891-3-19. PMID: 15496224; PMCID: PMC526387.

Duan Y, Zeng L, Zheng C, Song B, Li F, Kong X, Xu K. Inflammatory Links Between High Fat Diets and Diseases. Front Immunol. 2018 Nov 13;9:2649. Doi: 10.3389/fimmu.2018.02649. PMID: 30483273; PMCID: PMC6243058.

Efeyan A, Comb WC, Sabatini DM. Nutrient-sensing mechanisms and pathways. Nature. 2015 Jan 15;517(7534):302-10. doi: 10.1038/nature14190. PMID: 25592535; PMCID: PMC4313349.

Enkhmaa B, Surampudi P, Anuurad E, et al. Lifestyle Changes: Effect of Diet, Exercise, Functional Food, and Obesity Treatment on Lipids and Lipoproteins. [Updated 2018 Sep 11]. In: Feingold KR, Ahmed SF, Anawalt B, et al., editors. Endotext [Internet]. South Dartmouth (MA): MDText.com, Inc.; 2000-. Available from: https://www.ncbi.nlm.nih.gov/books/NBK326737/

Ennouri S, Daoud N, Berrazegua Y, El Benna H, Korbi S, Rachdi H, Mejri N, Labidi S, Boussen H. VARIATIONS IN DIETARY HABITS DURING CANCER TREATMENT: RESULTS OF A CROSS-SECTIONAL SURVEY. Acta Clin Croat. 2024 Apr;63(1):80-88. doi: 10.20471/acc.2024.63.01.10. PMID: 39959318; PMCID: PMC11827403.

Fagbohun OF, Gillies CR, Murphy KPJ, Rupasinghe HPV. Role of Antioxidant Vitamins and Other Micronutrients on Regulations of Specific Genes and Signalling Pathways in the Prevention and Treatment of Cancer. Int J Mol Sci. 2023 Mar 23;24(7):6092. doi: 10.3390/ijms24076092. PMID: 37047063; PMCID: PMC10093825.

Gibril BAA, Xiong X, Chai X, Xu Q, Gong J, Xu J. Unlocking the Nexus of Sirtuins: A Comprehensive Review of Their Role in Skeletal Muscle Metabolism, Development, and Disorders. Int J Biol Sci. 2024 Jun 3;20(8):3219-3235. Doi: 10.7150/ijbs.96885. PMID: 38904020; PMCID: PMC11186354.

Gomes AP, Blenis J. A nexus for cellular homeostasis: the interplay between metabolic and signal transduction pathways. Curr Opin Biotechnol. 2015 Aug;34:110-7. doi: 10.1016/j.copbio.2014.12.007. Epub 2015 Jan 3. PMID: 25562138; PMCID: PMC4490161.

Grune T, Lietz G, Palou A, Ross AC, Stahl W, Tang G, Thurnham D, Yin SA, Biesalski HK. Beta-carotene is an important vitamin A source for humans. J Nutr. 2010 Dec;140(12):2268S-2285S. Doi: 10.3945/jn.109.119024. Epub 2010 Oct 27. PMID: 20980645; PMCID: PMC3139236.

Handy DE, Castro R, Loscalzo J. Epigenetic modifications: basic mechanisms and role in cardiovascular disease. Circulation. 2011 May 17;123(19):2145-56. doi: 10.1161/CIRCULATIONAHA.110.956839. PMID: 21576679; PMCID: PMC3107542.

Hardie DG. AMP-activated protein kinase: an energy sensor that regulates all aspects of cell function. Genes Dev. 2011 Sep 15;25(18):1895-908. doi: 10.1101/gad.17420111. PMID: 21937710; PMCID: PMC3185962.

He L, Zhang J, Zhao J, Ma N, Kim SW, Qiao S, Ma X. Autophagy: The Last Defence against Cellular Nutritional Stress. Adv Nutr. 2018 Jul 1;9(4):493-504. Doi: 10.1093/advances/nmy011. PMID: 30032222; PMCID: PMC6054220.

Herzig S, Shaw RJ. AMPK: guardian of metabolism and mitochondrial homeostasis. Nat Rev Mol Cell Biol. 2018 Feb;19(2):121-135. doi: 10.1038/nrm.2017.95. Epub 2017 Oct 4. PMID: 28974774; PMCID: PMC5780224.

Houghton CA, Fassett RG, Coombes JS. Sulforaphane and Other Nutrigenomic Nrf2 Activators: Can the Clinician's Expectation Be Matched by the Reality? Oxid Med Cell Longev. 2016;2016:7857186. doi: 10.1155/2016/7857186. Epub 2016 Jan 6. PMID: 26881038; PMCID: PMC4736808.

Houtkooper RH, Pirinen E, Auwerx J. Sirtuins as regulators of metabolism and healthspan. Nat Rev Mol

Jewell JL, Guan KL. Nutrient signaling to mTOR and cell growth. Trends Biochem Sci. 2013 May;38(5):233-42. doi: 10.1016/j.tibs.2013.01.004. Epub 2013 Mar 1. PMID: 23465396; PMCID: PMC3634910.

Jiang J, Chen B, Tang B, Wei Q. Selenium in Prostate Cancer: Prevention, Progression, and Treatment. Pharmaceuticals (Basel). 2023 Sep 5;16(9):1250. doi: 10.3390/ph16091250. PMID: 37765058; PMCID: PMC10536940.

Jiao L, Flood A, Subar AF, Hollenbeck AR, Schatzkin A, Stolzenberg-Solomon R. Glycemic index, carbohydrates, glycemic load, and the risk of pancreatic cancer in a prospective cohort study. Cancer Epidemiol Biomarkers Prev. 2009 Apr;18(4):1144-51. doi: 10.1158/1055-9965.EPI-08-1135. Epub 2009 Mar 31. PMID: 19336549; PMCID: PMC2687095.

Kahn BB, Alquier T, Carling D, Hardie DG. AMP-activated protein kinase: ancient energy gauge provides clues to modern understanding of metabolism. Cell Metab. 2005 Jan;1(1):15-25. doi: 10.1016/j.cmet.2004.12.003. PMID: 16054041.

Kaur J, Khare S, Sizar O, et al. Vitamin D Deficiency. [Updated 2025 Feb 15]. In: StatPearls [Internet]. Treasure Island (FL): StatPearls Publishing; 2025 Jan-. Available from: https://www.ncbi.nlm.nih.gov/books/NBK532266/

Kawai T, Autieri MV, Scalia R. Adipose tissue inflammation and metabolic dysfunction in obesity. Am J Physiol Cell Physiol. 2021 Mar 1;320(3):C375-C391. doi: 10.1152/ajpcell.00379.2020. Epub 2020 Dec 23. PMID: 33356944; PMCID: PMC8294624.

Kennedy BK, Lamming DW. The Mechanistic Target of Rapamycin: The Grand ConducTOR of Metabolism and Ageing. Cell Metab. 2016 Jun 14;23(6):990-1003. doi: 10.1016/j.cmet.2016.05.009. PMID: 27304501; PMCID: PMC4910876.

Kersten S. Peroxisome proliferator-activated receptors and lipoprotein metabolism. PPAR Res. 2008;2008:132960. doi: 10.1155/2008/132960. PMID: 18288277; PMCID: PMC2220040.

Kiani AK, Dhuli K, Donato K, Aquilanti B, Velluti V, Matera G, Iaconelli A, Connelly ST, Bellinato F, Gisondi P, Bertelli M. Main nutritional deficiencies. J Prev Med Hyg. 2022 Oct 17;63(2 Suppl 3):E93-E101. doi: 10.15167/2421-4248/jpmh2022.63.2S3.2752. PMID: 36479498; PMCID: PMC9710417.

Lam HN, Lin SP, Nguyen DHN, Chen CM, Su CT, Fang TC, Li SC. Integrative Roles of Functional Foods, Microbiotics, Nutrigenetics, and Nutrigenomics in Managing Type 2 Diabetes and Obesity. Nutrients. 2025 Feb 7;17(4):608. doi: 10.3390/nu17040608. PMID: 40004938; PMCID: PMC11858703.

Lee HT, Oh S, Ro DH, Yoo H, Kwon YW. The Key Role of DNA Methylation and Histone Acetylation in Epigenetics of Atherosclerosis. J Lipid Atheroscler. 2020 Sep;9(3):419-434. doi: 10.12997/jla.2020.9.3.419. Epub 2020 Sep 21. PMID: 33024734; PMCID: PMC7521974.

Libretti S, Puckett Y. Physiology, Homeostasis. [Updated 2023 May 1]. In: StatPearls [Internet]. Treasure Island (FL): StatPearls Publishing; 2025 Jan-. Available from: https://www.ncbi.nlm.nih.gov/books/NBK559138/

Ling ZN, Jiang YF, Ru JN, Lu JH, Ding B, Wu J. Amino acid metabolism in health and disease. Signal Transduct Target Ther. 2023 Sep 13;8(1):345. doi: 10.1038/s41392-023-01569-3. PMID: 37699892; PMCID: PMC10497558.

Liu GY, Sabatini DM. mTOR at the nexus of nutrition, growth, ageing and disease. Nat Rev Mol Cell Biol. 2020 Apr;21(4):183-203. doi: 10.1038/s41580-019-0199-y. Epub 2020 Jan 14. Erratum in: Nat Rev Mol Cell Biol. 2020 Apr;21(4):246. doi: 10.1038/s41580-020-0219-y. PMID: 31937935; PMCID: PMC7102936.

Liu H, Wang S, Wang J, Guo X, Song Y, Fu K, Gao Z, Liu D, He W, Yang LL. Energy metabolism in health and disease. Signal Transduct Target Ther. 2025 Feb 18;10(1):69. doi: 10.1038/s41392-025-02141-x. PMID: 39966374; PMCID: PMC11836267.

Liu T, Zhang L, Joo D, Sun SC. NF-κB signalling in inflammation. Signal Transduct Target Ther. 2017;2:17023–. doi: 10.1038/sigtrans.2017.23. Epub 2017 Jul 14. PMID: 29158945; PMCID: PMC5661633.

Makarem N, Nicholson JM, Bandera EV, McKeown NM, Parekh N. Consumption of whole grains and cereal fibre in relation to cancer risk: a systematic review of longitudinal studies. Nutr Rev. 2016 Jun;74(6):353-73. doi: 10.1093/nutrit/nuw003. Epub 2016 May 5. PMID: 27257283; PMCID: PMC4892300.

Mei J, Qian M, Hou Y, Liang M, Chen Y, Wang C, Zhang J. Association of saturated fatty acids with cancer risk: a systematic review and meta-analysis. Lipids Health Dis. 2024 Jan 30;23(1):32. doi: 10.1186/s12944-024-02025-z. PMID: 38291432; PMCID: PMC10826095.

Mei Z, Zhang X, Yi J, Huang J, He J, Tao Y. Sirtuins in metabolism, DNA repair and cancer. J Exp Clin Cancer Res. 2016 Dec 5;35(1):182. doi: 10.1186/s13046-016-0461-5. PMID: 27916001; PMCID: PMC5137222.

Mentella MC, Scaldaferri F, Ricci C, Gasbarrini A, Miggiano GAD. Cancer and Mediterranean Diet: A Review. Nutrients. 2019 Sep 2;11(9):2059. doi: 10.3390/nu11092059. PMID: 31480794; PMCID: PMC6770822.

Mitra S, Emran TB, Chandran D, Zidan BMRM, Das R, Mamada SS, Masyita A, Salampe M, Nainu F, Khandaker MU, Idris AM, Simal-Gandara J. Cruciferous vegetables as a treasure of functional foods bioactive compounds: Targeting p53 family in gastrointestinal tract and associated cancers. Front Nutr. 2022 Aug 4;9:951935. doi: 10.3389/fnut.2022.951935. PMID: 35990357; PMCID: PMC9386315.

Mutha RE, Tatiya AU, Surana SJ. Flavonoids as natural phenolic compounds and their role in therapeutics: an overview. Futur J Pharm Sci. 2021;7(1):25. doi: 10.1186/s43094-020-00161-8. Epub 2021 Jan 20. PMID: 33495733; PMCID: PMC7816146.

Nagy S, Petrosky SN, Demory Beckler M, Kesselman MM. The Impact of Modern Dietary Practices on Cancer Risk and Progression: A Systematic Review. Cureus. 2023 Oct 7;15(10):e46639. doi: 10.7759/cureus.46639. PMID: 37937022; PMCID: PMC10627144.

Nakrani MN, Wineland RH, Anjum F. Physiology, Glucose Metabolism. [Updated 2023 Jul 17]. In: StatPearls [Internet]. Treasure Island (FL): StatPearls Publishing; 2025 Jan-. Available from: https://www.ncbi.nlm.nih.gov/books/NBK560599/

Nicastro HL, Trujillo EB, Milner JA. Nutrigenomics and Cancer Prevention. Curr Nutr Rep. 2012 Mar 1;1(1):37-43. doi: 10.1007/s13668-011-0007-6. PMID: 24910810; PMCID: PMC4047824.

O'Brien J, Hayder H, Zayed Y, Peng C. Overview of MicroRNA Biogenesis, Mechanisms of Actions, and Circulation. Front Endocrinol (Lausanne). 2018 Aug 3;9:402. doi: 10.3389/fendo.2018.00402. PMID: 30123182; PMCID: PMC6085463.

Oniang'o R, Maingi Z, Jaika S, Konyole S. Africa's contribution to global sustainable and healthy diets: a scoping review. Front Nutr. 2025 May 2;12:1519248. doi: 10.3389/fnut.2025.1519248. PMID: 40386220; PMCID: PMC12083016.

Orlich MJ, Singh PN, Sabaté J, Fan J, Sveen L, Bennett H, Knutsen SF, Beeson WL, Jaceldo-Siegl K, Butler TL, Herring RP, Fraser GE. Vegetarian dietary patterns and the risk of colorectal cancers. JAMA Intern Med. 2015 May;175(5):767-76. doi: 10.1001/jamainternmed.2015.59. PMID: 25751512; PMCID: PMC4420687.

Ortega MA, Fraile-Martinez O, de Leon-Oliva D, Boaru DL, Lopez-Gonzalez L, García-Montero C, Alvarez-Mon MA, Guijarro LG, Torres-Carranza D, Saez MA, Diaz-Pedrero R, Albillos A, Alvarez-Mon M. Autophagy in Its (Proper) Context: Molecular Basis, Biological Relevance, Pharmacological Modulation, and Lifestyle Medicine. Int J Biol Sci. 2024 Apr 22;20(7):2532-2554. doi: 10.7150/ijbs.95122. PMID: 38725847; PMCID: PMC11077378.

Pawlowska E, Szczepanska J, Blasiak J. Pro- and Antioxidant Effects of Vitamin C in Cancer in Correspondence to

Its Dietary and Pharmacological Concentrations. Oxid Med Cell Longev. 2019 Dec 24;2019:7286737. Doi: 10.1155/2019/7286737. PMID: 31934267; PMCID: PMC6942884.

Qian F, Riddle MC, Wylie-Rosett J, Hu FB. Red and Processed Meats and Health Risks: How Strong Is the Evidence? Diabetes Care. 2020 Feb;43(2):265-271. doi: 10.2337/dci19-0063. PMID: 31959642; PMCID: PMC6971786.

Reuter S, Gupta SC, Chaturvedi MM, Aggarwal BB. Oxidative stress, inflammation, and cancer: how are they linked? Free Radic Biol Med. 2010 Dec 1;49(11):1603-16. doi: 10.1016/j.freeradbiomed.2010.09.006. Epub 2010 Sep 16. PMID: 20840865; PMCID: PMC2990475.

Röder PV, Wu B, Liu Y, Han W. Pancreatic regulation of glucose homeostasis. Exp Mol Med. 2016 Mar 11;48(3):e219. doi: 10.1038/emm.2016.6. PMID: 26964835; PMCID: PMC4892884.

Ruban M, Pozhidaeva E, Bolotina L, Kaprin A. The Role of Diet and Nutrition in Cancer Development and Management: From Molecular Mechanisms to Personalised Interventions. Foods. 2025 May 18;14(10):1788. doi: 10.3390/foods14101788. PMID: 40428567; PMCID: PMC12110988.

Rumgay H, Murphy N, Ferrari P, Soerjomataram I. Alcohol and Cancer: Epidemiology and Biological Mechanisms. Nutrients. 2021 Sep 11;13(9):3173. doi: 10.3390/nu13093173. PMID: 34579050; PMCID: PMC8470184.

Saha SK, Lee SB, Won J, Choi HY, Kim K, Yang GM, Dayem AA, Cho SG. Correlation between Oxidative Stress, Nutrition, and Cancer Initiation. Int J Mol Sci. 2017 Jul 17;18(7):1544. doi: 10.3390/ijms18071544. PMID: 28714931; PMCID: PMC5536032.

Santarelli RL, Pierre F, Corpet DE. Processed meat and colorectal cancer: a review of epidemiologic and experimental evidence. Nutr Cancer. 2008;60(2):131-44. doi: 10.1080/01635580701684872. PMID: 18444144; PMCID: PMC2661797.

Saxton RA, Sabatini DM. mTOR Signalling in Growth, Metabolism, and Disease. Cell. 2017 Mar 9;168(6):960-976. doi: 10.1016/j.cell.2017.02.004. Erratum in: Cell. 2017 Apr 6;169(2):361-371. doi: 10.1016/j.cell.2017.03.035. PMID: 28283069; PMCID: PMC5394987.

Seiler A, Chen MA, Brown RL, Fagundes CP. Obesity, Dietary Factors, Nutrition, and Breast Cancer Risk. Curr Breast Cancer Rep. 2018 Mar;10(1):14-27. doi: 10.1007/s12609-018-0264-0. Epub 2018 Jan 19. PMID: 30662586; PMCID: PMC6335046.

Sengupta S, Peterson TR, Sabatini DM. Regulation of the mTOR complex 1 pathway by nutrients, growth factors, and stress. Mol Cell. 2010 Oct 22;40(2):310-22. doi: 10.1016/j.molcel.2010.09.026. PMID: 20965424; PMCID: PMC2993060.

Sharifi-Rad J, Rayess YE, Rizk AA, Sadaka C, Zgheib R, Zam W, Sestito S, Rapposelli S, Neffe-Skocińska K, Zielińska D, Salehi B, Setzer WN, Dosoky NS, Taheri Y, El Beyrouthy M, Martorell M, Ostrander EA, Suleria HAR, Cho WC, Maroyi A, Martins N. Turmeric and Its Major Compound Curcumin on Health: Bioactive Effects and Safety Profiles for Food, Pharmaceutical, Biotechnological and Medicinal Applications. Front Pharmacol. 2020 Sep 15;11:01021. Doi: 10.3389/fphar.2020.01021. PMID: 33041781; PMCID: PMC7522354.

Sharman R, Harris Z, Ernst B, Mussallem D, Larsen A, Gowin K. Lifestyle Factors and Cancer: A Narrative Review. Mayo Clin Proc Innov Qual Outcomes. 2024 Mar 4;8(2):166-183. doi: 10.1016/j.mayocpiqo.2024.01.004. PMID: 38468817; PMCID: PMC10925935.

Simpson A, Petnga W, Macaulay VM, Weyer-Czernilofsky U, Bogenrieder T. Insulin-Like Growth Factor (IGF) Pathway Targeting in Cancer: Role of the IGF Axis and Opportunities for Future Combination Studies. Target Oncol. 2017 Oct;12(5):571-597. doi: 10.1007/s11523-017-0514-5. PMID: 28815409; PMCID: PMC5610669.

Sivasubramanian BP, Dave M, Panchal V, Saifa-Bonsu J, Konka S, Noei F, Nagaraj S, Terpari U, Savani P, Vekaria PH, Samala Venkata V, Manjani L. Comprehensive Review of Red Meat Consumption and the Risk of Cancer. Cureus. 2023 Sep 15;15(9):e45324. doi: 10.7759/cureus.45324. PMID: 37849565; PMCID: PMC10577092.

Sung H, Ferlay J, Siegel RL, Laversanne M, Soerjomataram I, Jemal A, Bray F. Global Cancer Statistics 2020: GLOBOCAN Estimates of Incidence and Mortality Worldwide for 36 Cancers in 185 Countries. CA Cancer J Clin. 2021 May;71(3):209-249. doi: 10.3322/caac.21660. Epub 2021 Feb 4. PMID: 33538338.

Tiffon C. The Impact of Nutrition and Environmental Epigenetics on Human Health and Disease. Int J Mol Sci. 2018 Nov 1;19(11):3425. doi: 10.3390/ijms19113425. PMID: 30388784; PMCID: PMC6275017.

Traber MG, Stevens JF. Vitamins C and E: beneficial effects from a mechanistic perspective. Free Radic Biol Med. 2011 Sep 1;51(5):1000-13. doi: 10.1016/j.freeradbiomed.2011.05.017. Epub 2011 May 25. PMID: 21664268; PMCID: PMC3156342.

Vaughn AE, Deshmukh M. Glucose metabolism inhibits apoptosis in neurons and cancer cells by redox inactivation of cytochrome c. Nat Cell Biol. 2008 Dec;10(12):1477-83. doi: 10.1038/ncb1807. Epub 2008 Nov 23. PMID: 19029908; PMCID: PMC2626347.

Vuolo L, Di Somma C, Faggiano A, Colao A. Vitamin D and cancer. Front Endocrinol (Lausanne). 2012 Apr 23;3:58. Doi: 10.3389/fendo.2012.00058. PMID: 22649423; PMCID: PMC3355893.

Wang G, Chen L, Qin S, Zhang T, Yao J, Yi Y, Deng L. Mechanistic Target of Rapamycin Complex 1: From a Nutrient Sensor to a Key Regulator of Metabolism and Health. Adv Nutr. 2022 Oct 2;13(5):1882-1900. doi: 10.1093/advances/nmac055. PMID: 35561748; PMCID: PMC9526850.

Widmer RJ, Flammer AJ, Lerman LO, Lerman A. The Mediterranean diet, its components, and cardiovascular disease. Am J Med. 2015 Mar;128(3):229-38. doi: 10.1016/j.amjmed.2014.10.014. Epub 2014 Oct 15. PMID: 25447615; PMCID: PMC4339461.

Wu HJ, Wu E. The role of gut microbiota in immune homeostasis and autoimmunity. Gut Microbes. 2012 Jan-Feb;3(1):4-14. doi: 10.4161/gmic.19320. Epub 2012 Jan 1. PMID: 22356853; PMCID: PMC3337124.

Wu YL, Lin ZJ, Li CC, Lin X, Shan SK, Guo B, Zheng MH, Li F, Yuan LQ, Li ZH. Epigenetic regulation in metabolic diseases: mechanisms and advances in clinical study. Signal Transduct Target Ther. 2023 Mar 2;8(1):98. doi: 10.1038/s41392-023-01333-7. PMID: 36864020; PMCID: PMC9981733.

Yang J, Nishihara R, Zhang X, Ogino S, Qian ZR. Energy sensing pathways: Bridging type 2 diabetes and colorectal cancer? J Diabetes Complications. 2017 Jul;31(7):1228-1236. doi: 10.1016/j.jdiacomp.2017.04.012. Epub 2017 Apr 13. PMID: 28465145; PMCID: PMC5501176.

Yoon H, Shaw JL, Haigis MC, Greka A. Lipid metabolism in sickness and in health: Emerging regulators of lipotoxicity. Mol Cell. 2021 Sep 16;81(18):3708-3730. doi: 10.1016/j.molcel.2021.08.027. PMID: 34547235; PMCID: PMC8620413.

Ziello JE, Jovin IS, Huang Y. Hypoxia-Inducible Factor (HIF)-1 regulatory pathway and its potential for therapeutic intervention in malignancy and ischemia. Yale J Biol Med. 2007 Jun;80(2):51-60. PMID: 18160990; PMCID: PMC2140184.

Chapter 4

Chronic Inflammation and Carcinogenesis: Dietary Regulation of Inflammatory Pathways

Lokesh Kumar Mishra[1], Ng. Joykumar Singh[2*], Sheetanshu Gupta[3], and Praneeth Juvvi[4]

[1]Department of BPME, College of Agriculture, Central Agricultural University (CAU), Imphal, Manipur, India
[2]Department of Food Process Engineering, College of Food Technology, Central Agricultural University (CAU), Imphal, Manipur, India
[3]Department of Food Safety and Quality Assurance, College of Food Technology, Central Agricultural University (CAU), Imphal, Manipur, India
[4]Department of Food Processing Technology, College of Food Technology-Central Agricultural University, Imphal, Manipur, India

Abstract

Carcinogenesis gets driven heavily by chronic inflammation across various cancer types and facilitates erratic tumour growth in very wonky, unexpected ways. Dietary factors influence inflammatory pathways within bodily systems, exacerbating or mitigating the risk of various cancers profoundly over long periods sometimes. Cytokines and prostaglandins effectively promote tumourigenesis via molecular machinations that underlie inflammation-driven carcinogenesis scrutinized thoroughly in scientific literature lately. Certain dietary components are obviously very central activate NF-κB and JAK-STAT signalling pathways, quite frequently eliciting intense inflammatory responses. Chapter reviews dietary patterns alongside specific nutrients like omega-3 fatty acids and polyphenols that modulate inflammatory pathways, significantly reducing cancer risk. Certain dietary components like trans fats and refined carbohydrates, alongside processed meats, rather curiously foster tumour development via chronic inflammation. Diet modulates inflammation and carcinogenesis fairly broadly according to findings from various epidemiological studies and some preclinical mouse models, obviously. Cancer prevention strategies have been enhanced surprisingly by various dietary interventions that manage chronic inflammation very effectively nowadays in diverse ways.

Keywords: Chronic Inflammation, Carcinogenesis, Inflammatory Pathways, Dietary Bioactive Compounds, Cytokine Regulation, NF

DOI: 10.1201/9781042010387-4

1. Introduction

Prolonged inflammatory responses contribute significantly to tumour initiation and progression, and metastasis, quite critically in cancer pathogenesis these days. Inflammation arises spontaneously in reaction to infection or bodily harm orchestrated by various immune cells, promoting rapid recuperation subsequently. Chronic response gradually morphs into a driving force for debilitating disease, rather slowly over quite some time, apparently. Chronic inflammation plays a role in various cancer developments, such as liver cancer and breast cancer, among many other kinds. Dietary modulation of inflammatory pathways and their intricate role in carcinogenesis constitute a crucial research area vital for cancer prevention endeavours.

Cancer and chronic inflammation are linked through complex pathways within human physiology, rather obviously. Multiple mechanisms underlie inflammatory processes fostering carcinogenesis partly through the production of pro-inflammatory cytokines and reactive oxygen species, fuelling cellular proliferation and angiogenesis vigorously. Inflammatory tumour environments foster genetic instability eerily and facilitate tissue remodeling a hallmark of cancer, quite quintessentially. Chronic inflammation, rather frequently nowadays, fosters a tumour-friendly microenvironment amidst diseases like hepatitis, obesity and inflammatory bowel disease. Tumour cell proliferation and metastasis get boosted by sundry inflammatory mediators like interleukins, tumour necrosis factor-alpha, and especially COX-2 (Zhao et al, 2021).

Diet significantly influences inflammatory responses, and chronic inflammation's role in carcinogenesis has been fairly well substantiated in recent times. Specific nutrients and dietary patterns directly modulate the body's inflammatory state by altering gut microbiota or influencing various inflammatory signalling pathways. Dietary intervention offers a fairly significant chance of influencing cancer risk through inflammation regulation, providing a complementary preventive strategy alongside traditional therapies. Multiple inflammatory pathways play crucial roles quite centrally in carcinogenesis at the molecular level. The NF-kB pathway plays a crucial albeit oft-maligned role in regulating inflammation and encourages somewhat lacklustre immune responses frequently found hyperactivated in various very nasty cancers linked with chronic inflammatory conditions. It orchestrates gene expression deeply embedded in survival mechanisms and proliferation alongside angiogenesis occurring somewhat mysteriously and stealthy tactics of immune evasion (Soldati et al., 2018).

Activation of NF-kB persists and drives tumourigenesis largely in response to pro-inflammatory cytokines or various other stressors in many cancer types. COX-2 produces prostaglandins, heavily promoting tumour growth and fueling metastasis vigorously in various cancerous tissues very effectively. Dietary components profoundly influence inflammatory pathways, thereby effectively mitigating cancer risk and inflammation through assorted nutritional strategies, somewhat surprisingly. Modulation of inflammation through diet originates from the notion that specific nutrients and foods exacerbate or alleviate various bodily inflammatory processes very significantly. The Western diet, replete with processed comestibles and refined sugars, tends ramp up inflammation and boosts cancer risk very drastically at times. A Mediterranean diet replete with fruits, vegetables, whole grains and healthy fats prevalent in olive oil and nuts has been linked with reduced cancer risk and lowered inflammation levels substantially. Dietary components profoundly affect inflammatory pathways and cancer development significantly across diverse populations under various nutritional regimens (Zhang et al, 2020).

Diet regulates inflammation mainly through the consumption of bioactive compounds that interact heavily with mediators of various inflammatory responses quite frequently. Polyphenols found abundantly in fruits and tea possess anti-inflammatory properties and have been shown naturally to be very bioactive. Compounds such as resveratrol, found in grapes and red wine, and curcumin, derived from turmeric, have garnered considerable attention for modulating inflammatory pathways vigorously by inhibiting NF-kB activity deeply in cells. Epigallocatechin gallate EGCG sourced from green tea, also inhibits COX-2 activity. Resveratrol and curcumin have been studied extensively for their anti-inflammatory properties. They work fantastically well in many cases (Pandey and Rizvi, 2009).

Green tea has various health benefits, too. Tumour-promoting inflammation gets suppressed very effectively nowadays by these compounds, which decrease oxidative stress via reduced production of pro-inflammatory cytokines. Omega-3 fatty acids present in fish oil and flaxseeds exert profoundly anti-inflammatory effects by markedly reducing pro-inflammatory eicosanoid synthesis and modulating immune responses. Dietary fibre plays a rather pivotal role in regulating inflammation largely through quite significant effects on microbiota in the gut. Diets rich in fibre foster growth of beneficial bacteria in the gut, producing short-chain fatty acids that have anti-inflammatory properties systemically (Szulińska et al, 2017).

Butyrate, acetate and propionate serve as colonocyte energy sources, heavily modulating immune system functionality, rather quietly underneath epithelial layers normally. Such cases often see fairly significant mitigation of chronic inflammation linked with conditions such as colorectal cancer, very effectively. Antioxidants play a crucial role somewhat haphazardly in curbing rampant inflammation, and another vital facet exists quietly within dietary control. Prolonged inflammation spawns chronic oxidative stress, very badly damaging DNA and mutating various genes, thereby activating oncogenes recklessly. Antioxidants such as vitamin C scavenge free radicals very vigorously in cells and mitigate oxidative damage rather effectively (Ney et al, 2023). Oxidative damage linked with inflammation can be very effectively mitigated by consuming foods rich in antioxidants like leafy greens and berries. The gut microbiome plays a pivotal role in regulating inflammation and carcinogenesis alongside various nutrients that deeply influence both pathological processes. Research emerging rapidly now indicates that gut flora severely disrupted by junk food promotes inflammation fervently and fuels the development of cancer significantly. A diet rich in fibre and fermented foods fosters a balanced microbiome, modulating immune responses effectively and reducing inflammation quite substantially. Consumption of copious red meats and sugars readily fosters inflammation, and tumourigenesis is thereby supported vigorously in most cases naturally (Munteanu and Schwartz, 2024). Chronic inflammation drives carcinogenesis through various molecular mechanisms and cellular processes, focusing on key inflammatory pathways. Diet plays a crucial role in modulating certain cellular pathways, and emphasising potential dietary interventions significantly reduces inflammation, thereby lowering cancer risk overall. Very effectively, cancer prevention strategies can be harnessed by grasping intricate links between dietary habits and the occurrence of malignant tumours.

2. The Link between Chronic Inflammation and Cancer Development

Cancers metastasise partly owing to chronic inflammation, which gets increasingly recognised as a crucial factor in tumour initiation and neoplastic progression. Immune systems react quite instinctively with shield-like inflammation against stimuli that irritate or very damaging infections typically occur. Unrelenting inflammatory responses gone haywire can instigate diverse pathological cascades, including DNA degradation and rampant cell division, neovascularisation, and immunosuppression, crucial for tumourigenesis. Research highlighting intricate roles of chronic inflammation within tumour microenvironments has amassed over several decades, rendering it remarkably focal nowadays (Gonzalez et al, 2018).

Chronic inflammation arises from a prolonged immune response exacerbated by myriad factors such as obesity and poor dietary habits quite frequently. Production of inflammatory cytokines and obesity-related inflammation markedly heighten risk of various cancers, including liver, breast and colorectal cancer. Epigenetic tweaks inside immune cells alongside genetic leanings can crank up inflammatory reactions, thus heaping on the overall risk of cancer substantially. Malignant tumour progression stems largely from chronic inflammation, effectively influencing various inflammatory pathways and the initiation of cancer development significantly. Lifestyle choices and dietary factors can very frequently modulate inflammation in rather significant ways, thereby impacting cancer risk, obviously.

2.1. Mechanisms Linking Chronic Inflammation to Cancer

Cancer growth gets fueled by chronic inflammation through myriad convoluted routes operating surreptitiously within various signalling pathways and via inflammatory cells' cytokines. Persistent inflammation nurtures a precarious environment ripe for cancer by precipitating genetic aberrations and fueling tumour cell proliferation, subverting host immune surveillance. TNF-α and STAT3, alongside NF-κB, COX-2 and IL-6 signalling pathways, are heavily implicated in carcinogenesis triggered by inflammatory responses.

2.1.1 NF-κB Pathway: Central to Inflammation and Cancer

The NF-κB signalling pathway plays a crucial albeit somewhat obscure role in modulating immune response vigorously downstream of activated B cells. NF-κB activation spawns expression of pro-inflammatory cytokines and chemokines, facilitating the combat of infections effectively under fairly normal physiological conditions. Persistently activated NF-κB morphs into a driver of tumourigenesis. Relentless NF-κB activation gets fueled very significantly by chronic inflammation, resulting in the production of molecules enhancing cell proliferation and survival via angiogenesis (Liu et al, 2017). Tumour microenvironment conducive to cancer initiation and progression forms rapidly in situ with remarkable swiftness under peculiar circumstances therein. NF-κB pathway quashes apoptotic pathways, thereby allowing cells with mutations or genomic instability survive, a characteristic inherent in cancerous cells, prolifically. NF-κB activation persists chronically in various malignancies, including colon cancer, liver tumours, and lung cancers, as a paradigm of inflammatory turmoil, thereby making it a crucial target for therapeutic intervention (Liu et al, 2017).

2.1.2 COX-2 and Prostaglandins in Inflammation-Induced Cancer

Cyclooxygenase-2 plays a major role in cancers related to inflammation, despite being largely underexamined in development processes. COX-2 catalyzes production of prostaglandins very intricately, which are lipid mediators that regulate various inflammatory aspects within bodily tissues normally. PGE2 fosters tumour growth and immune evasion by boosting angiogenesis, supplying nutrients and oxygen to growing tumours, rather vigorously. Promoting immune tolerance, allowing tumours to evade immune surveillance and immune cell killing. Tumours evade immune surveillance and are killed less by immune cells due partly to the promotion of tolerance somewhat irregularly (Pang et al, 2016).

2.1.3 Cytokines and Inflammatory Signalling in Tumourigenesis

Pro-inflammatory cytokines play a pivotal role linking chronic inflammation and cancer with NF-κB activation and overexpression of COX-2 enzymes. Tumour necrosis factor-alpha and interleukin-6 cytokines heavily foster cancer initiation in tumour microenvironments where they are frequently overexpressed and progression occurs rapidly. Cytokines rapidly exert effects via diverse signalling pathways, modulating cell proliferation, apoptosis or inducing angiogenesis in certain contexts. IL-6 activates the STAT3 signalling pathway, promoting cell survival, proliferation and tumour progression. IL-6 vigorously ramps up STAT3 signalling very intensely, promoting cell survival mechanisms and proliferation, which leads rapidly to tumour progression (Nishida and Andoh, 2025).

TNF-α, another cytokine produced in response to inflammatory stimuli, can induce apoptosis under normal physiological conditions but may instead promote survival in tumour cells through chronic inflammatory responses. IL-6 plays a crucial role in breast cancer and prostate cancer, often manifesting with elevated cytokine levels alongside hepatocellular carcinoma. TNF-alpha induces cell death normally, yet promotes survival in tumour cells through chronic inflammation fairly frequently under some bizarre circumstances (Nishida and Andoh, 2025).

2.2. Diet, Obesity, and Chronic Inflammation in Cancer Risk

Diet profoundly influences chronic inflammation, thereby sparking intense investigation into cancer development and its underlying complex multifaceted effects. Diets laden with processed food and saturated fats tend to fuel inflammation, while ones rich in fruits and omega-3s may counteract cancer risk somewhat.

2.2.1 Obesity and Inflammation-Induced Cancer Risk

Obesity remains a remarkably strong link between cancer and chronic inflammation, everywhere. Adipose tissue overabundance spuriously churns out myriad inflammatory cytokines such as IL-6 and TNF-α alongside leptin, thereby fostering tumourigenesis via rampant obesity-induced inflammation. Molecules trigger inflammation stubbornly promoting tumour growth by fueling insulin resistance and genomic instability whilst fostering angiogenesis very vigorously. Obesity links strongly suddenly with various cancer types, including breast and colon, and certain rare liver cancers, very frequently nowadays. Postmenopausal women exhibit a strong correlation, and adipose tissue morphs into a primary estrogen source, fiercely fueling cancers like estrogen-driven breast cancer (Divella et al, 2016).

2.2.2 Anti-Inflammatory Foods and Cancer Prevention

Nutrients boasting anti-inflammatory properties in abundance within a diet can mitigate chronic inflammation very significantly and somewhat effectively lower cancer risk. Foods rich in omega-3 fatty acids, fibre, and antioxidants have been shown to markedly reduce markers of systemic inflammation, including C-reactive protein. Omega-3 fatty acids found abundantly in fatty fish such as salmon inhibit the expression of pro-inflammatory cytokines like IL-6 and TNF-α and can drastically reduce inflammation in tissues vulnerable to cancer. Dietary fibre has an indirect effect on inflammation by promoting gut health and altering the gut microbiota. Dietary fibre exerts an indirect influence on inflammation largely by encouraging gut health and significantly altering gut microbiota composition (Yu et al, 2024).

Omega-3 fatty acids found in fatty fish like salmon ostensibly inhibit pro-inflammatory cytokine expression and mitigate tissue inflammation quite significantly. Polyphenols present in green tea berries, and curcumin possess antioxidant properties that neutralise free radicals and reduce oxidative stress markedly in cancer cells (Yu et al, 2024).

2.3. Therapeutic Targeting of Inflammation in Cancer Prevention

Disrupting strong ties between chronic inflammation and cancer development naturally holds huge potential for cancer prevention via inflammatory pathway targeting. Celecoxib and etanercept are utilised for treating ailments like arthritis by inhibiting pivotal inflammatory molecules such as COX-2 and TNF-α. Aspirin and other non-steroidal anti-inflammatory drugs are very effective in lowering the risk of certain cancers, like colorectal cancer, by inhibiting COX-2 and dampening inflammatory responses in tumour microenvironments, amidst fervent research in various scientific circles nowadays. Their role in cancer therapy remains shrouded in mystery. Immune checkpoint inhibitors, which target immune suppression in the tumour microenvironment, may also help to reverse the effects of chronic inflammation and enhance the body's ability to mount an immune response against cancer cells (Wang et al, 2024).

Immune checkpoint inhibitors targeting immune suppression in the tumour microenvironment may help reverse the effects of chronic inflammation and boost the body's ability against cancer cells vigorously. Very effectively, certain cancer risks are mitigated by aspirin-like non-steroidal anti-inflammatory drugs inhibiting COX-2. Tumour microenvironment immune suppression targeted by certain inhibitors may reverse chronic inflammation effects and enhance cancer-fighting prowess in the body quite effectively. Profound genomic instability and tumour promotion are fueled quite irregularly by chronic inflammation acting as a key mediator of cancer development significantly (Wang et al, 2024).

3. Dietary Factors as Modulators of Inflammatory Pathways in Cancer

Cancer has become intricately linked with chronic inflammation in recent years, largely owing to its pivotal role in fostering tumourigenesis. Prolonged low-grade inflammatory response fuels carcinogenesis drastically over quite an extended period, altering the tumour microenvironment remarkably. Evidence recently highlighted a powerful influence of dietary factors on inflammatory pathways regulation, offering potential strategies for cancer prevention quite effectively. Nutritional elements significantly modulate underlying inflammatory processes effectively, thereby either exacerbating or greatly alleviating chronic inflammation through diet. NF-κB, STAT3, and COX-2 signalling pathways profoundly impact the pathogenesis of many cancers heavily influenced by inflammatory responses (Greten and Grivennikov, 2019).

Apoptosis and cell growth, along with angiogenesis, are inextricably linked with immune response in various pathways contributing heavily to downstream cancer processes. Modifying diet holds considerable promise for mitigating cancer risk and encourage effectiveness of current treatments via multiple biochemical routes. Bioactive compounds alongside macronutrients and micronutrients modulate inflammatory pathways associated with various cancers very significantly in numerous ways. Various nutritional approaches and therapeutic regimens will be discussed for mitigating cancer risk effectively by reducing inflammation somewhat through dietary interventions (Greten and Grivennikov, 2019).

3.1. Inflammatory Pathways in Cancer and Their Regulation by Diet

Chronic inflammation plays a somewhat paradoxical role in cancer development, apparently fostering both pathological and protective processes simultaneously. Inflammation may serve initially to repair damaged tissue quite rapidly and control various nasty infections very effectively. Chronic inflammation notoriously fosters genomic instability very rapidly and promotes immune evasion mechanisms under various physiological conditions, aiding tumour formation and metastasis. Multiple crucial inflammatory pathways get directly embroiled in such complex physiological processes suddenly and quite vigorously.

3.1.1 NF-κB Pathway: A Central Regulator of Inflammation and Cancer

The NF-κB pathway mediates inflammation vigorously as a crucial enhancer of activated B cells through multiple cellular processes simultaneously. NF-κB vigorously regulates myriad immune responses under normal circumstances and protects effectively against nasty pathogens causing very severe infections. Prolonged NF-κB activation correlates fairly strongly with the development of various cancers, including certain colorectal cancers and highly malignant breast cancers, in contexts of chronic inflammation. NF-κB activation triggers rapid production of pro-inflammatory cytokines and chemokines, stimulating tumour cell proliferation deep within affected tissue (Liu et al, 2017). Dietary factors modulate NF-κB activation under specific conditions very frequently, thereby altering tumour microenvironments effectively. Omega-3 fatty acids found abundantly in salmon inhibit NF-κB activation quite profoundly, reducing inflammation significantly. Curcumin has anti-inflammatory properties and can inhibit NF-κB activation, reducing tumour growth and invasion markedly in preclinical cancer models (Liu et al, 2017).

3.1.2 COX-2 and Prostaglandin Signalling in Inflammation

COX-2 enzyme facilitates the conversion of arachidonic acid into prostaglandins very quietly, fostering inflammatory responses and cancer progression slowly. COX-2 becomes overexpressed quite frequently in various types of malignancies, including colon cancer, breast cancer and occasionally lung cancer, apparently too. Elevated prostaglandin levels, particularly PGE2, significantly spur tumour cell growth and facilitate angiogenesis with various immune evasion mechanisms. Dietary factors wildly modulate COX-2 expression and its downstream signalling via nonsteroidal anti-inflammatory drugs like aspirin, which heavily inhibit COX-2 (Desai et al, 2018). Omega-3 fatty acids found in fish and polyphenols in green tea reduce COX-2 expression very significantly, providing some anti-inflammatory benefits. Aspirin, thereby reducing the risk of certain nasty cancers, especially very aggressive colorectal cancer, is commonly used. Nonsteroidal anti-inflammatory drugs can lower cancer risk, and COX-2 expression is reduced simultaneously with their usage (Desai et al, 2018).

3.1.3 IL-6 and TNF-α: Cytokines in Chronic Inflammation

Pro-inflammatory cytokines such as IL-6 and TNF-α are often overproduced in chronic inflammation, with intense simultaneous cellular responses happening vigorously. Cytokines spur cancer growth very rapidly underneath cellular surfaces by stimulating angiogenesis, which supplies increasing tumours with nutrients. They induce cell proliferation and suppress apoptosis or programmed cell death within tissues. Modulating the immune response often promotes immune suppression that allows tumours to evade detection and destruction. Tumours frequently evade destruction by hijacking immune response mechanisms that often entail profound suppression, allowing stealthy escape from detection.

3.1.4 The Role of STAT3 in Inflammation and Cancer

STAT3 pathway mediates inflammation robustly in various cancer settings, effectively acting as a crucial downstream regulator with significant oncogenic potential. STAT3 activation frequently correlates with metastasis and tumour progression via sundry mechanisms that facilitate immune evasion remarkably effectively in various cancers. STAT3 remains activated very frequently in various cancers such as breast cancer, lung cancer, and hepatocellular carcinoma, among others. Curcumin, present in turmeric, substantially inhibits STAT3 activation, thereby markedly reducing expression of various inflammatory cytokines and certain growth factors. Polyphenols like quercetin or resveratrol have been identified as natural compounds that downregulate STAT3 signaling providing anti-inflammatory effects and anticancer properties (Yu et al, 2009).

3.2. Bioactive Compounds in Diet and Their Impact on Inflammatory Pathways

Fats and proteins aside, various bioactive compounds abundant in fruits and veggies exert remarkably potent anti-inflammatory effects on cancer-linked pathways.

3.2.1 Polyphenols: Anti-Inflammatory Agents in Cancer Prevention

Polyphenols occur naturally in various foods, like fruits and veggies, and also in drinks such as tea or wine fairly often. Compounds have been studied rather extensively of late for anti-inflammatory effects and possess fairly significant antioxidant properties, meanwhile. Quercetin and kaempferol drastically suppress NF-κB activation in cancer cells, reducing COX-2 expression significantly. Resveratrol, found in red wine, has anti-inflammatory effects through inhibition of NF-κB and modulation of the PI3K/Akt pathway involved deeply in tumourigenesis and cell survival mechanisms. Resveratrol, found in red wine and grapes, exhibits anti-inflammatory properties by inhibiting NF-κB and modulating PI3K/Akt signalling pathway crucial for cell survival (Pandey and Rizvi, 2009).

3.2.2 Omega-3 Fatty Acids and Inflammation

Fatty fish, flaxseed and some walnuts contain EPA and DHA, namely omega-3 fatty acids, essentially found abundantly therein. Omega-3 fatty acids very effectively modulate multiple inflammatory pathways and exert anti-cancer effects through several mechanisms, inhibiting NF-κB activation downstream. Omega-3s very significantly downregulate inflammatory responses by reducing COX-2 expression and pro-inflammatory cytokines such as IL-6 and TNF-α. Production of anti-inflammatory eicosanoids like resolvins and protectins gets promoted, thereby counteracting pro-inflammatory eicosanoids derived from omega-6 fatty acids. Omega-3s spur production of anti-inflammatory eicosanoids like resolvins and protectins, which counter pro-inflammatory ones derived from omega-6 fatty acids vigorously (Rodriguez-Leyva et al, 2010).

3.2.3 Dietary Fibre and Gut Health

Fruits, legumes, and whole grains richly supplying fibre have been tied with markedly diminished inflammation and lower cancer risk. Fibre fosters the growth of beneficial bacteria deep within the gut microbiome, which ferment it into short-chain fatty acids like butyrate, possessing anti-inflammatory properties. Butyrate inhibits activation of NF-κB and reduces expression of pro-inflammatory cytokines, helping to protect against colon cancer driven by inflammation. Gut microbiota plays an integral role in modulating immune responses, with fibre-rich diets supporting a healthy microbiome that can help reduce systemic inflammation (Fu et al, 2022).

Gut microbiota modulates immune responses quite effectively, and fibre-rich diets foster a healthy microbiome that helps mitigate systemic inflammation very significantly. Butyrate suppresses NF-κB activation very significantly and diminishes pro-inflammatory cytokine expression, thereby helping fend off inflammation-driven cancers, namely colon cancer. Fibre-rich diets ostensibly foster a healthy microbiome, which mitigates systemic inflammation effectively, and gut microbiota modulates immune responses with considerable efficacy. Cancer onset spreads rapidly through complex biological pathways with alarming frequency, fueled by chronic inflammation under various circumstances. Modulating inflammatory pathways via diet presents a promising cancer prevention strategy alongside some potentially effective therapeutic management options (Fu et al, 2022).

4. Molecular Mechanisms

Chronic inflammation surfaces as a crucial factor in cancer initiation and metastasis, unfolding stealthily over prolonged periods beneath notice. Injury sparks protective inflammation via the immune system, but when gone awry, it nurtures a distinctly pro-tumourigenic microenvironment. Normal cells undergo malignant transformation via various signalling pathways within this environment, fueled by complex interactions between inflammatory cells and cytokines. Novel therapeutic strategies crucially hinge on deciphering molecular mechanisms underlying carcinogenesis related to inflammation with fairly high accuracy nowadays. Carcinogenesis is driven quite intricately by inflammation through molecular mechanisms that underlie genomic instability and proliferation of tumour cells alongside survival. Mutagenesis gets fueled by inflammatory mediators, and tumour progression metastasises rapidly, while targeting such pathways therapeutically might mitigate cancer risk very effectively (Rakoff-Nahoum S, 2006).

» To visualise a key mechanism discussed in the chapter, demonstrating that diet does not just act directly on cells, but also indirectly by shaping the gut microbiome, which in turn profoundly influences the body's inflammatory state.

4.1. Inflammation-Induced Genomic Instability: The Role of Oxidative Stress

Carcinogenesis is fueled remarkably by inflammation, largely through the generation of reactive oxygen species and reactive nitrogen species inside cells. Reactive molecules form quickly inside macrophages and neutrophils via inflammation and through pro-inflammatory signalling pathways like NF-κB activation pathways. Reactive oxygen species wreak havoc on DNA, causing single-strand breaks and base modifications fairly frequently in cells. Oxidative damage accumulates in DNA, leading to genomic instability, a hallmark frequently observed in cells that have suddenly become cancerous (Yu et al, 2022). Instability fosters epigenetic accumulation of mutations and chromosomal aberrations, rapidly driving normal cells towards frankly cancerous phenotypes with alarming speed. Chronic inflammation-induced ROS generation is closely linked to tumour initiation because DNA damage caused by ROS directly promotes mutations in critical tumour suppressor genes like TP53 and oncogenes like KRAS, leading to unchecked cell proliferation. ROS also contribute to epigenetic changes, such as DNA methylation and histone modification, which can silence tumour suppressor genes and activate oncogenes (Yu et al, 2022).

4.1.2 Nitric Oxide (NO) and Genomic Instability

Nitric oxide produced by inflammatory cells like macrophages, alongside ROS, can also heavily contribute to very significant DNA damage. NO reacts vigorously with superoxide, forming peroxynitrite, a highly potent mutagen that brutally induces DNA strand breaks, base modifications and nucleotide oxidations, leading rapidly to genetic mutations and cancer.

4.2. Immune Microenvironment and Tumour Promotion

Chronic inflammation drives genomic instability and fosters a tumour-promoting immune microenvironment deeply within affected tissues quite rapidly. Inflammatory response severely disrupts normal immune surveillance and facilitates immune evasion by rapidly proliferating tumour cells quite effectively. Mutated cells thrive and expand rapidly because normally, they would be readily obliterated by the immune system responses otherwise.

4.2.1 Immune Suppression and Tumour Escape

Tumours slyly recruit immunosuppressive cells like regulatory T cells and myeloid-derived suppressor cells amidst chronically nasty inflammation quite often. Tumour evasion occurs stealthily under immune suppression. Cytokines like IL-10 and TGF-β released during chronic inflammation facilitate recruitment of immunosuppressive cells into the tumour microenvironment. Tumour-associated macrophages (TAMs), which are often polarised to the M2 phenotype in the presence of inflammation, can promote tumour growth, angiogenesis, and metastasis through the secretion of pro-inflammatory cytokines and growth factors (Yang et al, 2020).

4.2.2 Tumour-Associated Macrophages and Tumour Growth

Macrophages play a pivotal role, deeply embedded in inflammatory responses unfolding vigorously within various bodily tissues, rather rampantly and extremely dynamically. M2 macrophages foster tumour progression partly by secreting VEGF and stimulating angiogenesis deeply within the tumour microenvironment. They produce matrix metalloproteinases, which degrade the extracellular matrix, facilitating tumour invasion and metastasis, rather quietly.

4.3. Chronic Inflammation and Tumour Cell Proliferation

Tumour cell proliferation and survival are driven by several key signalling pathways activated vigorously by chronic inflammation over time. Tumour growth gets a boost from these pathways, which also shield cancerous cells from apoptosis, thereby facilitating relentless proliferation amidst genomic mayhem.

4.3.1 NF-κB Pathway and Tumour Cell Proliferation

The NF-κB signalling pathway plays a crucial albeit oft-overlooked role nowadays in inflammation-driven cancer, quite frequently, apparently, in various contexts. NF-κB activation enables the body fight infection robustly under normal circumstances as part of innate immunity mechanisms effectively. Tumours with chronic NF-κB activation spur irregular expression of genes promoting cell survival and proliferation alongside somewhat aberrant angiogenesis. NF-κB directly upregulates pro-survival genes like Bcl-2 and Survivin, which inhibit apoptosis and promote survival, allowing cancer cells to evade programmed cell death normally. Additionally, NF-κB activates the expression of COX-2, IL-6, and TNF-α, all of which enhance tumour cell proliferation and invasiveness (Zhang et al, 2020).

4.3.2 JAK/STAT3 Pathway: Inflammation-Induced Tumour Progression

JAK/STAT3 signalling pathway critically regulates tumour cell proliferation within contexts of very frequent chronic inflammatory responses. IL-6 and TNF-α vigorously activate JAK/STAT3 signaling thereby substantially promoting tumourigenesis by enhancing cell proliferation and inhibiting apoptosis largely. Tumour growth and spread are facilitated by angiogenic factors and metastatic proteins whose expression is induced. Tumour growth spreads rapidly under certain conditions due to the expression of various angiogenic factors and metastatic proteins vigorously (Huang et al, 2020).

4.4. Inflammation and Angiogenesis in Cancer

Tumour progression relies heavily on angiogenesis, which involves the formation of new blood vessels, facilitating metastasis quite rapidly. Chronic inflammation promotes angiogenesis significantly via activation of several key inflammatory pathways.

4.4.1 Pro-angiogenic Mediators

Tumour cells and immune cells release inflammatory cytokines and growth factors abundantly in the tumour microenvironment, stimulating angiogenesis vigorously by inducing VEGF, FGF, and IL-8 expression, which acts on endothelial cells, promoting new blood vessel formation. Expression of matrix metalloproteinases gets enhanced, degrading the extracellular matrix, allowing endothelial cells to invade the tumour, further supporting angiogenesis robustly. Matrix metalloproteinases expression gets amplified quite vigorously, enabling endothelial cells surge into tumour tissues and further encourage angiogenesis robustly (Geindreau et al, 2022).

4.5. Inflammation and Metastasis

Chronic inflammation furthers tumour growth, and metastasis spreads cancer cells haphazardly into distant organs, often resulting in devastating consequences. Tumour cells display invasive behaviour mainly owing to inflammation-induced infiltration of immune cells and rapid, extensive remodelling of the ECM alongside swift angiogenesis.

4.5.1 Inflammatory Mediators in Tumour Metastasis

IL-6 and TNF-α play crucial roles in promoting the epithelial-to-mesenchymal transition (EMT), a key process in metastasis, where epithelial cells acquire migratory and invasive properties. Inflammatory cytokines such as IL-8 promote tumour cell migration and invasion, allowing cancer cells to detach from the primary tumour, invade the bloodstream, and establish secondary tumours in distant organs. IL-6 and TNF-α crucially promote epithelial-to-mesenchymal transition (EMT), a key metastasis process where epithelial cells acquire highly migratory properties. Inflammatory cytokines like IL-8 spur tumour cell migration and invasion, allowing cancer cells detach from the primary tumour and invade the bloodstream vigorously, establishing secondary tumours in distant organs (Xie et al, 2025).

IL-6 and TNF-α crucially promote epithelial-to-mesenchymal transition, or EMT, a key metastatic process wherein epithelial cells rapidly gain highly migratory mesenchymal properties. Tumour cell migration and invasion are heavily promoted by inflammatory cytokines like IL-8, facilitating the detachment of cancer cells from the primary tumour and invasion into the bloodstream, which eventually spawns secondary tumours deeply nestled in distant organs. Carcinogenesis is driven quite effectively by chronic inflammation, fueling initiation and progression of tumour through metastasis, underlying molecular mechanisms (Xie et al, 2025).

5. Nutritional Interventions in Chronic Inflammatory Diseases

Chronic inflammation frequently fuels various debilitating health issues nowadays, including autoimmune disorders and certain kinds of cancers very often. Inflammation becomes downright pernicious, persisting unabated in the absence of immediate threat and spawns a plethora of chronic diseases presently afflicting people everywhere. Evidence mounts that dietary factors remarkably sway inflammation across bodily systems, sometimes with profoundly unsettling long-term repercussions. Nutritional interventions silently exacerbate or mitigate inflammatory processes, offering fresh avenues for the prevention of chronic diseases effectively nowadays. Specific nutrients exacerbate inflammatory responses, whereas others attenuate them via intricate biochemical pathways modulated substantially by dietary influences. Bioactive compounds and various micronutrients alongside macronutrients potentially prevent chronic inflammatory diseases, with considerable benefits being examined very closely now.

5.1. The Role of Chronic Inflammation in Disease Pathogenesis

Chronic inflammation simmers quietly as the body releases pro-inflammatory molecules rapidly in response to stress and various environmental toxins persistently. Chronic inflammation slowly ravages tissue over time, disrupting normal cellular function and spurring diseases like cardiovascular ailments, such as atherosclerosis or heart attack, while fostering metabolic disorders, including obesity type 2 diabetes and insulin resistance. Activation of diverse immune cells, such as macrophages or T-cells, occurs alongside the release of various inflammatory cytokines like IL-6 and TNF-α and production of reactive oxygen species. Inflammation, promoting genomic instability and metastasis, spawns various diseases, including neurodegenerative conditions like Alzheimer's and autoimmune conditions such as rheumatoid arthritis or cancer. Molecules wreak havoc directly on cells and destroy tissues very slowly over a long period, leading to debilitating disease (Stone et al, 2025).

5.2. Nutritional Influences on Inflammatory Pathways

Specific nutrients and dietary patterns profoundly affect activity and expression of inflammatory mediators in bodily contexts with varying degrees of intensity. Certain foods ignite inflammation rather badly, while others wield an anti-inflammatory punch very effectively inside human systems fairly regularly. Crucially, nutrition profoundly impacts inflammatory pathways that underlie various chronic diseases, thereby facilitating the devising of effective dietary strategies.

5.2.1 Omega-3 Fatty Acids: Inflammation Modulators

Omega-3 fatty acids, especially EPA and DHA, are highly studied anti-inflammatory nutrients found in fatty fish such as salmon and certain plant sources. Polyunsaturated fatty acids suppress inflammation oddly by inhibiting NF-κB pathway a crucial regulator deeply inside various cellular responses. Production of pro-inflammatory cytokines and enzymes like COX-2 gets markedly reduced thereby converting into anti-inflammatory molecules called resolvins that actively promote resolution of inflammation. Suppressing the production of eicosanoids from omega-6 fatty acids, which are often pro-inflammatory. Production of eicosanoids derived from omega-6 fatty acids often pro-inflammatory in nature gets heavily suppressed (Calder PC, 2013).

5.2.2 The Role of Omega-6 Fatty Acids

Processed foods and sunflower oil as well as corn oil contain omega-6 fatty acids vital for wellbeing yet overconsumption heavily fuels chronic inflammation. Arachidonic acid derived from omega-6 fats rather quietly serves as precursor of pro-inflammatory eicosanoids like prostaglandins and leukotrienes downstream. Presence of such molecules excessively promotes chronic inflammation which heavily contributes to diseases like atherosclerosis obesity and type 2 diabetes. Western diets nowadays often display a glaring disparity stemming from a markedly elevated proportion of omega-6 fatty acids relative to omega-3. Such imbalance fosters chronic low-grade inflammation making dietary adjustments super critical for optimizing omega-3 intake and reducing excessive omega-6 consumption drastically (Mariamenatu et al, 2021).

5.2.3 Fibre and Gut Health:

Evidence accumulates rather quickly that fibre particularly from veggies, whole grains and various legumes, plays a crucial role in modulating inflammatory responses deeply via significant impacts on gut microbiome. Dietary fibre fuels beneficial gut bacteria very effectively, producing short-chain fatty acids like butyrate, acetate and propionate in the gut. SCFAs profoundly exert potent anti-inflammatory effects by inhibiting NF-κB activation and myriad inflammatory signalling pathways, effectively reducing production of pro-inflammatory cytokines like TNF-α and IL-6. Modulating immune cell function, particularly Treg cells, which help dampen inflammatory responses. Treg cells help dampen inflammatory responses significantly by modulating immune cell function effectively under various physiological conditions (Fu et al, 2022).

5.3. Micronutrients with Anti-Inflammatory Effects

Micronutrients like vitamins and certain minerals possess surprisingly well-documented anti-inflammatory properties, usually under specific physiological conditions. Vitamin D and magnesium play crucial roles in regulating immune responses deeply and modulating inflammation somewhat sloppily in various bodily tissues.

5.3.1 Vitamin D: Immune System Regulator

Vitamin D plays a pivotal role remarkably well in humans as a fat-soluble vitamin crucial for maintaining robust immune function very effectively. 1,25-dihydroxyvitamin D fervently inhibits pro-inflammatory cytokines and vigorously promotes differentiation of anti-inflammatory Treg cells in a very effective manner. Vitamin D deficiency strongly correlates with heightened inflammation and elevated risk of maladies like rheumatoid arthritis, multiple sclerosis, and cardiovascular disease. Vitamin D intake garnered sufficiently via sunlight or supplementation markedly betters clinical outcomes in those afflicted with various chronic debilitating conditions (Charoenngam and Holick, 2020).

5.3.2 Antioxidants: Vitamins C and E

Vitamin C and vitamin E act as potent antioxidants, shielding cells effectively from oxidative stress spawned by reactive oxygen species. Oxidative stress heavily fuels chronic inflammation, and antioxidants scavenge ROS, thereby remarkably dampening various inflammatory pathways very effectively in bodily tissues. Vitamin C markedly suppresses NF-κB expression, decreasing CRP levels significantly, and lowers production of pro-inflammatory cytokines. Meanwhile, vitamin E has similar effects, particularly in alpha-tocopherol form, inhibiting lipid peroxidation and NF-κB activation very effectively. The alpha-tocopherol form of vitamin E exerts fairly significant analogous effects by inhibiting lipid peroxidation and NF-κB activation very substantially (Traber and Stevens, 2011).

5.3.3 Magnesium: Modulator of Inflammatory Pathways

Magnesium plays a crucial role in numerous bodily functions, manifesting very much throughout bodily tissue in over 300 rather complex enzymatic reactions. Magnesium deficiency has been loosely tied quite tenuously to increased inflammation and onset of maladies like cardiovascular disease, type 2 diabetes, and metabolic syndrome. Magnesium significantly inhibits activation of NLRP3 inflammasome, quite crucially regulating various inflammatory responses and reduces production of TNF-α, IL-6 and CRP. Production of TNF-α and IL-6 alongside CRP drops very substantially (Al Alawi et al, 2018).

5.4. Bioactive Compounds with Anti-Inflammatory Effects

Various bioactive compounds found in plant-based foods possess remarkably strong anti-inflammatory properties alongside macronutrients and some very obscure micronutrients. Stuff like that gets listed here.

5.4.1 Polyphenols: Natural Anti-Inflammatory Agents

Polyphenols abound remarkably in fruits and tea, alongside vegetables and red wine, exhibiting quite extensive antioxidant and anti-inflammatory effects. Key polyphenolic compounds such as flavonoids and phenolic acids modulate inflammatory pathways deeply by inhibiting the activation of NF-κB signalling pathways vigorously. Pro-inflammatory cytokines like IL-6 and TNF-α are produced less. Promoting the resolution of inflammation by stimulating the production of anti-inflammatory molecules like resolvins (Singh et al, 2020).

5.4.2 Curcumin: A Powerful Anti-Inflammatory Compound

Curcumin has been extensively studied for its potent ability to suppress inflammation deeply within bodily tissues owing largely to its presence in turmeric roots. Curcumin exerts effects by inhibiting the NF-κB pathway and downregulating various pro-inflammatory cytokines quite effectively. It reduces the activity of COX-2 and other enzymes involved deeply in inflammation. COX-2 and LOX enzyme activity implicated in inflammatory responses gets diminished rapidly, significantly below normal levels over time (Kunnumakkara et al, 2023).

Curcumin reduces inflammation effectively in diseases like arthritis, colitis, and metabolic syndrome, particularly in various bodily systems. Eating specific nutrient-dense foods frequently may offer considerable promise for the prevention of ailments driven significantly by chronic underlying inflammation. Omega-3 fatty acids and bioactive compounds consumed in large quantities can modulate inflammatory pathways and lower the risk of chronic diseases developing slowly. Cutting down on processed food sugars and saturated fats very effectively mitigates chronic inflammation these days for most people (Kunnumakkara et al, 2023).

6. The Role of Inflammatory Cytokines in Diet-Related Cancer Risk

Cancer manifests as a complex disease largely shaped by heredity, surroundings and dietary habits, being a major modifiable risk factor. Mounting evidence rapidly underscores a pivotal role of chronic inflammation in fuelling the progression of cancer development haphazardly within bodily systems. Diet directly influences inflammatory pathways, thereby modulating levels of certain signalling proteins crucial for immune responses and cell communication effectively. Tumour necrosis factor-alpha and various interleukins play crucial roles in inflammatory responses and greatly contribute to tumourigenesis upon heavy dysregulation (Anand et al, 2008). Cancer risk relates intricately in a complex web of factors to diet and inflammatory cytokines very deeply. Pro-inflammatory diets ramp up inflammatory cytokines, thereby heightening cancer risk, while anti-inflammatory diets significantly mitigate such susceptibility very effectively. Inflammatory cytokines heavily modulate tumour progression via sundry molecular machinations, and very effective dietary interventions can be devised for cancer management, thereby.

6.1. Inflammatory Cytokines and Cancer

Inflammation functions rather precariously as a double-edged sword in cancer biology. Acute inflammation acts as a bodily defence mechanism against infection, but chronic inflammation silently fosters an environment conducive to carcinogenesis over time. Prolonged activation of immune responses can rapidly lead to genomic instability and fuel tumour progression silently over considerable time periods. Key inflammatory cytokines produced during chronic inflammation play pivotal roles somewhat quietly beneath myriad other ostensibly more prominent pathological processes.

6.1.1 Tumour Necrosis Factor-Alpha (TNF-α)

TNF-α plays a crucial role in cancer development stages and remains vastly studied as a pro-inflammatory cytokine in research nowadays. TNF-α gets produced irregularly by macrophages and T-cells, sometimes alongside adipocytes, playing a crucial role in various immune response regulations. TNF-α fosters tumour cell survival deeply inside tumour masses by activating the NF-κB pathway, which induces expression of various survival-related genes. Tumour cells often stubbornly activate this pathway enhanceed by TNF-alpha signaling which enhances resistance to chemotherapy and evades apoptosis. Angiogenesis occurs as TNF-alpha induces the expression of vascular endothelial growth factor, a crucial factor in forming new blood vessels. TNF-α induces vascular endothelial growth factor expression, thereby heavily contributing to the rapid formation of new blood vessels (Wang and Lin, 2008). T-regulatory cells and myeloid-derived suppressor cells get recruited by TNF-α, severely limiting the immune system's ability to destroy tumour cells. Tumour growth gets enhanced very significantly by a steady supply of nutrients and oxygen reaching it with remarkable consistency and speed. TNF-α fosters recruitment of immune-suppressive cells such as Tregs and MDSCs, severely hampering the ability of the immune system to destroy tumour cells (Wang and Lin, 2008).

6.1.2 Interleukins (IL-1, IL-6, IL-8)

Cytokines from the interleukin family, particularly IL-1, IL-6, and IL-8, are linked closely with inflammation and cancer very frequently these days. Multifarious stimuli induce production of cytokines by diverse immune and non-immune cells, including dietary factors, environmental toxins and sundry infections, slowly. IL-6 plays a crucial role in tumour progression found in breast, prostate, and colon cancer, amongst various others. IL-6 has been heavily implicated rather frequently nowadays in tumour progression across various cancers, including breast, prostate and colon cancer. IL-6 vigorously activates several signalling pathways, including JAK/STAT3, promoting tumour cell survival and proliferation and resisting apoptosis (Zhao et al, 2021).

NF-κB and MAPK signalling pathways get activated by IL-1, thereby substantially increasing the expression of pro-inflammatory cytokines and growth factors, facilitating cancer cell migration. The JAK/STAT3 pathway gets triggered by IL-6 encourage tumour cells to survive and proliferate. Pro-inflammatory cytokines are produced in abundance due to activation of NF-κB and MAPK pathways by IL-1. Tumour cells survive and migrate more due to several cascades triggered by IL-6 and IL-1 in the body. IL-8 is an important mediator of tumour angiogenesis and metastasis, as it promotes endothelial cell migration and blood vessel formation, enabling tumours to spread to distant organs. Tumour angiogenesis and metastasis rely heavily on IL-8, which promotes endothelial cell migration and blood vessel formation, enabling distant spread (Zhao et al, 2021).

6.1.3 Interferons (IFNs)

IFN-γ plays enigmatic multifaceted roles under certain conditions in various cancers with obvious complexity, rather quietly. Persistent cellular activation within tumour surroundings fosters immune dysregulation and enables surreptitious tumour advancement gradually over an extended period. IFN-γ vigorously boosts recruitment of inflammatory immune cells, thereby inducing production of pro-inflammatory cytokines and reactive oxygen species rather than promoting tumour growth. Diets heavy in pro-inflammatory foods markedly elevate IFN-γ levels while omega-3 fatty acid-rich diets effectively modulate expression somewhat (Jorgovanovic et al, 2020).

6.2. Diet-Related Modulation of Inflammatory Cytokines in Cancer

Dietary factors markedly sway cytokine profiles by altering pro-inflammatory mediators and somewhat eccentrically modulating the functionality of immune cells. Macronutrients such as proteins and carbohydrates, alongside micronutrients like vitamins, modulate inflammatory response, thereby significantly impacting the risk of various cancers.

6.2.1 The Role of Macronutrients in Modulating Inflammation

Dietary Fats: The consumption of saturated fats (found in red meats, processed foods, and certain oils) has been associated with increased levels of TNF-α, IL-6, and IL-1, which can foster an inflammatory environment conducive to cancer. Consumption of saturated fats found in red meats and processed foods has been linked with heightened TNF-α and IL-6 levels, fostering cancer. Diets rich in refined carbohydrates, such as sugar-sweetened beverages and pastries, trigger heightened secretion of IL-6 and CRP, fostering chronic inflammation. Consumption of saturated fats prevalent in red meats and processed foods correlates with elevated TNF-α and IL-6 levels, fueling inflammation (Watson et al, 2025).

6.2.2 Micronutrients and Bioactive Compounds

Vitamins and Minerals: Vitamin D is known to have immunomodulatory effects, and adequate levels can reduce TNF-α and IL-6 production, which in turn may reduce cancer risk. Vitamin D exhibits immunomodulatory effects, and adequate levels can decrease TNF-α production and lower IL-6, somewhat reducing cancer risk. Vitamin D exerts profoundly immunomodulatory effects, and sufficient levels of it significantly curb production of TNF-α and IL-6, thereby mitigating the risk of cancer. Magnesium markedly inhibits activation of pro-inflammatory pathways like NF-κB under diverse experimental settings. Polyphenolic compounds including flavonoids and resveratrol, found in fruits and tea, exhibit potent anti-inflammatory properties (Fenercioglu AK, 2024).

6.3. Strategies for Dietary Intervention to Modulate Inflammatory Cytokines in Cancer Prevention

Increasing knowledge nowadays of intricate links between dietary habits and cancer risk, inflammation opens the door somewhat effectively to novel preventive interventions. Modulating inflammatory cytokines effectively with diet can mitigate cancer risk or supplement traditional therapies by leveraging foods rich in omega-3 fatty acids. Foods high in fibre polyphenols, and antioxidants downregulate pro-inflammatory cytokines, thereby lowering cancer risk quite substantially with anti-inflammatory diets. Diets rich in omega-3 fatty acids heavily emphasize foods mitigating chronic inflammation, thereby downregulating pro-inflammatory cytokines somewhat effectively, and cancer risk is lowered very significantly. Reducing intake of processed foods and red meats elevates the chances of curbing chronic inflammation and mitigating cancer risk rather effectively. Supplementation: Nutritional supplements, such as omega-3 fatty acids, vitamin D, and curcumin, may also offer therapeutic benefits in modulating inflammatory pathways and complementing conventional cancer treatments (Han et al, 2023).

Nutritional supplements like omega-3 fatty acids, vitamin D, and curcumin may offer therapeutic benefits in modulating inflammatory pathways and encourage cancer treatments. Fruits, vegetables, nuts, seeds olive oil and fish are abundant in Mediterranean diet, which has rather strongly been linked to reduced inflammation. Cutting back on processed food, red meat, and refined sugars that boost pro-inflammatory cytokines can effectively curb chronic inflammation and mitigate cancer risk. Omega-3 fatty acids, vitamin D, and curcumin may therapeutically modulate inflammatory pathways alongside standard cancer treatments, offering various potential benefits (Han et al, 2023).

7. Exploring Anti-Inflammatory Diets for Cancer Prevention

Morbidity and mortality worldwide stem largely from cancer, heavily influenced by environmental factors alongside certain underlying genetic predispositions. Diet modulates physiological processes deeply, including inflammation and supplies crucial nutrients necessary for survival, thereby impacting cancer progression significantly. Emerging evidence suggests diet plays a pivotal role in heavily promoting or mitigating inflammatory responses, while chronic inflammation significantly drives carcinogenesis. Anti-inflammatory diets garner considerable attention lately within cancer prevention circles owing largely to the potential for mitigating inflammation, and they lower overall cancer risk subsequently. Specific nutrients modulate inflammatory pathways deeply within bodily tissues, and evidence strongly supports their profoundly protective anticancer effects.

7.1. The Link Between Inflammation and Cancer Development

Inflammation emerges spontaneously as a fervent immune reaction against damage or noxious stimuli flagged by bodily sentinels as perilous. Chronic inflammation can rather alarmingly contribute stealthily to a vast array of diseases, including cancer down the line. Chronic inflammation cultivates an environment that promotes genomic instability and tumour progression with severe immune suppression in affected tissues quite rapidly. It fosters secretion of pro-inflammatory cytokines and other mediators, driving cellular proliferation, survival, angiogenesis and metastasis rather vigorously in various ways. Key inflammatory pathways heavily implicated in various cancer developments include the NF-κB signalling pathway and JAK/STAT pathway alongside the MAPK pathway (Singh et al, 2019).

Pro-inflammatory cytokines TNF-α and IL-6 get upregulated quite vigorously, resulting from chronic pathway activation that promotes inflammation and facilitates tumour growth. Chronic inflammation fosters the accumulation of reactive oxygen species that induce DNA damage, essentially hallmarks of cancerous cellular transformations and nasty genetic mutations. Certain dietary patterns remarkably influence inflammation levels within various bodily tissues under specific physiological conditions, sometimes quite significantly. Diets heavy in junk foods and refined sugars have been strongly linked to increased inflammation, whereas specific eating habits may mitigate such responses naturally (Singh et al, 2019).

7.2. The Role of Anti-Inflammatory Diets in Cancer Prevention

Nutrients crucial for maintaining cellular health abound in diets loaded with anti-inflammatory food supporting immunity fairly effectively. Diets rich in fruits and veggies, along with whole grains, often incorporate lean proteins and healthy fats while minimising intake of processed foods. Diets geared towards mitigating inflammation often encompass a diverse array of food groups and nutrients remarkably well these days.

7.2.1 Omega-3 Fatty Acids

Extensively studied anti-inflammatory nutrients, omega-3 fatty acids are found primarily in fatty fish like salmon, mackerel and also in flaxseeds, chia seeds, and walnuts. Eicosapentaenoic acid and docosahexaenoic acid, found in omega 3 fatty acids, exert profoundly anti inflammatory effects by substantially inhibiting pro-inflammatory cytokine production. Eicosapentaenoic acid and docosahexaenoic acid substantially dampen cytokine expression, such as TNF-α and IL-6, by profoundly suppressing NF-κB pathway activation. Omega-3s boost production of anti-inflammatory resolvins and protectins that actively mitigate oxidative stress and quell inflammation (Mititelu et al, 2025).

Modulating immune responses: Omega-3 fatty acids promote the generation of regulatory T cells (Tregs), which suppress inflammation and prevent the chronic activation of the immune system. Omega-3 fatty acids enhance the generation of regulatory T cells, which suppress inflammation and prevent chronic immune system activation, rather effectively (Mititelu et al, 2025).

7.2.2 Fibre-Rich Foods and Gut Health

Diets rich in fibre comprising copious fruits and whole grains, exert profoundly significant anti-inflammatory effects overall on bodily functions. Gut bacteria metabolise fibre into short-chain fatty acids like butyrate, possessing surprisingly potent anti-inflammatory properties down there. SCFAs quite effectively suppress NF-κB activation by inhibiting pro-inflammatory pathways, thereby reducing production of various cytokines and inflammatory mediators. Meanwhile, a fibre-rich diet fosters a healthy gut microbiome, which plays a critical role in regulating immune responses and inflammation. Reducing inflammatory markers: Diets high in fibre have been associated with lower levels of systemic inflammatory markers like C-reactive protein (CRP) and IL-6. Diets rich in fibre correlate with significantly lower systemic inflammatory markers such as C-reactive protein and interleukin 6 very frequently (Fu et al, 2022).

7.2.3 Antioxidants and Polyphenols

Berries harbour antioxidants and polyphenols, fiercely combating cancer cells naturally, while leafy greens possess anti-inflammatory properties abundantly. Certain compounds very effectively quash reactive oxygen species, thereby mitigating oxidative stress under various physiological conditions and reducing inflammation markedly. Key antioxidants comprise vitamin C and vitamin E, alongside selenium, whereas polyphenolic compounds like curcumin exhibit potent anti-inflammatory effects. Curcumin, found in turmeric, has been extensively studied for suppressing inflammation by inhibiting NF-κB and MAPK signalling pathways vigorously, thus suppressing inflammation (Mileo et al, 2015). Resveratrol, found in grapes, red wine, and peanuts, modulates inflammatory cytokines, interfering with PI3K/Akt and NF-κB pathways, demonstrating anti-inflammatory and anticancer effects. Curcumin remarkably thwarts cancer initiation and progression in various models of colorectal, breast and very rare lung malignancies (Mileo et al, 2015).

7.2.4 Healthy Fats: The Role of Olive Oil and Avocados

Olive oil contains high levels of monounsaturated fats and polyphenols like oleocanthal, which possess decidedly anti-inflammatory and ostensibly anticancer properties naturally. Oleocanthal present in olive oil, has been shown to reduce the production of TNF-α and IL-6, somewhat similar to the effects of ibuprofen. Regular consumption of olive oil has been associated with a reduced risk of cancers, particularly breast and colon cancers. Avocados contain various compounds like vitamin E and carotenoids that act as anti-inflammatory agents alongside polyphenols quite effectively (González-Rodríguez et al, 2023).

7.3. The Mediterranean Diet

Fruits, vegetables, whole grains, legumes, olive oil and fish feature heavily in the Mediterranean diet, curbing the risk of various chronic diseases, including cancer . Omega-3 fatty acids and polyphenols exert remarkably potent anti-inflammatory effects in this diet, alongside monounsaturated fats, quite effectively. The Mediterranean diet supplies antioxidants and bioactive compounds that abundantly protect cells against oxidative damage and tumour initiation very effectively. Research shows people munching on Mediterranean food quite often develop relatively fewer cancers, like prostate cancer, breast cancer and lung tumours, surprisingly often. Gene expression pathways and immune system health are enhanced significantly nowadays by dietary influence very effectively in various cancer protection cases (Xiao et al, 2024). Dietary interventions ostensibly hold tremendous potential for thwarting cancer onset amidst chronic inflammation, modulating various inflammatory pathways effectively. Diets rich in omega-3 fatty acids and antioxidants can somewhat mitigate chronic inflammation and modulate immune function, decreasing cancer risk, oddly afterwards. Nowadays, people drastically limit pro-inflammatory foods and focus on whole foods to proactively reduce their risk of getting cancer. Nutritional oncology research evolves rapidly, making diet crucial in cancer prevention, and it will be increasingly pivotal in the forthcoming years. Precision cancer prevention approaches tailored around an individual's genetic blueprint and inflammatory responses may yield drastically better health outcomes for vulnerable populations (Xiao et al, 2024).

8. Diet-Induced Modulation of Inflammatory Signalling in Tumourigenesis

Inflammation plays a crucial albeit oft-overlooked role in sparking cancer initiation, followed subsequently by wildly erratic progression with fervour afterwards rapidly. Tumour microenvironment fosters genomic instability and rapid tumour growth alongside metastasis due to chronic inflammation manifesting crucially quite often. Various pro-inflammatory cytokines and enzymes drastically alter cellular behaviour in inflammatory signalling pathways, with quite significant effects on cells. Diet significantly alters inflammatory pathways, thereby occasionally mitigating or usually exacerbating cancer risk quite noticeably in various populations over time (Nishida and Andoh, 2025). Dietary components very significantly modulate pro-inflammatory cytokine levels and greatly influence the expression of various inflammatory enzymes and certain transcription factors. Diet heavily influences cancer risk progression by variously suppressing pathways or suddenly promoting them, thereby somewhat altering subsequent treatment response. Dietary components modulate inflammatory signalling intricately during tumourigenesis, offering insights into natural cancer prevention strategies quite effectively meanwhile (Nishida and Andoh, 2025).

8.1. Inflammatory Signalling Pathways and Tumourigenesis

Inflammation in cancer manifests at the molecular level through activation of key signalling pathways like NF-κB and JAK/STAT alongside MAPK and PI3K/Akt. Pathways intricately modulate expression of pro-inflammatory cytokines and immune mediators, fueling tumourigenic processes somewhat irregularly in various contexts.

8.1.1 NF-κB Pathway in Cancer

Nuclear factor-kappa B pathway remains a vastly studied inflammatory signalling mechanism deeply embedded in various cancerous tumours. NF-κB regulates the expression of genes deeply involved in inflammation and cell survival during fairly normal immune responses very frequently. NF-κB activation persists remarkably often in various cancer cells, surprisingly associating with tumour initiation and subsequent progression to metastasis rather frequently. NF-κB activation vigorously fuels tumour growth and angiogenesis by promoting pro-inflammatory cytokines TNF-α and IL-6 alongside growth factors like VEGF. Persistent chronic inflammatory stimuli drive sustained activation of NF-κB rather deeply within the tumour microenvironment (Zinatizadeh et al, 2020). Diet modulates this pathway effectively through various complex mechanisms under different circumstances, virtually every time with significant impact. Omega-3 fatty acids found in fish oil and flaxseeds inhibit the NF-κB pathway, thereby reducing inflammation, quite remarkably slowing the progression of cancers like colon or breast cancer. Diets replete with saturated fats and refined sugars spark NF-κB signaling which fuels inflammation very badly and drives tumour progression (Zinatizadeh et al, 2020).

8.1.2 JAK/STAT Pathway in Cancer

The Janus kinase/signal transducer and activator of transcription pathway plays a crucial albeit somewhat obscure role in inflammation underlying many types of cancer. Cytokines like IL-6 and IL-1 are often elevated in tumour microenvironments and very frequently activate JAK/STAT signalling pathways there. Activation of this pathway leads rather quickly to transcription of genes involved heavily in cell survival and proliferation, and also angiogenesis, which contribute significantly to tumour development. Curcumin and green tea polyphenols, alongside polyunsaturated fatty acids, effectively modulate the JAK/STAT pathway in diverse cellular contexts, remarkably. Curcumin, present in turmeric, very significantly hinders tumour growth in various cancer models by inhibiting the JAK/STAT3 signalling pathway and reducing levels of IL-6. A diet rich in saturated fats can activate JAK/STAT signaling thereby contributing quite inscrutably to the survival and proliferation of cancer cells extremely effectively (Bharadwaj et al, 2020).

8.1.3 MAPK Pathway in Tumourigenesis

Mitogen-activated protein kinase pathway plays a crucial role downstream in regulating inflammatory signaling very crucial in various cancer contexts. Cytokines like IL-6 and growth factors such as EGF activate this pathway, leading quickly downstream to activation of transcription factors regulating cell division. Tumour progression unfolds rapidly under persistent MAPK pathway activation, and intense chemoresistance festers deeply within cancer cells over prolonged periods. Various physiological conditions have pinpointed multiple dietary components as regulators of MAPK pathway activity effectively. Sulforaphane, a bioactive compound, very effectively inhibits MAPK signalling in cancer cells found abundantly in veggies like kale and broccoli. Diets heavy in trans and saturated fats, conversely, spur MAPK activation, thereby enhancing proliferation and invasion of tumour cells greatly (Munshi and Ramesh, 2013).

8.2. Dietary Modulators of Inflammatory Signaling in Tumourigenesis

Dietary interventions modulate key inflammatory pathways involved in cancer through various mechanisms quite effectively, apparently in many cases. Omega-3 fatty acids, alongside various micronutrients, profoundly influence signalling pathways, thereby exerting intensely anti-inflammatory effects deeply within bodily tissues. Naturally, certain dietary factors mitigate chronic inflammation quite significantly over time, thereby inhibiting cancer initiation and progression substantially.

8.2.1 Omega-3 Fatty Acids and Inflammatory Signalling

Omega-3 fatty acids, found mostly in fatty fish and seeds such as flaxseeds, possess very potent anti-inflammatory effects quite remarkably. Polyunsaturated fats very effectively modulate inflammatory signalling pathways by irregularly suppressing activation of NF-κB and JAK/STAT pathways mostly. Omega-3s spur the production of resolvins and protectins, very effectively downregulating inflammation via specialised molecules that actively quell it later on. Omega-3 fatty acids remarkably inhibit colon cancer cell proliferation in various tumour models and enhance apoptosis, shrinking tumour volume significantly. Chemotherapy efficacy improves via modulation of the tumour microenvironment and reduction of inflammatory cytokines heavily contributing to resistance in tumours (Calder PC, 2013).

8.2.2 Polyphenols: Modulators of Inflammatory Pathways

Polyphenolic compounds abundant in fruits and veggies have been studied rather extensively for anti-inflammatory properties found mostly in green tea. Extensively researched polyphenols curcumin, epigallocatechin gallate, and resveratrol modulate inflammatory signalling effectively in various cancers. Curcumin from turmeric inhibits the NF-κB pathway, reducing expression of pro-inflammatory cytokines IL-6 and TNF-α very significantly. Curcumin, a polyphenol derived from turmeric, markedly inhibits the NF-κB pathway, thereby considerably reducing downstream expression of pro-inflammatory cytokines such as IL-6 and TNF-α. EGCG found in green tea profoundly suppresses JAK/STAT and MAPK pathways, preventing tumour cell proliferation and angiogenesis effectively. Research suggests curcumin rapidly halts tumour growth in various malignancies such as colon cancer and highly aggressive forms of breast cancer (Cione et al, 2019).

8.2.3 Fibre and Short-Chain Fatty Acids

Dietary fibre present in whole grains, legumes, and veggies modulates inflammatory pathways heavily in various cancers fairly effectively nowadays. Gut microbiota ferments fibre producing short-chain fatty acids like butyrate that exert profoundly powerful anti-inflammatory effects deep within bodily tissues. SCFAs vigorously suppress activation of NF-κB and histone deacetylases, thereby fostering expression of genes with decidedly anti-inflammatory properties. High-fibre diets somewhat effectively mitigate the incidence of colorectal cancer by modulating inflammation in the gut and altering myriad immune responses effectively. Diets rich in fibre correlate with diminished levels of IL-6 and CRP markers of systemic inflammation, heavily linked to heightened risk of cancer (Fu et al, 2022).

8.2.4 Micronutrients and Anti-Inflammatory Effects

Vitamins and minerals deeply modulate various inflammatory pathways within bodily tissues and influence cellular processes crucially. Vitamin D remarkably inhibits NF-κB activation in various cellular contexts, substantially reducing pro-inflammatory cytokines and altering immune response dynamics. Vitamin D intake possibly mitigates the risk of colon and breast cancers by heavily modulating certain immune responses while reducing inflammation substantially. Selenium, a vital trace mineral, surprisingly enough inhibits the expression of pro-inflammatory cytokines and reduces oxidative stress, thereby offering protection against DNA damage. Vitamin E has demonstrated potent anti-inflammatory effects remarkably well by suppressing the production of pro-inflammatory cytokines like IL-6 and reactive oxygen species (Mitra et al, 2022).

Dietary factors significantly modulate inflammatory signalling pathways involved in tumourigenesis, and chronic inflammation vigorously drives cancer initiation with considerable force. People can very effectively slash cancer risk daily by wolfing down food rich in omega-3s and sundry obscure micronutrients. Nutritional approaches dense with whole grains and fruits effectively regulate various inflammatory pathways, offering potentially significant cancer prevention benefits. Deciphering intricate relationships between diet and malignant cell growth mechanisms yields valuable cancer prevention insights very evidently nowadays (Mitra et al, 2022).

9. Conclusion

Carcinogenesis is driven fundamentally by chronic inflammation, influencing nearly every tumour development stage, from initiation rapidly or metastatic promotion. Persistent oxidative stress and DNA damage alongside altered immune responses characterise a pro-tumourigenic environment fostered by chronic low-grade inflammation rather quietly. Diet emerges as a mighty modifiable factor capable of severely exacerbating or mercifully attenuating inflammatory pathways fairly strongly linked to heightened cancer risk. Molecular mediators such as NF-κB and prostaglandins are modulated rather quietly by various pro-inflammatory components and anti-inflammatory elements, fueling cancer and inflammation. Diets heavy in saturated fats and refined sugars alongside plenty of ultra-processed foods have been linked rather strongly to increased cancer risk.

Diets rich in omega-3 fatty acids and fibre exhibit potent anti-inflammatory effects within bodily responses often. Evidence strongly underscores that nutritional interventions profoundly influence systemic inflammation, thereby potentially altering carcinogenesis trajectory significantly over a considerable period. Copious consumption of fruits, vegetables, whole grains, legumes, olive oil and fish in the Mediterranean diet correlates significantly with greatly diminished inflammatory biomarkers. Bioactive compounds like curcumin and resveratrol exhibit remarkably promising anticancer effects in various experimental studies alongside some clinical trials. Incorporating anti-inflammatory dietary regimens into cancer prevention tactics holds significant promise well beyond current standard treatment modalities, quite naturally (Zivkovic et al, 2011).

Sizeable public health efforts are urgently needed to educate populations thoroughly about dietary choices severely impacting long-term inflammatory status and escalating cancer risk nationwide. Advancements in precision nutrition and biomarker-driven approaches offer potential for tailoring anti-inflammatory diets effectively for individual genetic profiles nowadays. Cancer prevention gets rather strategic with dietary changes targeting chronic inflammation and potentially amplifying overall care very effectively. Nutritional practices rooted deeply in inflammatory biology enhance overall health and reduce cancer risk remarkably, with intrinsic regulatory systems harnessed effectively.

References

Al Alawi AM, Majoni SW, Falhammar H. Magnesium and Human Health: Perspectives and Research Directions. Int J Endocrinol. 2018 Apr 16;2018:9041694. Doi: 10.1155/2018/9041694. PMID: 29849626; PMCID: PMC5926493.

Anand P, Kunnumakkara AB, Sundaram C, Harikumar KB, Tharakan ST, Lai OS, Sung B, Aggarwal BB. Cancer is a preventable disease that requires major lifestyle changes. Pharm Res. 2008 Sep;25(9):2097-116. doi: 10.1007/s11095-008-9661-9. Epub 2008 Jul 15. Erratum in: Pharm Res. 2008 Sep;25(9):2200. Kunnumakara, Ajaikumar B [corrected to Kunnumakkara, Ajaikumar B]. PMID: 18626751; PMCID: PMC2515569.

Bharadwaj U, Kasembeli MM, Robinson P, Tweardy DJ. Targeting Janus Kinases and Signal Transducer and Activator of Transcription 3 to Treat Inflammation, Fibrosis, and Cancer: Rationale, Progress, and Caution. Pharmacol Rev. 2020 Apr;72(2):486-526. doi: 10.1124/pr.119.018440. Erratum in: Pharmacol Rev. 2020 Jul;72(3):605. doi: 10.1124/pr.119.018440err. PMID: 32198236; PMCID: PMC7300325.

Calder PC. Omega-3 polyunsaturated fatty acids and inflammatory processes: nutrition or pharmacology? Br J Clin Pharmacol. 2013 Mar;75(3):645-62. doi: 10.1111/j.1365-2125.2012.04374.x. PMID: 22765297; PMCID: PMC3575932.

Charoenngam N, Holick MF. Immunologic Effects of Vitamin D on Human Health and Disease. Nutrients. 2020 Jul 15;12(7):2097. doi: 10.3390/nu12072097. PMID: 32679784; PMCID: PMC7400911.

Cione E, La Torre C, Cannataro R, Caroleo MC, Plastina P, Gallelli L. Quercetin, Epigallocatechin Gallate, Curcumin, and Resveratrol: From Dietary Sources to Human MicroRNA Modulation. Molecules. 2019 Dec 23;25(1):63. doi: 10.3390/molecules25010063. PMID: 31878082; PMCID: PMC6983040.

Desai SJ, Prickril B, Rasooly A. Mechanisms of Phytonutrient Modulation of Cyclooxygenase-2 (COX-2) and Inflammation Related to Cancer. Nutr Cancer. 2018 Apr;70(3):350-375. doi: 10.1080/01635581.2018.1446091. Epub 2018 Mar 26. PMID: 29578814; PMCID: PMC6309701.

Divella R, De Luca R, Abbate I, Naglieri E, Daniele A. Obesity and cancer: the role of adipose tissue and adipocytokines-induced chronic inflammation. J Cancer. 2016 Nov 26;7(15):2346-2359. doi: 10.7150/jca.16884. PMID: 27994674; PMCID: PMC5166547.

Fenercioglu AK. The Anti-Inflammatory Roles of Vitamin D for Improving Human Health. Curr Issues Mol Biol. 2024 Nov 26;46(12):13514-13525. doi: 10.3390/cimb46120807. PMID: 39727935; PMCID: PMC11674702.

Fu J, Zheng Y, Gao Y, Xu W. Dietary Fibre Intake and Gut Microbiota in Human Health. Microorganisms. 2022 Dec 18;10(12):2507. doi: 10.3390/microorganisms10122507. PMID: 36557760; PMCID: PMC9787832.

Geindreau M, Bruchard M, Vegran F. Role of Cytokines and Chemokines in Angiogenesis in a Tumour Context. Cancers (Basel). 2022 May 16;14(10):2446. doi: 10.3390/cancers14102446. PMID: 35626056; PMCID: PMC9139472.

Gonzalez H, Hagerling C, Werb Z. Roles of the immune system in cancer: from tumour initiation to metastatic progression. Genes Dev. 2018 Oct 1;32(19-20):1267-1284. doi: 10.1101/gad.314617.118. PMID: 30275043; PMCID: PMC6169832.

González-Rodríguez M, Ait Edjoudi D, Cordero-Barreal A, Farrag M, Varela-García M, Torrijos-Pulpón C, Ruiz-Fernández C, Capuozzo M, Ottaiano A, Lago F, Pino J, Farrag Y, Gualillo O. Oleocanthal, an Antioxidant Phenolic Compound in Extra Virgin Olive Oil (EVOO): A Comprehensive Systematic Review of Its Potential in Inflammation and Cancer. Antioxidants (Basel). 2023 Dec 14;12(12):2112. doi: 10.3390/antiox12122112. PMID: 38136231; PMCID: PMC10741130.

Greten FR, Grivennikov SI. Inflammation and Cancer: Triggers, Mechanisms, and Consequences. Immunity. 2019 Jul 16;51(1):27-41. Doi: 10.1016/j.immuni.2019.06.025. PMID: 31315034; PMCID: PMC6831096.

Han E, Lee E, Sukhu B, García J, López Castillo H. The relationship between dietary inflammatory potential and cancer outcomes among cancer survivors: A systematic review and meta-analysis of cohort studies. Transl Oncol. 2023 Dec;38:101798. doi: 10.1016/j.tranon.2023.101798. Epub 2023 Oct 10. PMID: 37826918; PMCID: PMC10582578.

Huang B, Lang X, Li X. The role of IL-6/JAK2/STAT3 signalling pathway in cancers. Front Oncol. 2022 Dec 16;12:1023177. Doi: 10.3389/fonc.2022.1023177. PMID: 36591515; PMCID: PMC9800921.

Jorgovanovic D, Song M, Wang L, Zhang Y. Roles of IFN-γ in tumour progression and regression: a review. Biomark Res. 2020 Sep 29;8:49. Doi: 10.1186/s40364-020-00228-x. PMID: 33005420; PMCID: PMC7526126.

Kunnumakkara AB, Hegde M, Parama D, Girisa S, Kumar A, Daimary UD, Garodia P, Yenisetti SC, Oommen OV, Aggarwal BB. Role of Turmeric and Curcumin in Prevention and Treatment of Chronic Diseases: Lessons Learned from Clinical Trials. ACS Pharmacol Transl Sci. 2023 Mar 6;6(4):447-518. doi: 10.1021/acsptsci.2c00012. PMID: 37082752; PMCID: PMC10111629.

Liu T, Zhang L, Joo D, Sun SC. NF-κB signalling in inflammation. Signal Transduct Target Ther. 2017;2:17023–. doi: 10.1038/sigtrans.2017.23. Epub 2017 Jul 14. PMID: 29158945; PMCID: PMC5661633.

Mariamenatu AH, Abdu EM. Overconsumption of Omega-6 Polyunsaturated Fatty Acids (PUFAs) versus Deficiency of Omega-3 PUFAs in Modern-Day Diets: The Disturbing Factor for Their "Balanced Antagonistic Metabolic Functions" in the Human Body. J Lipids. 2021 Mar 17;2021:8848161. Doi: 10.1155/2021/8848161. PMID: 33815845; PMCID: PMC7990530.

Mileo AM, Miccadei S. Polyphenols as Modulators of Oxidative Stress in Cancer Disease: New Therapeutic Strategies. Oxid Med Cell Longev. 2016;2016:6475624. doi: 10.1155/2016/6475624. Epub 2015 Nov 16. PMID: 26649142; PMCID: PMC4663347.

Mititelu, M., Lupuliasa, D., Neacșu, S. M., Olteanu, G., Busnatu, Ș. S., Mihai, A., Popovici, V., Măru, N., Boroghină, S. C., Mihai, S., Ioniță-Mîndrican, C.-B., & Scafa-Udriște, A. (2025). Polyunsaturated Fatty Acids and Human Health: A Key to Modern Nutritional Balance in Association with Polyphenolic Compounds from Food Sources. Foods, 14(1), 46. https://doi.org/10.3390/foods14010046

Mitra S, Paul S, Roy S, Sutradhar H, Bin Emran T, Nainu F, Khandaker MU, Almalki M, Wilairatana P, Mubarak MS. Exploring the Immune-Boosting Functions of Vitamins and Minerals as Nutritional Food Bioactive Compounds: A Comprehensive Review. Molecules. 2022 Jan 16;27(2):555. doi: 10.3390/molecules27020555. PMID: 35056870; PMCID: PMC8779769.

Munshi A, Ramesh R. Mitogen-activated protein kinases and their role in radiation response. Genes Cancer. 2013 Sep;4(9-10):401-8. doi: 10.1177/1947601913485414. PMID: 24349638; PMCID: PMC3863336.

Munteanu C, Schwartz B. Interactions between Dietary Antioxidants, Dietary Fibre and the Gut Microbiome: Their Putative Role in Inflammation and Cancer. Int J Mol Sci. 2024 Jul 28;25(15):8250. doi: 10.3390/ijms25158250. PMID: 39125822; PMCID: PMC11311432.

Ney LM, Wipplinger M, Grossmann M, Engert N, Wegner VD, Mosig AS. Short-chain fatty acids: key regulators of the local and systemic immune response in inflammatory diseases and infections. Open Biol. 2023 Mar;13(3):230014. doi: 10.1098/rsob.230014. Epub 2023 Mar 29. PMID: 36977462; PMCID: PMC10049789.

Nishida A, Andoh A. The Role of Inflammation in Cancer: Mechanisms of Tumour Initiation, Progression, and Metastasis. Cells. 2025 Mar 25;14(7):488. doi: 10.3390/cells14070488. PMID: 40214442; PMCID: PMC11987742.

Pandey KB, Rizvi SI. Plant polyphenols as dietary antioxidants in human health and disease. Oxid Med Cell Longev. 2009 Nov-Dec;2(5):270-8. doi: 10.4161/oxim.2.5.9498. PMID: 20716914; PMCID: PMC2835915.

Pang LY, Hurst EA, Argyle DJ. Cyclooxygenase-2: A Role in Cancer Stem Cell Survival and Repopulation of Cancer Cells during Therapy. Stem Cells Int. 2016;2016:2048731. doi: 10.1155/2016/2048731. Epub 2016 Nov 1. PMID: 27882058; PMCID: PMC5108861.

Rakoff-Nahoum S. Why cancer and inflammation? Yale J Biol Med. 2006 Dec;79(3-4):123-30. PMID: 17940622; PMCID: PMC1994795.

Rodriguez-Leyva D, Dupasquier CM, McCullough R, Pierce GN. The cardiovascular effects of flaxseed and its omega-3 fatty acid, alpha-linolenic acid. Can J Cardiol. 2010 Nov;26(9):489-96. doi: 10.1016/s0828-282x(10)70455-4. PMID: 21076723; PMCID: PMC2989356.

Singh A, Yau YF, Leung KS, El-Nezami H, Lee JC. Interaction of Polyphenols as Antioxidant and Anti-Inflammatory Compounds in the Brain-Liver-Gut Axis. Antioxidants (Basel). 2020 Jul 26;9(8):669. Doi: 10.3390/antiox9080669. PMID: 32722619; PMCID: PMC7465954.

Singh N, Baby D, Rajguru JP, Patil PB, Thakkannavar SS, Pujari VB. Inflammation and cancer. Ann Afr Med. 2019 Jul-Sep;18(3):121-126. doi: 10.4103/aam.aam_56_18. PMID: 31417011; PMCID: PMC6704802.

Soldati L, Di Renzo L, Jirillo E, Ascierto PA, Marincola FM, De Lorenzo A. The influence of diet on anti-cancer immune responsiveness. J Transl Med. 2018 Mar 20;16(1):75. doi: 10.1186/s12967-018-1448-0. PMID: 29558948; PMCID: PMC5859494.

Stone WL, Basit H, Zubair M, et al. Pathology, Inflammation. [Updated 2024 Aug 11]. In: StatPearls [Internet]. Treasure

Island (FL): StatPearls Publishing; 2025 Jan-. Available from: https://www.ncbi.nlm.nih.gov/books/NBK534820/

Szulińska M, Stępień M, Kręgielska-Narożna M, Suliburska J, Skrypnik D, Bąk-Sosnowska M, Kujawska-Łuczak M, Grzymisławska M, Bogdański P. Effects of green tea supplementation on inflammation markers, antioxidant status and blood pressure in NaCl-induced hypertensive rat model. Food Nutr Res. 2017 Mar 3;61(1):1295525. doi: 10.1080/16546628.2017.1295525. PMID: 28326006; PMCID: PMC5345575.

Traber MG, Stevens JF. Vitamins C and E: beneficial effects from a mechanistic perspective. Free Radic Biol Med. 2011 Sep 1;51(5):1000-13. doi: 10.1016/j.freeradbiomed.2011.05.017. Epub 2011 May 25. PMID: 21664268; PMCID: PMC3156342.

Wang M, Chen S, He X, Yuan Y, Wei X. Targeting inflammation as cancer therapy. J Hematol Oncol. 2024 Mar 22;17(1):13. doi: 10.1186/s13045-024-01528-7. PMID: 38520006; PMCID: PMC10960486.

Wang X, Lin Y. Tumour necrosis factor and cancer, buddies or foes? Acta Pharmacol Sin. 2008 Nov;29(11):1275-88. doi: 10.1111/j.1745-7254.2008.00889.x. PMID: 18954521; PMCID: PMC2631033.

Watson AE, Yusuf N. The Influence of Dietary Factors on Melanoma Development and Progression: A Comprehensive Review. Nutrients. 2025 May 31;17(11):1891. doi: 10.3390/nu17111891. PMID: 40507159; PMCID: PMC12157913.

Xiao Y, Xiao X, Zhang X, Yi D, Li T, Hao Q, Zhang F, Li X, Wang N. Mediterranean diet in the targeted prevention and personalised treatment of chronic diseases: evidence, potential mechanisms, and prospects. EPMA J. 2024 Apr 16;15(2):207-220. doi: 10.1007/s13167-024-00360-w. PMID: 38841625; PMCID: PMC11147989.

Xie Y, Wang X, Wang W, Pu N, Liu L. Epithelial-mesenchymal transition orchestrates tumour microenvironment: current perceptions and challenges. J Transl Med. 2025 Apr 2;23(1):386. doi: 10.1186/s12967-025-06422-5. PMID: 40176117; PMCID: PMC11963649.

Yang Q, Guo N, Zhou Y, Chen J, Wei Q, Han M. The role of tumour-associated macrophages (TAMs) in tumour progression and relevant advances in targeted therapy. Acta Pharm Sin B. 2020 Nov;10(11):2156-2170. doi: 10.1016/j.apsb.2020.04.004. Epub 2020 Apr 19. PMID: 33304783; PMCID: PMC7714989.

Yu H, Pardoll D, Jove R. STATs in cancer inflammation and immunity: a leading role for STAT3. Nat Rev Cancer. 2009 Nov;9(11):798-809. doi: 10.1038/nrc2734. PMID: 19851315; PMCID: PMC4856025.

Yu W, Tu Y, Long Z, Liu J, Kong D, Peng J, Wu H, Zheng G, Zhao J, Chen Y, Liu R, Li W, Hai C. Reactive Oxygen Species Bridge the Gap between Chronic Inflammation and Tumour Development. Oxid Med Cell Longev. 2022 Jun 28;2022:2606928. Doi: 10.1155/2022/2606928. PMID: 35799889; PMCID: PMC9256443.

Yu X, Pu H, Voss M. Overview of anti-inflammatory diets and their promising effects on non-communicable diseases. Br J Nutr. 2024 Oct 14;132(7):898-918. doi: 10.1017/S0007114524001405. Epub 2024 Oct 16. PMID: 39411832; PMCID: PMC11576095.

Zhang T, Ma C, Zhang Z, Zhang H, Hu H. NF-κB signalling in inflammation and cancer. MedComm (2020). 2021 Dec 16;2(4):618-653. doi: 10.1002/mco2.104. PMID: 34977871; PMCID: PMC8706767.

Zhao H, Wu L, Yan G, Chen Y, Zhou M, Wu Y, Li Y. Inflammation and tumour progression: signalling pathways and targeted intervention. Signal Transduct Target Ther. 2021 Jul 12;6(1):263. Doi: 10.1038/s41392-021-00658-5. PMID: 34248142; PMCID: PMC8273155.

Zinatizadeh MR, Schock B, Chalbatani GM, Zarandi PK, Jalali SA, Miri SR. The Nuclear Factor Kappa B (NF-kB) signalling in cancer development and immune diseases. Genes Dis. 2020 Jul 18;8(3):287-297. doi: 10.1016/j.gendis.2020.06.005. PMID: 33997176; PMCID: PMC8093649.

Zivkovic AM, Telis N, German JB, Hammock BD. Dietary omega-3 fatty acids aid in the modulation of inflammation and metabolic health. Calif Agric (Berkeley). 2011 Jul;65(3):106-111. doi: 10.3733/ca.v065n03p106. PMID: 24860193; PMCID: PMC4030645.

Chapter 5

Nutritional Epigenetics: Dietary Influences on Gene Expression and Genome Stability

Sarfraj Ahmad Siddiqui[1], Sheetanshu Gupta[2*], Ng. Joykumar Singh[3], and Praneeth Juvvi[4]

[1]Department of Biochemistry, King George's Medical University, U.P., India
[2]Department of Food Safety and Quality Assurance, College of Food Technology, Central Agricultural University (CAU), Imphal, Manipur, India
[3]Department of Food Process Engineering, College of Food Technology, Central Agricultural University (CAU), Imphal, Manipur, India
[4]Department of Food Processing Technology, College of Food Technology-Central Agricultural University, Imphal, Manipur, India

Abstract

Nutritional epigenetics drastically influences gene expression through epigenetic modifications like DNA methylation and histone alterations, amidst non-coding RNA regulatory machinations, getting entangled deeply. Dietary components profoundly modulate the epigenome within cells and influence cellular functions in a rather strikingly nuanced manner. Molecular mechanisms underlying nutrient interactions with epigenetic machinery shed light on the regulation of bodily processes like inflammation and metabolism, rather rapidly. Diet impacts genome stability profoundly, with folate and B vitamins orchestrating crucial DNA repair mechanisms normally under fairly typical conditions. Chronic nutrient deficiencies potentially precipitate aberrant epigenetic changes, thereby causing instability in the genomic framework and slowly promoting the progression of disease. Novel epigenetic reprogramming research suggests specific dietary adjustments could very effectively reverse gnarly epigenetic flubs and normalise gene expression radically. Next-generation sequencing heavily fuels the growing importance of personalised nutrition in health optimization alongside experimental studies for disease prevention, nowadays quite effectively. Dietary interventions' potential influence on the epigenome is highlighted here and sheds new light on nutrition's role in stabilising the human genome somewhat effectively.

Keywords: Epigenetics, Gene Expression, Nutrient Sensing, DNA Methylation, Histone Modification, Genome Stability

DOI: 10.1201/9781042010387-5

1. Introduction

Nutritional epigenetics has garnered considerable attention lately as scientists increasingly decipher how consumed foods subtly affect gene expression and overall human well-being. Epigenetics refers to the study of changes in gene activity not involving alterations to the underlying DNA sequence but rather chemical modifications genome-wide. DNA methylation and histone modification, alongside non-coding RNA regulation, can flip genes on or off, influencing various cellular functions heavily. Diet modulating epigenetic processes opens new avenues for understanding molecular mechanisms underlying health and multifaceted disease aetiology quite profoundly. This connection between nutrition and gene expression affords myriad opportunities to explore how dietary interventions can possibly prevent or reverse specific chronic maladies, including cancer.

Diet stands out as a profoundly impactful environmental factor influencing epigenetic modifications, alongside genetic predisposition, remarkably. Nutrients present in consumed food, including vitamins, minerals, fatty acids and bioactive compounds, directly influence molecular machinery governing epigenetic processes, altering gene expression very significantly. Certain nutrients serve as methyl donors, directly influencing DNA methylation, while others may tweak histone modification or production of small non-coding RNAs. Research has shown the epigenome to be remarkably responsive to dietary factors, particularly during critical periods of development, ageing, or disease onset lately. Dietary habits of an individual can have lasting consequences on gene expression and genome stability, potentially shaping the risk of various nasty diseases.

Early-life nutrition profoundly influences epigenetic marks, thereby affecting long-term health outcomes through nutritional programming, a concept within nutritional epigenetics. Prenatal and early postnatal nutrition starkly illustrate the maternal diet's profound influence on epigenetic regulation of metabolic and immune functions in offspring. A diet lacking essential nutrients like folate during pregnancy can lead to wonky DNA methylation patterns, increasing the risk of developmental disorders and cancer later. Exposure to pollutants during formative stages can have lasting epigenetic effects on individuals, contributing significantly to chronic disease onset later. Nutritional epigenetics holds considerable relevance amidst cancer research endeavours (Vickers MH, 2014).

Cancer manifests as a convoluted multi-stage malady driven by genetic mutations, alongside epigenetic alterations. Epigenetic changes are reversible and serve potentially as targets for various therapeutic interventions, unlike genetic mutations that result in permanent DNA sequence alterations. Evidence suggests dietary components influence cancer risk rather heavily by modulating various epigenetic mechanisms regulating tumour suppressor genes and oncogenes in cells. Nutrients such as folate and vitamin B12 play a key role in DNA methylation, influencing the expression of genes involved heavily in tumour progression. Compounds like curcumin and resveratrol, found in turmeric and grapes, respectively, have been shown often modify histones or alter DNA methylation (Coyle et al, 2017).

Diet plays a crucial role in maintaining genome stability outside cancer research realms. The genome constantly faces endogenous stresses and exogenous assaults that lead to mutations, chromosomal instability, and accumulation of DNA damage. Genome stability remains crucial in preventing disease because unstable genomes frequently spawn cancer and various other nasty genetic disorders. Antioxidants like vitamins C and E, alongside folate and zinc, help counteract oxidative stress and repair damaged DNA quite effectively. On the other hand, inadequate intake of such nutrients can ramp up the risk of DNA damage, genomic instability and the development of disease quite rapidly. Diets loaded with carcinogenic stuff like processed meats or food high in saturated fats disrupt the epigenome and jack up the risk of cancer (Fenech M, 2002).

Diet heavily influences key epigenetic modifications at the molecular level, including DNA methylation and chromatin remodeling rather extensively alongside histone modification. Methyl groups are added haphazardly to DNA molecules, mostly at cytosine bases, thereby silencing gene expression very effectively in many cases. Folate, vitamin B12, and choline play crucial roles in the methylation process, being vital components of one-carbon metabolism. Histone proteins enveloping DNA undergo addition or removal of diverse chemical moieties like acetyl groups and methyl substituents quite frequently. Such modifications can reconfigure chromatin structure, making DNA somewhat more or less transcriptionally accessible under fairly specific physiological conditions. Gene expression gets regulated largely through histone methylation, oddly influenced by dietary polyphenols, and crucial links exist with cancer (Tiffon C, 2018).

Recently, small non-coding RNA molecules known as microRNAs have come into sharp focus within nutritional epigenetics research, regulating gene expression post-transcriptionally. Certain microRNAs that regulate various genes involved in inflammation and apoptosis are modulated by dietary components such as omega-3 fatty acids and various flavonoids. Diet exerts effects markedly on gene expression via microRNA networks, influencing post-transcriptional regulation and histone modifications or DNA methylation epigenetically. Revealing intricate links between diet epigenetics and gene expression yields highly personalised nutrition plans based on unique genetic makeup, quite promising for optimising overall health (Ratti et al, 2020).

2. The Intersection of Diet and Epigenetic Regulation of Gene Expression

Epigenetics involves heritable changes in gene expression occurring, rather mysteriously these days, sans any underlying DNA sequence alterations whatsoever. Such changes can be reversed quite profoundly by environmental factors, including a person's dietary habits, of a person very rapidly. Epigenetic modifications play crucial roles nowadays in various biological processes, such as cell differentiation and cancer progression, very significantly. Diet intricately shapes epigenetic landscapes, influencing risk of various chronic diseases, including cancer, very significantly over time (Hamilton JP, 2011). Dietary habits intersecting with epigenetic processes offer rich terrain for investigating how lifestyle decisions remarkably impact gene expression and tumour formation subsequently. Bioactive compounds and nutrients from ingested food signal epigenetic fluctuations such as histone modification or non-coding RNA expression, rather effectively. Dietary factors heavily influence gene expression modulating cancer-related pathways and offering insights into some very novel therapeutic cancer prevention strategies (Hamilton JP, 2011).

2.1. Epigenetic Mechanisms

Gene expression gets regulated epigenetically through DNA methylation, histone tweaking, and non-coding RNA, primarily in three fundamental ways. Various mechanisms play crucial roles in cellular homeostasis maintenance while regulating the expression of genes intricately within cells.

2.1.1 DNA Methylation

Methyl group addition typically occurs onto the cytosine base in DNA molecules fairly frequently within CpG dinucleotides under normal conditions. DNA methylation typically silences genes under various circumstances across different cellular backgrounds. Hypermethylation of tumour suppressor genes or hypomethylation of certain oncogenes can significantly drive tumour initiation and progression very aggressively in various cancers. Hypermethylation of the p16^INK4A tumour suppressor gene occurs frequently in various cancers, fuelling unbridled cell division quite rapidly afterwards. Dietary components rather irregularly modulate DNA methylation patterns by supplying methyl groups or influencing enzyme activity responsible for epigenetic methylation processes (Lanata et al, 2018).

Folate, vitamin B12, and methionine act as pivotal methyl donors underlying one-carbon metabolism, thereby furnishing the requisite components for DNA methylation. Nutrient deficiencies may lead DNA methylation astray and heighten the risk of various cancers somewhat improperly and conversely with great frequency (Lanata et al, 2018).

2.1.2 Histone Modification

DNA wraps rather tightly around proteins known as histones, forming chromatin, very frequently in certain situations. Histone proteins get various post-translational modifications, including methylation, ubiquitination, and phosphorylation, that significantly alter chromatin structure and gene expression. Histone acetylation generally yields an open chromatin structure and activates gene expression variably, while histone methylation drastically modulates gene expression differently. Dietary compounds profoundly affect the activity of histone modification enzymes like histone acetyltransferases and histone deacetylases within diverse cellular settings quite dramatically. Butyrate, a short-chain fatty acid produced via fermentation of fibre by gut microbiota, acts as a potent HDAC inhibitor, thereby activating tumour suppressor genes. Polyphenols from green tea and curcumin modulate histone modifications quite effectively, promoting anti-cancer effects by reactivating tumour suppressor genes silenced epigenetically (Miller et al, 2013).

2.1.3 Non-Coding RNAs

Non-coding RNAs have emerged as crucial regulators of gene expression, encompassing microRNAs and long non-coding RNAs, surprisingly enough. MiRNAs bind messenger RNAs, prompting degradation or repressing translation, while lncRNAs tweak gene expression by interacting with chromatin and transcriptional machinery obscurely. Dysregulation of ncRNAs has been heavily implicated in various cancer stages, including initiation, metastasis, and also conferring drug resistance. Dietary components such as polyphenols influence the expression of specific miRNAs, which regulate tumour suppressors or oncogenes, rather effectively. Curcumin intricately governs miR-21 expression, a crucial miRNA tied deeply with cancerous cell proliferation, green tea catechins heavily modulate tumour suppressor miR-34a expression (Kaikkonen et al, 2011).

2.2. Diet and Epigenetic Modulation in Cancer

Diet plays a crucial role in modulating epigenetic mechanisms, thereby holding considerable promise for cancer prevention and treatment nowadays, quite effectively. Bioactive compounds and nutrients from various food sources subtly alter DNA methylation, histone modifications, and non-coding RNA expression quite heavily downstream. Devising novel cancer protocols involves elucidating the interplay between dietary factors and epigenetic modifications quite promising for prevention and treatment purposes.

2.2.1 Folate and One-Carbon Metabolism

Folate remains a vastly researched dietary component deeply influencing epigenetic regulation. Folate furnishes methyl groups crucial for methylation processes effectively in one-carbon metabolic pathways vital for DNA methylation reactions. Adequate folate intake crucially maintains normal DNA methylation fairly accurately throughout various cellular processes and bodily functions simultaneously. Folate deficiency precipitates hypomethylation of crucial genes, resulting in genomic instability and heightened cancer risk in humans normally. Folate supplementation very effectively prevents colorectal cancer in various animal models by maintaining DNA methylation patterns and reducing mutations in certain genes. High doses of folate, mainly from supplements, may fuel the growth of existing cancerous tumours, highlighting a need for cautious intake (Crider et al, 2012).

2.2.2 Polyphenols and Histone Modification

Polyphenolic compounds lurking in plant-based foods such as tea and spices heavily influence histone modification, and gene expression is markedly altered. Curcumin potently inhibits HDAC and induces histone acetylation, slowly activating tumour suppressor genes gradually in various cell types. Resveratrol, present in grapes and red wine, profoundly alters gene expression related to cell cycle regulation and apoptosis via histone methylation pattern modifications epigenetically. EGCG and quercetin present in green tea have been shown to regulate histone modifications that deeply influence gene expression involved in inflammatory pathways and cancer metastasis. Bioactive compounds wreak havoc on epigenetic regulation, thereby rendering them ostensibly promising candidates for novel cancer therapeutics very suddenly (Hassan et al, 2019).

2.2.3 Omega-3 Fatty Acids and DNA Methylation

Omega-3 fatty acids, especially EPA and DHA, present in fatty fish and flaxseeds, have been shown to modulate DNA methylation patterns. Omega-3s tweak the activity of DNA methyltransferases, which are enzymes responsible for slapping methyl groups onto specific DNA sequences very radically. Omega-3 fatty acids possibly downregulate DNA methylation of genes pivotal in cancer cell proliferation and metastasis, whilst fostering tumour suppressor gene expression irregularly. Omega-3 fatty acids very significantly dampen pro-inflammatory cytokine expression by modulating NF-κB signalling and messing with DNA methylation patterns. Omega-3 fatty acids potentially prevent cancer by modulating epigenetic marks quietly, alongside exerting an anti-inflammatory effect fairly effectively (Frankhouser et al, 2022).

2.2.4 The Gut Microbiome and Epigenetics

Gut microbiome emerges somewhat mysteriously from within bodily systems as a factor heavily influencing epigenetic regulation and cancer risk fairly significantly. Butyrate, produced rather quietly by fermenting dietary fibre in the gut, potently modulates gene expression through various histone acetylation mechanisms. Butyrate naturally functions as an HDAC inhibitor, often markedly increasing histone acetylation, subsequently activating various tumour suppressor genes very frequently. Research indicates this mechanism mitigates the risk of colorectal cancer and other gastrointestinal malignancies substantially over an extended period quite effectively. Gut bacteria strangely modulate gene methylation involved in immune response, thereby significantly impacting cancer risk under certain physiological conditions (Paul et al, 2015).

Promoting a healthy gut microbiome through dietary changes may hugely impact cancer prevention and epigenetic regulation across various bodily systems. Diet extensively influences epigenetic regulation within cellular environments profoundly under diverse physiological states and alters gene expression significantly. Dietary components intertwine with epigenetic marks such as DNA methylation and histone modification, offering promising new cancer treatment avenues quite surprisingly. Polyphenols and omega-3 fatty acids, alongside butyrate, somewhat heavily modulate epigenetic pathways rather irregularly during tumourigenesis processes (Paul et al, 2015).

3. Nutrient-Mediated Epigenetic Modifications

Epigenetics involves mystifying heritable changes in gene expression under diverse physiological conditions arising without alterations in the DNA sequence itself. Environmental factors often precipitously drive reversible changes, making them crucial alongside modifiable lifestyle factors like dodgy dietary habits and exercise regimes. Consumed food influences epigenetic marks like DNA methylation or histone modification and expression of non-coding RNAs very profoundly, it seems (Al Aboud et al, 2025).

Gene expression gets regulated by such modifications, thereby influencing various biological processes, including cellular metabolism, immune function, or sometimes cancer develops. Dietary components profoundly influence gene expression epigenetically, with significant implications for overall health promotion and disease prevention strategies downstream. Vitamins and minerals, alongside fatty acids and polyphenols, can trigger epigenetic changes heavily promoted or totally suppressed in rather obscure ways. Possibilities emerge rapidly for the development of dietary interventions that potentially stave off maladies like cancer or weird neurological disorders (Gu et al, 2020).

Nutrients mediate epigenetic modifications thoroughly, and massive implications exist for overall health downstream in bodily systems subsequently. Dietary interventions can epigenetically reprogram disease processes drastically, especially in cancer and chronic diseases, via nutrient-induced changes.

3.1. Epigenetic Mechanisms

Epigenetic regulation entails numerous biochemical tweaks of the genome that control gene expression without alteration of the DNA sequence. Epigenetic regulation involves various primary mechanisms, such as histone modification and non-coding RNA-associated gene silencing, everywhere.

3.1.1 DNA Methylation

Methyl group addition typically happens on cytosine residues in CpG dinucleotides deep within gene promoters, resulting in gene expression silencing. Hypermethylation of tumour suppressor genes or pervasive hypomethylation emerges rather frequently in diverse human cancers alongside various other diseases. Folate, vitamin B12, and methionine play a crucial role in one-carbon metabolism, significantly influencing the availability of methyl groups necessary for proper DNA methylation. Folate plays a crucial albeit oft underappreciated role in one-carbon metabolism, and its deficiency precipitates rather severe genomic instability, spurring diseases. Folate supplementation has been shown to reverse methylation defects, making it potentially useful for cancer prevention via diet. High folate consumption, particularly via dubious supplements, can rather quickly facilitate tumour expansion in the presence of pre-existing malignant lesions (Kulis and Esteller, 2010).

3.1.2 Histone Modifications

DNA wraps rather tightly around proteins known as histones, forming chromatin. Phosphorylation and ubiquitination drastically alter chromatin structure, subsequently influencing gene expression rapidly in various unexpected ways. Histone acetylation generally coincides with gene activation, while methylation variably modulates gene expression under diverse contextual conditions, repressing or activating genes erratically. Dietary components heavily influence histone modification enzymes like histone acetyltransferases and histone deacetylases in fairly complex biochemical processes daily. Butyrate, a short-chain fatty acid produced via dietary fibre fermentation, potently inhibits HDAC, thereby activating tumour suppressor genes and stifling cancer cell growth significantly. Curcumin and other polyphenolic compounds abundant in various fruits and spices modulate histone modifications, thereby affecting gene expression related to apoptosis and inflammation (Rossetto et al, 2012).

3.1.3 Non-Coding RNAs

Myriad non-coding RNAs, including microRNAs and rather recondite long non-coding RNAs, are being increasingly recognised as crucial regulators of gene expression. miRNAs can bind mRNA and spur degradation rapidly or inhibit translation into protein generally. lncRNAs, on the other hand interact heavily with chromatin and various transcription factors regulating gene expression machinery in a quite intricate manner. Polyphenols and fatty acids vividly influence the expression of specific miRNAs beneath cellular surfaces quite dynamically and ostensibly with a massive impact. Curcumin heavily regulates the expression of miR-21 associated with the proliferation of cancer cells. EGCG and other green tea catechins modulate the expression of tumour-suppressive miRNA miR-34a very effectively in various cancer cells naturally. Changes in miRNA expression tweak pathways vital for cell survival and heavily curb inflammation and tumour metastasis quite effectively downstream (Ling et al, 2013).

3.2. Dietary Factors Influencing Epigenetic Modifications

Several dietary factors influence epigenetic modifications by furnishing necessary nutrients for these processes or directly modulating epigenetic enzymes very effectively. Crucial nutrients playing pivotal roles epigenetically are mediated through various key dietary constituents, notably vitamins, minerals, and other vital bioactive compounds.

3.2.1 Folate and One-Carbon Metabolism

Folate has been studied extensively lately by various scientists in relation to epigenetics and ranks among the nutrients most heavily researched. Folate plays a crucial role somewhat irregularly in one-carbon metabolism, serving as a key methyl donor for DNA methylation. Folate deficiency precipitously leads to DNA hypomethylation, resulting in genomic instability, thereby substantially ratcheting up the risk of various cancers very quickly. Adequate folate intake has been linked very generally to healthier DNA methylation profiles, potentially lowering the risk of certain cancers, namely colorectal cancer. Folate and cancer risk have a rather weirdly intricate and mystifyingly complex linkage underlying their somewhat baffling association. Folate deficiency spurs aberrant DNA methylation and tumourigenesis, yet excessive folate intake via supplements has been linked quite alarmingly to tumour growth promotion in people with pre-existing cancerous lesions. Folate intake remains crucial for normal epigenetic regulation and cancer risk reduction under various physiological conditions (Crider et al, 2012).

3.2.2 Omega-3 Fatty Acids and Epigenetic Modifications

Fatty fish harbour abundant EPA and DHA omega-3s, which exert profoundly anti-inflammatory effects, occasionally found in walnuts or flaxseeds too. Omega-3 fatty acids heavily influence epigenetic changes very thoroughly by regulating DNA methylation, histone modifications, and expression of various non-coding RNAs. Omega-3 fatty acids drastically reduce DNA methylation of genes fueling inflammation, protecting quite effectively against cancer and myriad other maladies. Omega-3s very convincingly inhibit activation of pro-inflammatory pathways like NF-κB, which is often upregulated in many cancer cells. Omega-3 fatty acids very effectively quell chronic inflammation linked with cancer progression by modulating inflammatory gene expression in a rather significant manner (Zivkovic et al, 2011).

3.2.3 Polyphenols and Epigenetic Regulation

Polyphenols found abundantly in foods like exotic spices and certain fruits are potent antioxidants that modulate epigenetic pathways rather effectively. Curcumin remarkably inhibits HDAC derived from turmeric, spurring acetylation of histones, and tumour suppressor genes are suddenly activated suddenly. Modification has been shown quite effectively to curb proliferation and dissemination of cancerous cells in the breast liver and sundry malignancies. Resveratrol, present in grapes and red wine, tweaks histone modifications, thereby remarkably dampening the expression of various pro-inflammatory genes. EGCG and other green tea catechins significantly regulate epigenetic marks like tumour-suppressive microRNA miR-34a very substantially in various cellular processes. Polyphenols remarkably show promise as interventions that foster prevention of cancer and promote overall health quite effectively in diverse populations (Rajendran et al, 2022).

3.2.4 Amino Acids and Epigenetic Regulation

Methionine and other amino acids deeply entrenched in methylation processes play crucial, albeit often overlooked, roles in complex epigenetic regulatory mechanisms quietly. Methionine serves as a precursor for the synthesis of S-adenosylmethionine SAMe which donates methyl groups in various DNA methylation processes, and histone modifications occur. Methionine supplementation boosts DNA methylation greatly, promoting expression of tumour suppressor genes with a profoundly protective anticancer effect overall. Excessive methionine intake with high protein diet possibly supercharges methylation abnormally, thereby spurring tumour growth rapidly in certain individuals. Proper epigenetic regulation underpins health crucially, and balanced amino acid intake staves off disease very effectively (Zhang N et al, 2018).

3.3. Implications for Health: Epigenetics and Disease Prevention

Diet silently exerts profound influence on epigenetic regulation, harbouring far-reaching implications for health outcomes in diverse populations across lengthy periods. Nutrients tweak gene expression rather mysteriously by altering epigenetic markers and morphing cellular processes that play a pivotal role in disease onset. Nutrients heavily mediate epigenetic tweaks that influence cancer development profoundly by regulating genes controlling cell cycle, inflammation and various metabolic shenanigans within cells. Infusing epigenetic principles into public health strategies spawns potentially groundbreaking preventive measures that drastically overhaul diets to mitigate risk of chronic diseases. Polyphenols and omega-3 fatty acids significantly promote healthy epigenetic regulation with vitamins and essential minerals playing a crucial supporting role (Tiffon C, 2018).

Grasping intricate links between dietary habits and epigenetic modifications fosters modified nutritional approaches for enhanced wellbeing in people bearing distinct genetic makeups. Dietary factors profoundly impact epigenetic regulation thereby markedly altering gene expression cellular processes and disease susceptibility in surprisingly diverse manners. Diet substantially influences epigenetic marks representing a promising disease prevention avenue especially for nasty chronic conditions such as cancer. Knowledge of certain nutrients' effects on DNA methylation and histone modification facilitates creation of dietary guidelines that greatly enhance overall well-being. Modified medicine and proactive health strategies might get unlocked very quickly via emerging epigenetic reprogramming with certain nutritional interventions potentially (Asif et al, 2020).

4. How Diet Shapes DNA: The Role of Nutrients in Epigenetic Changes

Epigenetics involves scrutinizing heritable changes in gene expression largely without altering underlying DNA sequence configurations very profoundly . Modifications affecting chromatin structure and gene activity instigate changes that alter cellular processes rather profoundly and swiftly overnight . Dietary habits and environment intricately shape epigenetic marks thereby significantly influencing gene expression which ultimately determines how cells function under extreme stress. Scientific research has profoundly illuminated ways wherein dietary factors alter epigenetic pathways drastically making nutrition potentially key in preventing disease. Vitamins minerals and amino acids interact heavily with epigenetic machinery modulating DNA methylation and expression of various non-coding RNAs very significantly (Al Aboud et al, 2025).

Molecular events profoundly influence cell cycle regulation and DNA repair thereby linking disease development with cancer and various cardiovascular diseases quite intricately. Polyphenols and fatty acids tweak epigenetic machinery erratically enough to alter histone modification and modulate immune response somewhat unpredictably. Dietary factors drive epigenetic tweaks yielding novel nutrition plans that tweak gene expression very effectively and foster rather lasting wellness. Dietary factors weirdly affect epigenetic mechanisms via weird molecular routes sparking huge potential for prevention of various nasty diseases (Borsoi et al, 2022).

4.1. Epigenetic Mechanisms Modulated by Diet

Epigenetic regulation entails a multitude of convoluted processes governing gene expression rather intricately within cellular confines and chromatin structure simultaneously. Daily lifestyle choices alongside diet and environmental toxins cause wildly fluctuating processes with sometimes very unpredictable outcomes under varying circumstances. Epigenetic regulation involves DNA methylation and histone modifications very frequently through complex biochemical interactions with non-coding RNAs .

4.1.1 DNA Methylation

Methyl groups get added fairly extensively nowadays to DNA molecules typically at CpG dinucleotides within various gene promoter regions. Gene silencing happens fairly often when this addition hinders binding of sundry transcription factors and other regulatory proteins thereby halting expression. Dietary nutrients deeply supply methyl groups or modulate enzyme activity involved in cellular methylation processes rather normally within cells. Folate vitamin B12 and methionine play crucial roles in one-carbon metabolism cycle providing methyl groups for DNA methylation processes. Folate crucially maintains proper DNA methylation; deficiencies in related nutrients often lead to hypomethylation of tumour suppressor genes consequently. High doses of folate especially from supplements have been linked fairly convincingly to increased cancer risk in people with pre-existing lesions. Apparently balanced folate levels are crucial for overall health (Jang et al, 2017).

4.1.2 Histone Modifications

DNA wraps around proteins known as histones forming chromatin very intricately within cellular structures underneath various layers of nucleoplasm. Gene expression can be suppressed or vigorously promoted by histone modifications such as ubiquitination phosphorylation and acetylation methylation sometimes. Gene activation often correlates with histone acetylation very strongly because acetyl groups effectively neutralize positive charge on histone tails resulting in somewhat relaxed chromatin. Specific nutrients modify histone proteins effectively altering gene expression profoundly in various cellular contexts often with remarkably drastic outcomes. Butyrate a short-chain fatty acid produced from fermentation of dietary fibre in colon is known as potent HDAC inhibitor subsequently activating tumour-suppressing genes. Polyphenols found in turmeric and resveratrol extracted from specific grape varieties can alter histone modifications thereby offering a potential mechanism for dietary regimes influencing cancer-related pathways significantly (Mansisidor et al, 2022).

4.1.3 Non-Coding RNAs

MicroRNAs and long non-coding RNAs crucially regulate gene expression in cells alongside other non-coding RNAs very effectively. Small RNA molecules roughly 20-24 nucleotides long bind complementary mRNA sequences thereby degrading them or repressing translation into protein quite significantly. Long non-coding RNAs wield considerable influence over chromatin structure within cellular depths and subtly modulate gene transcription overall. Polyphenols and omega-3 fatty acids drastically alter expression of certain miRNAs involved in cancer progression very significantly in some cases. Resveratrol heavily regulates miR-21 an oft-overexpressed microRNA in various cancer types while green tea catechins modulate tumour-suppressive miR-34a with very decent efficacy generally (Ratti et al, 2020).

4.2. Key Nutrients that Influence Epigenetic Modifications

Several key nutrients evidently modulate epigenetic mechanisms very significantly within human cells and in various other bodily systems rather effectively. Nutrients profoundly affect DNA methylation and histone modifications significantly influencing non-coding RNA expression with major ramifications for overall health.

4.2.1 Folate and One-Carbon Metabolism

Folate a water-soluble B-vitamin crucially supports DNA methylation and maintains genomic stability remarkably in various cellular contexts normally. Folate deficiency connects genes implicated in cellular proliferation and DNA repair hypomethylation precipitating genomic instability thereby heightening risk of cancer significantly. Adequate folate intake helps maintain proper DNA methylation patterns rather effectively thereby potentially lowering risk of various cancers including colorectal cancer overall. Folate plays a part in cancer prevention yet has a dubious side beneath its oft acknowledged salutary effects on human bodily functions. High folate consumption mainly from sketchy dietary supplements correlates with elevated tumour growth risk in people harboring pre-existing malignant lesions rather alarmingly. Linking folate with cancer necessitates painstaking consideration during development of somewhat intricate dietary regimes very carefully under varying conditions (Crider et al, 2012).

4.2.2 Omega-3 Fatty Acids and Epigenetic Regulation

Oily fish contain EPA and DHA that play a vital albeit somewhat obscure role in maintaining cellular homeostasis very effectively. Fatty acids deeply entrench themselves in epigenetic tweaks by orchestrating enzyme activity for DNA methylation and histone manipulation very haphazardly. Omega-3s drastically reduce DNA methylation of pro-inflammatory genes and vigorously promote expression of anti-inflammatory tumour-suppressive genes via histone deacetylase suppression (Swanson et al, 2012).

4.2.3 Polyphenols and Epigenetic Mechanisms

Polyphenols derived from plants exhibit antioxidant properties remarkably and anti-inflammatory effects occur very naturally within human bodies. Polyphenols comprise curcumin found in turmeric and resveratrol sourced heavily from grapes while flavonoids abound remarkably in some fruits or vegetables. Bioactive compounds modulate epigenetic pathways effectively influencing histone modifications and DNA methylation in various cellular contexts with altered microRNA expression. Curcumin very effectively inhibits HDACs thereby promoting histone acetylation and activation of tumour suppressive genes in various murky cellular contexts. Resveratrol very significantly affects miRNA expression weirdly increasing miR-34a which inhibits various oncogenes and promotes apoptosis in cancer cells fairly rampantly (Pandey and Rizvi, 2009).

4.2.4 Vitamin D and Epigenetic Regulation

Vitamin D acquired largely through sunlight exposure and consuming fortified foods plays a crucial role in effectively regulating immune response mechanisms. Epigenetic regulation heavily involves it upstream of numerous complex biological processes occurring rather mysteriously beneath cellular surfaces. Vitamin D profoundly influences DNA methylation of genes related to immune response and cancer progression with research suggesting supplementation reduces methylation thereby encourage expression of tumour suppressor genes (Fetahu et al, 2014).

4.3. Implications for Health: Epigenetics, Disease Prevention, and Therapeutics

Dietary interventions hold considerable promise in prevention of chronic diseases like cancer through effective modulation of various epigenetic marks. Nutrients modulate gene expression intricately involved in cell cycle regulation immune response and inflammatory processes by altering DNA methylation patterns and histone modifications epigenetically. Modified nutrition plans infused with epigenetic principles potentially unlock novel pathways to mitigating disease and fostering better overall health outcomes remarkably. Nutritional interventions offer a potentially modifiable non-invasive approach nowadays for preventing disease by targeting distinct epigenetic pathways effectively (Bakrim et al, 2025).

Diet deeply alters epigenome dynamics through mechanisms like DNA methylation and histone tweaks alongside regulation of quirky non-coding RNAs thereby reshaping gene expression starkly inside cells. Folate and omega-3 fatty acids modulate epigenetic marks profoundly affecting health and potentially thwarting development of maladies like cancer entirely. Modified nutrition plans and therapeutic interventions emerge slowly that markedly improve health and mitigate risk of various nasty diseases effectively (Bakrim et al, 2025).

5. The Impact of Nutritional Deficiencies on Genome Stability

Maintaining genetic material wholeness throughout life spans and across successive generations remains vital for proper cellular operation and organismal well-being, basically. Genome instability spawns mutations and chromosomal aberrations, linking fairly frequently with cancer, ageing, and sundry neurodegenerative maladies. Nutritional deficiencies can significantly impact genome integrity, while exposure towards various carcinogens or high levels of radiation heavily contributes to instability. Severe deficiencies gravely impair biochemical processes crucial for DNA replication and maintenance of repair mechanisms, thereby significantly heightening the risk of genomic damage (Vijg et al, 2017).

Vitamins, minerals, amino acids and fatty acids play crucial albeit largely unappreciated roles in maintaining genomic stability under diverse physiological conditions. They act as cofactors for enzymes involved in DNA synthesis and repair, and chromatin remodelling processes really crucial for preserving genetic integrity. Genome integrity fails miserably when nutrients crucial for cellular homeostasis are scarce, thereby hastening mutagenesis and carcinogenesis quite significantly. Nutritional deficiencies significantly destabilise genome stability, partly due to insufficient intake of key nutrients that heighten the risk of cancer (Vijg et al, 2017).

5.1. The Role of Nutrients in Genome Maintenance

Genome stability relies heavily on quirky processes like DNA replication and repair mechanisms alongside epigenetic regulation, with chromatin remodelling occurring somewhat mysteriously. Nutrients fuel enzymatic machinery underlying these deeply complex processes, and deficiencies often severely impair overall effectiveness rather unpredictably. Folate and vitamin B12, alongside omega-3 fatty acids, significantly impact genome stability, with certain trace minerals like zinc helping moderately.

5.1.1 Folate and One-Carbon Metabolism

Folate, aka vitamin B9, plays a crucial albeit somewhat arcane role in one-carbon metabolism, furnishing methyl groups for DNA methylation and sundry cellular shenanigans. Folate deficiencies rather swiftly precipitate grossly impaired DNA replication and mutagenesis with chromosomal instability and tumourigenesis occurring concomitantly in a rather dramatic fashion. Folate deficiency triggers hypomethylation mostly of genes pivotal in cell cycle regulation and apoptosis, and badly hampers DNA repair, thereby substantially heightening the risk of chromosomal breakage or mutagenesis. Folate deficiency has notoriously been linked with heightened chromosomal instability in cases of colorectal cancer, with alarming frequency these days. Folate supplementation remarkably reverses certain effects, though excessive intake may prove very detrimental in individuals harbouring malignant lesions beforehand sometimes (Beetstra et al, 20050.

5.1.2 Vitamins B12 and B6 in DNA Synthesis and Repair

Cobalamin plays a significant role in amino acid metabolism alongside pyridoxine, which facilitates intricate processes of DNA synthesis. Vitamin B12 crucially facilitates remethylation of homocysteine into methionine, thereby yielding S-adenosylmethionine, a vital methyl donor for various DNA methylation processes. Sufficient vitamin B12 levels are crucial for maintaining stable gene expression and genomic integrity through proper DNA methylation patterns thereby. Vitamin B6 somewhat effectively enhance activity of enzymes mending oxidative DNA lesions and maintains stability of chromatin quite remarkably. Vitamin B6 deficiencies can very quickly ramp up genomic instability by disrupting repair of oxidative DNA damage leading potentially or mutations fueling cancer (Froese et al, 2019).

5.1.3 Omega-3 Fatty Acids in DNA Repair and Inflammation

Omega-3 fatty acids found mainly in fatty fish and flaxseed are crucial components of cell membranes facilitating anti-inflammatory responses very effectively. Modulating expression of repair enzymes such as poly ADP-ribose polymerase crucially impacts DNA repair machinery repairing single-strand DNA breaks effectively. Eicosapentaenoic acid and docosahexaenoic acid are omega-3 fatty acids that somewhat effectively mitigate oxidative stress and reduce DNA damage mostly through dampening inflammatory signaling. Omega-3 fatty acids may vigorously help shield against cancer initiation by damping down inflammation and boosting mechanisms that repair DNA. Omega-3 deficiencies may very significantly exacerbate oxidative damage hindering cellular ability to repair DNA and thereby rapidly increase likelihood of mutations and cancer progression (Calder PC, 2013).

5.1.4 Trace Minerals: Zinc, Iron, and Their Role in Genome Integrity

Zinc serves as a vital cofactor for enzymes crucial in DNA repair alongside antioxidant defense mechanisms while iron fuels replication basically. Zinc plays a crucial role in DNA polymerase function and repair enzymes such as DNA ligase extremely effectively alongside excision repair enzymes. Zinc deficiency tenuously links to heightened DNA damage fostering chromosomal instability characteristic of malignant cells with impaired repair mechanisms . Iron plays somewhat crucial albeit oft overlooked role in cellular metabolism and gets heavily involved in DNA synthesis subsequently undergoing repair processes. Excess iron can spur reactive oxygen species formation quite haphazardly over time and significantly contribute to oxidative DNA damage. Iron deficiency conversely hampers DNA replication leading to significant genomic instability and heightened susceptibility to various nasty diseases like nasty old cancer (Sharif et al, 2012).

5.2. The Consequences of Nutritional Deficiencies on Genome Stability

Nutritional deficiencies severely undermine bodily ability maintaining genome integrity vital for overall health and proper cellular functions get disrupted badly. Chronic nutritional deficiencies can lead to genomic instability characterized by loss of chromosomal integrity and increased frequency of mutagenic events occurring rapidly. Genomic instability manifests through myriad mechanisms including increased DNA damage from deficient intake of key nutrients like folate impairing DNA repair processes drastically. Key nutrients such as zinc play a crucial role in maintaining chromosomal integrity. Deficient intake of these nutrients can impair DNA repair. Mutagenic events occur frequently under such conditions. Nutrient deficiencies disrupt normal DNA repair processes or alter epigenetic regulation thereby heightening risk of cancer development precipitously under certain conditions suddenly. Genomic instability marked by loss of chromosomal integrity occurs quite frequently alongside heightened mutagenic events. Tumourigenesis manifests copiously in cancers such as colorectal cancer and breast cancer with wildly varying severity very frequently nowadays (Kiani et al, 2022).

5.3. Strategies for Preventing Nutrient-Induced Genomic Instability

Crucial nutrients play significant roles in maintaining genome stability somewhat reversing effects of glaring nutritional deficiencies through dietary interventions effectively. Ensuring sufficient intake of vitamins and omega-3 fatty acids through a very balanced diet teeming with antioxidants and various minerals fosters genomic stability somewhat effectively. Daily consumption of folate vitamin B12 zinc and omega-3 fatty acids must be ensured rigorously. Supplementation with specific vitamins or minerals becomes necessary in cases of glaring deficiencies to restore genomic maintenance. Glaring deficiencies necessitate supplementation with specific vitamins or minerals restoring genomic maintenance back somewhat normally (Gómez-Pinilla F, 2008).

Consuming diets rich in antioxidants like vitamin C and polyphenols reduces oxidative DNA damage protecting against reactive oxygen species. Folate or vitamin B12 supplements help restore proper DNA methylation thereby thwarting genomic instability in folks with glaring nutritional deficiencies very effectively. Eating foods rich in antioxidants such as vitamin C and polyphenols may somewhat mitigate DNA damage caused by oxidation and protect against reactive oxygen species quite effectively. Genomic instability arises partly due to egregious deficiencies in nutrients a critical factor in development of cancer and other chronic degenerative diseases. Folate alongside vitamins B12 and B6 and omega-3 fatty acids significantly support DNA synthesis repair and regulation, thereby maintaining genome integrity quite effectively with zinc (Gómez-Pinilla F, 2008).

6. Molecular Pathways: Dietary Signals and Epigenetic Reprogramming

Epigenetic reprogramming and dietary signals have simultaneously converged on a crucial research area in cancer biology and nutritional science lately. Epigenetics presents a riveting paradigm to grasp how external factors and diet sway the stability of genomes and the emergence of cancer quite profoundly. Epigenetic modifications display remarkably dynamic reversible characteristics, allowing organisms to be flexible towards adaptive responses under varying environmental conditions such as altered dietary habits. Macronutrients like proteins, fats, and carbohydrates exert diverse effects on epigenetic mechanisms that control gene expression profoundly in various ways (Supic et al, 2013).

Diet heavily influences cellular functions through epigenetic changes profoundly affecting health outcomes and risk of nasty diseases like cancer. Dietary signals drastically reprogram epigenome via obscure molecular mechanisms thereby influencing gene expression and altering cellular behavior rather unpredictably at times. Key dietary factors modulate cellular processes crucial for homeostasis and disease prevention by altering DNA methylation and histone modification significantly through non-coding RNA expression (Supic et al, 2013).

6.1. Epigenetic Mechanisms and Their Role in Health

Epigenetic regulation involves obscuringly complex mechanisms that control gene expression and maintain genome stability via DNA methylation, adding methyl groups heavily to cytosine residues. DNA methylation occurs typically within CpG dinucleotides and often results quietly in gene silencing beneath transcriptional machinery. Methyl groups are added to DNA fairly frequently through various mechanisms involving epigenetic modification processes. Gene silencing occurs typically via epigenetic tweaks, yielding substantial ramifications, and histone proteins undergo covalent alterations like acetylation and methylation quite frequently (Al Aboud et al, 2025).

Chromatin Remodelling: Structural changes in chromatin that affect gene transcription and cellular processes. Non-Coding RNAs: RNA molecules that regulate gene expression at the transcriptional and post-transcriptional levels without coding for proteins, including microRNAs (miRNAs) and long non-coding RNAs (lncRNAs). Chromatin undergoes radical restructuring entailing structural changes that deeply affect transcription of genes and various cellular processes (Al Aboud et al, 2025).

6.2. The Impact of Diet on Epigenetic Regulation

Dietary factors influence major epigenetic mechanisms, thereby contributing significantly to cellular homeostasis and possibly promoting or thwarting disease onset suddenly. Certain nutrients and bioactive compounds found in various foods modulate these processes quite effectively, with sometimes beneficial or downright detrimental effects.

6.2.1 DNA Methylation: A Critical Target of Dietary Modulation

DNA methylation ranks very high among epigenetic modifications that are fairly well understood nowadays. Folate and vitamin B12, together with methionine, supply methyl groups normally necessary for maintaining DNA methylation patterns very effectively. Nutrient deficiencies foster hypomethylation of tumour suppressor genes very significantly, thereby promoting instability in genomes and escalating cancer risk greatly. Folate crucially facilitates the synthesis of S-adenosylmethionine, a key methyl donor in numerous DNA methylation reactions occurring rather frequently. Low folate consumption fosters tumourigenesis fairly quickly under specific pathological states, leading to chromosomal instability and DNA hypomethylation. Folate supplementation restores normal DNA methylation patterns strikingly and slashes the risk of various cancers very noticeably in numerous cases. Excessive folate intake may ominously hasten tumour progression in people with undetected cancer cells lurking perilously inside their bodily systems (Crider et al, 2012).

6.2.2 Histone Modifications: Nutrients as Epigenetic Modulators

Histone modifications dynamically reconfigure chromatin thereby controlling gene expression in a rather reversible and somewhat unpredictable manner with significant reverberations on DNA accessibility. Specific nutrients drastically change histone marks, thereby influencing gene expression markedly under diverse physiological states with rather significant effects. Curcumin, present in turmeric, very strongly inhibits histone deacetylase activity, leading to significantly heightened histone acetylation and subsequent activation of gene expression. Curcumin, a polyphenol deep inside turmeric, vehemently inhibits histone deacetylase, heightening histone acetylation freely with gene activation ensuing subsequently quite rapidly (Molina-Serrano et al, 2019).

Resveratrol present in grapes and red wine heavily modulates histone acetylation and methylation affecting genes involved deeply in apoptosis tumour suppression pathways. This action somewhat significantly thwarts cancer cell proliferation and mysteriously promotes cell cycle arrest very effectively in many cases. Butyrate a short-chain fatty acid produced via gut microbes fermentation of dietary fibre very effectively inhibits HDAC and promotes histone acetylation thereby reducing risk of colorectal cancer by tweaking gene expression related to DNA repair and cell cycle regulation (Molina-Serrano et al, 2019).

6.2.3 Non-Coding RNAs: The Epigenetic Modulators of Gene Expression

Long non-coding RNAs and microRNAs emerge rapidly as crucial regulators of gene expression in response to diverse dietary cues apparently nowadays. Molecules bind mRNA transcripts very effectively, regulating gene expression at various transcriptional levels and some post-transcriptional ones, it seems. Gene expression gets regulated by small RNA molecules, typically 20-24 nucleotides long, binding mRNA sequences, leading to degradation or inhibiting translation. Rather tightly miRNAs bind complementary mRNA sequences, typically 20-24 nucleotides long, thereby degrading or inhibiting translation very effectively (Fernandes et al, 2019).

Several dietary compounds like green tea catechins epigallocatechin gallate and curcumin have been shown modulating miRNA expression extensively in various studies. LncRNAs are longer RNA molecules that play significant roles in regulating chromatin remodeling and transcriptional repression and post-transcriptional regulation occurs subsequently. EGCG effectively upregulates tumour-suppressive miRNAs such as miR-34a targeting oncogenes c-Myc and Bcl-2 thereby promoting apoptosis very effectively in various cancer cells (Fernandes et al, 2019).

6.3. Epigenetic Reprogramming and Cancer Prevention

Nutritional interventions present a substantial opportunity for effectively preventing cancer through epigenetic reprogramming influenced significantly by various dietary factors. Epigenetic mechanisms regulate myriad genes related to cancer, including some deeply entrenched in apoptosis and DNA repair processes, fairly irregularly. Folate plays a critical role in DNA methylation, heavily influencing cancer prevention while possibly reversing epigenetic alterations contributing significantly to tumour growth. Folate plays a critical role in DNA methylation, and nutrients like it help prevent cancer quite effectively sometimes. Polyphenols from green tea and turmeric and berries modulate histone acetylation and DNA methylation promoting activation of tumour suppressor genes and inhibition of oncogenes (Hardy and Tollefsbol, 2011).

Folate intake possibly averts DNA hypomethylation, silencing tumour suppressor genes, thereby markedly reducing cancer risk significantly in people generally. Polyphenols present in green tea and various berries heavily modulate histone acetylation and DNA methylation, thereby promoting activation of tumour suppressor genes. Polyphenols potentially exert a profoundly significant impact on cancer chemoprevention by subtly altering epigenetic pathways with remarkable efficacy downstream. Timing of dietary interventions poses a cancer prevention challenge, somewhat obviously due to factors like dosage (Hardy and Tollefsbol, 2011).

6.4. Future Directions and Therapeutic Implications

Novel avenues unfurl quite rapidly for modified nutrition and cancer therapeutics aimed squarely at prevention with deepening insight into the diet's epigenetic reprogramming nexus. Tackling gnarly problems stemming from variability in individual responses to dietary interventions requires putting knowledge into practical application quite effectively. Epigenome effects differ vastly among individuals largely due to genetic variances and variations in gut microbiota composition. Lifestyle factors play a rather significant role in such variability largely due to epigenetic reprogramming influenced by nutrients or their combinations effectively (Hardy and Tollefsbol, 2011).

Clinical trials: Well-designed clinical trials are essential to assess the long-term impact of dietary interventions on gene expression and cancer risk, as well as to determine the optimal dosage and timing of dietary compounds. Well-designed clinical trials are essential for assessing long-term impacts of dietary interventions on gene expression and cancer risk. Certain nutrients or unusual combinations thereof substantially influence epigenetic reprogramming and scrutinizing them meticulously may uncover effective strategies dietary in nature. Utterly essential nowadays are rigorously designed trials assessing the impact of dietary regimens on gene expression and subsequent cancer risk long-term (Hardy and Tollefsbol, 2011).

7. Epigenetic Mechanisms

Epigenetics has emerged rather forcefully as a lens whereby environmental factors conspire with gene expression in sundry cutting-edge scientific milieus nowadays. Genetics provides a rudimentary framework for traits, while epigenetics regulates gene expression strangely by tweaking factors beyond DNA sequence. Daily consumption of certain dietary components can drastically influence the epigenetic landscape, potentially altering gene expression that prevents disease and maintains overall health. Diet profoundly impacts epigenetic mechanisms unlocking novel pathways towards grasping links between nutrition and maladies like cancer or various heart diseases. Modulation of gene expression quietly bridges environmental signals and biological processes governing health and disease via dietary acts effectively. Dietary components impact molecular pathways quite significantly and irregularly affect epigenetic regulation hugely contributing to various disease prevention mechanisms thereby.

7.1. What is Epigenetics and Why Does It Matter?

Epigenetics involves somewhat mysterious alterations in gene expression not directly linked with changes in the underlying DNA sequence. Reversible modifications variably influence gene expression over fairly long periods of time. Epigenetic mechanisms crucially entail DNA methylation, whereby methyl groups, rather mysteriously, affix themselves on cytosine residues, silencing certain genes. DNA methylation plays a crucial role in cellular differentiation and X-inactivation while regulating tumour suppressor genes fairly effectively under normal circumstances. Histone modification involves chemical changes to histone proteins that DNA wraps around, altering chromatin structure and subsequently gene expression (Al Aboud et al, 2023).

Histone proteins undergo chemical modifications that drastically change chromatin structure and gene expression in tightly wrapped cells around these proteins. Small RNA molecules like microRNAs and long non-coding RNAs regulate gene expression at multiple levels. Gene expression fluctuates wildly at transcriptional levels and post-transcriptional levels under the influence of non-coding RNAs. Modifications such as histone methylation and acetylation frequently inhibit or promote gene transcription under certain specific physiological conditions. Small RNA molecules like microRNAs regulate gene expression somewhat weirdly at transcriptional levels and post-transcriptionally sometimes in peculiar ways (Al Aboud et al, 2023).

7.2. Diet as an Epigenetic Regulator

Macronutrients, micronutrients, and various bioactive compounds have been shown very convincingly to influence diverse epigenetic mechanisms greatly. The body interprets signals from food via nutrient-sensing pathways, and epigenome gets adjusted very drastically, thereby affecting gene expression patterns.

7.2.1 DNA Methylation and Nutrient Availability

Diet profoundly impacts DNA methylation, a notoriously studied epigenetic process in various cellular contexts and sometimes under peculiar environmental conditions. Folate and vitamin B12 fuel the one-carbon metabolism pathway, providing methyl groups necessary for DNA methylation reactions with considerable efficiency. Sufficient nutrients facilitate proper DNA methylation, helping regulate gene expression and genome stability is thereby maintained quite notably. Folate donates methyl groups crucial for DNA methylation processes unfolding mysteriously within cells during cellular metabolism and replication (Sobral et al, 2024).

Folate deficiency has been tenuously linked to hypomethylation, thereby eerily activating certain oncogenes and silencing tumour suppressor genes characteristic of cancer. DNA hypomethylation gets reversed by folate supplementation, thereby potentially lowering the risk of nasty diseases like colorectal cancer through dietary intervention. Methyl donors such as folate when overconsumed very quickly lead to DNA hypermethylation silencing tumour suppressor genes thus contributing ominously to cancer development. Methyl donors play a crucial role fairly often in maintaining epigenetic homeostasis very much throughout life (Sobral et al, 2024).

7.2.2 Histone Modifications: The Role of Nutrients in Gene Expression

DNA wraps around histone proteins very tightly forming chromatin a complex structure regulating gene expression and accessibility of genetic material. Histone proteins get heavily tweaked after translation via acetylation methylation and phosphorylation ubiquitination radically altering chromatin structure and silencing gene transcription or kickstarting it. Dietary factors heavily influence histone mods thereby significantly altering gene expression in cells under very unusual conditions very obviously. Curcumin a polyphenol found in turmeric very effectively acts as an HDAC inhibitor and promotes histone acetylation thereby facilitating various gene expressions (Shmueli et al, 2021).

Curcumin very effectively modulates histone acetylation linking it strongly with anti-cancer properties and potent anti-inflammatory effects. Resveratrol found in red wine influences histone acetylation and methylation thereby promoting activation of tumour suppressor genes. Resveratrol present in red wine remarkably sways histone acetylation and methylation thereby vigorously activating tumour suppressor genes. Butyrate a short-chain fatty acid produced by gut fermentation of dietary fibre is another natural HDAC inhibitor linked obliquely to regulation of histone modifications and gene expression notably in colorectal cancer prevention contexts. This mechanism very significantly contributes somewhat mysteriously in various studies against breast cancer and colon cancer with protective effects (Shmueli et al, 2021).

7.2.3 Non-coding RNAs: Dietary Regulation of miRNAs and lncRNAs

Non-coding RNAs particularly miRNAs and lncRNAs play crucial roles virtually everywhere in regulation of gene expression down the line . LncRNAs deftly orchestrate gene transcription with chromatin remodeling whereas MiRNAs modulate mRNA molecule stability and translation quite intricately afterwards. Dietary components tweak the expression of non-coding RNAs very radically in various cellular milieus, thereby altering gene expression further downstream somewhat eccentrically. Epigallocatechin gallate, present in green tea catechins, ostensibly modulates expression of several miRNAs, including miR-34a, which targets various oncogenic genes effectively (Ratti et al, 2020).

EGCG influences cancer cell growth rather curiously by altering the expression of various miRNAs and affecting survival quite markedly. Curcumin markedly influences lncRNA expression, thereby vigorously promoting activation of tumour suppressor genes and silencing specific oncogenes effectively. Curcumin profoundly impacts lncRNA expression, thereby activating tumour suppressor genes whilst silencing sundry oncogenes in malignant cells concurrently (Ratti et al, 2020).

7.3. Diet and Disease Prevention Through Epigenetic Modulation

Diet impacts epigenetic regulation, offering exciting possibilities for preventing diseases like cancer and cardiovascular disease quite effectively nowadays. Dietary interventions can thwart disease onset and advancement remarkably by tweaking crucial epigenetic routes like DNA methylation and histone modification radically.

7.3.1 Cancer Prevention

Certain dietary factors nowadays very effectively possess protective effects against various forms of cancer, influencing epigenetic mechanisms. Diets rich in fibre polyphenols, and various essential vitamins can significantly lower the risk of various cancers, including colorectal, breast and lung cancer. Gene expression mediates these effects largely through various regulatory mechanisms related to cellular proliferation, DNA repair, and apoptosis. Diets heavy in cruciferous veggies such as broccoli or cabbage, mostly comprising plant-based foods, have been associated with changes in DNA methylation, silencing various oncogenes (Montgomery et al, 2019).

7.3.2 Cardiovascular Disease and Metabolic Health

Epigenetic modifications crucially regulate genes deeply embedded in lipid metabolic pathways and insulin sensitivity under inflammatory conditions. Diets rich in unsaturated fats and fibre plus antioxidants mitigate the risk of atherosclerosis and obesity through epigenetic pathways regulating inflammation very effectively nowadays.

7.3.3 Neurodegenerative Diseases

Epigenetic changes drastically alter gene expression involved heavily in neuronal survival mechanisms and synaptic plasticity amidst various neurodegenerative diseases. Vitamin E and polyphenols modulate epigenetic mechanisms fairly extensively, protecting neurons rather effectively from oxidative stress, thereby reducing neurodegeneration risk. Deeper insight into complex relationships between diet and epigenetics yields fresh avenues for crafting modified nutritional strategies squarely aimed at disease prevention. Modified dietary tweaks can ameliorate health outcomes very effectively and reduce the risk of maladies like cancer or heart disease marginally. Food drastically alters gene expression via sundry molecular routes, and future precision nutrition entails modified dietary regimens leveraging epigenetic insights for sustained holistic wellness (Bertogliat et al, 2020).

8. Nutritional Interventions for Epigenetic Reprogramming and Genome Protection

Recently, nutrition and epigenetic regulation have become quite intricately entwined, sparking considerable interest largely for potentially thwarting various diseases and fostering overall wellbeing slowly. Epigenetic mechanisms weirdly orchestrate gene expression largely via histone modification and non-coding RNA regulation without tampering with the underlying DNA sequence. Modifications occur dynamically under varying environmental influences, such as dietary habits and patterns of nutrient consumption around individuals. Nutritional interventions very effectively modulate epigenetic pathways, offering promising strategies for genome protection alongside epigenetic reprogramming simultaneously.

8.1. Epigenetic Reprogramming: The Concept and Mechanisms

Epigenetic reprogramming entails drastic changes wrought by factors like nutrition that modify the epigenome, thereby altering gene expression patterns fairly reversibly under certain conditions. Epigenetic changes stay pliable throughout life and get shaped by dietary choices quite differently from permanent genetic mutations, basically. Key epigenetic modifications encompass DNA methylation, which involves adding methyl groups at cytosine residues, thereby typically silencing genes. Genomic stability relies heavily on proper DNA methylation, playing a crucial role in effectively regulating various tumour suppressor genes (Abraham et al, 2023).

Histone proteins get adorned with or stripped of sundry chemical groups like acetyl, methyl, or phosphate, altering chromatin structure and gene transcription patterns. Histone proteins undergo drastic alterations via the addition or removal of chemical groups such as acetyl or methyl, thereby changing chromatin structure. Non-coding RNAs like microRNAs and long non-coding RNAs regulate gene expression at multiple levels, including mRNA stability and translation. Gene expression is altered significantly by these molecules through chromatin remodelling and other obscure mechanisms simultaneously (Abraham et al, 2023).

Various non-coding RNAs play critical roles in gene regulation. They achieve this mostly through the stability of mRNA and translation. Chromatin remodelling occurs due to long non-coding RNAs very frequently. Alteration of chromatin structure drastically affects gene transcription. These molecules regulate gene expression very vigorously at many different obscure levels concurrently. Histone proteins undergo subtly nuanced tweaks that occasionally flip gene switches on or totally shut them down with sundry modifications (Abraham et al, 2023).

8.2. Nutrients as Epigenetic Modulators

Nutrients play crucial roles in epigenetic regulation, notably via DNA methylation and histone modification. Epigenetic modulators guide cellular processes, influencing health outcomes significantly. Roles of certain nutrients in the expression of non-coding RNAs have been observed in depth. Cellular processes are affected by nutrients acting as epigenetic regulators subtly. Non-coding RNAs expression is modulated epigenetically.

8.2.1 DNA Methylation and Nutrient Availability

DNA methylation stands as a primary epigenetic modification occurring very frequently in various cellular contexts and is heavily influenced by dietary intake. Folate, vitamin B12, methionine and choline crucially facilitate one-carbon metabolism, supplying methyl groups needed for S-adenosylmethionine synthesis, thereby facilitating DNA methylation heavily reliant on folate, a water-soluble B vitamin critical for methylation. Folate, a water-soluble B vitamin, participates crucially in DNA methylation processes thoroughly inside cells every day normally. Folate deficiency severely fuels cancer initiation by causing DNA hypomethylation, which activates oncogenes and silences tumour suppressor genes (Souza et al, 2025).

Vitamin B12 plays a crucial role in one-carbon metabolism and the regulation of DNA methylation patterns. Folate levels sufficiently high help maintain normal DNA methylation patterns, thereby preventing genomic instability very effectively in most genomes. Methionine, an essential amino acid, and choline, found plentifully in eggs and liver, are crucial for methyl group availability, ostensibly alongside vitamin B12. B12 deficiencies prevalent in vegetarian populations and elderly folks have been tied to DNA hypomethylation, which can spur cancer progression rapidly (Souza et al, 2025).

8.2.2 Histone Modifications: The Role of Dietary Components

Histone modifications alter DNA packaging within the nucleus very dynamically, determining gene accessibility for various transcriptional processes, almost always very subtly. Dietary compounds tweak gene expression heavily by altering chromatin structure through histone acetylation, methylation, or phosphorylation. Polyphenols found in fruits vegetables and beverages like green tea and red wine affect histone modifications very significantly. Polyphenols present in sundry fruits and drinks like green tea have been proven fairly definitively to induce histone modifications by circuitous means. Resveratrol promotes histone acetylation, thereby activating quiescent genes involved heavily in apoptosis and cell cycle regulation mechanisms in red wine (Pfluger and Wagner, 2007).

Curcumin, another well-known HDAC inhibitor found in turmeric, promotes histone acetylation very effectively. Uncontrolled cell growth, a hallmark of cancer, can be thwarted effectively quite often inside human bodies by this modification. Butyrate produced by gut microbiota during dietary fibre fermentation inhibits histone deacetylases, promoting histone acetylation and altering gene expression radically. Curcumin, another well-known HDAC inhibitor, promotes histone acetylation fairly effectively in various cellular contexts with very considerable potency (Pfluger and Wagner, 2007).

8.2.3 Non-Coding RNAs: Dietary Influence on Gene Regulation

Dietary compounds fairly frequently modulate expression of non-coding RNAs, including microRNAs and long non-coding RNAs, in various cellular contexts. RNAs wield significant influence epigenetically reprogramming cells by targeting specific genes, sometimes quite effectively, for activation or repression. Epigallocatechin gallate, a polyphenol found in green tea, has been shown to regulate miRNA expression. Polyphenol epigallocatechin gallate, or EGCG, abundant in green tea, regulates the expression of various miRNAs. EGCG upregulates miR-34a expression, a tumour suppressor miRNA that targets c-Myc and Bcl-2, heavily involved in cell proliferation and survival (Kumar et al, 2020).

Omega-3 fatty acids found in fatty fish, flaxseed, and walnuts influence miRNA expression very significantly. Curcumin rather rapidly spurs inhibition of cancer cell growth and tumour progression. Curcumin modulates lncRNA expression quite effectively, promoting activation of tumour suppressor genes while inhibiting expression of various oncogenes. Recently, omega-3 fatty acids present in walnuts and fatty fish have been shown to significantly influence miRNA expression in various studies (Kumar et al, 2020).

8.3. Epigenetic Reprogramming for Genome Protection

Epigenetic reprogramming helps shield genome integrity from mutations and instability that largely fuel cancer and various other chronic diseases. Genome protectors are substances that foster genomic stability and DNA repair, thereby maintaining cellular homeostasis quite crucially.

8.3.1 Antioxidants and DNA Protection

Antioxidants very effectively thwart oxidative stress damage to bodily cells daily with considerable gusto and varying degrees of protective success. Gross disparity between highly reactive free radicals spawned during normal metabolic processes and bodily neutralisation capacity precipitates considerable stress from environmental exposures. Free radicals accumulate rapidly inside cells, obliterating crucial cellular components like DNA, thereby facilitating mutations that spark the development of cancer. Nuts teem with antioxidants that rather handily stabilise free radicals by very quickly donating electrons, and veggies are similarly replete. Oxidative damage severely curtails proteins, lipids, and DNA, but this intricate process unfolding quietly underneath mitigates such harm rather effectively (Pizzino et al, 2017).

Selenium and vitamins C and E are among the heavily researched antioxidants studied extensively in various scientific endeavours globally these days. Selenium is a vital trace mineral necessary daily for certain enzymes battling oxidative damage vigorously inside human bodily cells. Vitamin C mops up free radicals vigorously in the cytosol, while vitamin E remarkably protects cell membranes from nasty lipid peroxidation quite effectively. Antioxidants very significantly help maintain genomic stability by safeguarding genetic material from oxidative stress, thus reducing mutagenesis risk substantially. This protective role hugely matters in the prevention of various cancers and other chronic diseases that develop insidiously over fairly long periods. A diet rich in antioxidant-containing foods obviously plays a vital role nowadays for maintaining long-term cellular health effectively (Pizzino et al, 2017).

8.3.2 Fibre and Gut Microbiota

Trillions of microorganisms residing in the human gut variably influence epigenetic mechanisms, thereby playing a crucial role in determining diverse health outcomes. Dietary fibre obtained mainly from whole grains, fruits, and veggies profoundly affects microbial composition and function in human guts. Fibre remains totally unprocessed by human digestive enzymes yet furnishes crucial substrate for vigorous fermentation by gut bacteria. Beneficial bacteria produce short-chain fatty acids like butyrate quite rapidly during fermentation in diverse nutritional settings and environments. Butyrate stands out remarkably in the epigenetic regulation of myriad cellular processes under various physiological conditions naturally. It functions as a histone deacetylase inhibitor modulating gene expression profoundly in various cellular contexts by altering chromatin structure dramatically (Fu et al, 2022). Epigenetic modulation quite effectively activates genes involved in anti-inflammatory responses and DNA repair under various highly stressful cellular conditions. Butyrate energetically enhance colon epithelial cell health and fortifies DNA integrity with markedly improved repair mechanisms operating very effectively. Such effects enhance genomic stability and may mitigate the risk of colorectal cancer substantially in populations genetically predisposed highly. Dietary fibre rather surreptitiously interacts with gut microbiota and host gene regulation in a feedback loop, maintaining intestinal health precariously. Very effectively high-fibre diets thwart disease onset via epigenetic routes mediated largely by surprisingly dynamic gut microbiome activity (Fu et al, 2022).

8.3.3 Polyphenols and Genome Protection

Polyphenols present in berries, green tea, and curcumin have shown the ability protecting genome stability by inducing various quirky DNA repair mechanisms. Such actions maintain genomic stability, effectively thwarting mutagenesis and offering fairly robust protection against cancer development over considerable time . Epigenetic reprogramming interventions and genome safeguarding tactics are evolving very rapidly nowadays as promising strategies for disease prevention. Crafting nutrition plans that enhance wellness and thwart maladies like cancer becomes plausible when grasping molecular mechanisms behind food's sway on genetic expression (Ferguson LR, 2001). Evidence accumulates slowly, indicating various dietary compounds from rather obscure micronutrients and fairly ubiquitous polyphenols epigenetically modify disease development and subsequently enhance bodily defences genomically against instability. Scientists strive mightily under diverse environmental conditions to tailor modified interventions specific to individual genetic makeup and wildly varying dietary habits. Nutrition swiftly becomes vital in thwarting maladies like cancer via epigenetic reprogramming of genes, yielding markedly superior health outcomes genetically.

9. Conclusion

Nutritional epigenetics offers transformative insight into the dynamic interplay between diet and gene expression, somewhat remarkably nowadays affecting genome stability rather profoundly. Epigenetic modifications like DNA methylation or histone modification can be reversed under specific environmental circumstances involving various dietary factors. Nutrition emerges crucially as a modulator epigenetically via complex mechanisms of plasticity that manifest significantly throughout various life stages with a lasting impact. Specific nutrients profoundly affect epigenetic processes governing cellular differentiation and DNA repair in various cellular contexts quietly. Folate, alongside vitamin B12 and choline serve as a methyl donor supporting DNA methylation, thereby maintaining gene silencing patterns properly (Bishop and Ferguson, 2015).

Polyphenols sulforaphane and sundry phytochemicals tweak histone acetylation and methylation, thereby drastically impacting chromatin structure, markedly and altering transcriptional activity. Various oncogene pathways and tumour suppressor gene networks are simultaneously regulated by non-coding RNAs, heavily influenced by dietary components. Interactions like these have rather alarmingly deep implications for human health and progression of many virulent diseases. Rapidly aberrant epigenetic modifications heavily contribute to cancer hallmarks by silencing tumour suppressor genes and activating various oncogenes very frequently. Nutritional interventions can therapeutically or preventively alter epigenetic patterns in specific contexts, playing a role rather obviously (Borsoi et al, 2022).

Maternal nutrition profoundly affects fetal epigenome development, illustrating long-term consequences of early dietary exposures rippling across generations in mystifying ways. Nutritional epigenetics harbours vast potential, yet several gnarly challenges stubbornly remain within this increasing field of research nowadays. Data interpretation becomes convoluted due to complex nutrient-gene interactions and substantial variability among individuals under wildly diverse environmental conditions. Epigenomic tech advancements coupled with systems biology slowly pave the way slowly for fairly precise personalised diets based on an individual's unique epigenetic makeup (Lee HS, 2015). Nutritional epigenetics emerges quite promisingly nowadays as an increasing frontier deeply integrating diet, molecular biology and disease prevention strategies effectively. Manipulating epigenetic mechanisms with dietary components enables the creation of modified nutritional regimens that markedly promote overall health and genome stability. Research advances rapidly, playing a crucial role in moulding modified dietary plans alongside proactive healthcare initiatives, hence positioning diet as a potent instrument.

References

Abraham MJ, El Sherbini A, El-Diasty M, Askari S, Szewczuk MR. Restoring Epigenetic Reprogramming with Diet and Exercise to Improve Health-Related Metabolic Diseases. Biomolecules. 2023 Feb 7;13(2):318. doi: 10.3390/biom13020318. PMID: 36830687; PMCID: PMC9953584.

Al Aboud NM, Tupper C, Jialal I. Genetics, Epigenetic Mechanism. [Updated 2023 Aug 14]. In: StatPearls [Internet]. Treasure Island (FL): StatPearls Publishing; 2025 Jan-. Available from: https://www.ncbi.nlm.nih.gov/books/NBK532999/

Asif S, Morrow NM, Mulvihill EE, Kim KH. Understanding Dietary Intervention-Mediated Epigenetic Modifications in Metabolic Diseases. Front Genet. 2020 Oct 15;11:590369. doi: 10.3389/fgene.2020.590369. PMID: 33193730; PMCID: PMC7593700.

Bakrim S, El Omari N, El Yaagoubi OM, Khalid A, Abdalla AN, Hamza SMA, Ibrahim SE, Atifi F, Zaid Y, Bouyahya A, El Fessikh M, Ming LC, Aanniz T. Epi-nutrients for cancer prevention: Molecular mechanisms and emerging insights. Cell Biol Toxicol. 2025 Jul 15;41(1):116. Doi: 10.1007/s10565-025-10054-2. PMID: 40663150; PMCID: PMC12263776.

Beetstra S, Thomas P, Salisbury C, Turner J, Fenech M. Folic acid deficiency increases chromosomal instability, chromosome 21 aneuploidy and sensitivity to radiation-induced micronuclei. Mutat Res. 2005 Oct 15;578(1-2):317-26. Doi: 10.1016/j.mrfmmm.2005.05.012. Epub 2005 Jul 11. PMID: 16005909.

Bertogliat MJ, Morris-Blanco KC, Vemuganti R. Epigenetic mechanisms of neurodegenerative diseases and acute brain injury. Neurochem Int. 2020 Feb;133:104642. doi: 10.1016/j.neuint.2019.104642. Epub 2019 Dec 12. PMID: 31838024; PMCID: PMC8074401.

Bishop KS, Ferguson LR. The interaction between epigenetics, nutrition and the development of cancer. Nutrients. 2015 Jan 30;7(2):922-47. doi: 10.3390/nu7020922. PMID: 25647662; PMCID: PMC4344568.

Borsoi FT, Neri-Numa IA, de Oliveira WQ, de Araújo FF, Pastore GM. Dietary polyphenols and their relationship to the modulation of non-communicable chronic diseases and epigenetic mechanisms: A mini-review. Food Chem (Oxf). 2022 Dec 13;6:100155. Doi: 10.1016/j.fochms.2022.100155. PMID: 36582744; PMCID: PMC9793217.

Calder PC. Omega-3 polyunsaturated fatty acids and inflammatory processes: nutrition or pharmacology? Br J Clin Pharmacol. 2013 Mar;75(3):645-62. doi: 10.1111/j.1365-2125.2012.04374.x. PMID: 22765297; PMCID: PMC3575932.

Coyle KM, Boudreau JE, Marcato P. Genetic Mutations and Epigenetic Modifications: Driving Cancer and Informing Precision Medicine. Biomed Res Int. 2017;2017:9620870. doi: 10.1155/2017/9620870. Epub 2017 Jun 8. PMID: 28685150; PMCID: PMC5480027.

Crider KS, Yang TP, Berry RJ, Bailey LB. Folate and DNA methylation: a review of molecular mechanisms and the evidence for folate's role. Adv Nutr. 2012 Jan;3(1):21-38. doi: 10.3945/an.111.000992. Epub 2012 Jan 5. PMID: 22332098; PMCID: PMC3262611.

Fenech M. Micronutrients and genomic stability: a new paradigm for recommended dietary allowances (RDAs). Food Chem Toxicol. 2002 Aug;40(8):1113-7. doi: 10.1016/s0278-6915(02)00028-5. PMID: 12067572.

Ferguson LR. Role of plant polyphenols in genomic stability. Mutat Res. 2001 Apr 18;475(1-2):89-111. doi: 10.1016/s0027-5107(01)00073-2. PMID: 11295156.

Fernandes JCR, Acuña SM, Aoki JI, Floeter-Winter LM, Muxel SM. Long Non-Coding RNAs in the Regulation of Gene Expression: Physiology and Disease. Noncoding RNA. 2019 Feb 17;5(1):17. doi: 10.3390/ncrna5010017. PMID: 30781588; PMCID: PMC6468922.

Fetahu IS, Höbaus J, Kállay E. Vitamin D and the epigenome. Front Physiol. 2014 Apr 29;5:164. Doi: 10.3389/fphys.2014.00164. PMID: 24808866; PMCID: PMC4010791.

Frankhouser DE, Steck S, Sovic MG, Belury MA, Wang Q, Clinton SK, Bundschuh R, Yan PS, Yee LD. Dietary omega-3 fatty acid intake impacts peripheral blood DNA methylation -anti-inflammatory effects and individual variability in a pilot study. J Nutr Biochem. 2022 Jan;99:108839. doi: 10.1016/j.jnutbio.2021.108839. Epub 2021 Aug 16. PMID: 34411715; PMCID: PMC9142761.

Froese DS, Fowler B, Baumgartner MR. Vitamin B12, folate, and the methionine remethylation cycle: biochemistry, pathways, and regulation. J Inherit Metab Dis. 2019 Jul;42(4):673-685. doi: 10.1002/jimd.12009. Epub 2019 Jan 28. PMID: 30693532.

Fu J, Zheng Y, Gao Y, Xu W. Dietary Fibre Intake and Gut Microbiota in Human Health. Microorganisms. 2022 Dec 18;10(12):2507. doi: 10.3390/microorganisms10122507. PMID: 36557760; PMCID: PMC9787832.

Gómez-Pinilla F. Brain foods: the effects of nutrients on brain function. Nat Rev Neurosci. 2008 Jul;9(7):568-78. doi: 10.1038/nrn2421. PMID: 18568016; PMCID: PMC2805706.

Gu M, Ren B, Fang Y, Ren J, Liu X, Wang X, Zhou F, Xiao R, Luo X, You L, Zhao Y. Epigenetic regulation in cancer. MedComm (2020). 2024 Feb 19;5(2):e495. doi: 10.1002/mco2.495. PMID: 38374872; PMCID: PMC10876210.

Hamilton JP. Epigenetics: principles and practice. Dig Dis. 2011;29(2):130-5. doi: 10.1159/000323874. Epub 2011 Jul 5. PMID: 21734376; PMCID: PMC3134032.

Hardy TM, Tollefsbol TO. Epigenetic diet: impact on the epigenome and cancer. Epigenomics. 2011 Aug;3(4):503-18. doi: 10.2217 /epi.11.71. PMID: 22022340; PMCID: PMC3197720.

Hassan FU, Rehman MS, Khan MS, Ali MA, Javed A, Nawaz A, Yang C. Curcumin as an Alternative Epigenetic Modulator: Mechanism of Action and Potential Effects. Front Genet. 2019 Jun 4;10:514. doi: 10.3389/fgene.2019.00514. PMID: 31214247; PMCID: PMC6557992.

Jang HS, Shin WJ, Lee JE, Do JT. CpG and Non-CpG Methylation in Epigenetic Gene Regulation and Brain Function. Genes (Basel). 2017 May 23;8(6):148. doi: 10.3390/genes8060148. PMID: 28545252; PMCID: PMC5485512.

Kaikkonen MU, Lam MT, Glass CK. Non-coding RNAs as regulators of gene expression and epigenetics. Cardiovasc Res. 2011 Jun 1;90(3):430-40. doi: 10.1093/cvr/cvr097. Epub 2011 May 9. PMID: 21558279; PMCID: PMC3096308.

Kiani AK, Dhuli K, Donato K, Aquilanti B, Velluti V, Matera G, Iaconelli A, Connelly ST, Bellinato F, Gisondi P, Bertelli M. Main nutritional deficiencies. J Prev Med Hyg. 2022 Oct 17;63(2 Suppl 3):E93-E101. doi: 10.15167/2421-4248/jpmh2022.63.2S3.2752. PMID: 36479498; PMCID: PMC9710417.

Kulis M, Esteller M. DNA methylation and cancer. Adv Genet. 2010;70:27-56. doi: 10.1016/B978-0-12-380866-0.60002-2. PMID: 20920744.

Kumar S, Gonzalez EA, Rameshwar P, Etchegaray JP. Non-Coding RNAs as Mediators of Epigenetic Changes in Malignancies. Cancers (Basel). 2020 Dec 5;12(12):3657. doi: 10.3390/cancers12123657. PMID: 33291485; PMCID: PMC7762117.

Lanata CM, Chung SA, Criswell LA. DNA methylation 101: what is important to know about DNA methylation and its role in SLE risk and disease heterogeneity. Lupus Sci Med. 2018 Jul 25;5(1):e000285. doi: 10.1136/lupus-2018-000285. PMID: 30094041; PMCID: PMC6069928.

Lee HS. Impact of Maternal Diet on the Epigenome during In Utero Life and the Developmental Programming of Diseases in Childhood and Adulthood. Nutrients. 2015 Nov 17;7(11):9492-507. doi: 10.3390/nu7115467. PMID: 26593940; PMCID: PMC4663595.

Ling H, Fabbri M, Calin GA. MicroRNAs and other non-coding RNAs as targets for anticancer drug development. Nat Rev Drug Discov. 2013 Nov;12(11):847-65. doi: 10.1038/nrd4140. PMID: 24172333; PMCID: PMC4548803.

Mansisidor AR, Risca VI. Chromatin accessibility: methods, mechanisms, and biological insights. Nucleus. 2022 Dec;13(1):236-276. doi: 10.1080/19491034.2022.2143106. PMID: 36404679; PMCID: PMC9683059.

Miller JL, Grant PA. The role of DNA methylation and histone modifications in transcriptional regulation in humans. Subcell Biochem. 2013;61:289-317. doi: 10.1007/978-94-007-4525-4_13. PMID: 23150256; PMCID: PMC6611551.

Molina-Serrano D, Kyriakou D, Kirmizis A. Histone Modifications as an Intersection Between Diet and Longevity. Front Genet. 2019 Mar 12;10:192. doi: 10.3389/fgene.2019.00192. PMID: 30915107; PMCID: PMC6422915.

Montgomery M, Srinivasan A. Epigenetic Gene Regulation by Dietary Compounds in Cancer Prevention. Adv Nutr. 2019 Nov 1;10(6):1012-1028. doi: 10.1093/advances/nmz046. PMID: 31100104; PMCID: PMC6855955.

Pandey KB, Rizvi SI. Plant polyphenols as dietary antioxidants in human health and disease. Oxid Med Cell Longev. 2009 Nov-Dec;2(5):270-8. doi: 10.4161/oxim.2.5.9498. PMID: 20716914; PMCID: PMC2835915.

Paul B, Barnes S, Demark-Wahnefried W, Morrow C, Salvador C, Skibola C, Tollefsbol TO. Influences of diet and the gut microbiome on epigenetic modulation in cancer and other diseases. Clin Epigenetics. 2015 Oct 16;7:112. doi: 10.1186/s13148-015-0144-7. PMID: 26478753; PMCID: PMC4609101.

Pfluger J, Wagner D. Histone modifications and dynamic regulation of genome accessibility in plants. Curr Opin Plant Biol. 2007 Dec;10(6):645-52. doi: 10.1016/j.pbi.2007.07.013. Epub 2007 Sep 19. PMID: 17884714; PMCID: PMC2140274.

Pizzino G, Irrera N, Cucinotta M, Pallio G, Mannino F, Arcoraci V, Squadrito F, Altavilla D, Bitto A. Oxidative Stress: Harms and Benefits for Human Health. Oxid Med Cell Longev. 2017;2017:8416763. doi: 10.1155/2017/8416763. Epub 2017 Jul 27. PMID: 28819546; PMCID: PMC5551541.

Rajendran P, Abdelsalam SA, Renu K, Veeraraghavan V, Ben Ammar R, Ahmed EA. Polyphenols as Potent Epigenetics Agents for Cancer. Int J Mol Sci. 2022 Oct 3;23(19):11712. doi: 10.3390/ijms231911712. PMID: 36233012; PMCID: PMC9570183.

Ratti M, Lampis A, Ghidini M, Salati M, Mirchev MB, Valeri N, Hahne JC. MicroRNAs (miRNAs) and Long Non-Coding RNAs (lncRNAs) as New Tools for Cancer Therapy: First Steps from Bench to Bedside. Target Oncol. 2020 Jun;15(3):261-278. doi: 10.1007/s11523-020-00717-x. PMID: 32451752; PMCID: PMC7283209.

Rossetto D, Avvakumov N, Côté J. Histone phosphorylation: a chromatin modification involved in diverse nuclear events. Epigenetics. 2012 Oct;7(10):1098-108. doi: 10.4161/epi.21975. Epub 2012 Sep 4. PMID: 22948226; PMCID: PMC3469451.

Sharif R, Thomas P, Zalewski P, Fenech M. The role of zinc in genomic stability. Mutat Res. 2012 May 1;733(1-2):111-21. doi: 10.1016/j.mrfmmm.2011.08.009. Epub 2011 Sep 16. PMID: 21939673.

Shmueli MD, Sheban D, Eisenberg-Lerner A, Merbl Y. Histone degradation by the proteasome regulates chromatin and cellular plasticity. FEBS J. 2022 Jun;289(12):3304-3316. doi: 10.1111/febs.15903. Epub 2021 May 13. PMID: 33914417; PMCID: PMC9292675.

Sobral AF, Cunha A, Silva V, Gil-Martins E, Silva R, Barbosa DJ. Unveiling the Therapeutic Potential of Folate-Dependent One-Carbon Metabolism in Cancer and Neurodegeneration. Int J Mol Sci. 2024 Aug 28;25(17):9339. doi: 10.3390/ijms25179339. PMID: 39273288; PMCID: PMC11395277.

Souza AP, Marinho V, Marques MR. The Fundamental Role of Nutrients for Metabolic Balance and Epigenome Integrity Maintenance. Epigenomes. 2025 Jul 9;9(3):23. doi: 10.3390/epigenomes9030023. PMID: 40700039; PMCID: PMC12286010.

Supic G, Jagodic M, Magic Z. Epigenetics: a new link between nutrition and cancer. Nutr Cancer. 2013;65(6):781-92. doi: 10.1080/01635581.2013.805794. PMID: 23909721.

Swanson D, Block R, Mousa SA. Omega-3 fatty acids EPA and DHA: health benefits throughout life. Adv Nutr. 2012 Jan;3(1):1-7. doi: 10.3945/an.111.000893. Epub 2012 Jan 5. PMID: 22332096; PMCID: PMC3262608.

Tiffon C. The Impact of Nutrition and Environmental Epigenetics on Human Health and Disease. Int J Mol Sci. 2018 Nov 1;19(11):3425. doi: 10.3390/ijms19113425. PMID: 30388784; PMCID: PMC6275017.

Vickers MH. Early life nutrition, epigenetics and programming of later life disease. Nutrients. 2014 Jun 2;6(6):2165-78. doi: 10.3390/nu6062165. PMID: 24892374; PMCID: PMC4073141.

Vijg J, Dong X, Milholland B, Zhang L. Genome instability: a conserved mechanism of ageing? Essays Biochem. 2017 Jul 11;61(3):305-315. doi: 10.1042/EBC20160082. PMID: 28550046; PMCID: PMC5988260.

Zhang N. Role of methionine on epigenetic modification of DNA methylation and gene expression in animals. Anim Nutr. 2018 Mar;4(1):11-16. doi: 10.1016/j.aninu.2017.08.009. Epub 2017 Sep 19. PMID: 30167479; PMCID: PMC6112339.

Zivkovic AM, Telis N, German JB, Hammock BD. Dietary omega-3 fatty acids aid in the modulation of inflammation and metabolic health. Calif Agric (Berkeley). 2011 Jul;65(3):106-111. doi: 10.3733/ca.v065n03p106. PMID: 24860193; PMCID: PMC4030645.

Chapter 6

Immune Surveillance and Nutritional Immunology in Oncology

Sheetanshu Gupta[1], Praneeth Juvvi[2*], Ng. Joykumar Singh[3], and Lokesh Kumar Mishra[4]

[1]Department of Food Safety and Quality Assurance, College of Food Technology, Central Agricultural University (CAU), Imphal, Manipur, India

[2]Department of Food Processing Technology, College of Food Technology-Central Agricultural University, Imphal, Manipur, India

[3]Department of Food Process Engineering, College of Food Technology, Central Agricultural University (CAU), Imphal, Manipur, India

[4]Department of BPME, College of Agriculture, Central Agricultural University (CAU), Imphal, Manipur, India

Abstract

Cancer immunotherapy modulation efforts lately pivot heavily on immune surveillance crucial for tumour cell detection and elimination mostly now. Dietary factors heavily influence various immune responses in a cancer context where dynamic relationships form between nutrition and immune function obviously. Malignant cells are combated effectively by innate immune cells and adaptive T-cells functioning vigorously with cancer defense mechanisms such as macrophages. Vitamin D and zinc profoundly alter activity of some immune cells thereby remarkably enhancing immune surveillance and changing cytokine profiles significantly. Tumour immunology gets significantly influenced by gut microbiome and efficacy of cancer treatments is impacted remarkably in myriad obscure strange ways. Superfood rich diets greatly enhance efficacy of standard cancer treatments markedly in oncology and patient outcomes improve significantly with anti-inflammatory regimens. Personalized nutrition remarkably holds promise in optimizing immune response based on genetic predispositions amidst diverse metabolic markers very quietly indeed nowadays. Cancer progression gets significantly shaped by nutrition and profoundly modulated immune surveillance according to various findings in clinical settings and preclinical research.

Keywords: Immune Surveillance, Nutritional Immunology, Tumour Immunity, Immunomodulation, Inflammation, Cytokine Regulation

DOI: 10.1201/9781042010387-6

1. Introduction

Cancer biology has relied heavily on immune surveillance, a process quite effectively detecting cells with cancerous potential for decades. Immune systems fervently detect aberrant cells morphing stealthily into tumours and eradicate them decisively before cancer festers deeply inside human bodies. Sometimes this immune defence is not entirely foolproof. Tumour cells often concoct surreptitious plans for evading immune detection and circumventing suppressive mechanisms, thereby thriving quite vigorously and proliferating uncontrollably. An increasing amount of data has recently underscored the influence of nutritional factors on immunological response, particularly within oncology contexts nowadays. Nutritional immunology emerges vigorously as a field exploring quite intensely links between dietary patterns and various immune responses, yielding novel cancer prevention therapy options (Swann and Smyth, 2007).

Cancer manifests multifacetedly through its rather intricate deeply intertwined connection with various components of human immune system . Harmful invaders including pathogens and cancerous cells are kept at bay very effectively always by immune system functions primarily. Actions of myriad cells and molecules including T cells B cells macrophages weirdly dendritic cells and natural killer cells make it operate. Immune cells scour bodily tissues rather stealthily identifying cells displaying aberrant antigens or proliferating uncontrollably and eliminate such threats with considerable haste. Cancer cells have evolved numerous furtive mechanisms evading detection by somewhat sluggish immune systems not perpetually on high alert (Sethi et al, 2012).

Tumour cells express proteins such as PD-L1 which bind PD-1 receptors on T cells and very effectively inhibit their activation downstream. Novel immunotherapies like immune checkpoint inhibitors that restore anticancer function have been studied keenly alongside tumour immune evasion strategies. Some cancers respond remarkably well to these therapies yet many stubborn tumours effectively thwart such treatments in quite a few cases. Nutritional intervention emerged fairly recently as a promising avenue after exploration of various adjunctive therapies ensued subsequently with some success. Specific nutrients play a crucial role in modulating human immune response remarkably well thereby supporting surveillance against various malignancies effectively (Han et al, 2020).

Nutritional immunology focuses heavily on grasping profound effects of certain nutrients upon development and remarkable activation of diverse immune cells. Proteins fats and carbohydrates alongside vitamins minerals and sundry bioactive compounds deeply influence myriad immune responses very profoundly in various ways. Vitamin D has long enhanceed innate immunity very effectively by spurring activation of macrophages and producing antimicrobial peptides that kill various microbes. Omega-3 fatty acids predominantly found in fish oils are renowned for anti-inflammatory properties and support function of various immune cells like T cells. Vitamins C and E flavonoids and polyphenols act as dietary antioxidants playing quite a significant role presently in nutritional immunology (Munteanu and Schwartz, 2022). Compounds exhibiting antioxidative properties effectively neutralize reactive oxygen species generated during immune responses that potentially damage cells. Antioxidants somewhat preserve immune cell function involved in cancer surveillance namely T cells and NK cells highly prone to oxidative cellular damage. Antioxidants somewhat effectively mitigate chronic inflammation by modulating inflammatory pathways like NF-kB in bodily processes and COX-2 (Jomova et al, 2023).

Nutritional immunology research nowadays reveals dietary fibre significantly impacts gut microbiome and thereby profoundly influences immune function in a very major way. Emerging research strongly suggests fibre-rich diets markedly promote growth of beneficial gut bacteria enhancing systemic immune responses quite significantly in humans. Butyrate and other short-chain fatty acids produced by fermenting dietary fibre in colon have markedly anti-inflammatory properties and boost immune surveillance vigorously. A balanced microbiome thwarts systemic inflammation very effectively which can otherwise greatly impede immune surveillance and rather swiftly facilitate cancer progression (Fu et al, 2022).

Discernment of normal cells from aberrant ones by immune system plays a crucial albeit oft underrated role evidently in oncology research nowadays. Modulation of antigen presentation via dietary means becomes pertinent in this context rather quietly. Dendritic cells crucially instigate anti-tumour immunity by snagging tumour antigens and presenting them moderately well to T cells subsequently. Crucial for proper dendritic cell function effectively vitamin A is found abundantly in carrots and sweet potatoes activating T cells. Zinc plays a crucial role in development of immune cells particularly in seafood consumers where it fosters adaptive immunity remarkably well. Zinc deficiency has been tenuously linked with impaired T cell functionality and heightened susceptibility to various cancer forms quite evidently (Wang et al, 2020).

Inflammation manifests rather problematically in cancer biology being simultaneously beneficial yet glaringly detrimental across various contexts. Acute inflammation manifests as protective bodily response against tissue damage and infection but chronic inflammation often precipitates cancer progression very rapidly. Chronic low-grade inflammation apparently stems from very risky eating habits loaded with abundant processed junk and lots of seriously unhealthy fats. Tumour initiation and subsequent growth are heavily influenced by this kind of inflammation that fosters an immunosuppressive microenvironment very effectively nowadays. Diets rich in anti-inflammatory foods like fruits and veggies alongside healthy fats can somewhat restore immune function by counteracting chronic inflammation.

Profound implications exist for oncology research regarding cancer prevention treatment and post treatment recovery linked intricately with dietary habits and immune response. Proper nutrition significantly enhance immune response against tumour cells and markedly improves efficacy of various immunotherapies potentially alleviating grueling side effects of chemotherapy. Nutritional strategies carefully designed modulate immune function holding considerable promise as complementary approaches in cancer care boosting body defenses (Janakiram et al, 2016).

Immune evasion functions somewhat secretly with immune surveillance in oncology contexts while nutritional modulation fluctuates rather mysteriously alongside them. Vitamins and bioactive compounds robustly support immune function vigorously around tumour sites and significantly modulate inflammation quite effectively. Emerging evidence on dietary interventions complementing traditional cancer therapies will be highlighted offering quite a holistic cancer prevention strategy. Fresh perspectives on diet's role in cancer prevention are furnished quite deliberately in this chapter as a potent immune system enhanceer.

2. The Role of Immune Surveillance in Cancer Detection and Prevention

Genetic mutations spark uncontrolled cell growth, and environmental factors aggressively fuel cancer progression at an alarming rapid pace. The immune system plays a crucial role in detecting cancerous cells and eliminating them before they wildly proliferate into utterly nasty tumours. Immune surveillance involves the eradication of aberrant cells harbouring malignant tendencies stealthily under perpetual vigilance in rather complex bodily mechanisms. Cancerous cells get eliminated vigorously through various mechanisms, as immune surveillance plays a crucial role in detection and prevention.

2.1. Immune Surveillance

Lewis Thomas and Sir Macfarlane Burnet floated the notion of immune surveillance rather quietly back in the 1950s, surprisingly enough, it appears. Immune systems possibly recognize then eliminate cancer cells emerging during normal cellular turnover or under stress from various environmental carcinogens rapidly. Cancer cell surfaces express tumour-associated antigens aberrantly, which immune system functionality thwarts via various very obscure mechanisms normally very effectively. Innate immunity forms a crucial defense mechanism entailing natural killer cells macrophages and dendritic cells functioning rather enigmatically beneath the surface. NK cells play a crucial role in pinpointing and liquidating malignant cells having undergone transformation, especially since they detect the absence of MHC I molecules on tumour cells frequently in various cancerous cell types (Corthay A, 2014).

Malignant cells are readily recognised by macrophages and dendritic cells which foster phagocytosis through obscure mechanisms operating simultaneously. T lymphocytes and B cells play essential roles in targeted responses against cancer. T lymphocytes and B cells facilitate targeted responses against cancer quite effectively alongside innate immune cells naturally in most cases. Cytotoxic T lymphocytes readily kill cancer cells displaying specific tumour antigens on their surface with considerable effectiveness and rather high precision. Helper T cells stimulate other immune cells vigorously and boost CTL activity thereby playing a crucial albeit somewhat obscure role in orchestrating overall immune response effectively (Corthay A, 2014). Immune system remarkably harnesses diverse checkpoints somewhat irregularly besides merely identifying foreign entities or tumour cells in human bodies. T cells usually express various immune checkpoint proteins such as PD-1 and CTLA-4 acting very much as molecular brakes on rampant immune responses. Clever cancers hijack immune mechanisms effectively evading detection with notable secrecy and effectively under various circumstances (Shibru et al, 2021).

2.2. Mechanisms of Immune Evasion in Cancer

Cancer cells devise intricate evasion tactics beneath radar of immune surveillance while ostensibly being annihilated by host defense mechanisms rapidly. Tumours often downregulate certain tumour-associated antigens on cell surfaces thereby becoming stealthy and far less recognizable by various immune cells. Tumours evade cytotoxic T cells by stealthy maneuvers highly effectively and upregulate PD-L1 immune checkpoints rather successfully in many cases. Tumours frequently hijack immune checkpoints like PD-L1 very effectively suppressing cancer-fighting ability of immune system rather thoroughly in many cancer cases. Tumour microenvironment plays a rather critical role underground in evading various rather obscure immune responses quite effectively (Kim and Cho, 2022).

Tumours inhibit T cell activation effectively by upregulating checkpoint proteins, promoting tolerance which enables cancer cells evade destruction very stealthily. Cancer cells thrive amidst a tumour microenvironment that masterfully engineers profoundly immunosuppressive conditions thereby facilitating sly immune evasion mechanisms. Tolerance mechanisms induced copiously in certain instances may cause the immune system to fail recognizing cancer cells as foreign entities. Cancer cells cunningly recruit immunosuppressive cells such as Tregs and MDSCs which vigorously suppress immune response and foster tumour-friendly microenvironment very effectively (Kim and Cho, 2022).

2.3. Enhancing Immune Surveillance through Nutrition

Emerging research rather quietly highlights profound impacts of nutrition on immune function and enhances mechanisms underlying cancer prevention efforts very effectively. A diet replete with vital nutrients fosters immunity and boosts the capacity to eradicate malignant cells remarkably quickly in most cases effectively.

Nutrient deficiencies severely impair immune function thereby compromising bodily ability quite effectively and responding sluggishly against cancerous cells rapidly. Several nutrients remarkably impact immune response and enhance immunity greatly amidst varying dietary elements with considerable potential benefits overall.

2.3.1 Antioxidants and Immune Function

The immune system plays a crucial role in defending the body against pathogens and infections or abnormal cell growth, including certain forms of cancer, quite effectively. Oxidative stress severely compromises immune responses heavily implicated in cancer development, and dysfunction occurs alongside rampant inflammation very frequently. Antioxidants very effectively counteract harmful conditions by neutralizing free radicals thereby protecting immune cells from oxidative stress and damage. Highly reactive molecules are generated naturally during metabolism and produced copiously due to environmental stressors like pollution or UV radiation. Unchecked molecules ravage crucial immune cell components like proteins lipids and DNA thereby seriously impairing function and greatly diminishing capacity for detecting cancerous cells or destroying infected ones (Pizzino et al, 2017).

Crucial for surveillance under certain conditions are T lymphocytes and natural killer cells obviously quite pivotal for response. Beta-carotene works alongside vitamin C and selenium naturally mitigating oxidative stress through bodily mechanisms rather effectively on a daily basis. Vitamin C somewhat mysteriously enhance sundry immune cells by augmenting antibody production and fostering inflammation that remains healthy rapidly. Vitamin E as a fat-soluble antioxidant remarkably stabilizes immune cell membranes very effectively keeping them intact and remaining functional. Selenium backs antioxidant enzymes fairly effectively preventing oxidative cellular damage of DNA and various other cellular components remarkably inside cells (Pizzino et al, 2017).

Naturally occurring compounds such as curcumin directly affect immune cells abundant in turmeric extracts having been shown previously. Curcumin markedly amplifies activity of NK cells and T lymphocytes boosting their ability to target cancer cells very effectively nowadays. Antioxidants play a vital role in encourage robust immunity by maintaining bodily well-being effectively and possibly staving off various forms of cancer.

2.3.2 Polyphenols and Immune Modulation

Polyphenols encompass myriad phytochemicals displaying robust antioxidant properties and profoundly anti-inflammatory effects with immunomodulatory activities underlying their peculiar benefits. Polyphenols remarkably support immune function quite extensively in fruits and tea and also in dark chocolate every single day. Compounds subtly tweak immune cell activity and markedly amplify responses while modulating inflammatory pathways crucial for cancer prevention and balanced immune response apparently. Resveratrol a highly studied polyphenol is found mainly in red wine and some rather exotic grapes or berries quite unusually. Resveratrol effectively modulates immune cell activity by substantially enhancing T cell proliferation and significantly improving cytokine production (Yahfoufi et al, 2018).

Requisite immune responses get activated thereby enabling body to subsequently recognize and eradicate cells harboring viral infections or cancerous mutations effectively. Resveratrol substantially reduces inflammation playing another crucial albeit somewhat enigmatic role in immunomodulation down the line very effectively. Resveratrol quite effectively enhance overall immune surveillance and discourages tumour growth by suppressing pro-inflammatory cytokine expression in an immune environment. Epigallocatechin gallate (EGCG) mostly found in green tea exhibits very potent immunomodulatory effects and has been fairly extensively researched already (Yahfoufi et al, 2018).

EGCG profoundly boosts activity of T lymphocytes and natural killer cells that recognize tumour cells and annihilate them very rapidly. EGCG substantially enhance secretion of cytokines activating immunity and helps activate cellular pathways protective against cancer metastasis very effectively. Polyphenols such as resveratrol eradicate cancerous cells effectively while compounds like EGCG enhance immune function and significantly reduce inflammation naturally. Polyphenol-rich foods remarkably foster optimal health and thwart cancer development by modulating immune response quite effectively in various ways (Singh et al, 2011).

2.3.3 Omega-3 Fatty Acids and Immune Activation

Omega-3 fatty acids form a crucial category of polyunsaturated fats utterly vital for cellular processes and surprisingly promoting overall health remarkably down life's path. Fatty fish like sardines and mackerel teem with essential fats and plant-based sources such as walnuts and flaxseeds contain them abundantly. Omega-3 fatty acids remarkably support brain health and heart function significantly while encourage overall immune system functionality quite nicely underwater. Research suggests omega-3 fatty acids somewhat enhance T cell activation which plays a crucial role in defense against various pathogens. Omega-3s heavily modulate production of cytokines, small signaling proteins that regulate various immune responses deeply inside bodily tissues often (Krupa et al, 2024).

Omega-3s very effectively foster production of certain anti-inflammatory cytokines and suppress pro-inflammatory ones, maintaining a fairly balanced immune response. Essential balance averts chronic inflammation, which stealthily fosters immune dysfunction and spawns diseases like cancer when festering darkly unresolved in bodily tissues. Tumour growth thrives in environments fostered by chronic inflammation, playing a crucial role in the progression of various aggressive cancers rapidly (Krupa et al, 2024). Eicosapentaenoic acid and docosahexaenoic acid, namely omega-3 fatty acids, reduce the production of pro-inflammatory cytokines like tumour necrosis factor-alpha, very effectively suppressing immune activity. Omega-3s revive immune function very effectively by quashing inflammation chronically and spurring activation of immunity, making body ridiculously well-equipped to detect cancer cells readily now. Eating foods rich in omega-3 remarkably boosts immune surveillance and substantially decreases cancer risk over time very effectively (Tan et al, 2018).

2.3.4 Vitamin D and Immune Response

Vitamin D plays a crucial role in immune function regulation alongside various other nutrients fairly mysteriously. Emerging research reveals significant effects on the immune system, which plays a crucial role remarkably well in maintaining bone health. Vitamin D profoundly impacts numerous immune cells, such as T cells, macrophages and B cells, crucial for detecting infections and abnormal cancerous cells. T cells tasked with directly targeting infected or abnormal cells function very optimally with sufficient vitamin D levels, basically. Vitamin D profoundly influences macrophages and these immune cells rapidly engulf pathogens, with cancer cells occasionally getting digested in the process (Aranow C, 2011).

Vitamin D boosts the ability of certain immune cells to recognise malignant cells rapidly and eliminates them, thereby supporting the body's natural cancer-fighting mechanisms effectively. Vitamin D plays a crucial role in modulating the production of various immune mediators like cytokines and chemokines that help orchestrate somewhat complex immune responses. Vitamin D fosters anti-inflammatory cytokines thereby maintaining immune balance and stifling pro-inflammatory ones, which can prevent cancer development slowly over time. People with elevated vitamin D levels often tend to display a significantly lower risk of various cancers including breast colorectal and prostate cancer (Aranow C, 2011). Vitamin D regulates cell growth and programmed cell death, thereby preventing uncontrollable cell proliferation, a hallmark typically found in various cancerous malignancies. Vitamin D deficiency may markedly increase cancer progression risk in various populations and very significantly heighten metastasis odds. Supplementation or dietary changes can enhance immune response effectively while mitigating risk of certain cancers very significantly over time (Carlberg and Velleuer, 2022).

2.3.5 Probiotics and Gut Health

Trillions of bacteria fungi and other microorganisms constituting gut microbiota play a pivotal role nowadays in somewhat effectively regulating immune function. Diverse microbiome profoundly shapes local gut immunity and systemic responses maintaining overall immune health effectively amidst various physiological fluctuations. Gut microbiota profoundly impacts immune surveillance which detects abnormal cells quickly and eliminates cancerous ones under various physiological conditions normally. Maintaining a healthy gut microbiome effectively reduces disease risk and enhance immune function very obviously beneath surface level . Consuming diverse fermented foods daily supports gut health very effectively with a diet extremely rich in prebiotics and probiotics (Belkaid and Hand, 2024).

Non-digestible fibres reside abundantly in whole grains and sundry fruits or veggies, nourishing beneficial gut bacteria rather effectively. Beneficial microbes very commonly inhabit foods like yogurt or fermented veggies and thrive inside gloopy kefir with relative frequency. Prebiotics and probiotics conjointly promote gut microbiota equilibrium, thereby significantly encouraging immune responses in many individuals to a considerable extent. Probiotics fairly effectively stimulate production of antibodies and quite vigorously enhance the activity of natural killer cells in various instances. Crucial immune cells quite vigorously detect cancer cells in various parts of human body and eliminate them rapidly (Belkaid and Hand, 2024). Some probiotics alter cytokine production, fostering a very favourable immune environment for cancer detection and prevention quite effectively nowadays. Probiotics fairly effectively reduce chronic inflammation in bodily systems, thereby mitigating the risk of immune dysfunction and tumour development quite significantly. Probiotics may profoundly impact gut-associated lymphoid tissue, deeply nestled within gut walls a crucial component of overall immune function. GALT plays a critical role in recognising pathogens and abnormal cells, thereby supporting overall immune surveillance bodily functions fairly effectively nowadays. Prebiotics and probiotics get consumed quite frequently thereby fostering robust gut microbiota and significantly encourage overall health or cancer prevention efforts markedly (Śliżewska et al, 2020).

2.4. Immune Surveillance, Cancer Immunotherapy, and Nutrition

Cancer treatment nowadays relies heavily on immune surveillance owing largely in part to immunotherapy breakthroughs such as CAR-T cell therapy and certain immune checkpoint inhibitors. Therapies vigorously block checkpoints like PD-1 or genetically modify cells to enhance immune system's ability and attack cancer cells effectively. Nutritional interventions enhance immune function significantly reducing inflammation and fairly remarkably enhancing effectiveness of immunotherapy in certain cases. Food loaded with antioxidants and anti-inflammatory compounds remarkably boosts efficacy of immunotherapy while somewhat mitigating its nasty unintended side effects (Kong et al, 2024).

Crucial immune surveillance prevents cancer largely, and emerging evidence underscores the importance of nutrition in bodily functions for eliminating malignant cells rapidly. Antioxidants alongside omega-3 fatty acids and vitamin D appear to beneficially modulate immune function,, somewhat fostering robust antitumour responses very effectively. Nutritional factors intricately influence the body's innate defence against cancer as complexities of diet and immune system interactions gradually surface. Diets rich in immune-boosting foods can rather effectively enhance surveillance and reduce overall cancer risk with anti-inflammatory compounds present (Kong et al, 2024).

3. Nutritional Modulation of Immune Responses in Cancer Therapy

Cancer immunotherapy has emerged remarkably as a cornerstone in the treatment of diverse malignancies utilizing body's intricate immune system quite effectively these days. Various immunotherapeutic approaches have revolutionised cancer care very significantly lately, with stuff like immune checkpoint inhibitors and adoptive T cell therapy emerging but such treatments often have significant side effects and aren't universally effective. Growing interest lies heavily in figuring out how nutrition might tweak immune systems, thereby enhancing cancer therapy effectiveness and ameliorating patient outcomes very significantly. The immune system plays a critical role in recognizing cancerous cells and eliminates them from the body quite effectively.

Cancer cells devise fiendishly sneaky mechanisms underground, allowing tumours and metastases to flourish rapidly, evading detection by immune cells. Strangely enough, recent studies suggest tweaks in diet rev up immune responses quickly and reduce nasty inflammation very effectively nowadays. Nutritional modulation of immune responses plays a vital role in cancer therapy, synergising effectively with various treatments and encouraging immunotherapy.

3.1. Immune Modulation and Cancer Therapy:

Cancer therapies such as chemotherapy target tumour cells indirectly with varying degrees of specificity and moderate efficacy these days obviously. Tumour success hinges very effectively on cunning ability under various circumstances evading immune response with remarkable stealth quite often. Immunotherapy vigorously stimulates immune systems recognizing malignant cells and subsequently launches a ferocious attack on them with unrelenting fervor. Nasty immune-related side effects emerge suddenly and severely limit treatment success amidst immunosuppressive tumour microenvironments and intricate tumour immune evasion mechanisms (Anand et al, 2024).

Efficacy of cancer therapies hinges significantly on immune status of patients under diverse medical conditions and various other circumstances. Malignant cells severely hinder efficacy of treatment protocols in an immune-suppressed system that falters mounting response rather badly overall. Bioactive compounds and micronutrients variably modulate components of immune response quite profoundly impacting immune function in surprisingly diverse ways effectively. Cancer therapy gets optimized quite effectively nowadays by subverting various evasive immune mechanisms via nutrition-based strategies holding considerable promise underground (Anand et al, 2024).

3.2. The Role of Nutrients in Modulating Immune Function

Nutrients play a vital role deeply in regulating immune function influencing body's ability vigorously to respond infections and abnormal cell growth. T lymphocytes macrophages natural killer cells and dendritic cells require specific nutrients functioning optimally within a very complex environment. Nutrient deficiencies or imbalances can drastically weaken immune systems over time making body rather susceptible to a plethora of diseases very rapidly. Essential vitamins and minerals enhance immune responses fairly effectively supporting bodily functions in abnormal cell detection quite naturally. Nutrients crucial nowadays for immune health include vitamins, minerals, fatty acids, antioxidants and various phytochemicals remarkably enough (Munteanu and Schwart, 2022).

Vitamins like vitamin C and vitamin E crucially maintain immune cell function and reduce oxidative stress while minerals such as selenium activate various immune responses. Omega-3 fatty acids present in fatty fish and flaxseeds foster somewhat obscure anti-inflammatory responses and boost detection of malignant cells very effectively. Stuff like fruits and nuts contain antioxidants that help neutralize free radicals thereby protecting immune cells from rather severe oxidative cellular damage. Oxidative stress gravely impairs immune cell function fueling chronic inflammation very ominously which drives cancer progression in a rather nasty manner (Munteanu and Schwart, 2022).

Polyphenols in tea and dark chocolate exhibit anti-inflammatory properties enhancing immune cell activity vigorously while promoting cellular surveillance remarkably well. Collectively these nutrients form a convoluted entity that supports immune cells and regulates responses whilst balancing overall inflammation maintaining vibrant health. Nutrient-rich diets play a crucial role in ensuring optimally functioning immunity and lowering risk of chronic maladies such as cancer very effectively nowadays (Yan et al, 2020).

3.2.1. Omega-3 Fatty Acids: Enhancing Antitumour Immunity

Omega-3 polyunsaturated fatty acids found mostly in fatty fish and occasionally in flaxseeds possess extensively documented anti-inflammatory properties and modulate several immune responses quite effectively. Research suggests eicosapentaenoic acid and docosahexaenoic acid found in omega-3 fatty acids modulate T lymphocytes activity quite vigorously and effectively. Omega-3 fatty acids rather effectively sensitize tumours by promoting cytotoxic T cell responses and encourage immune checkpoint inhibitors activity in cancer therapy (Weylandt et al, 2015). Omega-3 fatty acids modulate the tumour microenvironment rather effectively and reduce chronic inflammation, thereby fostering a somewhat favorable milieu for various immune cells. Omega-3 fatty acids possibly amplify the effectiveness of radiotherapy remarkably by encourage immune response significantly in certain contexts very effectively. Omega-3s may drastically boost chemotherapy drugs and immune cells into tumour sites by reducing vascularity greatly and lowering tumour permeability (Weylandt et al, 2015).

3.2.2. Antioxidants

Cancer treatments such as chemotherapy induce oxidative stress arising from imbalance between production of reactive oxygen species and antioxidant defenses in body. Reactive oxygen species are very nasty molecules that can severely damage cellular components like DNA and proteins or lipids extensively over time. Oxidative stress gets harnessed haphazardly killing tumour cells but badly damages surrounding tissues, including various immune cells, thereby impairing cancer cell elimination effectively. Cancer treatment efficacy gets torpedoed rather quickly and body becomes extremely vulnerable to opportunistic infections when immune system gets severely battered (Yang et al, 2018).

Selenium and zinc quite effectively enhance immune function by safeguarding cells from oxidative damage while vitamins C and E play crucial supporting roles. Antioxidants enhance immune cells' functionality including natural killer cells T cells and macrophages which play pivotal roles in warding off cancerous cells effectively. Vitamin C boosts cytotoxic activity of NK cells and T cells enabling them to rather effectively recognize malignant cells and annihilate them quite readily. Vitamin E remarkably stabilizes cell membranes largely due to its fat-soluble antioxidant properties and profoundly exhibits anti-inflammatory effects. Antioxidants very vigorously help modulate inflammatory responses that crudely accompany cancer treatments alongside various nasty bodily reactions and side effects (Yang et al, 2018).

Debilitating fatigue frequently besets patients suffering nasty side effects from chronic inflammation like nausea and neutropenia severely impacting lives. Antioxidants fairly effectively mitigate nasty side effects by significantly lowering oxidative damage thereby noticeably enhancing overall effectiveness of various cancer therapies. Antioxidants shield immune cells from oxidative stress damage playing a crucial albeit understated role in fostering somewhat balanced immune responses thereby encourage cancer therapy recovery rather effectively.

3.2.3. Vitamin D: Immune Regulation and Cancer Therapy

Vitamin D plays a crucial role in regulating immune responses effectively through various intricate cellular mechanisms mostly quite profoundly. 1,25-dihydroxyvitamin D influences differentiation of various immune cells including T cells and profoundly impacts activation of macrophages and dendritic cells. Vitamin D significantly modulates immune surveillance by facilitating detection and elimination of cancer cells through various crucial immune mechanisms essentially. Sufficiently high vitamin D levels appear linked very cryptically to enhanceed immunity and very markedly better outcomes in some cancer therapies (Aranow C, 2011).

Vitamin D deficiency gravely debilitates bodily defenses leaving it woefully unprepared fend off nasty tumours somewhat over lengthy periods naturally. Severe vitamin D deficiency quite possibly impairs immune cells' capacity drastically and destroys cancerous cells thereby diminishing effectiveness of cancer treatments significantly. Optimal vitamin D levels enhance cytotoxic activity of T cells and natural killer cells crucial for immune system tumour cell elimination. Vitamin D becomes crucial occasionally for tumour suppression mediated by immune systems thereby improving overall outcomes significantly in such dire cases. Vitamin D supplementation somewhat effectively boosts efficacy of cancer treatments including immunotherapy in various regimens with very decent results (Aranow C, 2011).

Checkpoint inhibitors may work way more effectively in patients with higher vitamin D levels by blocking proteins that normally suppress immune response mechanisms. Vitamin D may possibly make tumours vulnerable fairly effectively to destruction by immune systems reversing immune resistance in them very effectively. Vitamin D's therapeutic potential in cancer treatment gets highlighted effectively by surmounting tumour immune evasion mechanisms with considerable efficacy obviously. Maintaining sufficient vitamin D nowadays may offer a valuable strategy for effectively encourage outcomes of cancer treatment through supplementation or sun exposure (Lao et al, 2022).

3.2.4. Polyphenols: Bioactive Compounds with Anticancer Properties

Polyphenols encompass myriad phytochemicals richly embedded in sundry plant-derived foods like fruits veggies tea and surprisingly dark chocolate. Compounds have been rather extensively studied lately owing largely to markedly beneficial impacts on overall health and on immunity against cancer cells. Polyphenols heavily support immune responses via antioxidant properties and may significantly impact prevention or treatment of various cancers greatly. Resveratrol a polyphenol found mostly in red wine boosts immunity quite effectively and has rather impressive capabilities overall. Tumour cell recognition and elimination relies heavily on activation of immune cells such as T lymphocytes and natural killer cells occurring effectively (Pandey and Rizvi, 2009).

Resveratrol very effectively boosts production of key cytokines like tumour necrosis factor-alpha thereby significantly enhancing immune response against various cancers nowadays. Resveratrol quite effectively enhance bodily defenses against tumours by very subtly modulating a myriad of immune pathways normally. Epigallocatechin gallate a potent polyphenol found abundantly in green tea decidedly exhibits markedly antioxidant properties and yields profoundly anti-inflammatory effects. EGCG markedly enhances chemotherapy and immunotherapy efficacy by reducing oxidative stress and vigorously promoting activation of immune cells. Cancer treatments become remarkably more effective largely thanks to its propensity for modulating immune responses thereby rendering oncology quite valuable (Pandey and Rizvi, 2009).

Polyphenols may help surmount resistance related to immune checkpoint a mechanism tumours utilize rather frequently evading immune surveillance very effectively. Polyphenols ostensibly influence immune checkpoints such as PD-1 or CTLA-4 that tumours hijack very effectively suppressing immune responses vigorously. Polyphenols make tumours rather susceptible to immune attack by tinkering with checkpoints thus potentially greatly enhancing effectiveness of various immune-based therapies. Polyphenols enhance immune function and synergize quite effectively with conventional cancer therapies greatly improving outcomes in most patients naturally (Wang et al, 2022).

3.2.5. Probiotics and Gut Microbiota in Cancer Therapy

Recent studies underscore gut microbiota's profound impact on various immune responses during some very unconventional cancer treatments quite remarkably. Dysbiosis severely impairs immune function hindering cancer therapy significantly under certain obscure conditions as gut microbiome interacts very intricately with immune system. Probiotics harbouring live microbes bestow health benefits onto people by substantially tweaking gut flora and markedly impacting diverse immune responses. Probiotics vigorously stimulate production of antibodies and activate T cells thereby enhancing NK cell activity effectively eradicating cancer cells. Probiotics boost effectiveness of immune checkpoint inhibitors remarkably within various cancer immunotherapy contexts nowadays with surprising efficacy and heightened potency. They effectively accomplish this feat by fostering activation of immune systems and dampening inflammation within tumour microenvironments surrounding cancer cells (Gopalakrishnan et al, 2018).

A healthy gut microbiota greatly lessens toxic side effects of cancer treatment and improves overall quality of life for patients undergoing treatment. Modulating immune responses remarkably well nowadays offers a potentially efficacious strategy for encourage effectiveness of cancer therapy through nutrition's varied capacity. Omega-3 fatty acids and antioxidants alongside vitamin D polyphenols probiotics can be incorporated rather effectively into regimens for treating cancer nowadays. Cancer therapies get augmented by nutritional interventions which mitigate rather nasty side effects and reduce overall risk remarkably improving patient outcomes. Cancer treatment regimens infused with nutritional strategies provide a holistic approach underscoring significance of balanced diets supporting various bodily functions thoroughly. Nutritional oncology research evolves quickly and becomes integral with cancer immunotherapy in modified treatment regimens enhancing life quality and long-term survival prospects for numerous patients (Gopalakrishnan et al, 2018).

4. Diet and Immune System Function

Body's defense mechanism against infections operates quite effectively normally within human physiology serving as primary shield. Ongoing tumour surveillance enables immune system to vigilantly identify aberrant cells and eliminate them thereby mostly thwarting proliferation into cancers. Genetics and lifestyle choices drastically shape this process amidst sundry environmental exposures and very significantly too under normal circumstances. Nutritional intake markedly modulates immune system function with growing evidence suggesting tumour surveillance mechanisms are impaired or significantly enhanced thereby. Nutrients surprisingly exert influence on immune surveillance and tumourigenesis through both direct pathways and relatively obscure dietary mechanisms. Biological mechanisms underlying complex interactions are reviewed alongside impact of certain dietary components on various immune cell functions and broader cancer survivorship implications.

4.1. Tumour Surveillance: The Immune System at Work

Tumour surveillance enables body to identify abnormal cells often called neoplastic cells with fairly high propensity for becoming cancerous very rapidly. Immune system deploys multifaceted strategy detecting cells subtly via innate responses and adaptive ones maintaining cellular integrity preventing tumour formation quietly. Innate immunity operates rapidly from outset as a swift non-specific defense mechanism against tumour cells very effectively. Dendritic cells and macrophages recognize stressed tumour cells with altered morphology on their surface quite naturally and with great specificity. NK cells destroy tumour cells with altered MHC I molecules very frequently observed in transformed cells exhibiting quite abnormal behavior (Swann and Smyth, 2007).

Immune cells recognize patterns of abnormality on tumour cells like upregulated stress proteins and mutated surface markers distinguishing them from healthy cells. Tumour cells frequently dodge innate immunity with stealth and very soon adaptive immune response retaliates with vehemence quite rapidly. Response gets tailored rather meticulously around unique tumour characteristics with high specificity. Cytotoxic T cells ravage bodily tissues swiftly killing tumour cells by targeting tumour-associated antigens present uniquely on cancerous cell surfaces. CD4+ helper T cells greatly facilitate activation of various immune cells thereby mostly ensuring a somewhat coordinated response effectively. B lymphocytes produce antibodies flagging tumour cells for destruction and further vigorously enhancing elimination mediated by various immune responses (Swann and Smyth, 2007).

Malignant cells have quietly spawned numerous furtive strategies under radar of elaborate immune responses mounted against them by human bodies. Tumours often drastically downregulate tumour antigen expression making them far less recognizable by various immune cells lingering ominously in vicinity. Cytokines with immunosuppressive properties are secreted and a rather hostile microenvironment gets created or molecules like PD-L1 express immune checkpoint functions. Tumours evade detection and proliferate relentlessly under such strategies starkly highlighting complexity of cancer immunoevasion in diverse murky contexts. Tumour surveillance and evasion mechanisms must be thoroughly grasped for therapies that remarkably boost cancer treatment outcomes by enhancing immune recognition (Kallingal et al, 2023).

4.2. How Diet Affects Immune System Function

Diet plays a crucial role in shaping immune system functionality and certain dietary components directly affect immune responses potentially enhancing tumour surveillance quite remarkably. Diet influences immunity in various primary ways notably through subtle yet crucial bodily adjustments and physiological responses.

4.2.1. Macronutrients and Immune Health

Proteins fats and carbohydrates play a vital role quite crucially in encourage immune function vital for thwarting nasty tumours effectively overall. Optimal immune responses are ensured and bodily defenses enhanceed very effectively against rogue cells including cancerous ones with a well-balanced intake. Proteins serve as fundamental building blocks of immune systems being required quite extensively for synthesis of various antibodies and cytokines or T cells. Tumourous entities are destroyed quite swiftly by cells playing a crucial role in recognition and elimination of cancer cells rapidly. Amino acids vitally function down there as basic units of proteins crucial for immune cell activity. Glutamine and arginine crucially support immune cells like T cells requiring these amino acids for optimal functionality in a rather complex manner (Munteanu and Schwartz, 2022).

Deficiency in essential amino acids precipitates markedly weakened immune responses impairing bodily ability fighting off nasty tumours rather vigorously and opportunistic infections. Adequate protein intake fosters robust immunity capable of vigorously detecting malignant cells and mounting potent counterattacks fairly effectively. Dietary fats profoundly impact immune function variably based on type and quantity consumed recklessly over some period naturally in most individuals. Omega-3 polyunsaturated fatty acids found in fatty fish and in walnuts have profoundly anti-inflammatory properties that occur very naturally.

Omega-3s enhance activity of natural killer cells that play a pivotal role in immune surveillance and destroy tumour cells very vigorously. Omega-6 fatty acids abundant in processed foods and deep-fried food can very significantly promote chronic inflammation and suppress immune response badly. Western diets typically involve gorging on omega-6 fats which may badly hamper immunity from detecting rogue cells thereby facilitating tumour growth unimpeded (Munteanu and Schwartz, 2022).

Veggies and whole grains rich in fibre help regulate blood sugar levels remarkably and enhance immune function quite ordinarily. Fibre enhance gut health remarkably linking it to very strong immune responses and boosting bodily resilience quite vividly overall. Consuming copious amounts of refined sugars and simple carbs sparks systemic inflammation compromising immune function and fostering cancer growth very readily. Elevated glucose concentrations foster chronic inflammation thereby creating an environment strangely conducive to tumourigenesis and crippling immune surveillance of malignant cellular entities rapidly. Macronutrient balance plays a pivotal role in supporting immune health, with each nutrient strongly influencing the activity of immune cells and overall surveillance mechanisms. Diets rich in protein and complex carbohydrates with healthy fats maintain strong immunity and significantly reduce the risk of certain cancers (Alahmari LA, 2024).

4.2.2. Micronutrients and Immune Support

Vitamins and minerals play a crucial role in naturally supporting immune function very effectively throughout the human body with utmost efficacy. Vitamin D plays a crucial role in regulating immune responses effectively amidst various micronutrients that significantly enhance tumour surveillance mechanisms. Vitamin D remarkably enhance T cell differentiation, and macrophage function gets boosted somewhat while pro-inflammatory cytokines get somewhat counterbalanced by anti-inflammatory ones. Low vitamin D levels might significantly hamper immune function, thereby potentially elevating the risk of various cancers quite substantially over quite some time. Vitamin D supplementation has been linked mostly in cancer research to markedly improved immune responses, especially in breast cancer (Mitra et al, 2022).

Retinoic acid derived from vitamin A plays a crucial role in regulating immune responses by fostering T cell maturation and encourage activity of dendritic cells vigorously. Retinoic acid derived from vitamin A fosters T cell maturation quite effectively and enhance activity of dendritic cells very significantly. Vitamin A deficiency has been tenuously linked to woefully impaired immune responses and surging susceptibility to nasty infections or cancer. Both vitamins C and E possess antioxidant properties, protecting immune cells from oxidative damage. Vitamin A's impact on immunity underscores considerable significance in thwarting cancer benefiting from dietary sources like carotenoids found quite abundantly in rather colorful veggies (Mitra et al, 2022).

Vitamin C and E fiercely possess antioxidant properties protecting immune cells from oxidative damage quite effectively within human bodies. Zinc supports immune function by vigorously promoting T cell proliferation. Essential trace element Selenium enhance macrophage activity very significantly. Vitamin C activates T cells whereas vitamin E rather substantially boosts activity of NK cells very deeply in the body. Vitamins collectively maintain immune homeostasis remarkably well and enhance antitumour responses quite effectively in a rather unusually synergistic manner (Traber and Stevens, 2011).

4.2.3. Bioactive Compounds and Their Role in Immune Modulation

Bioactive compounds present in various plant-based foods emerge rather powerfully as potent regulators of immune function in tumour surveillance modulation lately. Polyphenols flavonoids and sulforaphane garner attention rapidly for encourage immune responses and mitigating inflammation significantly improving overall bodily capacity. Polyphenols abundant in tea wine and various fruits possess potent antioxidant properties and exhibit remarkably strong anti-inflammatory effects normally. Polyphenols studied extensively include resveratrol present in red wine and grapes curcumin derived from turmeric and EGCG extracted mainly from green tea. Compounds tweak signalling pathways inside immune cells thereby boosting T cell activity and unleashing natural killer cells that spot tumour cells with ease effectively (Rivero-Pino and Montserrat-de la Paz, 2024).

Polyphenols recently found to downregulate expression of immunosuppressive cytokines within tumour microenvironments rendering cancer cells rather vulnerable to immune cell destruction. Polyphenols synergize effectively with conventional cancer treatments by enhancing immune function and suppressing inflammation significantly in various bodily contexts very nastily. Flavonoids a subclass of polyphenols exist abundantly very much everywhere in foods such as berries onions and dark chocolate. Compounds have been shown enhancing function of dendritic cells crucially involved in antigen presentation vigorously promoting activation and proliferation of T cells. Quercetin and similar flavonoids exhibit profoundly anti-inflammatory properties helping create a somewhat conducive milieu for destruction of cancer cells mediated by immune responses. Flavonoids very effectively enhance immune defense against tumours by supporting dendritic cell function and they enhance T cell responses robustly (Rivero-Pino and Montserrat-de la Paz, 2024).

Sulforaphane present remarkably in cruciferous veggies like broccoli and kale possibly enhances immune surveillance significantly as a mighty bioactive compound. Sulforaphane boosts antioxidant production quite rapidly and triggers Nrf2 transcription factor very effectively shielding cells from oxidative damage meanwhile. Sulforaphane very effectively curbs chronic inflammation which can spur tumour growth downstream and hinder various immune responses in a major way . Sulforaphane very significantly ramps up activity of immune cells and fosters a healthy inflammatory response thereby supporting bodily ability to eradicate cancerous cells. Bioactive compounds function synergistically modulating immune response rather vigorously enhancing surveillance greatly supporting efforts for cancer prevention (Ruhee and Suzuki, 2020).

4.3. The Impact of Diet on Tumour Microenvironment and Immune Escape Mechanisms

Tumours have spawned myriad crafty tactics evading immune surveillance effectively a process whereby cancer cells get detected then subsequently eliminated. Such strategies facilitate tumour growth very vigorously despite fervent bodily defenses kicking in against them with considerable countervailing force. Upregulation of immune checkpoint molecules like PD-L1 happens very frequently and they bind PD-1 receptors on various immune cells thereby inhibiting their activity heavily. Tumours covertly hijack regulatory T cells gradually suppressing immunity and fostering an immunosuppressive milieu eerily around their periphery. Tumours stealthily induce tolerance in immune systems rendering them woefully unable to recognize malignant cells utterly for destruction (Swann and Smyth, 2007).

Dietary factors potentially mitigate remarkably immunosuppressive environment within tumour microenvironments fairly well under rather specific physiological conditions. Tumours exhibit significantly lower pro-inflammatory cytokine levels when subjected to diets abundant in polyphenols and omega-3 fatty acids. Omega-3 fatty acids present in fatty fish or flaxseeds very significantly quell inflammation and rather effectively promote function of immune cells potentially counteracting tumour-induced immune suppression. Polyphenols like resveratrol exhibit profoundly antioxidant effects markedly reducing tumour-associated inflammation and thereby very significantly enhancing diverse immune responses (Swann and Smyth, 2007).

Vitamin D and curcumin may modulate immune checkpoints effectively under diverse physiological states rather surprisingly in many different contexts. Vitamin D has been shown downregulating PD-L1 expression on tumour cells rendering them quite susceptible to a ferocious attack by immune cells. Turmeric's curcumin has been shown vigorously influencing certain checkpoint molecules and ramping up immune response against tumours remarkably. Targeted nutritional regimens may render tumour microenvironments more vulnerable to immune system destruction and enhance various cancer treatments (Tsuji et al, 2023).

4.4. Integrating Diet into Cancer Prevention and Therapy

Integrating nutrition into cancer prevention and therapy becomes increasingly vital strategy amidst mounting evidence diet very significantly modulates immune function. Prevention entails consuming a nutrient rich diet fairly balanced and supportive of immune health thereby enhancing bodily tumour surveillance mechanisms significantly reducing overall cancer risk. Consuming copious amounts of fruits whole grains lean proteins and healthy fats regularly optimizes immune function and mitigates cancer risk substantially. Nutritional interventions adjunct to therapy may enhance effectiveness of immunotherapies and conventional cancer treatments fairly significantly (Janakiram et al, 2016).

Nutritional interventions may enhance effectiveness of immunotherapies and traditional cancer treatments quite significantly alongside therapy post-treatment survivorship hinges precariously on dietary choices. Diet remains a critical health component during survivorship. Nutrition can very significantly ameliorate patient outcomes during therapy by mitigating side effects like oxidative stress and inflammation quite effectively. Diet stays remarkably vital afterwards for overall health maintenance post-treatment during survivorship very well. Nutritious diet rich in essential nutrients supports immune function thereby reducing recurrence risk and fostering long-term health quite effectively preventing secondary malignancies. Dietary factors play quite crucial role in proper functioning of immune system effectively enhancing its tumour surveillance capacity remarkably (Janakiram et al, 2016).

5. Nutritional Interventions to Enhance Immune Defense Against Cancer

Breakthroughs in detection and therapeutic interventions have substantially boosted survival odds globally yet cancer still kills loads of people recently. Cancer biology remains stubbornly complex nowadays with tumour cells evading immune surveillance and presenting challenges for effective treatment despite advancements. Nutritional interventions targeting malignant cells enhance immune defense mechanisms very effectively enhancing cancer therapy markedly these days in various oncology settings. Nutrition plays a crucial role sustaining immune function meanwhile mounting evidence suggests tweaks in diet can significantly boost capacity for detecting cancerous cells very effectively.

Abnormal cells get recognized then subsequently removed by various immune system mechanisms that thwart morphing into full-blown cancerous entities effectively. Cancer cells rapidly devise clandestine mechanisms and grow uncontrollably deep within bodily tissues metastasizing with stealthy aggression underground. Nutritional interventions potentially surmount diverse evasive maneuvers employed by immune systems and significantly amplify effectiveness of various cancer treatments with considerable activation. Nutrition plays a complex role in enhancing cancer immune defense via specific exotic dietary patterns and bioactive compounds with various nutrients (Messerschmidt et al, 2016).

5.1. The Role of the Immune System in Cancer Defense

Multiple facets of immunity work assiduously behind the scenes safeguarding bodily functions from sundry pathogens and neoplasms remarkably well daily. T lymphocytes and natural killer cells alongside macrophages and dendritic cells play crucial roles frequently in various tumour surveillance mechanisms. Cells function critically detecting and eliminating cancerous cells arising within bodily tissues usually very rapidly and extremely effectively . Tumours evade immune responses very effectively and remain significant barriers for cancer elimination by various immune systems rather often nowadays. Cancer cells thwart immune responses via sundry dodgy mechanisms including expression of peculiar immune checkpoint molecules that stifle T cell activation very effectively (Masmoudi et al, 2025).

Production of immunosuppressive cytokines like TGF-β and IL-10 curtails function of various immune cells severely under certain pathological conditions. Regulatory T cells or Tregs recruitment substantially dampens overall immune responses thereby rendering immune cells ineffective at recognizing cancer cells. Mechanisms collectively sabotage immune cells' ability to target cancerous cells for destruction quite effectively in many cases apparently. Certain strategies vigorously enhance immune responses against tumours through some dietary interventions that modulate immune function quite effectively (Masmoudi et al, 2025).

5.2. Nutritional Components That Modulate Immune Function

Abnormal cell growths including certain cancers are thwarted nowadays by immune system which plays crucial role in defending body very effectively. Nutritional components directly impact immune system's ability for recognizing cancer cells swiftly under certain conditions physiologically. Nutrients enhance defense mechanisms significantly by modulating immune cell function and remarkably enhance effectiveness of various cancer treatments. Proteins and constituent amino acids play a crucial role rather fundamentally in function of various immune cells almost everywhere in bodily tissues. Body requires amino acids for synthesizing crucial immune system components like antibodies cytokines T lymphocytes and B lymphocytes very effectively. Amino acids like glutamine play crucial roles in maintaining activity of T cells that detect tumour cells and kill them very swiftly (Coventry and Henneberg, 2016).

Adequate protein intake ensures immune cells function optimally with requisite tools vigorously mounting effective cancer defense mechanisms very robustly. Omega-3 fatty acids play crucial roles in effectively modulating immune function under certain physiological conditions very quietly . Omega-3 polyunsaturated fatty acids present abundantly in fatty fish and certain walnuts surprisingly support natural killer cell activity very effectively. Processed food rife with omega-6 fatty acids fuels chronic inflammation suppressing immune function and spurring cancer progression quite rapidly nowadays. Omega-3 fatty acids and omega-6 fatty acids must be kept in essential balance to prevent tumour growth and maintain immune balance. Vitamins such as vitamin C or vitamin E coupled with antioxidants somewhat effectively play a crucial role in encourage immune function (Coventry and Henneberg, 2016).

Vitamin C enhance immune function significantly by augmenting T cells and natural killer cells whereas vitamin E exerts deeply anti-inflammatory effects . Vitamin D remarkably stands out for regulating differentiation of sundry immune cells thereby encourage body's cancer-fighting prowess with considerable effectiveness down the line. Antioxidants radically neutralize highly reactive oxygen species that ravage immune cells thereby safeguarding their capacity to detect and destroy cancerous cells effectively (Carr and Maggini, 2017).

Flavonoids and polyphenols in plants modulate immune function quite effectively nowadays within various physiological contexts. Resveratrol and epigallocatechin gallate possess potent antioxidant properties enhancing T cells and NK cells activity significantly in red wine and green tea respectively. Bioactive compounds help suppress expression of immunosuppressive cytokines within tumour microenvironment making it rather conducive for immune surveillance and destruction occurs of cancerous cells. Consuming nutritionally balanced meals rich in proteins vitamins and bioactive compounds furnishes essential nutrients necessary for optimizing immunity and encourage capacity to eradicate cancerous cells quite effectively. Nutrients play crucial roles very effectively in modulating various immune responses subtly for cancer prevention and enhancing therapeutic efficacy (Montané et al, 2020).

5.2.1. Omega-3 Fatty Acids: Promoting Antitumour Immunity

Eicosapentaenoic acid and docosahexaenoic acid are polyunsaturated fats found mainly in fatty fish like salmon or in flaxseeds very quietly underground. Essential fats have garnered significant attention recently owing largely to their profoundly anti-inflammatory properties in cancer prevention therapy . Omega-3 fatty acids enhance immune response largely by supercharging activity of T cells crucial for recognizing tumour cells and they eliminate them rather rapidly. Omega-3s vigorously ramp up T cell activation and very rapidly proliferation happens ultimately leading to robust immune response against cancerous cells. Omega-3s enhance bodily defenses rather effectively by activating cytotoxic T cells thereby markedly enhancing eradication of cancerous rogue cells quickly (Rodriguez-Leyva et al, 2010).

Omega-3 fatty acids substantially enhance activity of natural killer cells adept at recognizing cancer cells and killing them quite effectively. Research has shown omega-3s significantly boost natural killer cell activity thereby substantially enhancing their capacity to detect tumour cells and kill them rapidly. Tumour surveillance gets boosted by enhanced NK cell function markedly amplifying immune system's defense against neoplastic growth with great vigor suddenly. Omega-3 fatty acids somewhat effectively modulate immune response daily through various biochemical pathways inhibiting production of pro-inflammatory cytokines. Tumour microenvironment harboring chronic inflammation fosters conditions that suppress immune activity thereby allowing tumours to effectively evade immune surveillance (D'Eliseo and Velotti, 2016).

Omega-3s foster a propitious milieu somewhat for immune cells attacking cancer cells by diminishing pro-inflammatory molecules significantly in bodily fluids. Counteraction of immune suppression occurs, thereby vigorously boosting bodily ability, effectively mounting rather defensive responses under various circumstances quite rapidly. Omega-3 supplementation crudely sensitises stubborn tumours towards chemotherapy and immunotherapy, potentially according to findings from sundry recent studies. Omega-3s ramp up immune cell activity very vigorously and modulate inflammation, thereby heightening treatment efficacy, making tumour cells rather susceptible to immune response mediated destruction now. Dietary intake of omega-3 fatty acids may yield significant immune-boosting benefits during various cancer therapies and cancer prevention efforts quite effectively. Omega-3s remarkably enhance bodily defences against cancer very effectively by enhancing the function of immune cells and reducing tumour-induced inflammation (D'Eliseo and Velotti, 2016).

5.2.2. Antioxidants: Supporting Immune Function and Tumour Defence

Chemotherapy and similar cancer treatments wildly boost reactive oxygen species production while bodily neutralisation mechanisms remain somewhat impaired under stress. Oxidative stress ravages tumour cells and concomitantly debilitates immune function, thereby rendering eradication of cancer cells a very formidable task entirely. Antioxidant nutrients crucially safeguard immune cells from oxidative stress, thereby keeping the immune system robust and responsive against cancer effectively. Vitamin C a potent antioxidant maintains immune health vitally during cancer treatments that induce extremely high oxidative stress levels. Vitamin C shields T cells and natural killer cells from oxidative stress thereby preserving capacity for robust immune surveillance and vigorously thwarting tumour cell proliferation (Yang et al, 2018).

Vitamin C effectively regenerates immune cells supporting proliferation very significantly in various studies and boosts cytotoxic activity remarkably well too. Vitamin C very significantly enhances phagocytic activity of macrophages encourage overall immune response against cancer extremely effectively. Vitamin E somewhat effectively reduces oxidative damage in cellular membranes thereby protecting immune cells from severe stress-induced dysfunction quite remarkably. NK cells and macrophages play a pivotal role in recognizing cancer cells effectively and destroying them with considerable vigor subsequently. Vitamin E fosters longevity in certain immune cells thereby making them rather effective against tumour cells quite remarkably under various conditions. Vitamin E modulates inflammatory cytokines effectively thereby creating a favorable milieu for cancer-fighting immune cells that perform optimally under certain conditions (Yang et al, 2018).

Selenium crucially enables activity of glutathione peroxidase an antioxidant enzyme, fairly effectively neutralising ROS in various cellular contexts. Selenium plays a vital role in maintaining immune cell integrity during cancer treatment because oxidative stress severely impairs normal immune function. Selenium levels hovering just above deficiency marks correspond with sluggish immune responses but supplementation boosts NK cell activity rapidly and fortifies T cell-mediated immunity. Selenium remarkably enhance immune system function by enhancing antioxidant defenses and facilitates capacity to vanquish cancerous cells with great effectiveness thereby. Selenium and vitamins C and E mitigate oxidative stress greatly, thereby safeguarding immune cells and fostering tumour destruction via mediation of immunity. Crucial roles surface haphazardly during cancer therapies fostering oxidative stress which enables immune systems keenly detect tumour cells rather precisely. Integrating foods rich in antioxidants or certain supplements into regimens for cancer therapy may significantly enhance immune response and promote destruction of tumours (Lee et al, 2025).

5.2.3. Vitamin D: Enhancing Immune Surveillance

Vitamin D plays a crucial role in maintaining bone health while its newly discovered function in immune regulation has sparked intense cancer research recently and 1,25-dihydroxyvitamin D interacts very vigorously with various immune cells like T cells and macrophages promoting activation down the line very effectively. Vitamin D crucially modulates immune response making it an essential nutrient in body's defense against various cancers quite remarkably every day. Vitamin D very significantly enhance immune defense by supercharging T cell differentiation remarkably inside bodies of humans very effectively. T cells play a pivotal role in orchestrating an immune response against malignant cells thereby facilitating tumour surveillance remarkably well amidst various obstacles (Bikle DD, 2010).

Vitamin D facilitates differentiation of naive T cells into cytotoxic T cells that very effectively target cancer cells killing them. Vitamin D fosters T cell activation thereby enabling immune system recognition of aberrant cells which are subsequently destroyed before morphing into full-blown cancer. Vitamin D's effects target macrophages heavily and they engulf pathogens and cancer cells quite vigorously with rather reckless abandon. Vitamin D activates macrophages making them somewhat more adept at recognizing tumour cells and phagocytosing them vigorously afterwards with increased efficacy. Activation boosts bodily capacity quite effectively for clearing cancerous cells and contributes significantly to overall enhanced immune surveillance. Vitamin D plays a crucial albeit somewhat obscure role in maintaining an intricate balance between pro-inflammatory cytokines and their anti-inflammatory counterparts effectively (Bikle DD, 2010).

Crucial equilibrium maintains immune response steadfast avoiding perilous vacillation between supine tolerance letting malignancies stealthily escape surveillance and frenzied hyperactivity wreaking havoc indiscriminately. Vitamin D modulates cytokine production quite effectively helping foster an optimal immune milieu for thwarting cancer onset and encourage overall immune function. Numerous studies recently conducted worldwide showed vitamin D deficiency linked with impaired immune function and elevated cancer risk very frequently. Deficient vitamin D levels cripple bodily ability to summon effective immune response and cancer cells evade detection stealthily most times. Vitamin D supplementation enhance immune responses very significantly and augments efficacy of various cancer therapies mostly in breast cancer and colon cancer. Vitamin D plays crucial role in immune function regulation and sufficient levels are vital for robust cancer responses effectively. Vitamin D supplementation offers very significant adjunctive benefits for boosting immune response and amplifying effectiveness of various cancer therapies these days (Bikle DD, 2010).

5.2.4. Polyphenols: Bioactive Compounds for Immune Enhancement

Polyphenols have garnered significant attention remarkably for anti-inflammatory effects in various plant-based foods such as exotic fruits and green tea. Diverse natural compounds very significantly enhance immune function and facilitate cancer combat through modulation of several key immune response aspects effectively. Resveratrol quite frequently shows up in red wine grapes and various berry types rather apparently. Resveratrol has been shown to activate T cells crucial for recognizing cancerous cells and very vigorously attacking them in several different studies. Resveratrol very significantly boosts cytokine production and stimulates an antitumour immune response encouraging T cells targeting cancerous cells for eventual destruction rapidly. Adaptive immunity gets enhanceed quite effectively by such an immunomodulatory effect that recognizes cancer-associated antigens and responds rather specifically (El Oirdi M, 2024).

Naturally curcumin possesses profoundly potent anti-inflammatory properties and exhibits remarkably strong antioxidant effects being a polyphenol abundant in turmeric. Curcumin modulates immune checkpoints such as PD-L1 which tumours frequently hijack very effectively to evade various immune surveillance mechanisms. Curcumin suppresses specific checkpoints rendering tumours rather susceptible to immune onslaught and substantially augmenting immune system's ability to detect cancer cells. Curcumin inhibits tumour growth significantly and reduces metastasis making it a valuable adjunct in cancer therapies very effectively nowadays. Epigallocatechin gallate abounds quietly in green tea remarkably boosting natural killer cells and tweaking T cells regulatory functions somewhat (El Oirdi M, 2024).

EGCG significantly amplifies natural killer cells' activity which play crucial roles in targeting cancer cells effectively within immune system. EGCG stimulates NK cells and reduces suppressive effects of Tregs slyly recruited by various tumours to entirely dodge immune mechanisms. EGCG facilitates tumour destruction by dampening Treg activity subsequently skewing immune response balance heavily toward eradication of cancer cells very effectively. Polyphenols such as resveratrol curcumin and EGCG modulate tumour microenvironment very effectively with markedly varied potency. Compounds create hostile microenvironments suppressing immunity fairly ineffectively and rendering conditions very conducive for very active immune cells (Talib et al, 2024).

Enhancement of overall immune response against tumours naturally enhance immune surveillance and effectively supports various cancer therapies simultaneously. Incorporating polyphenol-rich foods into one's diet may somewhat effectively offer a complementary strategy supporting cancer prevention endeavors alongside immune system function. Polyphenolic compounds furnish valuable backing for cancer therapies and offer routes for nutritional interventions geared towards substantial immune enhancement.

5.3. Probiotics and Gut Microbiota

Diverse microorganisms residing within gastrointestinal tract have emerged rather quietly as crucial players in immune regulation encompassing tumour surveillance mechanisms. Gut microbiome profoundly influences activity of various immune cells thereby significantly shaping cancer response in body through myriad complex mechanisms. Fermentation of dietary fibre yields short-chain fatty acids and other metabolites which play a pivotal role in quietly modulating immune function . Fruits and whole grains rich in fibre foster growth of beneficial gut bacteria producing SCFAs like butyrate subsequently in the colon. SCFAs act as an energy source profoundly influencing various aspects of immune cell function in human body fairly deeply (Zhao et al, 2023).

SCFAs markedly amplify natural killer cells' activity and T cells crucially pinpoint cancerous cells rather effectively eliminating them swiftly. Fibre and its microbiota-driven metabolites enhance immune surveillance by spurring differentiation and activation of certain immune cells more effectively targeting tumour cells. Live beneficial microorganisms conferring health benefits upon consumption in adequate amounts play a vital role in modulating various immune responses greatly. Tumours frequently hijack immune checkpoint molecules such as PD-1 or CTLA-4 to dodge detection by various immune cells apparently. Probiotics can markedly boost effectiveness of immunotherapies such as checkpoint inhibitors that revive immune system's tumour-fighting capabilities by tweaking key molecular checkpoints (Zhao et al, 2023).

Probiotics modulate production of anti-inflammatory cytokines thereby helping reduce systemic inflammation fairly quietly amidst various bodily functions underneath. Modulation fosters a very propitious tumour microenvironment rendering tumours fairly unlikely to flourish and immune cells more likely eradicate them vigorously. Evidence mounts quickly that tweaks like boosting fibre consumption or injecting probiotics into gut can significantly juice up immune function very rapidly. Microbiota-targeted interventions are potentially pivotal in some cutting-edge cancer treatment regimens presently underscoring a increasing trove of research findings. A healthier gut microbiome might remarkably enhance immune system function and very significantly enhance effectiveness of cancer therapies such as immunotherapy. Gut microbiota emerges rather promisingly as a frontier in cancer immunity. Probiotics and fibre-rich diets may offer novel cancer treatment options by significantly modulating tumour microenvironment and influencing immune cell function (Mazziotta et al, 2023).

5.4. Dietary Patterns for Enhancing Immune Defense

Dietary patterns play a pivotal role in maintaining optimal immune function within contexts of cancer prevention and assorted therapeutic regimens. Whole foods loaded with fruits and lean proteins significantly enhance immune health by dialing down chronic inflammation very substantially over time. Malignant cells are obliterated with heightened vigilance and precision naturally by eating habits that foster a remarkably robust immune system. Plethora of research underscores Mediterranean diets as remarkably efficacious in encourage immune function very well across sundry populations worldwide nowadays. This diet heavily emphasizes consumption mostly of vegetables fruits and legumes alongside healthy fats from olive oil and various nuts. Fatty fish laden with omega-3 acids possess anti-inflammatory properties boosting immunity moderately in people consuming them somewhat regularly (Golonko et al, 2024).

Studies reveal adherence to Mediterranean diets correlates strongly with suppressed inflammation and significantly enhanceed immune function against a myriad of cancer types. Tumour immunity gets a potent boost from Mediterranean diet comprising antioxidant-rich foods heart-healthy fats and sizeable amounts of omega-3 fatty acids. Diets comprising mainly plants teeming with fibre antioxidants, and polyphenols enhance gut microbiota very effectively and foster fairly robust immune health. Fibre from fruits and whole grains nourishes gut microbes very richly, producing metabolites that modulate immune response in a highly positive manner. Phytonutrients like flavonoids and polyphenols abound in plant-based diets exhibiting potent antioxidant properties and very effective anti-inflammatory effects (Golonko et al, 2024).

Dietary components modulate immune response effectively lowering cancer risk and encourage responses amidst gruelling chemotherapy sessions very notably. Nutritional tweaks can enhance bodily defenses against cancer quite remarkably as we probe nuanced interplay between diet and immune function nowadays deeply. Omega-3 fatty acids and antioxidants rich in polyphenols can be harnessed effectively in cancer treatment strategies optimizing immune responses remarkably well. Dietary modifications might surprisingly emerge as a crucial cornerstone of personalized cancer care when used alongside various effective immunotherapies in clinical cancer treatment. Boosting immunity remarkably enhances life quality and patient outcomes exhibit much better treatment tolerance with significantly lower risks of recurrence afterwards (Janakiram et al, 2016).

6. Immune Evasion Mechanisms in Cancer and the Role of Nutrition

Cancer cells fervently deploy myriad clandestine subterfuges beneath radar and evade destruction with stealthy precision by immune systems ordinarily. Immune system functions with remarkable finesse identifying aberrant cells and eradicating them rather quickly usually with great success almost always. Tumours hijack immune pathways deploying various clandestine tactics and cultivate an immunosuppressive microenvironment fostering unbridled growth and dubious survival mechanisms simultaneously. Cancer cells often upregulate immune checkpoint molecules like PD-L1 or CTLA-4 thereby evading surveillance by immune system very effectively nowadays. Tumour cells and surrounding cells in tumour microenvironment express proteins that rather vigorously inhibit activation of T cells and natural killer cells. Cancer cells stealthily evade detection under immune system's radar by engaging checkpoints and effectively turning off various immune responses suddenly (Costoya and Arce, 2023).

Cancer cells secrete immunosuppressive cytokines such as TGF-β very effectively dampening immune responses and further hindering tumour surveillance . Tumours induce immune tolerance making it rather arduous for various immune systems to mount an efficacious defense rather effectively inside body tissues. New findings nowadays suggest nutritional interventions effectively counteract immune evasion playing a rather pivotal role with surprising frequency in research lately. Diets rich in polyphenols enhance immune pathways significantly within tumour microenvironment and reduce inflammatory burden very substantially with omega-3 fatty acids present. Curcumin has been shown modulating immune checkpoints rather effectively thereby potentially reversing resistance in diverse immune systems very irregularly nowadays. Omega-3 fatty acids ostensibly mitigate inflammation quite profoundly and NK cell efficacy gets a considerable boost subsequently making cancer cells vulnerable (Yang et al, 2010).

Antioxidants like vitamin C or vitamin E help protect immune cells very radically from oxidative stress so they remain fairly effective. Diets rich in fibre curiously enhance gut microbiome very effectively thereby influencing immune system function and cultivating environment conducive to tumour destruction. Grasping nuances of immune evasion mechanisms is vital nowadays for devising very potent treatments against cancer effectively with significant nutritional impact. Strategically incorporating specific nutritional interventions may possibly reverse immune suppression and greatly enhance effectiveness of various cancer treatments including cutting-edge immunotherapy. Nutrients modulate immune function effectively nowadays offering complementary strategies for overcoming cancer's evasive mechanisms through diverse dietary patterns (Munteanu et al, 2024).

6.1. Immune Evasion Mechanisms in Cancer

Cancer cells employ myriad dodgy tactics evading detection by immune systems allowing utterly uncontrolled growth and very chaotic metastasis subsequently. Several key strategies can be broadly categorized from immune cell activation onwards involving mechanisms that facilitate tumour cell destruction gradually.

6.1.1. Immune Checkpoint Inhibition

Tumours evade immune detection rather effectively through upregulation of specific checkpoints and myriad other clandestine mechanisms very naturally. Crucial regulatory proteins ordinarily maintain immune tolerance beneath stringent thresholds and prevent autoimmunity with controlled immune responses effectively. Cancer cells frequently hijack such checkpoints and suppress immune activation stealthily persisting deep within various bodily tissues over prolonged periods normally. Programmed cell death protein 1 (PD1) along with its ligand PD-L1 are studied extensively amidst plethora of immune checkpoint molecules apparently (Kim et al, 2022).

PD-1 manifests as inhibitory receptor on T cells' surface whereas PD-L1 often materializes on cancer cells amidst tumour microenvironment very frequently. PD-L1 binding transmits an inhibitory signal rather stealthily to T cells which then dampen their frantic activity very effectively afterwards. Tumours cleverly evade onslaught from immune system through this pivotal interaction fueling proliferation amidst plethora of surrounding immune cells. CTLA-4 or cytotoxic T-lymphocyte-associated protein 4 constitutes another crucial immune checkpoint remarkably alongside PD-1 and PD-L1 axis. CTLA-4 exerts remarkably potent inhibitory effects on T cells significantly dampening activation of various immune responses quite profoundly. It ostensibly outcompetes co-stimulatory molecule CD28 hindering full activation of T cells responding vigorously against various kinds of tumour cells (Kim et al, 2022).

Overexpression of certain immune checkpoints occurs frequently in cancer creating novel therapeutic opportunities thereby leading to ICI development. ICIs block interaction between checkpoint molecules such as PD-1 or PD-L1 and CTLA-4 restoring T cell activation and boosting immune system ability substantially to recognize tumour cells. Nivolumab alongside ipilimumab have rather remarkably revolutionized treatment of cancers such as melanoma or non-small cell lung cancer yielding very durable responses (Kim et al, 2022).

6.1.2. Recruitment of Regulatory T Cells (Tregs)

Cancer cells vigorously exploit regulatory T cells and create an immunosuppressive tumour microenvironment allowing quite effective immune evasion with help from other molecules. Tregs play crucial role in maintaining immune tolerance mainly by throttling aberrant responses thereby precluding autoimmunity quite effectively under various physiological conditions. Tumours co-opt regulatory function directing Tregs toward tumour sites and very vigorously suppress anti-tumour immune responses over fairly lengthy periods. Tregs amass inside tumour microenvironments through numerous signaling pathways mediated mostly by various cell surface receptors and some soluble factors. Tumour cells spew forth various chemokines and cytokines locally recruiting Tregs which can subsequently suppress activity of cancer recognizing immune cells (Chaudhary and Elkord, 2016).

Tregs mostly suppress effector T cells comprising cytotoxic T lymphocytes skilled at directly killing tumour cells within diverse cancerous tissue environments. Tregs effectively foster an environment conducive for proliferation of cancer cells by suppressing T cell activation and function very aggressively. Tregs suppress immune responses very effectively largely through secretion of immunosuppressive cytokines like transforming growth factor-beta and some interleukin-10. Cytokines surprisingly dampen activity of NK cells and macrophages further contributing significantly quite profoundly to overall immune suppression. Tregs express CTLA-4 which throttles activation of effector T cells and directly offs immune cells through granzyme B and perforin rather quietly (Chaudhary and Elkord, 2016). Tregs accumulate within tumour microenvironments ultimately blunting immune response thereby facilitating progression rather quickly and fostering occurrence of metastasis. Treg-targeted therapies are being explored vigorously nowadays and may eventually yield better outcomes in cancer treatment with reversed immunosuppressive state. Researchers hope anti-tumour immunity gets enhanced and tumours become sensitized to existing therapies by depleting Tregs or hindering suppressive action markedly (Chaudhary and Elkord, 2016).

6.1.3. Secretion of Immunosuppressive Cytokines

Tumours utilize immunosuppressive cytokines very effectively evading immune surveillance and crushing responses targeting rogue cancer cells alongside regulatory T cells. Cytokines quietly reshape tumour microenvironment drastically favoring tolerance of immune systems and hindering activation of effective responses. Tumour cells secrete key immunosuppressive cytokines most notably Transforming Growth Factor-beta a potent cytokine that lurks quietly within tumour microenvironment. TGF-β functions mightily as suppressor of immune response largely behind the scenes. It exerts inhibitory effects mainly by downregulating activity of cytotoxic T cells and natural killer cells, crucial for killing rogue cancer cells. TGF-β furthers the differentiation of regulatory T cells, namely Tregs thereby heavily contributing to effective suppression of various immune responses. TGF-β quite skillfully helps tumours evade detection by suppressing activation of various effector immune cells with immense effectiveness (Tie et al, 2022).

Elevated TGF-β levels in tumour microenvironment frequently portend poor outcomes by facilitating swift tumour proliferation and metastasis at distant sites. IL-10 another immunosuppressive cytokine quite effectively helps create an environment conducive to growth of tumours very readily. It suppresses activity of pro-inflammatory cytokines culpable for vigorously activating immune cells and fighting tumours under certain pathological conditions. IL-10 heavily inhibits production of crucial cytokines thereby profoundly dampening activation and function of effector T cells and macrophages. IL-10 markedly dampens immune system efficacy thereby facilitating tumour proliferation largely unhindered by strong antitumour responses in a rather natural way. Indoleamine 2 3-dioxygenase or IDO efficiently catalyzes degradation of tryptophan which many immune cells including T cells need for proper functioning (Tie et al, 2022).

IDO effectively suppresses T cell activation and proliferation by depleting tryptophan deeply within tumour microenvironments leading to profound tolerance. Tryptophan deficiency stemming from this process fosters expansion of Tregs further dampening immune responses very substantially in various ways. IDO-mediated immune suppression crucially fuels tumour immune resistance and abets escape from immune surveillance rather effectively in various metastatic cancers. Tumour cells evade destruction via highly immunosuppressive cytokines that synergize fairly often and create an environment inhibiting immune cells effectively. Secretion of certain cytokines within tumour microenvironments facilitates immune evasion and blocking such factors presents a promising avenue for cancer immunotherapy. Reinvigorating those pathways might significantly boost effectiveness of immune checkpoint inhibitors and other assorted cancer treatments quite remarkably (Munn et al, 2016).

6.1.4. Antigen Loss and Tumour Heterogeneity

Tumour cells surreptitiously employ various shifty strategies evading immune detection and loss of tumour-associated antigens emerges as a remarkably insidious mechanism. Tumour cells often mutate rapidly becoming genetically unstable and exhibiting wildly divergent antigen expression profiles over fairly short periods sometimes. Tumour cell surfaces display diverse antigens and antigenic variation poses significant problems for immune system functionality relying heavily on specific recognition. Tumour cells stealthily evade immune cells entirely by shedding certain antigens and downregulating others thereby becoming imperceptible. Antigen loss happens via myriad mechanisms including gene mutations and epigenetic tweaks that warp surface molecule expression like MHC class I drastically (Vesely and Schreiber, 2013).

Cytotoxic T lymphocytes largely fail recognizing altered self antigens on tumour cells subsequently in most cancer cases. Unchecked proliferation and tumour persistence transpire when immunity falters badly at eradicating tumours effectively under certain circumstances. Tumour heterogeneity further complicates immune surveillance variably under selective pressure across disparate tumour subpopulations alongside antigen loss.

Malignant cells embedded deep within a tumour frequently display considerable genomic heterogeneity and generate a motley assortment of aberrant cellular morphologies. Intratumoural heterogeneity precipitates emergence of cancer cell subpopulations exhibiting wildly diverse antigen sets remarkably variably within disparate tumour microenvironments (Vesely and Schreiber, 2013).

Some subpopulations retain original antigens while others evolve rapidly over time losing or drastically altering expression of cellular markers. Immune cells target tumour cells effectively but some cancerous cells slip through undetected resulting in tumour persistence and eventual recurrence. Tumour masses exhibit considerable diversity rendering comprehensive immune responses somewhat challenging largely due to heterogeneity of tumour cells present therein. Cancer cells slyly undergo immune editing with time adapting rapidly or downregulating antigen expression entirely morphing their molecular makeup under immense pressure. Tumours often evade immune recognition and grow increasingly resistant very quickly to various therapies, like some checkpoint inhibitors or certain tumour vaccines (Vesely and Schreiber, 2013).

Crucial understanding of tumour heterogeneity persists in cancer immunotherapy, devising gnarly strategies that can effectively overcome antigen loss variably. Tumour subpopulations are targeted by modified cancer vaccines and T cell therapies that enhance recognition of broader antigenic spectra very effectively. Strategies thereby aim very significantly at encouraging efficacy of novel immunotherapies and mitigating the likelihood of relapse in various tumour cases.

6.2. The Role of Nutrition in Modulating Immune Evasion Mechanisms

Cancer cells have developed myriad cunning strategies evading immune detection, rather thoroughly already as outlined in preceding chapters with much elaboration. Dietary interventions offer promising countermeasures against immune evasion largely due to the sheer complexity of various underlying pathological factors. Emerging research starkly highlights nutrition's direct sway on immune response irregularly while overall health hangs precariously in an uncertain delicate balance. Certain nutrients and bioactive compounds present in foods can effectively boost immune surveillance and possibly surmount tumour resistance now quite effectively. Certain dietary factors vigorously enhance immune cell activity, reducing chronic inflammation significantly, and encourage modulation of immune checkpoints very effectively in cancer prevention therapy (Kim et al, 2022).

Polyphenols and omega-3 fatty acids modulate immune responses fairly effectively supporting tumour immunity in many quite obscure, mysterious ways alongside vitamins. Polyphenols such as resveratrol, curcumin, and epigallocatechin gallate EGCG present in various fruits, tea and red wine exhibit remarkably potent antioxidant properties. Tumours heavily exploit PD-1 expression on various immune cells and PD-L1 to suppress their activity, but these novel compounds vigorously boost T cell responses. Polyphenols effectively boost immune surveillance by targeting specific pathways and render tumours highly susceptible to intense immune onslaught. Fatty fish like salmon harbour eicosapentaenoic acid and docosahexaenoic acid, which substantially reduces chronic inflammation with omega-3 fatty acids present abundantly. Omega-3s vigorously promote T cell activation and significantly enhance natural killer cell activity whilst downregulating pro-inflammatory cytokines like TNF-α very substantially (Kim et al, 2022).

Omega-3s render tumours extremely responsive to diverse immune interventions and chemo or immunotherapies by drastically dampening inflammation around tumour sites. Vitamins such as vitamin D play crucial yet understated roles normally beneath the surface level in the regulation of immune responses quietly. Vitamin D boosts cytotoxic activity of T cells and NK cells while regulating immune checkpoints, vigorously maintaining a fairly balanced immune response. Vitamin C protects immune cells effectively from oxidative stress induced by brutal cancer therapies like chemotherapy or intense radiation, thereby significantly enhancing overall immune function. Vitamin E offers protection by mitigating oxidative damage, thereby boosting immune cell activity vigorously inside a largely favourable tumour microenvironment. Presence of naturally occurring microbes therein fosters robust immune function and tumour suppression through profoundly enhanced responses against malignant cells (Zhao et al, 2021).

Probiotics harbouring live beneficial microbes stimulate NK cells and T cells whilst regulating various immune checkpoint molecules, effectively modulating cytokine production in an anti-inflammatory environment. Fibre-rich prebiotics further enhance the growth of beneficial microbes, thereby quietly helping maintain a fairly robust immune system in the background. A diet teeming with probiotics and prebiotics markedly enhances gut health and significantly improves immune responses, possibly amplifying the effectiveness of some cancer therapies greatly. Certain dietary tweaks may potentially augment tumour defence and enhance immune surveillance for cancer patients and individuals seeking reduced cancer risk (Zhao et al, 2021).

Nutritional interventions paired alongside conventional cancer therapies might remarkably restore weakened immune functionality and significantly enhance overall treatment outcomes. Personalised nutrition plays a crucial role in oncology care regimens nowadays, with emerging research increasingly highlighting its quite significant potential. Deciphering links between dietary patterns and immune system evasion yields keen insights into forging novel nutritional interventions for thwarting cancer onset remarkably well.

6.2.1. Omega-3 Fatty Acids: Enhancing T Cell Function

Fatty fish such as salmon or mackerel teem with eicosapentaenoic acid and docosahexaenoic acid, rich polyunsaturated fats also found abundantly in flaxseeds. Emerging evidence nowadays suggests they play a pivotal role in modulating immune function by encouraging T cell activity and thwarting cancer's evasive tactics effectively. Omega-3 fatty acids remarkably boost activation and cytotoxicity of T cells, crucial players in targeting cancer cells with heightened efficacy. T cells play a crucial role in adaptive immunity and obliterate tumour cells with remarkable efficacy during surveillance under specific pathological conditions. Cancer cells evade detection by manipulating various checkpoints and create a profoundly immunosuppressive microenvironment around themselves with great cunning, very effectively (Mititelu et al, 2024).

Omega-3s might enhance immune response rather effectively by facilitating swift recognition of malignant cells and subsequently triggering their eradication directly. Omega-3s reduce the expression of PD-L1, a protein that various tumours overexpress quite effectively suppressing T cell activity. PD-L1 binds PD-1 receptor on T cells quite effectively and dampens their vigor rather rapidly thereby reducing their ability to attack cancer cells. Omega-3s markedly boost T cell cytotoxicity by inhibiting that pathway and significantly enhance immune system capacity for destroying tumours vigorously. Omega-3 fatty acids very significantly ramp up natural killer cell activity thereby effectively encourage immune response against various forms of cancer. NK cells belong to innate immunity and readily kill tumour cells when T cell activity falters under certain heinous pathological conditions obviously (Gutiérrez et al, 2019).

Omega-3s enhance NK cell function remarkably fostering very effective immune responses against tumours with various evasive tactics employed by cancer cells. Omega-3 fatty acids modulate inflammatory pathways rather deeply inside various bodily tissues and shift immune response towards an anti-inflammatory profile very effectively. Tumour progression gets boosted substantially by chronic inflammation within tumour microenvironment and fosters stubborn resistance against many treatments very effectively. Omega-3s might restore balance inside immune systems very effectively by diminishing inflammation and strengthening immune response rendering tumours fairly susceptible. Omega-3 fatty acids present a potentially efficacious cancer treatment approach by markedly encourage immune responses under diverse clinical settings effectively (Gutiérrez et al, 2019).

Omega-3s might ramp up T cell activation very vigorously inside tumours and enhance NK cell activity somewhat while squelching immune checkpoints thereby rendering them rather vulnerable to chemo and immunotherapy treatments. Omega-3-rich foods and supplements might play a crucial role very significantly in cancer prevention regimens optimizing various immune responses.

6.2.2. Vitamin D

Vitamin D crucially modulates immune responses and plays a pivotal role in overall bodily function beyond bone health remarkably. 1,25-dihydroxyvitamin D interacts with myriad immune cells including T cells and macrophages effectively enhancing responses against certain cancers. Vitamin D proves valuable for cancer prevention and therapy by boosting immune surveillance that detects abnormal cells very effectively and eliminates them. Vitamin D's potency stems partly from starkly enhancing T cell differentiation remarkably in a crucial manner with considerable efficacy apparently. T cells play a crucial role in adaptive immunity recognizing malignant cells and orchestrating elimination with great specificity quite effectively . Vitamin D fosters differentiation of CD8+ cytotoxic T cells that play a crucial albeit oft underappreciated role in decimating tumour cells remarkably well. It boosts activation of CD4+ helper T cells which orchestrate immune response vigorously and augment function of other immune cells like macrophages (Aranow C., 2011).

Vitamin D promotes macrophage activation fairly effectively thereby enabling cells to recognize cancer cells and subsequently destroy them quite rapidly inside tissues. Macrophages play crucial role in innate immunity by rapidly identifying tumour cells and eliminating them effectively via early cancer defense mechanisms. Vitamin D substantially enhance overall immune response from within by very significantly enhancing macrophages' functional efficacy. Vitamin D plays a crucial role in thwarting immune suppression within tumour microenvironments and significantly impacts T cell functionality very deeply. Tumours frequently hijack regulatory T cells that suppress sundry immune responses thereby facilitating evasion of detection by host immune surveillance mechanisms. Vitamin D inhibits recruitment of immunosuppressive Tregs fairly quickly thereby helping restore quite effective immune onslaught against various tumour cells (Aranow C., 2011).

Tumours heavily produce immunosuppressive cytokines such as TGF-β and IL-10 which vitamin D has been shown to reduce expression of thereby somewhat vigorously dampening immune responses. TGF-β fosters Treg differentiation and inhibits T cell function thereby suppressing immune activity further downstream with mighty immunosuppressive potency. Vitamin D reverses some shrewd immune evasion tactics employed by cancer cells by drastically lowering levels of certain rogue cytokines rendering cells rather susceptible. Vitamin D deficiency correlates with markedly heightened risk of breast cancer and prostate cancer risk simultaneously alongside colon cancer. Vitamin D deficiency gravely hinders mounting immune response resulting in lackluster defense against cancer slowly over prolonged period. People lacking vitamin D face bleaker cancer prevention odds and subsequent treatment regimens unfold rather dismally under such deficient circumstances unfortunately (Thepmalee et al, 2018).

Vitamin D supplementation holds promise for encourage immune function in individuals battered by grueling chemotherapy and intense radiotherapy regimens simultaneously. Supplementation robustly boosts immune responses nowadays potentially improving treatment efficacy and enhancing overall patient outcomes very effectively under certain conditions. Vitamin D plays multifaceted roles somewhat irregularly in cancer defense by promoting activation of T cells and enhancing functionality of macrophages. Vitamin D somewhat effectively helps counteract cancer cells' immune evasion tactics by tilting balance toward pro-inflammatory signals very favorably. Boosting vitamin D levels through dietary sources or supplements and maybe even sunlight exposure possibly amplifies immune system's prowess at eliminating cancer cells (Thepmalee et al, 2018).

6.2.3. Polyphenols

Polyphenols a diverse group of bioactive compounds are found very abundantly in various plant-based foods such as exotic fruits and red wine exhibiting potent antioxidant properties. Tumours utilize diverse immune evasion tactics which some compounds may flip and thereby remarkably enhance overall immunity in a significant way. Resveratrol and EGCG show remarkably promising antitumour effects under complex conditions enhancing immunity very vigorously with varied success rates apparently. Curcumin heavily researched for potent antioxidant properties functions by modulating immune checkpoints and diminishing accumulation of Treg cells significantly in various tissues. Cancer cells evade detection rather effectively under certain conditions by inhibiting expression of key molecule PD-L1 in immune system. PD-L1 binds PD-1 quite effectively on diverse immune cells thereby fostering substantial immune suppression and consequently facilitating tumour cell persistence remarkably (Pandey and Rizvi, 2009).

Curcumin fosters a vigorous immune reaction against tumour cells by diminishing PD-L1 expression fairly effectively in various cellular contexts. Curcumin remarkably reduces Treg accumulation in tumour microenvironment and exerts quite varied effects on several immune checkpoints simultaneously. Tregs effectively thwart activation of effector immune cells like cytotoxic T cells and natural killer cells crucial for killing cancer cells. Curcumin restores immune activity somewhat vigorously by diminishing Treg cells presence thereby making tumours extremely vulnerable to fierce surveillance and brutal bodily attack. Resveratrol present naturally in many types of grapes and various berries exhibits significant immunomodulatory effects as a polyphenolic compound. Resveratrol has been shown very effectively to activate NK cells essential for recognizing and destroying tumour cells. NK cells wield significant influence over innate immunity staunchly defending against various malignancies before full activation of adaptive immune responses occurs (Pandey and Rizvi, 2009).

Resveratrol markedly amplifies T cell responses boosting CD4+ helper T cells and CD8+ cytotoxic T cells vital for targeting cancer cells very effectively. Resveratrol effectively fosters activation and proliferation of certain immune cells surmounting tumour-induced immune evasion via mediation by immune cells. Epigallocatechin gallate or EGCG a primary polyphenol found predominantly in green tea remarkably exhibits potent antioxidant properties and profound anti-inflammatory effects. EGCG remarkably boosts macrophage function enhancing ability of immune cells recognizing and destroying tumour cells very effectively inside body. Macrophages play a pivotal role in fostering tumour-specific immune responses and facilitate early detection of various tumours quite effectively nowadays. EGCG has been found rather effectively counteracting immunosuppressive cells such as Tregs within tumour microenvironment (Shan et al, 2023).

EGCG ramps up immune responses against cancer cells quite effectively by tweaking Treg activity fostering a pro-inflammatory environment and boosting chemotherapy effectiveness. Polyphenols modulate immune checkpoint molecules effectively and counteract various immunosuppressive factors thereby rendering them valuable dietary compounds in cancer prevention strategies. Polyphenols subtly alter tumour microenvironment quite radically and help overcome key immune evasion tactics employed by malignant cells. Polyphenols such as curcumin and resveratrol help restore immune system ability potentially improving outcomes badly for cancer patients recognizing tumour cells. Polyphenols found in diets may quite effectively complement cancer prevention efforts alongside chemotherapy radiation and various immunotherapy treatment modalities (Shan et al, 2023).

Polyphenols wield potent immunomodulatory and antioxidant properties effectively enhancing immune system's ability to vanquish cancer with remarkable efficacy underground. Bioactive compounds very effectively crank up bodily defenses against tumours by activating NK cells and boosting macrophage activity with lots of energy. Foods rich in polyphenol such as green tea or berries may enhance cancer prevention naturally by effectively enhancing mechanisms of immune surveillance.

6.2.4. Fibre and Gut Health

Gut microbiome has emerged very significantly as a key modulator of immune function via various intricate pathways influencing systemic immunity. Diets rich in fibre from fruits and whole grains curiously foster growth of beneficial gut bacteria that produce short-chain fatty acids like butyrate having profoundly various immune-enhancing effects. SCFAs very effectively foster differentiation of regulatory T cells or Tregs thereby preventing excessive inflammation in various bodily contexts normally. Microbiome modulates immunotherapy effectiveness heavily via intricate immune checkpoints and T cell responses that vary somewhat mysteriously (Wastyk **et al**, 2021).

Fermented foods coupled with a diet rich in fibre may enhance immune surveillance reducing cancer progression by thwarting immune evasion rather effectively. Tumour cells deploy intricate maneuvers stealthily escaping immune surveillance posing a hurdle in cancer treatment efforts with eradication proving highly elusive. Nutritional interventions can rather convincingly modulate immune system function significantly improving outcomes in various cancer treatments with emerging overwhelming evidence. Certain nutrients enhance bodily defenses against cancer naturally by modulating gut health and generally enhancing activation of various immune cells vigorously. Rapidly expanding research on nutrition interplay with immune function may lead to dietary interventions becoming crucial in personalized cancer therapy offering non-invasive rather cost-effective approaches that significantly enhance treatment efficacy and patient survival (Wastyk **et al**, 2021).

7. Targeting Immune Pathways

Novel immunotherapeutic strategies have emerged quite rapidly and interplay between diet and immune system regulation has become a critical oncology research area. Immunotherapy relies heavily on host immune systems detecting malignant cells swiftly with wonky immune checkpoint inhibitors and adoptive cell transfer being utilized. Novel therapeutic interventions are substantially influenced by dietary factors that significantly modulate immune function according to recent compelling evidence. Amino acids and vitamins significantly impact numerous immune pathways such as cytokine production and T-cell activation in various intricate ways obviously. Gut microbiome plays a pivotal role regulating systemic immunity shaped rather intricately by various dietary factors and numerous other obscure elements obviously (Lafont et al, 2021).

Diets consisting of plenty fibre and nutrients sourced from plants robustly promote growth of commensal bacteria which vigorously enhance antitumour immunity effectively. Diets ridiculously high in fat and heavily processed may drastically disrupt balance of gut microbes thereby fostering environments that breed tumour progression and nasty inflammation. Emerging clinical trials alongside preclinical studies suggest dietary interventions can markedly enhance responsiveness in patients undergoing various immune-based therapies nowadays. Ketogenic diets and fasting-mimicking regimens have shown considerable promise in modulating tumour microenvironments rather effectively encourage T-cell mediated cytotoxic responses significantly (Lafont et al, 2021).

Findings highlight potential for integrating dietary strategies somewhat effectively as adjuncts alongside existing cancer therapies in various clinical settings. Incorporating nutritional practices into oncological treatment protocols presents remarkably a novel noninvasive therapeutic approach enhancing patient outcomes significantly. Optimal dietary regimens tailored around individual tumour types necessitate further mechanistic studies and fairly well-designed clinical trials really urgently. Precision nutrition could become a cornerstone of personalized cancer care as understanding of tumour biology deepens rapidly offering fresh possibilities longterm for survivorship (Mercier et al, 2022).

7.1. Immune System and Cancer: A Delicate Balance

Aberrant cells get eliminated by immune cells via a vigilant surveillance mechanism that serves as a crucial bulwark against oncogenic transformations stealthily. Cytotoxic T lymphocytes and natural killer cells along with macrophages detect tumour cells with varying efficacy and destroy them rapidly. Cells thwart tumour initiation and progression under fairly normal physiological circumstances quite effectively sometimes. Malignant cells surreptitiously garner capacity for stealthy evasion and utter suppression of immune system's detection mechanisms in a twisted evolutionary pursuit. Tumours effectively exploit various immunosuppressive mechanisms by upregulating immune checkpoint molecules and recruiting regulatory T cells or myeloid-derived suppressor cells. Immunotherapy has fairly remarkably revolutionized cancer treatment by very effectively harnessing immune systems targeting a wide variety of nasty tumours (Masmoudi et al, 2025).

Chimeric antigen receptor T-cell therapies and immune checkpoint inhibitors blocking inhibitory receptors such as PD-1 or CTLA-4 exhibit remarkable efficacy quite often in various solid tumours lately. Patients fail treatments or develop resistance gradually over quite some time nonetheless in significant proportion. Immune-related adverse events still loom ominously underscoring necessity for novel adjunctive approaches rather than haphazardly augmenting treatment rather optimistically nowadays. Diet plays a crucial role nowadays in modulating fairly significant immune responses within diverse physiological contexts very much everywhere. Nutritional status profoundly influences systemic immunity in complex ways and tumour microenvironment heavily obviously through specific dietary components very dynamically (Masmoudi et al, 2025).

Diet may enhance immunotherapy by subtly tweaking effector immune cells or nudging gut microbiota towards radically different profiles that strongly favour robust immunity. Modified dietary regimens amplify antitumour immunity remarkably while mitigating resistance to treatment thereby unfolding novel avenues for cancer therapeutics.

7.2. Diet and Immune Pathways

Cancer treatment nowadays hinges precariously on intricate interplay between diet and immune function recognized increasingly as vital factor in effective therapies. Dietary elements seem influential on certain immune pathways combating cancer effectively over time in surprisingly robust ways under specific conditions. Chronic inflammation modulation happens alongside shifts in gut microbiota makeup and metabolic regulation occurs simultaneously within diverse immune cellular populations. Diet quietly modulates inflammation within bodily systems every day largely influencing immune function through subtle fluctuations in internal bodily processes. Tumour initiation and progression are driven quietly by chronic low-grade inflammation that fosters metastasis within affected tissues over considerable time periods. Consuming food rich in super refined sugars and processed meats can crank inflammation way up and aggressively foster development of cancer (Golonko et al, 2024).

Diets rich in fruits whole grains and omega-3 fatty acids potentially slow tumour growth by reducing systemic inflammatory response somewhat effectively. Omega-3 fatty acids present in fatty fish such as salmon and some nuts exhibit markedly anti-inflammatory properties within human bodies . Fatty acids frequently downregulate pro-inflammatory cytokines like IL-6 and TNF-α that play a role in progression of various nasty cancers. Omega-3s might substantially enhance cancer-fighting prowess of immune system by fairly effectively dialing down sundry inflammatory mediators very remarkably. Polyphenols and vitamin

C found in various fruits help fight oxidative stress thereby upholding immune cell integrity remarkably well inside human bodies (Golonko et al, 2024).

7.3. The Gut Microbiome and Cancer Immunity

Diet profoundly affects immune pathways mainly through its significant impact on composition of gut microbiome and functionality overall . Diverse microorganisms flourish within human hosts forming a complex ecosystem crucial for effectively modulating immune responses beneath the surface. Gut microbiome imbalance has been tenuously linked to various health issues including sundry forms of cancer rather mysteriously and suddenly. Gut microbiome plays a crucial role modulating effectiveness of immunotherapies like checkpoint inhibitors and heavily influencing overall immune response against tumours. Diet exerts a surprisingly direct profound influence on gut microbiome composition rather quickly within a normal human body. Fibre-rich whole grains and legumes and various fruits and vegetables foster growth of beneficial microbes producing SCFAs like butyrate very abundantly (Zhang P, 2022).

SCFAs enhance immune function remarkably amidst reduced inflammation and somewhat vigorously promote anti-tumour immunity. A balanced microbiome fosters development of immune cells such as T helper cells and regulatory T cells which help maintain tolerance effectively stalling cancer progression. Diets crammed with copious animal fats and sugars yet woefully deficient in fibre foster proliferation of heinous microbes that spawn inflammation teeming with carcinogenic pathogens. Nutritional adjustments very effectively ramp up immune responses against cancer these days by encourage a robust microbiome (Zhang P, 2022).

7.4. Targeting Immune Checkpoints with Diet

Monoclonal antibodies targeting PD-1 and its ligand PD-L1 or CTLA-4 show remarkable efficacy under immune checkpoint blockade in diverse malignancies. Tumours cunningly exploit certain inhibitory pathways evading detection and therapies disrupt such pathways thereby very effectively facilitating immune destruction. Immune checkpoint inhibitors achieve considerable success albeit being hampered heavily by wildly varied patient responses and multifaceted resistance mechanisms alongside severe adverse effects related to immunity. Growing interest lies in adjunctive strategies potentiating ICI efficacy somewhat while mitigating toxicity and diet emerges as surprisingly promising candidate (Wojtukiewicz et al, 2021).

Ketogenic diets strangely modulate metabolism of immune cells, thereby influencing therapeutic response significantly, and overall immune function gets altered very radically. Fasting-mimicking diets apparently crank up effector T cells' activation very significantly, whilst diminishing regulatory T cells' immunosuppressive action quite markedly alongside myeloid-derived suppressor cells. Such interventions may vigorously upregulate expression of stress-related ligands on tumour cells, making them rather susceptible to immune-mediated destruction. Ketogenic diet induces a drastic metabolic shift favoring production of ketone bodies, reducing glycolytic flux, thereby somewhat irregularly influencing T lymphocyte function (Wojtukiewicz et al, 2021).

Preclinical studies hint that a ketogenic metabolic state significantly enhance cytotoxic capacity of CD8+ T cells and renders the tumour microenvironment less profoundly immunosuppressive. This dietary approach nowadays may substantially decrease the likelihood of autoimmune toxicity associated with checkpoint blockade by reducing systemic inflammation. These findings effectively support dietary modulation as a potentially useful adjunct for immune checkpoint therapy adjunctively overall quite successfully. Ongoing clinical studies probe ways these strategies might be heavily tailored for improving outcomes in various immuno-oncology research contexts very effectively nowadays.

7.5. Micronutrients and Cancer Immunity

Essential vitamins and trace minerals vitally enhance bodily defense against cancer maintaining immune competence remarkably under various physiological conditions. Evidence underscores their pivotal role in encourage general immune function and modulating antitumour responses very effectively augmenting cancer treatment outcomes lately. Vitamin D plays quite a pivotal role in immune system regulation possessing fat-soluble secosteroid hormonal properties oddly enough. It substantially boosts innate immunity and adaptive immunity by fostering T lymphocytes differentiation and activity alongside macrophages very effectively. Vitamin D signaling has been very deeply tied into diminishing chronic inflammation and encourage antigen presentation against tumour cells rather effectively . Heightened incidence of various malignancies like colorectal cancer and prostate cancer correlates strongly with low serum vitamin D levels often yielding dismal prognosis (Stefanache et al, 2023).

Vitamin D supplementation gets examined as adjunct therapy alongside immunotherapy with early findings hinting at slightly boosted efficacy and mitigated harsh side effects. Zinc and selenium simultaneously play crucial roles vital for maintenance of immune cell structure and function in a rather intricate manner. Zinc fuels activity of numerous enzymes involved in DNA repair or apoptosis playing a crucial role in thymic development and T-cell differentiation slowly. Selenium exerts potent antioxidant effects through incorporation into selenoproteins that shield immune cells from oxidative damage amidst intense inflammation (Stefanache et al, 2023).

Micronutrient deficiencies severely cripple immune response and amplify vulnerability to heinous infections whilst eroding bodily capacity for tumour suppression rather drastically. Micronutrients from diet significantly impact tumour-immune interactions through numerous cellular mechanisms and pathways apparently altering their interface markedly. Micronutrients offer promising avenues for integration into comprehensive cancer care by heavily modulating immune responses and regulating oxidative stress. Optimizing micronutrient status rather impressively enhance treatment responses and significantly improves patient outcomes over a remarkably long term.

8. Linking Nutrition and Immunity: A Strategy for Cancer Prevention and Treatment

Aberrant cells are detected by immune system quite effectively playing a pivotal role in surveillance of tumours and prevention of cancer. Cancer therapies like chemotherapy remain crucial and surgery stays essential but modulation through specific nutritional interventions greatly influences development outcomes. Recent studies indicate certain nutrients profoundly interact with immune systems thereby influencing cancer onset and responsiveness to treatment very significantly. Cancer cells deftly sidestep immune surveillance through myriad covert tactics involving upregulation of checkpoint molecules and metabolic pathway reprogramming within tumour microenvironments. Such alterations nurture a profoundly immunosuppressive microenvironment that rather vigorously impairs effective immunity and facilitates neoplastic proliferation with unusual ferocity (Coventry and Henneberg, 2015).

Diet potentially counteracts these effects by modulating inflammation heavily and encourage cytotoxic immune cell function thereby restoring somewhat underground immune surveillance. Omega-3 fatty acids alongside assorted polyphenols and certain vitamins exert profoundly immunomodulatory effects with dietary fibre very effectively. Fibre-rich diets ramp up gut microbiota very significantly influencing systemic immunity and sparking inflammation elsewhere in rather surprising ways sometimes. Polyphenols present in sundry fruits and some veggies exhibit markedly anti-inflammatory properties and antioxidant effects that thwart cancer-promoting pathways quite effectively (Coventry and Henneberg, 2015).

Nutritional strategies such as caloric restriction and ketogenic diets effectively reprogrammed immune metabolism very robustly favoring decidedly anti-tumour activity in various contexts. Nutritional strategies incorporated into cancer treatment regimens somewhat effectively mitigate malignancy risk and boost efficacy of various immunotherapies noticeably. Nutritional immuno-oncology evolves rapidly paving way for modified dietary interventions that support long-term survivorship alongside very standard cancer treatments.

8.1. The Role of Inflammation in Cancer

Chronic inflammation plays a critical role fairly often in tumour initiation and progression deep beneath layers of obscure cellular response mechanisms. Chronic inflammation fosters a protracted pro-tumourigenic milieu rather quickly marked by release of reactive oxygen species and inflammatory cytokines. Inflammatory cells sneaking into tumour microenvironment remarkably enhance tumour cell proliferation and survival facilitating immune evasion and further invasion. Diet acts as potent modulator of inflammation representing a key factor in cancer prevention effectively through various lifestyle modifications . Polyunsaturated omega-3 fatty acids and certain phytochemicals can robustly counteract deeply rooted inflammatory molecular processes quite effectively inside human bodies (Nishida and Andoh, 2025).

Eicosapentaenoic acid and docosahexaenoic acid present in fatty fish and flaxseed get absorbed very quickly into cellular membranes influencing eicosanoid production significantly. Fatty acids have shown ability to downregulate nuclear factor-kappa B signaling a crucial transcription factor in various oncogenic inflammatory pathways heavily downstream. Fruits rich in carotenoids and vitamin C very effectively scavenge free radicals thereby reducing oxidative stress and mitigating DNA damage somewhat. Phytochemicals like curcumin and resveratrol deeply inhibit pro-inflammatory enzymes COX-2 and cytokines inside an anti-tumour immune environment thereby contributing greatly. Diets heavy in ultra-processed food and replete with saturated fats curiously jack up cancer risk and foster chronic inflammatory responses. Anti-inflammatory dietary strategies may serve as preventive therapeutic tools in comprehensive cancer management and adjunctive ones too in some manner (Nishida and Andoh, 2025).

8.2. The Gut Microbiome and Cancer Immunity

Trillions of microorganisms inhabit gastrointestinal tract forming complex ecosystem that plays pivotal role in regulating immune response effectively maintaining homeostasis. Evidence emerging rapidly underscores microbiome's pivotal role in modulating innate and adaptive immune responses yielding subsequent far-reaching implications for cancer therapy development. Microbial dysbiosis sparks chronic inflammation and malignancies whereas diverse gut microbiota enhance antitumour activity and enhances immune surveillance remarkably. Diet heavily influences gut microbiota composition remarkably across various populations with significant effects on overall health obviously (Talapko et al, 2022).

Diets rich in dietary fibre from whole grains legumes fruits and veggies promote proliferation of commensal bacteria that ferment fibre into short-chain fatty acids like acetate propionate butyrate. Butyrate stands out among them largely due to potent anti-inflammatory properties and its immunoregulatory effects have been extensively researched. Butyrate functions very quietly as a potent histone deacetylase inhibitor modulating gene expression significantly in various immune cells rather drastically. Effector T cells and regulatory T cells differentiation gets markedly enhanced while epithelial barrier integrity improves significantly supporting antitumour immunity involving dendritic cells. Diets heavy in saturated fats and sugars but woefully lacking fibre utterly disrupt microbial balance fostering very much a pro-inflammatory environment (Talapko et al, 2022).

Harsh conditions may severely impair maturation of immune cells deep within bodily tissues and facilitate tumour-promoting pathways variously. Targeted dietary interventions modulate gut microbiota thereby offering a potentially efficacious approach for encourage immune response substantially and mitigating oncogenic risks. Microbiota composition significantly impacts efficacy of immune checkpoint inhibitors and microbiome-targeted nutrition might optimize outcomes of immunotherapy rather markedly. Breakthroughs in research could potentially thrust dietary adjustments targeting microbiome firmly into oncologic treatment as vital component of highly personalized cancer prophylaxis strategies.

8.3. Immunomodulatory Effects of Phytochemicals

Phytochemicals present abundantly in various fruits and veggies along with other plant-based edibles garner considerable attention owing largely to anti-cancer properties. Compounds intricately modulate signaling networks within immune systems and tumour microenvironments encourage cancer prevention and furnishing therapeutic support very effectively . Several obscure compounds naturally possess notable phytochemicals like curcumin resveratrol and epigallocatechin gallate EGCG exhibiting rather significant immunological activity. Curcumin from Curcuma longa heavily inhibits key signaling pathways like nuclear factor kappa B and STAT3 exhibiting potent immunomodulatory effects. Pathways often get dysregulated in cancer and are linked with chronic inflammation tumour cell survival and deeply entrenched immune suppression (Yuan et al, 2022).

Curcumin boosts cytotoxic activity of CD8+ T cells and natural killer cells while simultaneously reducing production of tumour-promoting cytokines like interleukin-6. Resveratrol exerts profoundly multi-faceted effects on immune responses in various foods like berries and peanuts quite effectively nowadays apparently. Tumour angiogenesis gets suppressed quietly by downregulating vascular endothelial growth factor and promoting apoptosis in cancer cells through several wonky immune mechanisms. Resveratrol very effectively restores immune surveillance by encourage maturation of dendritic cells and modulating activity of several kinds of T cells vigorously (Yuan et al, 2022).

EGCG predominantly present in green tea exhibits anti-cancer properties by heavily influencing T regulatory cell function and crippling cancer cell proliferation rather noticeably. EGCG inhibits NF-κB and sundry transcriptional regulators rather similarly curcumin or resveratrol does in inflammation pathways and cell survival mechanisms. Phytochemicals collectively represent a distinct class of dietary agents that effectively reprogram immune responses and radically alter tumour microenvironment profoundly. Phytochemicals may serve as adjunctive agents slowly in cancer immunotherapy significantly contributing to highly personalized diet-based treatment approaches eventually.

8.4. Nutrients and Immune Cell Function

Micronutrients play a crucial role encourage immune system's ability to detect cells with cancerous characteristics and eliminate them very effectively nowadays. Vitamins and trace minerals such as vitamin D or zinc play a crucial role in maintaining immune responses rather effectively. Key nutrient deficiencies rapidly precipitate immune dysfunction and markedly heighten susceptibility to a plethora of egregious malignancies rather frequently nowadays. Vitamin D exerts profoundly significant immunomodulatory effects very much everywhere as a secosteroid hormone soluble in fats within bodily tissues. It enhance innate immunity very effectively by fostering intense antimicrobial activity inside macrophages and dendritic cells crucial for antigen presentation. Vitamin D quite effectively regulates T cell differentiation in adaptive immune system and inhibits pro-inflammatory Th17 cells proliferation remarkably well (Gombart et al, 2020).

Heightened risk of various malignancies such as colorectal cancer breast cancer and prostate cancer often correlates strongly with low serum vitamin D levels. Supplementation in deficient individuals possibly enhance immune efficacy very effectively and may substantially enhance response to cancer immunotherapy. Zinc serves as a crucial micronutrient needed quite mysteriously for thymic development and T cell maturation alongside natural killer cell functionality properly. It acts as a cofactor in numerous enzymes deeply embroiled in cellular signaling DNA repair and apoptosis processes all at once simultaneously. Zinc deficiency precipitates lymphopenia and reduces T cell-mediated cytotoxicity somewhat thereby severely compromising anti-tumour immunity variably in physiological contexts (Gombart et al, 2020).

Selenium gets incorporated into selenoproteins that serve mainly as antioxidants protecting immune cells vigorously from damage induced by oxidative stress during inflammation. T cell activity gets augmented rather robustly via redox mechanisms while tumour progression remains suppressed and NK cell function stays enhanced somewhat. Very much always micronutrient levels suffice for encourage general immune health and resistance against cancer development mediated by immune responses . Nutritional assessment and intervention serve valuably as adjuncts in comprehensive cancer management protocols nowadays with fairly obvious beneficial effects (Huang et al, 2012).

8.5. Caloric Restriction and Immune Enhancement

Caloric restriction sans malnutrition has been probed extensively for salubrious effects on prolonging lifespan and it thwarts cancer effectively . CR significantly reduces cancer incidence and progression in various preclinical animal models by heavily modulating immune function and altering systemic metabolic pathways. CR exerts anticancer effects partly via attenuation of chronic inflammation and enhance immune surveillance effectively under diverse physiological conditions normally. Intermittent fasting entails periodic fasting spells and has garnered significant attention recently for potentially encourage cancer therapy outcomes quite substantially (Longo and Fontana, 2010).

Protocols that diminish pro-inflammatory cytokines like interleukin-6 or tumour necrosis factor-alpha are often elevated in cancer patients and foster tumour-promoting inflammation heavily. CR and IF ostensibly stimulate activity of various effector immune cells like cytotoxic T lymphocytes and natural killer cells thereby markedly enhancing body's ability to destroy malignant cells. CR may profoundly sensitize tumour cells to chemotherapy and immunotherapy by precipitating significant metabolic turmoil and recasting tumour microenvironment thereby encourage drug efficacy substantially (Longo and Fontana, 2010).

Caloric restriction might impede proliferation of cancer cells and spare function of immune cells that rely heavily on oxidative metabolic processes. Complex interplay between tumour immunity and dietary components highlights considerable advantages of supplementary nutritional approaches fairly well in modern oncology settings. Tailored dietary interventions could drastically cut cancer risk and markedly improve patient outcomes by supplying vital nutrients and cultivating a robust gut microbiome. Personalized diet-based therapies may emerge vital in cancer care providing non-invasive cost-effective complements alongside conventional treatments very slowly over time.

9. Conclusion

Nutrition interplay with immune system represents a critical axis deeply embedded nowadays in various cancer biology contexts fairly obviously. Nutritional status profoundly influences immune surveillance a complex mechanism for detecting cells turned malignant or abnormal within bodily tissues quietly. Cancer evolves complex strategies evading immune detection slowly leveraging principles of nutritional immunology which offers a rather compelling new therapeutic approach. Bioactive dietary compounds and various nutrients effectively modulate aspects of immune surveillance under fairly specific physiological conditions quite remarkably. Sufficient intake of vitamins A, C, D, E, selenium, zinc and omega-3 fatty acids vitally maintains integrity of innate and adaptive immune responses effectively (Munteanu and Schwartz, 2022).

Nutrients intricately modulate myriad immune responses including antigen presentation and cytokine signaling with activation of lymphocytes and cytotoxic natural killer cell activity. Dietary components radically alter metabolism of immune cells and differentiation thereby shifting balance quite dramatically between pro-inflammatory and anti-inflammatory states. Diets rich in anti-inflammatory compounds like polyphenols and short-chain fatty acids derived from fibre reduce chronic inflammation very markedly. Nutritional status impacts immunotherapy responses significantly, and fairly recently, this therapy has emerged as a promising advancement in oncology. Certain dietary patterns are intricately linked, and obesity and metabolic syndrome can significantly impair immune function quite drastically, alongside reducing the efficacy of immune checkpoint inhibitors (Noor et al, 2021).

Personalised nutritional interventions incorporated into cancer treatment protocols remarkably boost therapeutic responsiveness and quality of life alongside significantly enhanced immune competence. Challenges persist stubbornly in morphing nutritional immunology into viable clinical practice amidst glimmers of promising yet sporadic new insight. Treatment modality and patient condition influence outcomes variably alongside tumour type and nutrient metabolism differences found in most cases. Quite frankly, fairly novel evidence-based nutritional strategies complementing cancer therapies require collaboration among oncologists, immunologists, and various nutrition scientists (Wang et al, 2022).

Nutrition modulates immune surveillance very effectively and serves as a crucial determinant of resilience against cancer in oncology settings. Nutritional immunology principles potentially unlock remarkably robust immune function supporting long-term survivorship via an integrative path for cancer prevention and treatment.

References

Alahmari LA. Dietary fibre influence on overall health, with an emphasis on CVD, diabetes, obesity, colon cancer, and inflammation. Front Nutr. 2024 Dec 13;11:1510564. doi: 10.3389/fnut.2024.1510564. PMID: 39734671; PMCID: PMC11671356.

Anand U, Dey A, Chandel AKS, Sanyal R, Mishra A, Pandey DK, De Falco V, Upadhyay A, Kandimalla R, Chaudhary A, Dhanjal JK, Dewanjee S, Vallamkondu J, Pérez de la Lastra JM. Cancer chemotherapy and beyond: Current status, drug candidates, associated risks and progress in targeted therapeutics. Genes Dis. 2022 Mar 18;10(4):1367-1401. doi: 10.1016/j.gendis.2022.02.007. Erratum in: Genes Dis. 2024 Jan 20;11(4):101211. doi: 10.1016/j.gendis.2024.101211. PMID: 37397557; PMCID: PMC10310991.

Aranow C. Vitamin D and the immune system. J Investig Med. 2011 Aug;59(6):881-6. doi: 10.2310/JIM.0b013e31821b8755. PMID: 21527855; PMCID: PMC3166406.

Belkaid Y, Hand TW. Role of the microbiota in immunity and inflammation. Cell. 2014 Mar 27;157(1):121-41. doi: 10.1016/j.cell.2014.03.011. PMID: 24679531; PMCID: PMC4056765.

Bikle DD. Vitamin D: newly discovered actions require reconsideration of physiologic requirements. Trends Endocrinol Metab. 2010 Jun;21(6):375-84. doi: 10.1016/j.tem.2010.01.003. Epub 2010 Feb 10. PMID: 20149679; PMCID: PMC2880203.

Carlberg C, Velleuer E. Vitamin D and the risk for cancer: A molecular analysis. Biochem Pharmacol. 2022 Feb;196:114735. doi: 10.1016/j.bcp.2021.114735. Epub 2021 Aug 16. PMID: 34411566.

Carr AC, Maggini S. Vitamin C and Immune Function. Nutrients. 2017 Nov 3;9(11):1211. doi: 10.3390/nu9111211. PMID: 29099763; PMCID: PMC5707683.

Chaudhary B, Elkord E. Regulatory T Cells in the Tumour Microenvironment and Cancer Progression: Role and Therapeutic Targeting. Vaccines (Basel). 2016 Aug 6;4(3):28. doi: 10.3390/vaccines4030028. PMID: 27509527; PMCID: PMC5041022.

Corthay A. Does the immune system naturally protect against cancer? Front Immunol. 2014 May 12;5:197. Doi: 10.3389/fimmu.2014.00197. PMID: 24860567; PMCID: PMC4026755.

Costoya JA, Arce VM. Cancer cells escape the immune system by increasing stemness through epigenetic reprogramming. Cell Mol Immunol. 2023 Jan;20(1):6-7. doi: 10.1038/s41423-022-00953-3. Epub 2022 Nov 15. PMID: 36380095; PMCID: PMC9794797.

Coventry BJ, Henneberg M. The Immune System and Responses to Cancer: Coordinated Evolution. F1000Res. 2015 Aug 12;4:552. doi: 10.12688/f1000research.6718.3. PMID: 33365125; PMCID: PMC7735224.

D'Eliseo D, Velotti F. Omega-3 Fatty Acids and Cancer Cell Cytotoxicity: Implications for Multi-Targeted Cancer Therapy. J Clin Med. 2016 Jan 26;5(2):15. doi: 10.3390/jcm5020015. PMID: 26821053; PMCID: PMC4773771.

El Oirdi M. Harnessing the Power of Polyphenols: A New Frontier in Disease Prevention and Therapy. Pharmaceuticals (Basel). 2024 May 27;17(6):692. doi: 10.3390/ph17060692. PMID: 38931359; PMCID: PMC11206774.

Fu J, Zheng Y, Gao Y, Xu W. Dietary Fibre Intake and Gut Microbiota in Human Health. Microorganisms. 2022 Dec 18;10(12):2507. doi: 10.3390/microorganisms10122507. PMID: 36557760; PMCID: PMC9787832.

Golonko A, Pienkowski T, Swislocka R, Orzechowska S, Marszalek K, Szczerbinski L, Swiergiel AH, Lewandowski W. Dietary factors and their influence on immunotherapy strategies in oncology: a comprehensive review. Cell Death Dis. 2024 Apr 9;15(4):254. doi: 10.1038/s41419-024-06641-6. PMID: 38594256; PMCID: PMC11004013.

Gombart AF, Pierre A, Maggini S. A Review of Micronutrients and the Immune System-Working in Harmony to Reduce the Risk of Infection. Nutrients. 2020 Jan 16;12(1):236. doi: 10.3390/nu12010236. PMID: 31963293; PMCID: PMC7019735.

Gopalakrishnan V, Helmink BA, Spencer CN, Reuben A, Wargo JA. The Influence of the Gut Microbiome on Cancer, Immunity, and Cancer Immunotherapy. Cancer Cell. 2018 Apr 9;33(4):570-580. doi: 10.1016/j.ccell.2018.03.015. PMID: 29634945; PMCID: PMC6529202.

Gutiérrez S, Svahn SL, Johansson ME. Effects of Omega-3 Fatty Acids on Immune Cells. Int J Mol Sci. 2019 Oct 11;20(20):5028. doi: 10.3390/ijms20205028. PMID: 31614433; PMCID: PMC6834330.

Han Y, Liu D, Li L. PD-1/PD-L1 pathway: current research in cancer. Am J Cancer Res. 2020 Mar 1;10(3):727-742. PMID: 32266087; PMCID: PMC7136921.

Huang Z, Rose AH, Hoffmann PR. The role of selenium in inflammation and immunity: from molecular mechanisms to therapeutic opportunities. Antioxid Redox Signal. 2012 Apr 1;16(7):705-43. doi: 10.1089/ars.2011.4145. Epub 2012 Jan 9. PMID: 21955027; PMCID: PMC3277928.

Janakiram NB, Mohammed A, Madka V, Kumar G, Rao CV. Prevention and treatment of cancers by immune-modulating nutrients. Mol Nutr Food Res. 2016 Jun;60(6):1275-94. doi: 10.1002/mnfr.201500884. Epub 2016 Mar 9. PMID: 26833775; PMCID: PMC6038926.

Jomova K, Raptova R, Alomar SY, Alwasel SH, Nepovimova E, Kuca K, Valko M. Reactive oxygen species, toxicity, oxidative stress, and antioxidants: chronic diseases and aging. Arch Toxicol. 2023 Oct;97(10):2499-2574. doi: 10.1007/s00204-023-03562-9. Epub 2023 Aug 19. PMID: 37597078; PMCID: PMC10475008.

Kallingal A, Olszewski M, Maciejewska N, Brankiewicz W, Baginski M. Cancer immune escape: the role of antigen presentation machinery. J Cancer Res Clin Oncol. 2023 Aug;149(10):8131-8141. doi: 10.1007/s00432-023-04737-8. Epub 2023 Apr 9. PMID: 37031434; PMCID: PMC10374767.

Kim SK, Cho SW. The Evasion Mechanisms of Cancer Immunity and Drug Intervention in the Tumour Microenvironment. Front Pharmacol. 2022 May 24;13:868695. doi: 10.3389/fphar.2022.868695. PMID: 35685630; PMCID: PMC9171538.

Kong X, Zhang J, Chen S, Wang X, Xi Q, Shen H, Zhang R. Immune checkpoint inhibitors: breakthroughs in cancer treatment. Cancer Biol Med. 2024 May 24;21(6):451–72. doi: 10.20892/j.issn.2095-3941.2024.0055. PMID: 38801082; PMCID: PMC11208906.

Krupa KN, Fritz K, Parmar M. Omega-3 Fatty Acids. [Updated 2024 Feb 28]. In: StatPearls [Internet]. Treasure Island (FL): StatPearls Publishing; 2025 Jan-. Available from: https://www.ncbi.nlm.nih.gov/books/NBK564314/

Lafont V, Lucas S, Bonnefoy N. Editorial: Novel Strategies for Cancer Immunotherapy: Targeting Immune-Mediated Suppressive Mechanisms. Front Immunol. 2021 May 3;12:691899. doi: 10.3389/fimmu.2021.691899. PMID: 34012459; PMCID: PMC8128245.

Lao Y, Shen D, Zhang W, He R, Jiang M. Immune Checkpoint Inhibitors in Cancer Therapy-How to Overcome Drug Resistance? Cancers (Basel). 2022 Jul 22;14(15):3575. doi: 10.3390/cancers14153575. PMID: 35892835; PMCID: PMC9331941.

Lee JG, Jang JY, Baik SM. Selenium as an Antioxidant: Roles and Clinical Applications in Critically Ill and Trauma Patients: A Narrative Review. Antioxidants (Basel). 2025 Feb 28;14(3):294. doi: 10.3390/antiox14030294. PMID: 40227249; PMCID: PMC11939285.

Longo VD, Fontana L. Calorie restriction and cancer prevention: metabolic and molecular mechanisms. Trends Pharmacol Sci. 2010 Feb;31(2):89-98. doi: 10.1016/j.tips.2009.11.004. Epub 2010 Jan 25. PMID: 20097433; PMCID: PMC2829867.

Masmoudi D, Villalba M, Alix-Panabières C. Natural killer cells: the immune frontline against circulating tumour cells. J Exp Clin Cancer Res. 2025 Apr 10;44(1):118. doi: 10.1186/s13046-025-03375-x. PMID: 40211394; PMCID: PMC11983744.

Mazziotta C, Tognon M, Martini F, Torreggiani E, Rotondo JC. Probiotics Mechanism of Action on Immune Cells and Beneficial Effects on Human Health. Cells. 2023 Jan 2;12(1):184. doi: 10.3390/cells12010184. PMID: 36611977; PMCID: PMC9818925.

Mercier BD, Tizpa E, Philip EJ, Feng Q, Huang Z, Thomas RM, Pal SK, Dorff TB, Li YR. Dietary Interventions in Cancer Treatment and Response: A Comprehensive Review. Cancers (Basel). 2022 Oct 20;14(20):5149. doi: 10.3390/cancers14205149. PMID: 36291933; PMCID: PMC9600754.

Messerschmidt JL, Prendergast GC, Messerschmidt GL. How Cancers Escape Immune Destruction and Mechanisms of Action for the New Significantly Active Immune Therapies: Helping Nonimmunologists Decipher Recent Advances. Oncologist. 2016 Feb;21(2):233-43. doi: 10.1634/theoncologist.2015-0282. Epub 2016 Feb 1. PMID: 26834161; PMCID: PMC4746082.

Mititelu M, Lupuliasa D, Neacșu SM, Olteanu G, Busnatu ȘS, Mihai A, Popovici V, Măru N, Boroghină SC, Mihai S, Ioniță-Mîndrican CB, Scafa-Udriște A. Polyunsaturated Fatty Acids and Human Health: A Key to Modern Nutritional Balance in Association with Polyphenolic Compounds from Food Sources. Foods. 2024 Dec 27;14(1):46. doi: 10.3390/foods14010046. PMID: 39796335; PMCID: PMC11719865.

Mitra S, Paul S, Roy S, Sutradhar H, Bin Emran T, Nainu F, Khandaker MU, Almalki M, Wilairatana P, Mubarak MS. Exploring the Immune-Boosting Functions of Vitamins and Minerals as Nutritional Food Bioactive Compounds: A Comprehensive Review. Molecules. 2022 Jan 16;27(2):555. doi: 10.3390/molecules27020555. PMID: 35056870; PMCID: PMC8779769.

Montané X, Kowalczyk O, Reig-Vano B, Bajek A, Roszkowski K, Tomczyk R, Pawliszak W, Giamberini M, Mocek-Płóciniak A, Tylkowski B. Current Perspectives of the Applications of Polyphenols and Flavonoids in Cancer Therapy. Molecules. 2020 Jul 23;25(15):3342. doi: 10.3390/molecules25153342. PMID: 32717865; PMCID: PMC7435624.

Munn DH, Mellor AL. IDO in the Tumour Microenvironment: Inflammation, Counter-Regulation, and Tolerance. Trends Immunol. 2016 Mar;37(3):193-207. doi: 10.1016/j.it.2016.01.002. Epub 2016 Jan 31. PMID: 26839260; PMCID: PMC4916957.

Munteanu C, Schwartz B. Interactions between Dietary Antioxidants, Dietary Fibre and the Gut Microbiome: Their Putative Role in Inflammation and Cancer. Int J Mol Sci. 2024 Jul 28;25(15):8250. doi: 10.3390/ijms25158250. PMID: 39125822; PMCID: PMC11311432.

Munteanu C, Schwartz B. The relationship between nutrition and the immune system. Front Nutr. 2022 Dec 8;9:1082500. doi: 10.3389/fnut.2022.1082500. PMID: 36570149; PMCID: PMC9772031.

Nishida A, Andoh A. The Role of Inflammation in Cancer: Mechanisms of Tumour Initiation, Progression, and Metastasis. Cells. 2025 Mar 25;14(7):488. doi: 10.3390/cells14070488. PMID: 40214442; PMCID: PMC11987742.

Noor S, Piscopo S, Gasmi A. Nutrients Interaction with the Immune System. Arch Razi Inst. 2021 Dec 30;76(6):1579-1588. doi: 10.22092/ari.2021.356098.1775. PMID: 35546980; PMCID: PMC9083862.

Pandey KB, Rizvi SI. Plant polyphenols as dietary antioxidants in human health and disease. Oxid Med Cell Longev. 2009 Nov-Dec;2(5):270-8. doi: 10.4161/oxim.2.5.9498. PMID: 20716914; PMCID: PMC2835915.

Pizzino G, Irrera N, Cucinotta M, Pallio G, Mannino F, Arcoraci V, Squadrito F, Altavilla D, Bitto A. Oxidative Stress: Harms and Benefits for Human Health. Oxid Med Cell Longev. 2017;2017:8416763. doi: 10.1155/2017/8416763. Epub 2017 Jul 27. PMID: 28819546; PMCID: PMC5551541.

Rivero-Pino F, Montserrat-de la Paz S. The Role of Bioactive Compounds in Immunonutrition. Nutrients. 2024 Oct 10;16(20):3432. doi: 10.3390/nu16203432. PMID: 39458428; PMCID: PMC11510454.

Rodriguez-Leyva D, Dupasquier CM, McCullough R, Pierce GN. The cardiovascular effects of flaxseed and its omega-3 fatty acid, alpha-linolenic acid. Can J Cardiol. 2010 Nov;26(9):489-96. doi: 10.1016/s0828-282x(10)70455-4. PMID: 21076723; PMCID: PMC2989356.

Ruhee RT, Suzuki K. The Integrative Role of Sulforaphane in Preventing Inflammation, Oxidative Stress and Fatigue: A Review of a Potential Protective Phytochemical. Antioxidants (Basel). 2020 Jun 13;9(6):521. doi: 10.3390/antiox9060521. PMID: 32545803; PMCID: PMC7346151.

Sethi G, Shanmugam MK, Ramachandran L, Kumar AP, Tergaonkar V. Multifaceted link between cancer and inflammation. Biosci Rep. 2012 Feb;32(1):1-15. doi: 10.1042/BSR20100136. PMID: 21981137.

Shan G, Minchao K, Jizhao W, Rui Z, Guangjian Z, Jin Z, Meihe L. Resveratrol improves the cytotoxic effect of CD8 +T cells in the tumour microenvironment by regulating HMMR/Ferroptosis in lung squamous cell carcinoma. J Pharm Biomed Anal. 2023 May 30;229:115346. doi: 10.1016/j.jpba.2023.115346. Epub 2023 Mar 15. PMID: 37001272.

Shibru B, Fey K, Fricke S, Blaudszun AR, Fürst F, Weise M, Seiffert S, Weyh MK, Köhl U, Sack U, Boldt A. Detection of Immune Checkpoint Receptors - A Current Challenge in Clinical Flow Cytometry. Front Immunol. 2021 Jul 1;12:694055. doi: 10.3389/fimmu.2021.694055. PMID: 34276685; PMCID: PMC8281132.

Singh BN, Shankar S, Srivastava RK. Green tea catechin, epigallocatechin-3-gallate (EGCG): mechanisms, perspectives and clinical applications. Biochem Pharmacol. 2011 Dec 15;82(12):1807-21. doi: 10.1016/j.bcp.2011.07.093. Epub 2011 Jul 30. PMID: 21827739; PMCID: PMC4082721.

Śliżewska K, Markowiak-Kopeć P, Śliżewska W. The Role of Probiotics in Cancer Prevention. Cancers (Basel). 2020 Dec 23;13(1):20. doi: 10.3390/cancers13010020. PMID: 33374549; PMCID: PMC7793079.

Stefanache A, Lungu II, Butnariu IA, Calin G, Gutu C, Marcu C, Grierosu C, Bogdan Goroftei ER, Duceac LD, Dabija MG, Popa F, Damir D. Understanding How Minerals Contribute to Optimal Immune Function. J Immunol Res. 2023 Nov 1;2023:3355733. doi: 10.1155/2023/3355733. PMID: 37946846; PMCID: PMC10632063.

Swann JB, Smyth MJ. Immune surveillance of tumours. J Clin Invest. 2007 May;117(5):1137-46. doi: 10.1172/JCI31405. PMID: 17476343; PMCID: PMC1857231.

Talapko J, Včev A, Meštrović T, Pustijanac E, Jukić M, Škrlec I. Homeostasis and Dysbiosis of the Intestinal Microbiota: Comparing Hallmarks of a Healthy State with Changes in Inflammatory Bowel Disease. Microorganisms. 2022 Dec 5;10(12):2405. doi: 10.3390/microorganisms10122405. PMID: 36557658; PMCID: PMC9781915.

Talib WH, Awajan D, Alqudah A, Alsawwaf R, Althunibat R, Abu AlRoos M, Al Safadi A, Abu Asab S, Hadi RW, Al Kury LT. Targeting Cancer Hallmarks with Epigallocatechin Gallate (EGCG): Mechanistic Basis and Therapeutic Targets. Molecules. 2024 Mar 20;29(6):1373. doi: 10.3390/molecules29061373. PMID: 38543009; PMCID: PMC10976257.

Tan A, Sullenbarger B, Prakash R, McDaniel JC. Supplementation with eicosapentaenoic acid and docosahexaenoic acid reduces high levels of circulating proinflammatory cytokines in aging adults: A randomized, controlled study. Prostaglandins Leukot Essent Fatty Acids. 2018 May;132:23-29. doi: 10.1016/j.plefa.2018.03.010. Epub 2018 Apr 3. PMID: 29735019; PMCID: PMC5941937.

Thepmalee C, Panya A, Junking M, Chieochansin T, Yenchitsomanus PT. Inhibition of IL-10 and TGF-β receptors on dendritic cells enhances activation of effector T-cells to kill cholangiocarcinoma cells. Hum Vaccin Immunother. 2018 Jun 3;14(6):1423-1431. doi: 10.1080/21645515.2018.1431598. Epub 2018 Feb 21. PMID: 29420117; PMCID: PMC6037468.

Tie Y, Tang F, Wei YQ, Wei XW. Immunosuppressive cells in cancer: mechanisms and potential therapeutic targets. J Hematol Oncol. 2022 May 18;15(1):61. doi: 10.1186/s13045-022-01282-8. PMID: 35585567; PMCID: PMC9118588.

Traber MG, Stevens JF. Vitamins C and E: beneficial effects from a mechanistic perspective. Free Radic Biol Med. 2011 Sep 1;51(5):1000-13. doi: 10.1016/j.freeradbiomed.2011.05.017. Epub 2011 May 25. PMID: 21664268; PMCID: PMC3156342.

Tsuji A, Yoshikawa S, Morikawa S, Ikeda Y, Taniguchi K, Sawamura H, Asai T, Matsuda S. Potential tactics with vitamin D and certain phytochemicals for enhancing the effectiveness of immune-checkpoint blockade therapies. Explor Target Antitumour Ther. 2023;4(3):460-473. doi: 10.37349/etat.2023.00145. Epub 2023 Jun 30. PMID: 37455830; PMCID: PMC10344894.

Vesely MD, Schreiber RD. Cancer immunoediting: antigens, mechanisms, and implications to cancer immunotherapy. Ann N Y Acad Sci. 2013 May;1284(1):1-5. doi: 10.1111/nyas.12105. PMID: 23651186; PMCID: PMC3648872.

Wang Q, Yang B, Wang N, Gu J. Tumour immunomodulatory effects of polyphenols. Front Immunol. 2022 Nov 24;13:1041138. doi: 10.3389/fimmu.2022.1041138. PMID: 36505462; PMCID: PMC9729837.

Wang X, Zeng H, Li L, Fang Z, Xu L, Shi W, Li J, Qian J, Tan X, Li J, Qian Y, Xie L. Personalized nutrition intervention improves nutritional status and quality of life of colorectal cancer survivors in the community: A randomised controlled trial. Nutrition. 2022 Nov-Dec;103-104:111835. doi: 10.1016/j.nut.2022.111835. Epub 2022 Aug 28. PMID: 36183482.

Wang Y, Xiang Y, Xin VW, Wang XW, Peng XC, Liu XQ, Wang D, Li N, Cheng JT, Lyv YN, Cui SZ, Ma Z, Zhang Q, Xin HW. Dendritic cell biology and its role in tumour immunotherapy. J Hematol Oncol. 2020 Aug 3;13(1):107. doi: 10.1186/s13045-020-00939-6. PMID: 32746880; PMCID: PMC7397618.

Wastyk HC, Fragiadakis GK, Perelman D, Dahan D, Merrill BD, Yu FB, Topf M, Gonzalez CG, Van Treuren W, Han S, Robinson JL, Elias JE, Sonnenburg ED, Gardner CD, Sonnenburg JL. Gut-microbiota-targeted diets modulate human immune status. Cell. 2021 Aug 5;184(16):4137-4153.e14. doi: 10.1016/j.cell.2021.06.019. Epub 2021 Jul 12. PMID: 34256014; PMCID: PMC9020749.

Weylandt KH, Serini S, Chen YQ, Su HM, Lim K, Cittadini A, Calviello G. Omega-3 Polyunsaturated Fatty Acids: The Way Forward in Times of Mixed Evidence. Biomed Res Int. 2015;2015:143109. doi: 10.1155/2015/143109. Epub 2015 Aug 2. PMID: 26301240; PMCID: PMC4537707.

Wojtukiewicz MZ, Rek MM, Karpowicz K, Górska M, Polityńska B, Wojtukiewicz AM, Moniuszko M, Radziwon P, Tucker SC, Honn KV. Inhibitors of immune checkpoints-PD-1, PD-L1, CTLA-4-new opportunities for cancer patients and a new challenge for internists and general practitioners. Cancer Metastasis Rev. 2021 Sep;40(3):949-982. doi: 10.1007/s10555-021-09976-0. Epub 2021 Jul 8. PMID: 34236546; PMCID: PMC8556173.

Yahfoufi N, Alsadi N, Jambi M, Matar C. The Immunomodulatory and Anti-Inflammatory Role of Polyphenols. Nutrients. 2018 Nov 2;10(11):1618. doi: 10.3390/nu10111618. PMID: 30400131; PMCID: PMC6266803.

Yan Z, Zhong Y, Duan Y, Chen Q, Li F. Antioxidant mechanism of tea polyphenols and its impact on health benefits. Anim Nutr. 2020 Jun;6(2):115-123. doi: 10.1016/j.aninu.2020.01.001. Epub 2020 Jan 23. PMID: 32542190; PMCID: PMC7283370.

Yang H, Villani RM, Wang H, Simpson MJ, Roberts MS, Tang M, Liang X. The role of cellular reactive oxygen species in cancer chemotherapy. J Exp Clin Cancer Res. 2018 Nov 1;37(1):266. doi: 10.1186/s13046-018-0909-x. PMID: 30382874; PMCID: PMC6211502.

Yang L, Pang Y, Moses HL. TGF-beta and immune cells: an important regulatory axis in the tumour microenvironment and progression. Trends Immunol. 2010 Jun;31(6):220-7. doi: 10.1016/j.it.2010.04.002. Epub 2010 Jun 1. PMID: 20538542; PMCID: PMC2891151.

Yuan M, Zhang G, Bai W, Han X, Li C, Bian S. The Role of Bioactive Compounds in Natural Products Extracted from Plants in Cancer Treatment and Their Mechanisms Related to Anticancer Effects. Oxid Med Cell Longev. 2022 Feb 15;2022:1429869. Doi: 10.1155/2022/1429869. PMID: 35211240; PMCID: PMC8863487.

Zhang P. Influence of Foods and Nutrition on the Gut Microbiome and Implications for Intestinal Health. Int J Mol Sci. 2022 Aug 24;23(17):9588. doi: 10.3390/ijms23179588. PMID: 36076980; PMCID: PMC9455721.

Zhao H, Wu L, Yan G, Chen Y, Zhou M, Wu Y, Li Y. Inflammation and tumour progression: signalling pathways and targeted intervention. Signal Transduct Target Ther. 2021 Jul 12;6(1):263. Doi: 10.1038/s41392-021-00658-5. PMID: 34248142; PMCID: PMC8273155.

Zhao LY, Mei JX, Yu G, Lei L, Zhang WH, Liu K, Chen XL, Kołat D, Yang K, Hu JK. Role of the gut microbiota in anticancer therapy: from molecular mechanisms to clinical applications. Signal Transduct Target Ther. 2023 May 13;8(1):201. doi: 10.1038/s41392-023-01406-7. PMID: 37179402; PMCID: PMC10183032.

Chapter 7

Metabolic Reprogramming in Cancer: Dietary Modulation of Tumour Bioenergetics

Praneeth Juvvi[1], Lokesh Kumar Mishra[2], Sarfraj Ahmad Siddiqui[3], Sheetanshu Gupta[4]

[1]Department of Food Processing Technology, College of Food Technology-Central Agricultural University, Imphal, Manipur, India
[2]Department of BPME, College of Agriculture, Central Agricultural University (CAU), Imphal, Manipur, India
[3]Department of Biochemistry, King George's Medical University, U.P., India
[4]Department of Food Safety and Quality Assurance, College of Food Technology, Central Agricultural University (CAU), Imphal, Manipur, India

Abstract

Cancer cells reprogram metabolism quite radically, thereby supporting rapid proliferation amidst dense nutrients often found under very low oxygen levels. Warped cancer cell metabolism and potential interventions undergo very frequent scrutiny nowadays through dietary modulation that alters tumour bioenergetics rather effectively. Tumour cells display warped metabolic traits and heightened glycolytic activity under hypoxic conditions, sustaining energy production very effectively. Glucose fuels profound metabolic shifts that significantly influence crucial pathways, such as glycolysis, in various cellular processes alongside lipids and oxidative phosphorylation. Ketogenic diets, ridiculously low in carbs and fabulously high in fats, drastically alter tumour metabolism, slowing cancer progression by hammering metabolic vulnerabilities deep within cancer cells. Calorie restriction and intermittent fasting potentially emerge as strategies for modulating tumour bioenergetics, thereby enhancing the effectiveness of conventional cancer therapies very significantly. Emerging research highlights a wildly complex interaction between the gut microbiome and host metabolic processes irregularly within tumour growth patterns. Dietary interventions radically reshape cancer metabolism, offering fresh trajectories for cancer prevention and care quite starkly nowadays. Ultimately, it underscores the necessity of thoroughly grasping the metabolic requirements of diverse tumours for devising innovative therapeutic strategies rooted in nutrition.

Keywords: Metabolic Reprogramming, Tumour Bioenergetics, Glycolysis, Mitochondrial Function, Dietary Interventions, Oncogenic Metabolism

DOI: 10.1201/9781042010387-7

1. Introduction

Malignant cells exhibit aberrant bioenergetic flux and undergo erratic metabolic reprogramming, thereby sustaining frenzied growth amidst inhospitable surroundings with harsh tissue conditions. Tumour cells diverge from normal metabolic pathways used by healthy cells, exhibiting quite dramatic alterations known as metabolic reprogramming fundamentally. Tumour cells thrive quite haphazardly by leveraging various unusual metabolic routes, fueling rapid expansion and circumventing mortality with stubborn resistance. Malignant cells often drastically switch over to aerobic glycolysis for their energy needs while normal cells rely heavily on oxidative phosphorylation. A metabolic shift furnishes ATP and crucial intermediates for anabolic processes such as nucleotide synthesis and lipid production vital for sustaining extremely rapid growth (Schiliro and Firestein, 2021).

Tumourigenesis gets driven partly by quirky metabolic rewiring that oncology metabolism breakthroughs have underscored as a simultaneously crucial outcome and weird catalyst. Cancer cells rapidly reconfigure their bioenergetic profile amidst progressively hypoxic tumour microenvironments largely due to aberrant oncogenic signaling and tumour suppressor dysfunction. Metabolic shifts in cells foster a pro-inflammatory milieu significantly encourage cancer progression further under various pathological conditions quite ominously (Herst et al, 2022).

Reprogramming cellular metabolism enables tumour cells thriving under harsh conditions which makes this a crucial area for snagging potential therapeutic targets. Evidence emerging rather surprisingly suggests dietary interventions via specific nutrients and bioactive compounds modulate tumour bioenergetics effectively providing a novel relatively non-toxic cancer therapy approach. Diet links intricately with metabolic reprogramming in cancer, exhibiting complex phenomena manifesting multifaceted characteristics remarkably within tumour microenvironments. Diet furnishes raw materials for cellular metabolism and modulates crucial signaling pathways controlling enzyme activity in glycolysis, oxidative phosphorylation and fatty acid breakdown processes simultaneously. Glucose alongside microelements and lipids directly impacts cancer cell bioenergetics by influencing key metabolic enzymes through various regulatory pathways energetically (Nong et al, 2020).

Tumour cells are heavily fueled by glucose a primary energy source whose uptake is very frequently upregulated by oncogenes like PI3K/AKT and MYC. Fatty acids derived from dietary fats play a crucial role in synthesising membranes and signaling molecules, and storing energy requisite for tumour proliferation vigorously. Glutamine and serine alongside glutamate play crucial roles fueling diverse biosynthetic pathways upholding redox homeostasis precariously inside cancerous cells. Dietary patterns heavily influence tumour metabolism sparking keen interest amongst researchers studying relationships between diet and cancer prevention very closely. Evidence abounds that tumourigenesis gets a significant boost from Western diets loaded with heaps of processed food and saturated fats (Yang et al, 2023).

Fostering somewhat balanced metabolism diets rich in veggies and whole grains akin to Mediterranean cuisine have been loosely tied to lowered cancer risk. Novel research indicates caloric restriction and intermittent fasting profoundly alter tumour bioenergetics by markedly shifting metabolic pathways toward oxidation of fatty acids. Research focuses increasingly on bioactive compounds in foods that potentially modulate tumour metabolism and alter cellular bioenergetics rather profoundly. Compounds sourced from turmeric like curcumin and resveratrol present in grapes deeply affect metabolic pathways by inhibiting specific enzymes naturally (Mentella et al, 2019).

Crucial roles are played by these compounds in regulating metabolic gene expression via epigenetic mods like DNA methylation and histone modification reprogramming tumour metabolism potentially.

Omega-3 fatty acids present in fish and flaxseeds convincingly alter lipid metabolism in cancer cells shifting them radically toward oxidative metabolic states (Huo et al, 2021).

Mitochondrial function plays a crucial role deeply within cancer's metabolic reprogramming and recent research highlights mitochondria's complex dual role as key energy producers and vital signaling hubs. Mitochondria regulate ATP production and various cellular processes including apoptosis autophagy and ROS production rather intricately deep within eukaryotic cells. Tumours often exhibit aberrant mitochondrial dynamics with heightened biogenesis occurring alongside respiration processes somewhat altered simultaneously in many cases. Cancer cells' metabolic flexibility relies heavily on remodeling mitochondrial function fairly rapidly in response to wildly fluctuating nutrient availability (Du et al, 2025).

Provision of vitamins C or E and other antioxidants holds promise for improving mitochondrial function through nutritional interventions aimed somewhat irregularly. Coenzyme Q10 therapies potentially reinstate equilibrium somewhat irregularly within bodily systems. Tumour cells exhibit wildly fluctuating bioenergetics somewhat erratically limiting their proliferation ability under certain conditions rather unpredictably. Dietary interventions are gaining traction nowadays as potentially effective therapeutic strategies targeting tumour metabolism rapidly and surprisingly quite effectively. Reprogramming metabolic pathways enables cancer cells sustain rapid growth and survival while efficacious dietary interventions potentially thwart malignant processes somewhat effectively (Alexandru et al, 2024).

Ketogenic diets drastically curtail glucose availability thereby potentially starving tumours of preferred fuel and instead encouraging alternative utilization of fatty acids and ketone bodies. Pharmacological agents mimicking certain dietary components' effects are being explored as potential therapies that markedly enhance dietary intervention effects. Metabolic reprogramming mechanisms in cancer have profound bioenergetic implications for tumours and can be somewhat modulated by various dietary interventions (Poffet al, 2019). Tumour growth relies heavily on glucose metabolism and fatty acid metabolism for survival under diverse physiological stresses alongside amino acid catabolism. Emerging evidence on dietary patterns potentially preventing cancer by effectively modulating tumour metabolism will be discussed very thoroughly nowadays. Cancer biology intersects intriguingly with dietary habits and metabolic pathways in profoundly complex manners shedding light on modified nutritional interventions supplementary.

2. The Metabolic Shift in Cancer Cells: Understanding Tumour Bioenergetics

Malignant cells reprogram metabolism extensively beneath stress for survival and swift proliferation amidst diverse tumour microenvironments often under highly abnormal conditions. Cells prefer glycolysis fervently as primary ATP production pathway despite being enveloped by copious oxygen levels ordinarily surrounding them. Differentiated cells mostly rely heavily on mitochondrial oxidative phosphorylation under aerobic settings yielding ATP very efficiently with considerable effectiveness. Cancer cells derive several benefits from relying heavily on glycolysis which proves energetically inefficient yet remains strangely advantageous in many weird obscure ways. It facilitates swift production of metabolic intermediates necessary for biosynthesis of nucleotides, amino acids and lipids crucial for rapid cell growth (Schiliro and Firestein, 2022).

Glycolysis churns out lactate rapidly acidifying tumour microenvironment very vigorously thereby heavily promoting tissue invasion and immune evasion alongside angiogenesis. Cancer cells thrive quite haphazardly amidst wildly gyrating oxygen concentrations and uneven nutrient distribution within dense tumour masses owing largely to metabolic reprogramming. Cancer cells drastically alter glutamine metabolism and fatty acid synthesis alongside glucose metabolism sustaining proliferation under oxidative stress very effectively. Tumour progression gets enhanceed by sundry metabolic tweaks fostering metastasis and resistance therapies like chemotherapy that target proliferating cells or crank out reactive oxygen species (Schiliro and Firestein, 2022).

Tumour metabolism presents a promising avenue nowadays for novel interventions quite effectively in cancer research facilities globally with considerable potential. Agents disrupting anabolic pathways and modulators of mitochondrial function alongside inhibitors of glycolytic enzymes face intense scrutiny exploiting metabolic vulnerabilities inherent in cancer cells. Metabolic reprogramming deeply affects immune cell functionality within tumour microenvironments facilitating radically new combination strategies markedly enhancing immunotherapy efficacy. Rapidly emerging novel interventions stem from ongoing cancer bioenergetics research advances offering hope for lately more efficacious personalized treatment options (Tufail et al, 2024).

2.1. The Warburg Effect and its Implications

Otto Warburg initially observed cancer cells displaying heightened glycolytic rates under aerobic conditions in 1920s sparking interest in aerobic glycolysis. Mitochondria churn out energy very efficiently under normal circumstances via oxidative phosphorylation producing a whole lot more ATP per glucose molecule. Glycolysis gets weirdly upregulated in cancer cells even with oxygen around leading quickly to lactate production fairly rapidly. Tumour cells derive numerous benefits from heavily shifting metabolic pathways towards glycolysis enabling swift ATP production and biosynthesis of necessary macromolecules for rapid proliferation. Tumour microenvironment changes alongside genetic mutations and altered oncogene signaling ostensibly drive Warburg effect (Liberti and Locasale, 2016).

Tumour cells often harbor mutations in genes like PIK3CA or KRAS and TP53 that drastically heighten glucose demand altering metabolic pathways. Tumour environments with hypoxic conditions vigorously promote activation of transcription factors like HIF-1α upregulating various glycolytic enzymes and glucose transporters further. Cancer cells ferment glucose quickly into lactate even when oxygen is available diminishing mitochondrial oxidative phosphorylation very rapidly. Unbridled cell division necessitates rampant bioenergetic and anabolic activity that cancer cells tap into with facility at astonishing speed very quickly. Tumour microenvironment lactate accumulation fosters an acidic milieu that promotes invasion and metastasis by weakening surrounding tissues very rapidly (Liberti and Locasale, 2016).

2.2. Metabolic Reprogramming Beyond Glycolysis

Tumours display aberrant biosynthetic pathways and bioenergetic flux amidst a broader metabolic shift not limited merely to glycolytic upregulation in cancerous cells. Tumour cells undergo significant weird changes quite frequently in various metabolic pathways including lipid metabolism or altered mitochondrial function . Alterations vigorously support energy production and synthesis of key biomolecules needed for tumour growth under various harsh conditions obviously. Cancer cells often exhibit markedly elevated fatty acid synthesis and lipid uptake crucial for rapidly forming new membranes and storing energy (Phan et al, 2014).

Lipid metabolism becomes intricately entangled with regulation of various signaling pathways that control cell proliferation and survival remarkably well. Fatty acid metabolism ramps up acetyl-CoA production fueling activation of enzymes that acetylate proteins and thereby dynamically modulate gene expression. Metabolism of amino acids such as glutamine or serine gets drastically altered rather frequently in various types of cancer cells . Glutamine fuels biosynthesis vigorously supplying nitrogen for various cellular processes and remarkably boosts energy production under diverse physiological states (Fu et al, 2020).

Glutamine converts fairly extensively into α-ketoglutarate feeding TCA cycle under certain conditions thereby supporting mitochondrial energy production quite robustly. Serine metabolism remarkably fuels synthesis of nucleotides and proteins crucial for cancer cell proliferation very effectively under certain conditions. Cancer cells rely heavily on glycolysis for energy production yet mitochondria play crucial roles in supporting various metabolic processes normally in cells (Jin et al, 2023).

Mitochondrial dysfunction or reprogramming in cancerous cells remarkably maintains metabolic balance under various physiological conditions favoring growth quite anomalously. Mitochondria churn out biosynthetic intermediates such as NADPH and acetyl-CoA regulating cell survival pathways very crucially in cells. Mitochondria play a role in apoptotic resistance very effectively, another ghastly hallmark of cancerous cells facilitating evasion of cell death (Księżakowska-Łakoma et al, 2014).

2.3. Tumour Metabolism and Therapeutic Targeting

Peculiar biochemical quirks of malignant cells are grasped nowadays unlocking fresh, remarkably groundbreaking treatment avenues very quickly. Several metabolic enzymes and sundry biochemical pathways are being flagged very rapidly as potential targets for developing novel drugs these days. Key glycolytic enzymes such as hexokinase 2 and pyruvate kinase M2 have inhibitors being explored very actively nowadays as potential therapeutic agents. Inhibitors quite vigorously disrupt glycolytic pathways in tumour cells, effectively starving them by thwarting energy and biosynthetic intermediate production. Glutamine metabolism has rather surprisingly emerged as a novel therapeutic target deeply rooted and firmly established in oncology research endeavours (Kumar et al, 2022).

Glutaminase inhibitors have shown considerable promise in preclinical cancer models, effectively blocking the conversion of glutamine into glutamate quite remarkably. Tumour cells might be starved of a crucial nutrient necessary for survival by severely limiting glutamine availability through this rather unorthodox approach. Metabolic reprogramming therapies strive quite desperately to restore very normal metabolic function in malignant cells, rendering them fairly susceptible to treatments like chemotherapy. Therapies promote cell death by targeting metabolic vulnerabilities and reduce inflammation associated with tumours in diverse microenvironments very effectively. Malignant cells undergo drastic metabolic rewiring, allowing tumours surreptitiously flourish in nutrient-scarce and very hypoxic conditions with aplenty chaotic molecular signalling (Yang et al, 2021).

Malignant cells thrive at an astonishing rate under rather inhospitable circumstances by reconfiguring metabolic routes effectively enough for boosted viability. Novel cancer treatments emerge quite effectively nowadays from grasping the intricate energy needs of malignant tumours with considerable pathological precision. Researchers craft novel tactics capitalising on the frailties inherent in cancer cells, thereby boosting survival rates significantly with current regimens complemented. Tumour bioenergetics research profoundly propels cancer therapy forward and sheds critical light on obscure facets of cancer metabolism's fundamental biology (Krzyszczyk et al, 2018).

3. Dietary Influences on Cancer Cell Metabolism and Growth

Malignant cells exhibit profoundly altered metabolic reprogramming, manifesting as a pronounced shift from mitochondrial oxidative phosphorylation towards heightened glycolysis under aerobic conditions. Tumour cell proliferation happens swiftly, and survival gets enhanced by metabolic adaptation within a very rough tumour microenvironment under intense biosynthetic demands. Tumour cells become heavily reliant on nutrients such as glucose and glutamine rapidly fueling anabolic processes and sustaining redox balance somewhat irregularly. Evidence accumulating rapidly suggests certain dietary factors modulate tumour growth remarkably whereas traditional cancer therapies interfere heavily with metabolic processes (Zhang et al, 2020).

Dietary nutrients profoundly impact cancer cell bioenergetics by modulating systemic metabolism hormonal cascades and gut microbiota configuration rather indirectly or directly. Low carb diets or caloric restriction regimens drastically curtail glucose supply fueling glycolytic tumour cells thereby starving them of vital energy sources. Ketogenic diets ridiculously high in fats and lowish in carbs have been shown in preclinical models shifting systemic metabolism towards fatty acid oxidation very effectively making cancer cells reliant on glucose quite vulnerable. Polyphenols and omega-3 fatty acids exhibit an ability rather curiously to interfere with cancer-associated metabolic pathways like glycolysis and fatty acid synthesis heavily (Caprara et al, 2025).

Tumour microenvironment gets profoundly tweaked by dietary changes that mess with immune cell metabolism and inflammatory signaling linked rapidly to tumour progression. Findings underscore diet as a modifiable factor complementing conventional cancer treatments by targeting bioenergetics of tumours very effectively nowadays. Ongoing research in oncology care endeavors quite vigorously elucidating precise and intensely scrutinized nutrition interventions effective in highly modified treatment plans (Bader et al, 2020).

3.1. Metabolic Reprogramming and Cancer Growth

Mitochondria efficiently crank out energy via oxidative phosphorylation under normal conditions using oxygen and glucose very quickly . Aerobic metabolism fuels various cellular functions remarkably efficiently overall with little waste being produced. Cancer cells often exhibit aberrant metabolic reprogramming known as Warburg effect characterized by markedly favoring aerobic glycolysis over oxidative phosphorylation for abundant ATP generation. Tumour cells proliferate rapidly and survive off metabolic reprogramming that generates biosynthetic precursors and energy at a frenzied pace. Mutations in genes like PIK3CA or KRAS often dysregulate signaling pathways such as PI3K/AKT/mTOR driving metabolic switch largely in cancerous cells (Zheng J, 2012).

Activation of these pathways yields upregulation of glycolytic enzymes and glucose transporters which facilitates very increased glucose uptake rather quickly and enhances glycolysis somewhat. Cancer cells dividing rapidly have bioenergetic demands met by this shift and it supports anabolic processes producing intermediates essential for biosynthesis of nucleotides lipids and amino acids. Dietary intake markedly alters tumour metabolic phenotype under certain conditions and significantly influences various complex metabolic pathways quite profoundly. Macronutrients such as carbs and proteins alongside micronutrients including antioxidants effectively modulate signaling pathways involved in cancer metabolism (Zheng J, 2012).

Diets deprived of simple sugars or replete with anti-inflammatory fats like omega-3 fatty acids may impede tumour progression and metabolic reprogramming somewhat. Antioxidants in various fruits or veggies can mitigate oxidative stress thereby significantly influencing tumour growth and modulating diverse immune responses rapidly. Diet stands out as a mutable factor capable of either supercharging or stifling metabolic flux in cancer cells highlighting prospects for modified nutritional regimens and improved clinical results (Yu et al, 2024).

3.2. Glucose and Glycolytic Pathways

Glucose fuels glycolysis a primary metabolic pathway that many cancer cells hijack rather haphazardly supporting rapid proliferation and survival very vigorously. Gobbling refined sugars and high-glycemic-index foods surges dietary glucose intake thereby vigorously fueling tumour growth from within bodily tissues rapidly. Glucose consumption at a high level often cultivates insulin resistance systemically and triggers hyperinsulinemia quite abnormally in certain people suddenly. Insulin acts vigorously as a potent mitogenic factor beyond metabolic roles by activating insulin and insulin-like growth factor signaling pathways. IGF-1 receptor activation sparks multiple downstream cascades involving PI3K/AKT/mTOR pathway fueling cancer cell proliferation and inhibiting apoptosis rather heavily (Cunha et al, 2023).

Modulating glucose availability through diet emerges as a promising strategy that influences tumour metabolism effectively under some physiological circumstances. Ketogenic diets have garnered considerable interest lately for starving tumours of glucose very effectively by depriving them of energy suddenly. Ketogenic diets drastically curtail carbohydrate intake often plunging below 10 percent of total caloric intake and ramping up fat consumption very significantly inducing ketosis. Systemic energy metabolism shifts decidedly away from glucose oxidation toward fatty acid oxidation and ketone body utilization remarkably quickly. Ketogenic diets very significantly hinder growth of certain tumour types by reducing glycolytic flux and starving cancer cells dependent on glycolysis (Cunha et al, 2023).

Ketone bodies exert profoundly anti-tumour effects by modulating various cellular signaling pathways and inhibit AKT/mTOR axis leading to apoptosis in tumour cells. Ketogenic diets rather effectively sensitize tumours to standard therapies like chemotherapy or radiation by altering cellular bioenergetics very profoundly. Very much emerging clinical data substantiate roles of glucose restriction in diet and metabolic reprogramming as strategies for adjunctive cancer management (Talib et al, 2021).

3.3. Fatty Acids and Lipid Metabolism

Cancer cells drastically reconfigure lipid metabolism rapidly under wildly aberrant circumstances for survival and cell proliferation occurs somewhat haphazardly. Lipid biosynthesis generates cellular membranes crucial for tumour growth and produces signaling molecules vital for energy storage mechanisms . Fatty acids serve crucially as blocks for phospholipid synthesis and substrates for β-oxidation providing surplus ATP for cancer cells quietly. Certain fatty acids can profoundly affect cancer cell metabolism under specific physiological conditions or surprisingly alter it in subtle ways. Monounsaturated and polyunsaturated fats found in olive oil nuts and fatty fish remarkably modulate expression and activity of crucial lipogenic enzymes (Fu et al, 2020).

FASN catalyzes synthesis of long-chain fatty acids necessary in membrane biogenesis fairly often in various types of cancerous cells. Diets rich in unsaturated fats potentially alter tumour lipid metabolism and growth by impacting activity of FASN quite significantly nowadays. Diets rich in saturated fats found in red meat and processed foods correlate with heightened inflammatory markers and greater risk of various cancers suddenly. Saturated fatty acids activate sterol regulatory element-binding protein 1 or SREBP-1 which subsequently upregulates genes involved in lipid synthesis quite vigorously. Enhanced SREBP-1 activity vigorously ramps up de novo lipogenesis fueling tumour proliferation and enhance survival mechanisms rather effectively in cancer cells. Omega-3 polyunsaturated fatty acids found copiously in fatty fish and quite plentifully in flaxseeds lately have garnered much attention for markedly anti-inflammatory effects (Menendez et al, 2024).

Fatty acids disrupt lipid rafts rich with cholesterol in cancer cell plasma membranes which serve as crucial microdomains for signal transduction apparently. Omega-3 PUFAs drastically modify lipid raft composition thereby thwarting PI3K/AKT/mTOR pathway activation suppressing tumour growth quite markedly and diminishing metastasis potential. Omega-3 fatty acids dampen pro-inflammatory cytokines thus modulating tumour milieu further encourage therapeutic potential remarkably in various cancerous contexts. Findings underscore importance of dietary fatty acid composition in cancer lipid metabolism and highlight potential for nutritional interventions modulating tumour progression slowly (Menendez et al, 2024).

3.4. Amino Acids and Cancer Cell Proliferation

Amino acids frantically serve as precursors for nucleotides and glutathione in cancer cells undergoing rapid chaotic protein synthesis. Glutamine plays quite a pivotal role in tumour metabolism deeply within cells. Glutamine furnishes vital carbon and nitrogen rather haphazardly for various anabolic processes in cancer contexts being dubbed a conditionally essential amino acid. Glutamine serves as vital nitrogen donor in nucleotide biosynthesis and fuels energy production replenishing tricarboxylic acid cycle intermediates via conversion to α-ketoglutarate. Glutamine metabolism rather quietly influences cell growth signaling pathways directly beyond its biosynthetic role somewhat mysteriously. Glutamine vigorously activates mechanistic target of rapamycin pathway crucial for cellular growth and subsequent proliferation occurs (Liu et al, 2024).

mTOR signaling dysregulation manifests as hallmark of various cancers intricately linking tumour progression with nutrient availability very deeply. Tumour growth gets markedly modulated by dietary glutamine in cancers with pronounced glutamine addiction like some very aggressive pancreatic tumours and lymphomas. Tumour growth and survival in highly malignant cancer cells can be enhanced rapidly with increased glutamine availability under certain conditions quite effectively. Tumours are being starved of critical nutrient by depriving them of glutamine and inhibiting transporters such as ASCT2 through various therapeutic strategies. Serine glycine and cysteine vigorously fuel nucleotide synthesis in cancer progression alongside methylation reactions and redox balance very energetically (Harachi et al, 2018).

Certain amino acids crucially play a role sustaining DNA replication and encourage cellular redox homeostasis via glutathione synthesis naturally in cells. Diets rich in animal proteins tend to furnish copious amounts of these amino acids potentially fuelling tumour growth rather vigorously. Plant-based proteins usually flaunt a motley crew of amino acids and lower glycemic index possibly exerting rather subdued stimulatory effects on cancer metabolism. Tumour growth intertwines intricately with amino acid metabolism revealing novel avenues for oncology therapies via dietary modulation of targeted metabolic pathways (Harachi et al, 2018).

3.5. Micronutrients and Antioxidants

Essential vitamins and minerals play crucial roles normally in sustaining immune function and mitigating oxidative stress deeply within bodily tissues. Vitamin D and A alongside trace elements such as selenium rather effectively modulate immune responses and protect cellular homeostasis with some efficacy. Vitamin D a secosteroid hormone gets studied extensively nowadays globally for anti-cancer properties in various research studies every single year. Vitamin D receptor profoundly influences genes involved in tumour suppression downstream and affects cell proliferation and apoptosis in a rather significant manner. Vitamin D markedly boosts immune surveillance by promoting cytotoxic T lymphocytes activity and macrophages thus honing immune system's prowess eliminating malignant cells effectively (Mitra et al, 2022).

Vitamin D deficiency strongly correlates with higher incidence of cancers like colorectal cancer and dismal prognosis in prostate malignancies or breast cancer. Antioxidants plentiful in fruits and veggies crucially neutralize reactive oxygen species that violently ravage DNA and proteins very badly. Oxidative damage foments carcinogenesis haphazardly via sundry mutations and genomic instability thereby promoting tumour growth further with erratic fervor. Phytochemicals like flavonoids and vitamins C and E very effectively scavenge free radicals thereby reducing oxidative stress within tumour cells and surrounding microenvironment. Selenium serves as cofactor remarkably well for glutathione peroxidase and other antioxidant enzymes maintaining redox balance against DNA damage effectively. Adequate selenium levels have been linked with remarkably reduced cancer risk and enhanceed immune function very well in numerous studies (Gupta et al, 2011).

Dietary components profoundly impact cancer cell metabolism and growth under various physiological conditions in sometimes strongly contradictory ways. Glucose and saturated fats fuel glycolysis thereby fuelling tumour proliferation rapidly while omega-3 fatty acids thwart tumour progression somewhat haphazardly. Dietary factors intricately modulate various metabolic pathways offering a promising complementary strategy remarkably for enhancing efficacy of chemotherapy and radiation therapy effectively. Cancer prevention efforts through nutritional interventions offer a potentially holistic approach as research steadily deepens into diet and cancer metabolic interplay. Precise evidence-based dietary guidelines must be developed for cancer patients optimizing immune function and overall metabolic health potentially improving outcomes greatly (Gupta et al, 2011).

4. Metabolic Reprogramming: A Key Feature of Cancer Progression

Tumour cells thrive in hostile environments owing largely to remarkable metabolic reprogramming that underpins their prolific survival capabilities quite remarkably. Reprogramming entails drastic shifts in cellular metabolism fueling extremely high bioenergetic demands and frenzied biosynthetic needs tied with rapid cell division. Cells display a bizarre affinity for glycolytic routes even when oxygen supply seems plentiful thereby manifesting a warped metabolic anomaly dubbed Warburg effect. Normal differentiated cells produce ATP mainly via mitochondrial oxidative phosphorylation a fairly efficient bioenergetic process that fully oxidizes glucose into water and carbon dioxide. Malignant cells deliberately shunt glucose metabolism toward glycolysis converting glucose into lactate even when oxygen surrounds them in abundance nearby (Schiliro and Firestein, 2021).

Glycolysis yields fewer ATP molecules than OXPHOS but remarkably confers several crucial benefits on proliferating cancer cells under very specific physiological conditions. Metabolic adaptation spawns ATP rapidly meeting urgent energy demands yielding crucial intermediates for synthesizing key macromolecules like nucleotides, amino acids, lipids necessary for biomass accrual and cell proliferation. Cancer cells thrive in hypoxic tumour regions with low oxygen levels by heavily shifting metabolic processes towards decidedly glycolytic pathways. Tumour microenvironment acidifies substantially with lactate accumulation thereby promoting angiogenesis and invasion while cytotoxic immune cell activity gets dampened slowly (Zheng J, 2012).

Ongoing oncogenic mutations intricately orchestrate metabolic reprogramming upregulating glycolytic enzymes through dysregulated signaling pathways like hypoxia-inducible factor 1-alpha pathways becomes: Oncogenic mutations reprogram metabolism quite intricately by upregulating glycolytic enzymes via aberrant signaling pathways involving hypoxia-inducible factor 1-alpha. Cancer cells shift metabolic gears dynamically in response to various cues and foster tumour progression robustly under diverse environmental conditions thereafter. Metabolic reprogramming plays a crucial role in cancer development and researchers devise new tactics aimed at exploiting various inherent vulnerabilities squarely in cancer cells. Modulating lipid biosynthesis and inhibiting glycolysis or disrupting glutamine metabolism starves tumour cells of energy sources promising improved treatment outcomes effectively (Zheng J, 2012).

4.1. The Warburg Effect: A Metabolic Signature of Cancer Cells

Otto Warburg initially pinpointed a bizarre metabolic tweak in cancer cells during 1920s whereby they inexplicably harness glycolysis for energy despite surrounding oxygen abundance. Mitochondria produce up to 36 ATP molecules per glucose molecule efficiently under normal physiological conditions via oxidative phosphorylation primarily. Cancer cells rely heavily on glycolysis a rather inefficient metabolic pathway that yields merely 2 ATP molecules per glucose molecule. Glycolysis yields relatively low ATP yet confers significant advantages on rapidly dividing tumour cells under peculiar circumstances rather anomalously.

Biosynthetic precursors build up swiftly through this process facilitating synthesis of nucleotides, amino acids and lipids crucial for cell growth and proliferation rapidly (Liberti and Locasale, 2016).

Cancer cells shunt glycolytic intermediates into anabolic pathways, sustaining proliferation's remarkably high metabolic demands at a very fast rate. Mutant oncogenes and tweaked tumour suppressor genes orchestrate metabolic recalibration towards glycolysis, not merely in cancerous cells. Mutations in genes such as KRAS and TP53 very aggressively ramp up signalling cascades, promoting expression of glycolytic enzymes and glucose uptake. Tumour microenvironment hypoxia induces stabilisation of hypoxia-inducible factor 1-alpha, a master regulator upregulating genes encoding glycolytic enzymes, heavily driving flux. Enhanced glycolysis triggers lactate production, rampantly acidifying the tumour microenvironment severely with rather drastic consequences nearby (Hammoudi et al, 2011).

Acidic environments ferociously facilitate cancer cell invasion by degrading the extracellular matrix, thus enabling metastasis formation in distant locales very quickly. Lactate accumulation severely impairs cytotoxic immune cells like T lymphocytes and natural killer cells, enabling tumour evasion of immune surveillance effectively. Grasping the Warburg effect sheds crucial light on tumour biology nowadays, highlighting metabolic vulnerabilities that can be rather therapeutically exploited (Liberti and Locasale, 2016).

4.2. Altered Amino Acid Metabolism in Cancer Cells

Cancer cells rapidly proliferating in harsh nutrient-deprived environments undergo drastic changes in amino acid metabolism, with reconfigured glucose metabolism occurring simultaneously. Glutamine emerges as a crucial nutrient furnishing carbon and nitrogen liberally for myriad biosynthetic processes vital to rapid tumour growth. Malignant cells drastically enhance glutamine uptake and subsequent breakdown via an obscure metabolic pathway known as glutaminolysis somewhat irregularly. Glutamine converts into glutamate, subsequently morphing into α-ketoglutarate, a vital intermediate that replenishes tricarboxylic acid cycle via anaplerotic pathways energetically. Cancer cells exhibiting metabolic flexibility produce ATP and biosynthetic precursors via sustained TCA cycle activity under glucose-scarce conditions (Cluntun et a, 2017).

Glutaminolysis very effectively fuels the synthesis of various nucleotides and amino acids, thereby facilitating cell proliferation and survival mechanisms quite rapidly. The serine-glycine biosynthesis pathway often goes haywire in cancer cells, amidst wildly aberrant glutamine metabolism very frequently underground. Serine and glycine play crucial roles in one-carbon metabolism, fueling nucleotide biosynthesis very effectively while maintaining redox homeostasis with methylation reactions happening simultaneously. Phosphoglycerate dehydrogenase catalyzes conversion of 3-phosphoglycerate to serine and is frequently overexpresses in aggressive cancers such as melanoma or glioblastoma. Elevated PHGDH expression boosts serine production, which supercharges nucleotide synthesis turbocharging tumour growth rapidly these days in various cancer types (Cluntun et a, 2017).

Tumour cells display aberrant amino acid metabolism quite remarkably under harsh conditions sustaining bioenergetic demands and supporting anabolic processes very effectively. Metabolic plasticity offers fresh avenues down cancer therapy pathways becoming increasingly pivotal in devising novel treatments rapidly nowadays. Pharmacological inhibitors of glutaminase are being investigated quite slowly nowadays in various research studies for their potential therapeutic effects. Disrupting tumour-specific metabolic dependencies very effectively in serine biosynthesis pathway by targeting enzymes like PHGDH represents promising therapeutic options squarely. Tumour progression gets a significant boost from altered amino acid metabolism and very innovative treatments can capitalize on resultant metabolic vulnerabilities (Do et al, 2025).

4.3. Lipid Metabolism and Cancer Progression

Lipids play a fundamental role alongside glucose and amino acids in cancer cell metabolism supporting proliferation quite effectively very rapidly. Fatty acids serve as crucial precursors in synthesizing cellular membranes essential suddenly during cell division and rapid cellular expansion occurs. Cancer cells vigorously upregulate fatty acid synthesis pathway satisfying heightened demand for membrane lipids with FASN acting as a key enzyme. Aggressive cancers such as triple-negative breast cancer and ovarian cancer quite frequently exhibit pronounced upregulation of diverse lipid biosynthesis pathways. Metabolic reprogramming often coincides with buildup of lipid droplets inside cells that serve as reservoirs protecting cancer cells from oxidative stress very effectively (Fu et al, 2020).

Tumour cell survival gets markedly enhanced correlating with presence of lipid droplets and heightened metastatic potential alongside chemotherapy resistance emerging fairly frequently. Lipids play crucial roles somewhat mysteriously in oncogenic signaling modulation and serve as fundamental structural components very frequently. Sphingolipids and phosphoinositides serve as bioactive molecules intricately regulating key intracellular signaling pathways deeply embedded in cell growth and motility . Phosphoinositides flagrantly enable PI3K/AKT/mTOR pathway activation a major cancer cell proliferation driver and survival mechanism fairly quickly. Lipid metabolism plays a crucial role in cancer progression and represents a tantalizing target for novel therapeutic interventions (Fu et al, 2020).

FASN inhibitors efficaciously disrupt lipid synthesis in preclinical models thereby stunting cancer cell proliferation and impairing membrane formation quite significantly. Inhibiting fatty acid synthesis rather effectively sensitizes cancer cells to therapies like chemotherapy and radiation by very significantly reducing metabolic adaptability. Reprogramming lipid metabolism supports facets of cancer progression quite vigorously from membrane biogenesis and signaling right through chemoresistance making intervention therapeutically critical (Chen et al, 2025).

4.4. Mitochondrial Function and Metabolic Flexibility

Mitochondria remains vital for tumour cell metabolism survival even though cancer cells rely very heavily on glycolysis for producing energy. Mitochondria rapidly fuel cancer progression by generating crucial biosynthetic precursors needed for synthesis of nucleotides lipids and various amino acids. Crucial role played by them maintaining cellular redox homeostasis proves vital for mitigating oxidative stress and sustaining viability of cancer cells under harsh conditions. Mitochondrial dysfunction plays a precariously ambivalent role in cancer biology with somewhat paradoxical consequences often emerging rather quietly. Mitochondrial dysfunction precipitously leads to overproduction of reactive oxygen species that foster genetic instability via induction of DNA damage rather haphazardly. Genomic instability rapidly drives tumour evolution and somewhat fuels heterogeneity down line, markedly increasing malignancy with enhanced ferocity over time (Phan et al, 2014).

High ROS levels ramp up signaling pathways fostering swift tumour growth and mediating stubborn resistance to cell death under specific circumstances. Tumour cells dynamically switch between glycolysis and oxidative phosphorylation under varying conditions with fluctuating oxygen levels and nutrient availability . Cancer cells remarkably thrive under wildly fluctuating conditions such as hypoxia within poorly vascularized tumours and scarcity of various nutrients. Cancer cells drastically alter their reliance on mitochondrial oxidative metabolism for energy production when glucose becomes suddenly severely limited. Tumour cells remarkably withstand therapeutic stressors due to metabolic adaptability fueling resistance against various treatments very effectively (Aggarwal et al, 2019).

Disrupting mitochondrial function has emerged rather promisingly as therapeutic strategy by targeting metabolic flexibility with some considerable efficacy lately. Cancer cells may get sensitized to chemotherapy and radiation by agents that mess with mitochondrial respiration or ramp up ROS production metabolically . Glycolysis dominates cancer metabolism yet mitochondria persist stubbornly supporting biosynthesis and maintaining precarious redox homeostasis fueling tumour progression thereby (Aggarwal et al, 2019).

4.5. Therapeutic Implications of Targeting Metabolic Reprogramming

Novel therapeutic strategies disrupting unique tumour cell metabolic dependencies have emerged very rapidly owing largely recognition of metabolic reprogramming as fundamental driver of cancer. Tumour growth gets selectively thwarted by targeting certain crucial enzymes crucial for cancer cells' energy production sparing normal cells from harsh effects. Glycolysis inhibition has garnered considerable attention recently owing largely cancer cells' heavy reliance on aerobic glycolysis crudely dubbed Warburg effect. Hexokinase 2 inhibitors and lactate dehydrogenase catalysts of crucial glycolytic steps are being explored vigorously nowadays for starving rapidly proliferating cancer cells. Suppressing LDH activity reduces lactate accumulation thereby somewhat normalizing tumour microenvironment and encourage functionality of immune cells quite significantly (Zhao et al, 2011).

Cancer cells display intense reliance on glutamine fairly frequently making glutaminase a potentially promising target therapeutically for novel strategies . Glutaminase inhibitors face intense scrutiny for blocking glutamine-driven anaplerosis and biosynthesis thus severely disrupting proliferation of cancer cells. Aberrant lipid biosynthesis plays crucial roles in membrane formation and signaling deeply within cancer cells spreading very rampantly. FASN inhibitors and other lipogenesis crucial enzymes are being developed at a rapid pace thereby limiting tumour growth noticeably and enhancing chemosensitivity. Cancer cells display remarkable metabolic plasticity and targeting mitochondrial function offers supplementary anticancer strategy with quite astonishing effectiveness generally (Yang et al, 2021).

Certain agents markedly impair mitochondrial respiration or boost ROS production thereby sensitizing tumours and diminishing adaptability of cancer cells. Metabolic inhibitors coupled with conventional treatments such as chemotherapy alongside dodgy molecular therapies hold tremendous promise for efficacy therapeutically (Yang et al, 2021). Assailing cancer cells on multiple metabolic genetic and immune fronts simultaneously yields synergistic effects thereby surmounting various mechanisms of resistance to therapy.

5. Nutritional Strategies for Targeting Tumour Metabolism

Cancer cells undergo profound metabolic reprogramming sustaining rapid growth very much and ensuring their survival through some very weird cellular mechanisms . Tumours burgeon energetically by hijacking metabolic pathways favoring glycolysis with oxygen galore and concurrently tweak amino acid and lipid metabolism recklessly. Metabolic vulnerabilities being recognized has opened up new rather unusual avenues for therapeutic approaches cleverly designed to starkly alter tumour metabolism. Dietary interventions modulate nutrient availability perturbing metabolic pathways in myriad ways hindering tumour growth and amplifying effectiveness of conventional cancer therapies somewhat vigorously (Schiliro et al, 2021).

Nutritional strategies craft a metabolic milieu inhospitable for cancer progression slyly by tweaking nutrient composition and timing of intake quite effectively. Drastically cutting glucose intake via ketogenic diets starves glycolysis-dependent tumour cells of fuel rather effectively in certain examined nutritional strategies. Tumour energy metabolism gets impaired somewhat effectively by restriction and insulin signaling that fuels cancer cell proliferation decreases sensitizing tumours to chemotherapy meanwhile. Biosynthesis and growth of cancer cells gets disrupted rather effectively upon restricting dietary glutamine or inhibiting uptake of serine and glycine. Diets rich in plant-based nutrients having varied amino acid compositions may greatly influence tumour metabolism starkly differently than animal-based regimens. Unsaturated and omega-3 fatty acids found in sources such as olive oil nuts and fatty fish may hinder tumour growth very substantially (Schiliro et al, 2021).

Lowering saturated fat consumption possibly diminishes pro-tumourigenic signaling intricately linked with lipid biosynthesis amidst multifaceted biological mechanisms meanwhile. Minerals and antioxidants consumed adequately enhance immune function and curb oxidative stress that fuels tumour development at an alarming rate quickly. Fasting regimens and caloric restriction protocols significantly enhance efficacy of cancer therapies by modulating inflammatory pathways in various preclinical models very effectively. Harnessing interplay between diet and tumour metabolism offers a low-cost non-invasive complement alongside other therapies quite promisingly to traditional cancer treatments. Further clinical research becomes essential amidst varying tumour characteristics for establishing evidence-based dietary guidelines tailored highly for individual patient needs.

5.1. The Role of Diet in Cancer Cell Metabolism

Malignant cells siphon off vital nutrients and energy sources furnished mainly by dietary intake fueling frenzied growth and reinforcing survival tactics very effectively. Glucose and micronutrients directly impact metabolic pathways crucial for cancer cells making diet a potent modulator of tumour biology effectively. Nutrients fuel glycolysis and glutaminolysis pathways thereby boosting cancer cell proliferation with unusually heightened resistance against various therapies. High glucose intake stimulates glycolytic flux rather vigorously and activates growth-promoting insulin signaling alongside IGF-1 pathways under some peculiar circumstances (Doaei et al, 2019).

Consumption of certain amino acids and saturated fats fuels biosynthesis very aggressively and inflammatory pathways thereby favoring tumour progression quite rapidly. Tweaking metabolic impact or restricting crucial nutrients severely disrupts metabolism of cancerous cells with drastic consequences for their survival and growth. Restricting carbs cuts glucose supply and glycolytic activity heavily while consumption of anti-inflammatory fatty acids such as omega-3s powerfully counteracts pro-tumour lipid signals. Elevating nutrient levels furiously strengthens bodily defenses and fortifies immunity thereby somewhat effectively helping check aberrant cell proliferation down somewhat (Doaei et al, 2019).

Dietary approaches may act synergistically with conventional cancer treatments like chemotherapy and radiation by sensitizing tumour cells remarkably well. Nutrition plays a somewhat complementary role nowadays underscoring huge potential for integration of very personalized dietary strategies into fairly comprehensive cancer treatment plans effectively.

5.2. Low-Carbohydrate and Ketogenic Diets

Ketogenic diet has garnered considerable attention lately by rather effectively exploiting metabolic vulnerabilities inherent in various types of cancer cells these days. Ketogenic diet entails consuming copious amounts of fat alongside moderate protein and very low carbs inducing fat oxidation and producing ketone bodies largely. Cancer cells hooked on glycolysis suddenly find themselves bereft of their go-to energy supply as blood glucose plummets sharply from metabolic upheaval. Ketogenic diet severely restricts glucose availability thereby starving tumour cells slowly and hindering their proliferation fairly effectively overall in most cases (Tan-Shalaby J et al, 2017).

Fat metabolism yields ketone bodies such as β-hydroxybutyrate and acetoacetate which serve as alternative energy sources for normal cells yet many cancer cells metabolize them sluggishly thereby creating a disadvantageous metabolic milieu for tumours. Ketogenic diets possibly thwart cancer progression in gliomas breast cancer and prostate cancer by drastically curtailing glycolytic flux and heightening oxidative stress deeply within tumour cells. Ketogenic diet has shown unusual promise nowadays in markedly enhancing efficacy of cancer therapies like chemotherapy and radiation therapy very remarkably. Tumour cells get sensitized possibly through tumour microenvironment modulation which reduces inflammation and exacerbates oxidative stress thereby improving outcomes therapeutically. Ketogenic diet emerges as promising adjunctive strategy in comprehensive cancer care partly due to severely restricting nutrient intake with dual effect (Tan-Shalaby J et al, 2017).

5.3. Caloric Restriction and Intermittent Fasting

Cancer metabolism and tumour progression have been quite vigorously studied under caloric restriction with extensively beneficial effects in recent years apparently. CR markedly lowers circulating insulin levels and insulin-like growth factor while slowing various cellular processes including DNA replication quite significantly. Collectively these effects suppress tumour growth significantly and may yield markedly improved cancer outcomes overall under fairly specific contexts sometimes. Cycles of eating and fasting emerge rather promisingly alongside continuous caloric restriction as a dietary tactic targeting metabolism of tumours quite effectively (Longo and Fontana, 2010).

Fasting periods drastically deplete glucose and amino acids, forcing cancer cells towards reliance on fatty acids or ketone bodies very rapidly. Metabolic stress ravages tumours heavily reliant on glycolysis, while normal cells exhibiting greater flexibility adapt rapidly under stringent fasting regimens. Intermittent fasting triggers vital cellular processes such as autophagy, which rids cells of dysfunctional organelles and proteins, thereby fostering cellular homeostasis and possibly inducing death in tumour cells. IF can modulate the tumour microenvironment rather effectively and enhance the immune system, enhancing the efficacy of chemotherapy significantly alongside certain kinds of immunotherapy (Longo and Fontana, 2010). Intermittent fasting drastically impedes cancer cells' proliferation disrupting crucial metabolic pathways they depend on heavily for sustenance making cancer therapy rather promising.

5.4. Amino Acid Restriction and Targeting Glutamine Metabolism

Amino acids crucially facilitate proliferation of cancer cells by furnishing precursors for protein synthesis and nucleotide production very essentially. Glutamine surprisingly plays a pivotal role amidst various amino acids in cancer metabolism rather quietly. Cancer cells frequently exhibit glutamine dependency fueling rapid proliferation energetically through various biosynthetic pathways and energy production mechanisms. Glutamine metabolism deeply maintains cellular function under various physiological conditions within tricarboxylic acid cycle playing a crucial role. Glutamine converts into α-ketoglutarate a crucial intermediate that feeds straight into the TCA cycle thereby helping generate ATP very effectively, maintaining cellular energy homeostasis (Liu et al, 2024).

Glutamine serves as a vital nitrogen source, synthesising nucleotides rapidly essential for DNA production and RNA synthesis during frenetic cell division. Tumour cells proliferating at a frantic pace require glutamine crucially for unchecked growth and utterly depend on it for survival. Targeting glutamine metabolism presents a potentially game-changing therapeutic strategy overall in cancer treatment nowadays, very clearly. Dietary glutamine restriction being investigated very thoroughly, could potentially starve tumour cells of an essential nutrient fairly effectively nowadays. Certain glutaminase inhibitors have been proposed severely limit glutamine supply, thereby thoroughly disrupting key metabolic pathways cancer cells rely heavily upon (Liu et al, 2024).

Research emerging into glutaminase inhibition and glutamine restriction has yielded promising results, particularly when amalgamated with traditional therapies and chemotherapy. Depriving tumour cells of glutamine severely impairs growth and survival significantly in various types of cancerous tissue under certain conditions. Glutamine restriction leveraged alongside chemotherapy enhances treatment efficacy by inducing tumour cell death and overcoming resistance mechanisms rapidly.

5.5. Fatty Acids and Lipid Metabolism

Lipid metabolism remarkably supports cancer cell growth and fuels survival rapidly under diverse physiological states with varying intensity. Tumour cells often drastically reprogram lipid metabolism under surging demands for membrane biogenesis and energy production remarkably. Fatty acid synthesis gets ramped up very heavily during reprogramming, and fatty acid synthase FASN is found overexpressed in many cancerous cells. FASN enables the synthesis of long-chain fatty acids, crucial for building cellular membranes and generating energy in lipid form with remarkable efficiency. FASN inhibition or disruption of key lipid metabolism enzymes might conceivably retard tumour growth, rendering lipid metabolism a fairly tantalising therapeutic target. Tumour metabolism gets heavily impacted by dietary fats in cancer cases, with varied lipid pathways being affected very obviously (Fu et al, 2020).

Omega-3 fatty acids, abundant in sources like fish oils and flaxseeds, have garnered considerable attention recently for potentially profound anti-cancer effects. Fatty acids vigorously exert potent anti-inflammatory effects that may help mitigate chronic inflammation, fueling metastasis and proliferation of cancer cells rapidly. Omega-3 fatty acids have been shown to profoundly alter lipid membrane composition, thereby disrupting metabolic processes tumours rely on for fairly rapid growth. Omega-3s can subvert the PI3K/Akt/mTOR signalling pathway very effectively, and it drives cell survival in many cancers rapidly. Omega-3 fatty acids may hinder cancer cell proliferation very substantially and markedly heighten sensitivity to treatments by inhibiting cellular pathways. Fats rich in saturated fats found mostly in red meat and highly processed foods correlate with inflammation and oftentimes fairly rapid growth of tumours (Fu et al, 2020).

Consuming copious amounts of saturated fats ostensibly sparks pro-inflammatory pathways that quite aggressively fuel tumour growth and enhance metastasis significantly. Ramping up consumption of healthy fats from sources like avocados and olive oil may thwart cancer growth and boost chemo effectiveness significantly. Modifying lipid metabolism in cancerous cells through specific diets or certain pharmaceutical interventions could potentially provide an additional stratagem for conventional cancer therapies. Targeting FASN to inhibit lipid biosynthesis or manipulating cellular membranes with certain fatty acids very significantly weakens tumour metabolic support and impairs vigorous metastasis. Ramping up omega-3 intake and slashing saturated fats alongside traditional treatments might foster very hostile environments for tumour cells encourage normal functions meanwhile.

5.6. Micronutrients and Antioxidants

Vitamins and minerals maintain metabolic balance remarkably well inside bodily systems and regulate numerous cellular processes ordinarily with great efficacy. Certain micronutrients exert a profound influence over immune response and oxidative stress mitigation in various cancerous contexts, alongside obscure DNA repair processes. Vitamin D plays a crucial role in modulating immune responses profoundly, while various studies demonstrate its ability to suppress cancer cell proliferation significantly in numerous cases. Tumour-suppressor genes get activated, and the immune system's capacity ferrets out malignant cells very rapidly, annihilating them with great efficacy. Vitamin D levels sufficiently high correlate with substantially lower risk of various cancers, including colorectal and breast cancer (Stefanache et al, 2023).

Retinoic acid, a very potent derivative of vitamin A, plays a crucial role in cell differentiation and programmed cell death, somewhat surprisingly. Tumour growth gets throttled significantly in various cancer models while immune responses are modulated quite effectively under certain conditions. Retinoic acid quite effectively thwarts cancer development by regulating abnormal cell growth and staving off damage from oxidation very thoroughly. Selenium acts rapidly as an antioxidant, enhancing immune function, being a trace mineral in the human body, somewhat effectively. Selenium supplementation might very effectively mitigate cancer risk by thwarting oxidative DNA damage and regulating cellular stress responses rather effectively within cells. Certain enzymes activated partly by it remarkably reduce cancer risk further in liver cells, where detoxification processes unfold vigorously (Stefanache et al, 2023).

Highly reactive molecules known as reactive oxygen species induce oxidative stress, damaging DNA, proteins and lipids found within cells. Tumours growing at breakneck speed frequently exhibit elevated ROS levels, fueling swift genomic instability and aggressively promoting cancer progression very rapidly nowadays. Antioxidants neutralising ROS are very interesting in contexts like these. Fruits rich in vitamin C contain natural antioxidants shielding normal cells from oxidative harm very effectively amidst considerable biochemical turmoil, apparently. Antioxidants very significantly reduce inflammation and help prevent cancer initiation by mopping up reactive oxygen species extremely effectively inside bodily tissues. Antioxidants play quite a complex role, somewhat paradoxically, in cancer therapy, rather often nowadays with varying degrees of success, apparently (Zhao et al, 2023).

Antioxidants may shield normal cells from harm and potentially thwart the efficacy of treatments inducing oxidative stress, such as chemotherapy, killing cancer cells. Large amounts of certain antioxidant supplements could undermine cancer therapies by mitigating oxidative stress that helps eradicate tumour cells gradually. Antioxidants play a crucial role in thwarting cancer onset but require cautious utilisation during treatment regimens for highly malignant tumour formations. Vigorously promoting antioxidant activity in healthy tissues while permitting oxidative stress to occur fairly freely remains a critical research area for targeting cancer cells effectively. Tumour metabolism responds remarkably well to dietary interventions nowadays, thereby significantly encourage efficacy of various cancer treatment protocols effectively. Tumour proliferation may be stunted by specific nutritional interventions that sensitise cancer cells to therapy by limiting crucial energy sources like glucose (Zhao et al, 2023).

Cutting dietary glucose remarkably impacts the Warburg effect and slashes reliance on glycolysis in tumour cells under fairly typical conditions. Ketogenic diets severely curtail carb intake, precipitating ketosis and forcing cells burn fat-derived ketones rather than glucose for fuel, thereby starving nasty tumours. Restricting certain amino acids, like glutamine, a crucial nutrient for myriad cancer cells, can curb tumour growth in a somewhat unpredictable manner. Experimental therapies are probing glutaminase inhibitors deeply for disrupting glutamine metabolism in various tumour types quite aggressively nowadays. Omega-3 fatty acids sourced from fatty fish and flaxseeds very effectively enhance chemotherapy effects by disrupting PI3K/Akt/mTOR signalling pathways (Poff et al, 2019).

Dietary strategies targeting tumour metabolism remarkably enhance cancer treatment effectiveness alongside traditional therapies very significantly every single day. Dietary interventions drastically modify the tumour microenvironment, offering a holistic cancer care approach alongside chemotherapy and radiation therapy effectively.

6. Energy Metabolism in Cancer: The Role of Diet in Tumourigenesis

Cancer cells undergo wildly aberrant metabolic rewiring rather quickly to meet the biosynthetic demands of rapid growth or proliferation somewhat drastically. Cancer cells bizarrely opt for aerobic glycolysis over oxidative phosphorylation for energy production in oxygen-rich environments inexplicably. Cancer cells rapidly produce ATP via a metabolic shift despite oxygen being readily available, and it furnishes essential biosynthetic intermediates necessary for division. Otto Warburg initially observed cancer cells converting glucose furiously into lactate under aerobic conditions way back in the 1920s. Glycolysis enables cancer cells rapidly produce key metabolites like nucleotides and lipids necessary for macromolecular synthesis and cell proliferation quite sloppily. Glycolysis gets favoured surprisingly even with oxygen around and brings cancer cells some very handy advantages, basically (Liberti et al, 2016).

Glycolysis rapidly churns out ATP, fueling the frenzied biosynthetic demands of cells dividing at an alarming rate under intensely anabolic conditions. Intermediates spawned by glycolysis trickle into crucial biosynthetic pathways necessary for cell growth, notably nucleotide biosynthesis for DNA production and lipid biosynthesis processes in membrane formation. Tumour cells in solid tumours often endure low oxygen levels or hypoxia quite frequently beneath surface regions somewhat irregularly. Cells thrive in oxygen-deprived environments, daily relying heavily on glycolysis and lacking sufficient oxygen supply very often. Glycolysis spawns lactate and other acidic metabolic byproducts, which acidify the tumour microenvironment, severely impairing various immune cells' function and facilitating tumour cells' escape from immune surveillance (Liberti et al, 2016).

Dietary factors profoundly impact cancer cell metabolism, and nutrition plays a crucial role therein with considerable intricacy. Dietary interventions can very effectively modulate metabolic pathways exploited by cancer cells for growth by altering nutrient availability. Cancer cells feed on glucose from carb-rich diets, fueling glycolysis liberally and influencing tumour growth significantly in many metabolic processes. Tumour metabolism gets affected rather profoundly by glucose availability. Tumour cells consume glucose very voraciously. Certain diets impact tumour metabolism in obscure ways through glycolysis and other largely unknown biochemical pathways very significantly (Liberti et al, 2016).

Ketogenic diets severely restrict glucose availability, thereby forcing tumour cells into frantic scavenging for fatty acids or ketones as energy sources. Ketogenic diets are remarkably low in carbs and rich in healthy fats, which induce ketosis, providing an alternate energy source in the form of β-hydroxybutyrate ketone bodies. Ketones potentially fuel normal cells but starve cancer cells heavily reliant on glucose for survival. Cancer cells frequently ramp up fatty acid synthesis via enzymes like fatty acid synthase FASN fueling their surging demand for membrane biogenesis and energy production. Diets rich in omega-3 fatty acids present in fatty fish and flaxseeds disrupt metabolic processes cancer cells rely heavily on for survival. Omega-3 fatty acids profoundly disrupt lipid membrane composition, thereby forcing tumour cells to labour intensely, sustaining vital signalling functions prolifically for sheer survival (Tan-Shalaby J, 2017).

Omega-3 fatty acids possibly thwart crucial oncogenic signalling pathways like PI3K/Akt/mTOR that regulate various metabolic processes in cancer cells fairly effectively. Glutamine, a vital amino acid, plays a crucial role in the metabolism of cancer cells, often dubbed glutamine-addicted, rather mysteriously. Glutamine fuels the TCA cycle vigorously and supports the biosynthesis of various nucleotides and amino acids, thereby somewhat energetically promoting cell division. Cancer therapy gains traction slowly, with glutaminase inhibitors targeting glutamine metabolism or dietary glutamine being restricted very heavily nowadays. It can severely hamper growth and render them rather sensitive to chemotherapy treatments involving various toxic compounds normally used (Tan-Shalaby J, 2017).

Vitamins and minerals crucially regulate metabolic pathways and shield against oxidative stress, often found rampantly inside tumour cells. Vitamin D inhibits cancer cell proliferation very effectively and activates tumour suppressor pathways, while selenium superbly regulates redox balance and shields cells from nasty DNA damage. Antioxidants present in luscious fruits and veggies quite effectively neutralise reactive oxygen species, protecting normal cells from oxidative onslaught. Excessive antioxidant supplementation might interfere significantly with oxidative stress induced by treatments like chemotherapy, making their role in cancer treatment complicated, rather often nowadays (Sheeley et al, 2022).

6.1. The Warburg Effect and Cancer Cell Metabolism

Cancer cells bizarrely manifest a peculiar metabolic anomaly known as the Warburg effect, heavily relying on glycolysis for energy production instead of oxidative phosphorylation. A plethora of genetic mutations alongside oncogenic signalling pathways irregularly drives phenomenon first spotted by Otto Warburg way back in the 1920s. Cancer cells strangely favour glycolysis, producing ATP, which results in lactate accumulating as a byproduct, while normal cells typically utilise oxidative phosphorylation very efficiently. Tumour cells rapidly proliferating in quite hostile environments ostensibly garner multiple survival advantages from such a rather dramatic shift in energy metabolism. Anabolic processes and biomass accumulation rely heavily on biosynthetic intermediates essentially supplied by the Warburg effect during rapid cell proliferation (Wu and Zhao, 2013).

Glycolysis churns out ATP and critical metabolites crucial for synthesising nucleotides, amino acids, lipids and other essential building blocks for vigorous cell division rapidly. Upregulation of glucose transporters drastically ramps up glucose uptake in cancer cells, fueling rapid proliferation quite significantly under varied conditions. Tumour microenvironment struggles under hypoxia and acidic conditions alongside scarcity of nutrients, thereby markedly heightening dependence on glycolysis under harsh circumstances. Lactate accumulation drastically lowers extracellular pH, thereby vigorously promoting tumour cell invasion and metastasis while erecting a robust barrier against immune cells (Wu and Zhao, 2013).

Reprogramming energy metabolism enables cancer cells to thrive remarkably well inside hostile environments with significant stress, and they thrive very quickly. Therapeutically targeting the Warburg effect presents an ostensibly attractive strategy for limiting cancer cell survival very effectively in some contexts. Blocking crucial glycolytic enzymes or glucose transporters might deprive tumour cells of vital nutrients, thereby impairing their proliferation ability quite significantly. Pairing metabolic inhibitors with chemo boosts tumour sensitivity substantially, thereby yielding a very promising new cancer treatment trajectory.

6.2. Dietary Influence on Glucose Metabolism

Glucose fuels cancer cell metabolism remarkably well, making dietary interventions aimed at restricting it a crucial consideration in cancer patient care nowadays. Refined sugars and simple carbs in diets elevate blood glucose levels, furnishing cancer cells with copious fuel, directly benefiting them greatly. Tumour cells manifesting the Warburg effect rely heavily on glycolysis for energy production amidst an abundance of oxygen and plenty of nutrients. Cancer cells exhibit extreme sensitivity to fluctuations in blood glucose, largely owing to reliance on glucose for producing energy rapidly. Diets rich in glucose heavily spur insulin secretion, and tumour growth gets exacerbated very quickly in some very nasty cases. Insulin, a potent growth factor, vigorously activates several intracellular signalling pathways similar to IGF-1, stimulating cell proliferation and fostering cancer cell survival (Qian et al, 2022).

Ketogenic diets severely limit carbs quite effectively, thereby offering therapeutic potential against cancer cell proliferation in various cases. A ketogenic diet very effectively induces a profound metabolic shift towards fat-derived ketone bodies for energy production, with carbs severely restricted. Cancer cells get starved of glucose, their primary energy source, and burn alternative fuel rather haphazardly with noticeably poor efficiency. Gross nutrient deficiencies severely afflict cancer cells, thereby grossly hampering proliferation and triggering ordinarily dormant cell death pathways (Qian et al, 2022). Ketogenic diets can markedly amplify the effectiveness of traditional cancer therapies like chemotherapy and radiation beyond just rapidly reducing glucose.

Ketogenic diets rather effectively sensitise tumour cells to treatments by markedly ramping up oxidative stress and triggering autophagy at a fairly rapid pace. Diets rich in certain nutrients can quite effectively curb the growth and spread of tumours by reducing systemic inflammation characteristic of many cancers. Super low-carb ketogenic diets aimed at tweaking glucose metabolism offer a potentially game-changing way to drastically slow the growth of tumours.

6.3. Amino Acid Metabolism and Tumourigenesis

Amino acids act as vital precursors fueling the rapid proliferation of cancer cells under diverse physiological states, rather mysteriously. Amino acids furnish crucial precursors for nucleotide biosynthesis and lipid synthesis necessary very much necessary for swift cell division and tumour growth. Glutamine surfaces rather quietly as a key player in cancer cell metabolism amidst various amino acids. Energy production occurs vigorously through oxidative phosphorylation inside cells and is fueled by α-ketoglutarate, a pivotal intermediate in the tricarboxylic acid cycle. Glutamine furnishes nitrogen essential for the synthesis of nucleotides and amino acids crucial to rapidly proliferating tumour cells amidst diverse settings (Ge et al, 2025).

Cancer cells heavily rely on external sources very frequently to meet their surging metabolic needs driven by glutamine addiction. Certain individuals may intensify glutamine reliance significantly under various physiological stressors, possibly due to peculiar eating habits fairly regularly. Tumours get plenty of glutamine from diets heavy in glutamine-rich food like meat and dairy, and some grains, furthering growth spurts rapidly. Novel therapeutic strategies potentially efficacious involve restricting dietary glutamine or certain pharmacological interventions that inhibit glutamine metabolism very effectively (Ge et al, 2025).

Cancer cells might be starved of energy and biosynthetic precursors slowly over time by restricting glutamine, thereby totally impairing proliferative capacity. Serine and glycine, alongside proline, energise anabolic processes vigorously in cancer cells with glutamine, abundantly fueling cellular activity. Amino acids fuel protein synthesis remarkably and heavily participate in nucleotide formation and lipid biosynthesis with surprisingly great efficacy. Diets heavy in animal protein and bursting with amino acids may supercharge tumour growth by furnishing abundant resources for rapid cell proliferation (Jiang et al, 2019).

Plant-based proteins harbour unique amino acid signatures and exhibit lower glycemic indices, thereby potentially cultivating metabolic milieus less hospitable for tumour growth. Rapid tumour cell growth might not be sufficiently fueled by plant proteins, and a diet replete with such nutrients could confer cancer protection. Tumour cells heavily rely on specific amino acids and glutamine for energy production and biosynthesis, revealing glaring metabolic vulnerabilities that are exploitable therapeutically. Restricting certain amino acids through dietary manipulations or pharmaceutical interventions might emerge nowadays as a rather promising strategy for treating cancer.

6.5. Fatty Acids and Lipid Metabolism in Cancer

Lipids play a crucial role energetically in cancer cell metabolism, supporting rapid proliferation through various complex biochemical pathways. Tumours grow rapidly inside cells, undergoing frequent division, and cellular membranes must be synthesised quickly in a somewhat haphazard manner. Membrane biogenesis demand surges and fuels upregulation of fatty acid synthesis, crucial for producing lipids rapidly needed for new membrane formation. Fatty acid synthase, a crucial enzyme in producing fatty acids, gets overexpressed frequently in breast cancer and various other malignancies, including liver cancers. Elevated FASN expression fuels lipid biosynthesis rapidly furnishing tumour cells with precursors necessary for membrane formation and signaling molecule production (Fu et al, 2020).

Certain fats trigger rapid tumour growth and alter cancer cell metabolism drastically with different types of dietary fat consumed ordinarily. Saturated fats lurk surreptitiously in red meat and certain processed foods or oils and have been linked alarmingly enough to various heightened cancer risks including breast cancer. Copious saturated fats foster systemic inflammation that fuels cancer progression rapidly by augmenting cellular proliferation and survival very quickly alongside metastasis. Saturated fats trigger inflammatory pathways festering deep inside tumour microenvironments and drastically alter cellular processes quite profoundly therein becomes (Fu et al, 2020).

Fats rich in saturation trigger inflammatory cascades deep within tumour microenvironments altering various cellular processes very profoundly. Omega-3 fatty acids present in fatty fish and flaxseeds naturally display profoundly anti-inflammatory properties playing somewhat protective role in cancer prevention. Omega-3 fatty acids somewhat effectively hinder cancer cell proliferation and metastasis via impacting crucial PI3K/Akt/mTOR pathways for cell survival. Fatty acids hinder inflammatory processes cancer cells rather frequently exploit and very much unchecked growth ensues in various bodily tissues (Rodriguez-Leyva et al, 2010). Modulating lipid metabolism very effectively via dietary tweaks represents a rather promising cancer prevention strategy alongside innovative therapeutic modalities. Abundance of omega-3 fatty acids might effectively retard tumour growth very significantly in people who drastically cut back on saturated fats. Tweaking diet possibly enhances traditional cancer therapies by altering lipid profiles of tumour cells and slowing progression quite markedly in some cases.

6.6. Micronutrients and Energy Regulation

Cancer cell metabolism relies heavily on glucose and amino acids and lipids for fuel yet various micronutrients play a crucial supporting regulatory role. Vitamin D profoundly impacts mitochondrial functionality and enhance immune efficacy in detecting malignant cells fairly effectively annihilating them quite rapidly. Vitamin D profoundly impacts energy metabolism by modulating genes deeply involved in oxidative phosphorylation within mitochondria primarily for ATP production. Vitamin D further amplifies cytotoxic prowess of immune cells such as T cells and natural killer cells vital for annihilating cancerous cells effectively. Low levels of vitamin D correlate with heightened risk of sundry cancers including colorectal cancer and breast cancer suggesting protection against tumourigenesis through adequate dietary intake (Sheeley et al, 2021).

Antioxidants found rather abundantly in numerous fruits and veggies play a crucial role in energy metabolism by neutralizing reactive oxygen species fairly effectively. Tumultuous mitochondrial electron transport chain processes trigger ravaging of cellular components like lipids and proteins and DNA by excessive ROS accumulation. High ROS levels inside cancer cells often nurture genetic mutations vigorously and drive tumour growth swiftly over a prolonged period. Antioxidants like vitamin C or selenium can mitigate ROS-induced damage in normal cells and foster apoptosis very readily in tumour cells. A diet rich in antioxidants can weirdly shield normal cells from oxidative damage and abet oxidative stress in cancer cells enhancing eradication of them (Sheeley et al, 2021).

Energy metabolism nowadays forms a cornerstone very fundamental in cancer cell biology obviously. Tumour cells rapidly hijack metabolic pathways involving glucose, lipids, and amino acids for high-energy biosynthetic demands during rapid cell proliferation. Targeting specific pathways, dietary interventions hold promise in cancer prevention alongside treatment, with substantial benefits accumulating rapidly nowadays. Low-carb diets severely limit glucose availability, and glutamine restriction hinders tumour growth, boosting treatment outcomes fairly significantly through such nutritional deprivation. Vitamin D and antioxidants modulate cellular responses subtly and rather effectively, supporting immune function across diverse metabolic milieus nowadays. Dietary strategies may serve as adjuncts offering new opportunities for personalised cancer care and potentially improve outcomes significantly in modern oncology practice nowadays.

7. The Warburg Effect and Dietary Modulation in Cancer Cells

Cancer cells strangely prefer glycolysis for producing energy even when plenty of oxygen is available, a phenomenon Otto Warburg initially observed. Cancer cells usually exhibit a pronounced shift towards aerobic glycolysis yielding lower ATP but encourage rapid tumour growth remarkably. Glycolysis churns out crucial biosynthetic intermediates like nucleotides and lipids essential for synthesizing new cell components needed for tumour cells dividing rapidly. Glycolysis churns out lactate, accumulating around tumours and fostering an acidic microenvironment that very effectively promotes invasion and metastasis. Metabolic rewiring occurs quite dynamically under regulation by various oncogenes and tumour suppressors alongside some microenvironmental factors very actively (Liberti and Locasale, 2016).

Tumour cells thrive quite vigorously in hypoxic environments often facilitated by a glycolytic shift typical of various solid tumour microenvironments. HIF-1α activates transcription of glycolytic enzymes and glucose transporters, thereby further reinforcing a metabolic shift under severely hypoxic conditions. Research increasingly uncovers dietary interventions influencing the rapid progression of peculiar metabolic shifts fueling cancer growth in many people nowadays. Tumour growth gets modulated quite effectively by diet through clever manipulation of glucose and amino acid availability. Ridiculously high glucose intake fuels glycolysis, thereby vigorously promoting tumour cell proliferation fairly quickly in some cases, obviously (Liberti and Locasale, 2016). Ketogenic diets drastically curtail glucose intake, thereby severely impairing energy sources fueling glycolysis and stunt growth of tumours reliant on glucose for survival. Cancer cells often flail about helplessly, unable to tap into ketone bodies derived from fat breakdown for sustenance or energy production. Disrupting glutamine metabolism or serine-glycine biosynthesis very effectively messes with the biosynthetic needs of rapidly dividing cancer cells or others. Tumour growth may be drastically slowed by restricting key amino acids via dietary changes or certain pharmacological interventions, apparently (Liberti and Locasale, 2016).

Dietary manipulation of metabolic pathways within malignant cells presents a novel stratagem encourage conventional oncological treatments rather effectively nowadays. Ketogenic regimens or low-glucose diets combined with radiation or chemotherapy possibly heighten tumour sensitivity significantly under some peculiar conditions. Boosting omega-3 fatty acids and slashing saturated fats might modulate lipid metabolism, a crucial feature rampant in cancer cell proliferation, somewhat erratically. Elucidating intricate relationships between the Warburg effect and dietary patterns ostensibly paves the way for modified nutritional interventions melded with mainstream cancer therapies targeting cancer cell metabolic Achilles' heels.

7.1. The Warburg Effect

Energy production occurs mostly through oxidative phosphorylation deep inside mitochondria of normal cells, remarkably under healthy physiological conditions. OXPHOS generates a high energy yield very efficiently by fully oxidizing glucose and fatty acids in presence of oxygen. Cancer cells often undergo alterations very frequently in this process. Cancer cells weirdly favor aerobic glycolysis even when oxygen abounds a process that converts glucose into pyruvate and subsequently lactate very quickly. Cancer cell metabolism exhibits a hallmark involving peculiarly adopting somewhat mysteriously a metabolic shift known obscurely as Warburg effect. Warburg effect originates suddenly from reconfigured signaling pathways within cells displaying quirky behaviors rather than malfunctioning mitochondria essentially (Zheng J, 2012).

Mutations within oncogenes like PIK3CA spur changes by activating key pathways downstream of HIF-1α via PI3K/Akt/mTOR signaling quite vigorously. Pathways facilitate glycolysis vigorously under oxygen-rich surroundings thereby furnishing tumour cells a decided growth edge quite remarkably always. Cancer cells reap numerous benefits from heavy reliance on aerobic glycolysis under surprisingly various circumstances. Glycolysis churns out nucleotides, lipids and amino acids crucial for tumour cells' rapid frenzied growth in a rather haphazard manner quite energetically. Such intermediates facilitate synthesis of macromolecules and cell proliferation essential for rapid tumour expansion in various tissues quite aggressively (Zheng J, 2012).

Glycolysis produces lactate which gets secreted into tumour microenvironment lowering pH very significantly thereby creating quite an acidic ambiance. Tumour invasion gets boosted significantly in acidic environments enhancing cancer cell mobility very substantially and promoting extracellular matrix degradation allowing surrounding tissue invasion and rapid cancer spread. Cancer cells acquire a survival edge fairly often deep within solid tumours beset by grossly insufficient vascular supply under extremely hypoxic circumstances. Glycolysis enables tumour cells producing ATP rapidly sustaining growth vigorously even when oxidative phosphorylation falters in hypoxic environments very badly sometimes (Zheng J, 2012). Warburg effect enables cancer cells remarkably adapt under hostile tumour microenvironments and thrive fairly well in low-oxygen conditions contributing significantly to resistance. Grasping reprogramming of metabolic processes crucially underpins development of therapeutic strategies that target inherent vulnerabilities in cancerous cells quite effectively.

7.2. Dietary Influence on Glucose Metabolism in Cancer

Glucose fuels aberrant metabolism of cancer cells largely via Warburg effect where aerobic glycolysis gets utilized preferentially for producing energy . Nutritional tactics modulating glucose supply remarkably influence cancer treatment outcomes since glucose fuels a major metabolic reprogramming quite effectively. Gorging on heaps of sugary stuff can spark off wildly high blood glucose levels very darn quickly in most cases. Elevated glucose levels furnish cancer cells with copious energy thereby fostering proliferation swiftly and frenetic growth spurts remarkably often underneath cellular surfaces. High glucose levels spur production of insulin and insulin-like growth factor 1 or IGF-1 quite potently downstream in cells remarkably (Liberti and Locasale, 2016).

Factors intricately activate key signaling pathways namely PI3K/Akt and mTOR regulating cell growth survival and metabolism in a very complex manner. Tumour growth gets a vigorous boost from high-glucose diets under certain physiological conditions by fueling cancer cells' anabolic demands very effectively. Ketogenic diet proves quite effective in targeting Warburg effect as certain dietary approaches severely restrict carbohydrate intake with promising results. Ketogenic diet involves drastically high fat intake and remarkably low carb consumption, shifting bodily metabolism towards fatty acid degradation suddenly. Cancer cells are drastically deprived of the primary energy source by severely reducing glucose availability, which could hinder proliferation and sustain abnormal growth patterns (Liberti and Locasale, 2016).

Fat metabolism produces ketone bodies such as β-hydroxybutyrate and acetoacetate, serving as alternative energy sources for cells under certain peculiar conditions. Cancer cells often flail wildly at efficiently utilising ketones thereby making them unusually susceptible to starvation in absence of glucose. Research indicates a ketogenic diet amplifies oxidative stress, thereby damaging cancer cells, and systemic inflammation that fuels tumour progression gets reduced, inducing autophagy. Such effects render cancer cells extremely susceptible to treatments with surprisingly great efficacy, ridiculously fast under certain conditions.

A ketogenic diet quite frequently amplifies the efficacy of conventional therapies like chemotherapy and radiation therapy, making tumours more responsive rather noticeably. Ketogenic diet potentially limits tumour growth and boosts efficacy of cancer therapies by modulating glucose metabolism through strict dietary interventions. Further research into dietary tweaks effectively integrable into oncology management is sorely needed as underscored by cancer treatment outcomes lately.

7.3. Amino Acid Metabolism and Cancer Cells

Amino acids rapidly fuel proliferation of cancer cells providing key building blocks for synthesis of proteins and lipids crucial for cell division. Cancer cells exhibit drastic metabolic shifts in amino acid usage fueling rampant biosynthetic demands amidst rapid tumour growth and proliferation remarkably. Cancer cells aberrantly reprogram glutamine metabolism representing a very critical metabolic shift with profoundly significant consequences downstream . Glutamine becomes vital for tumour cells largely due to its pivotal role in cellular energy production and various biosynthetic pathways. It serves as primary source of carbon fueling the synthesis of glutamate and α-ketoglutarate and other intermediates driving tricarboxylic acid cycle with nitrogen (Liu et al, 2024).

Crucial intermediates form readily for ATP production and generation of other vital metabolites necessary for biosynthesis of nucleotides and various lipids. Glutamine addiction manifests strikingly in various cancers and tumour cells overexpress glutamine transporters very actively facilitating glutamine metabolism with glutaminase. Glutamine metabolism presents a tantalizing therapeutic target largely owing to its crucial albeit somewhat obscure role in fuelling cancer cell proliferation processes. Glutamine restriction has shown promise in preclinical models of various cancer types including glioblastoma lymphoma and breast cancer via dietary modification or glutaminase inhibitors. Tumour cells get starved of glutamine a very crucial nutrient and their growth get hindered significantly deep inside bodily tissue (Liu et al, 2024).

Glutaminase inhibitors effectively block conversion of glutamine into glutamate shrinking tumour volume and sensitizing cancer cells quite profoundly chemotherapy treatments. Besides glutamine serine and glycine two other amino acids vitally fuel irregular metabolic processes in cancer cells very oddly. They both play roles somewhat crucially in one-carbon metabolism which synthesizes nucleotides very fundamentally. Rapidly proliferating cancers markedly ramp up biosynthesis of serine and glycine as cell division demands these amino acids for synthesizing nucleic acid. Tumours with unusually high demand for such amino acids often rely heavily on serine-glycine biosynthesis pathways making them potentially viable metabolic targets for intervention. Altering certain nutrients that influence bioavailability of specific amino acids could possibly result in entirely new treatment approaches (Liu et al, 2024).

Diets rich in plants tend to have less serine and glycine than animal-derived proteins and may somewhat starve cancer cells of nutrients effectively. Restricting specific amino acids in plant-based diets possibly hinders tumour growth and enhance efficacy of conventional therapies for cancer treatment remarkably. Diets packed with animal proteins can fuel cancer progression rapidly by supplying loads of amino acids for tumour biosynthesis. A crucial hallmark in cancer cell biology remains reprogramming amino acid metabolism specifically glutamine and serine/glycine pathways very evidently. Tumour growth can be significantly inhibited and efficacy of current treatments boosted through dietary changes or certain pharmacological interventions very effectively. Further obscure cancer research is sorely needed alongside devising dietary regimens very effectively for oncology therapeutics and amino acid metabolic pathways.

7.4. Lipid Metabolism in Cancer Cells and Diet

Lipid metabolism crucially facilitates cancer cell survival and proliferation during very rapid cell division for synthesizing new cell membranes. Fatty acids alongside phospholipids play crucial roles in membrane structure while participating significantly in cellular signaling and energy storage vital for most cancer cells. Fatty acid synthase regulates lipid metabolism quite effectively in various tumours through de novo fatty acid synthesis. FASN frequently shows markedly elevated expression in various malignancies, including breast, prostate cancer and liver tumours, thereby making it a putative therapeutic target. FASN upregulation enables cancer cells to produce lipids necessary for constructing new cell membranes as they rapidly proliferate quite uncontrollably and aggressively (Fu et al, 2020).

Dietary fats profoundly impact lipid metabolism within cancer cells under certain quirky conditions, very dramatically in a multitude of cellular contexts. Omega-3 fatty acids sourced mainly from fatty fish like salmon and occasionally mackerel exert profoundly varied anti-cancer effects through flaxseeds. Omega-3 fatty acids trigger key metabolic regulators, such as AMPK or PPAR-α robustly in diverse cellular environments. Molecules crucially inhibit lipogenesis and foster oxidative stress which thwarts tumour growth effectively while simultaneously reducing inflammation very radically (Fu et al, 2020).

Omega-3 fatty acids effectively suppress signalling pathways that drive lipid biosynthesis and cell proliferation by activating downstream AMPK. Tumour cells become substantially more susceptible to oxidative damage, thereby very significantly enhancing the effectiveness of conventional cancer therapies like radiation. Red meat and processed food are rife with saturated fats tenuously linked to heightened inflammation and stubborn tumour progression resisting most therapy. Elevated consumption of saturated fats hyperactivates PI3K/Akt/mTOR pathway thereby significantly enhancing cellular proliferation and markedly fortifying survival mechanisms (Fu et al, 2020).

Dysregulation of this pathway occurs frequently in various cancers and it significantly contributes to metabolic rewiring characteristic of tumours. Saturated fats may further exacerbate Warburg effect by greatly boosting glycolytic shift in cancer cells and furnishing a supplementary energy source. Lipid metabolism gets tweaked by dietary changes offering potential therapeutic strategies for cancer cells which rely heavily on lipids metabolically. Drastic dietary overhauls or supplementation hikes omega-3 fatty acid intake thereby somewhat counterbalancing pro-tumourigenic effects of saturated fats and encourage cancer treatment efficacy substantially. Downstream tumourigenesis driven by pro-inflammatory and metabolic processes gets inhibited quite effectively possibly by reducing consumption of foods rich in saturated fats.

Cancer cells peculiarly favor aerobic glycolysis over oxidative phosphorylation even when oxygen abounds exhibiting warped metabolism very characteristically . Rapid tumour cell proliferation gets fueled by metabolic reprogramming that somewhat surprisingly boosts glucose uptake and glycolysis meeting biosynthetic demands. Cancer cells churn out lactate under fairly aerobic conditions thus fueling a rather acidic microenvironment that facilitates metastasis very aggressively. Dietary interventions targeting key metabolic pathways in glucose amino acid and lipid metabolism hold significant potential for modulating cancer progression through Warburg effect. Ketogenic diets drastically slash glucose availability thereby starving cancer cells of primary fuel and severely curtailing malignant growth very significantly (Liberti et al, 2016).

Cancer cells heavily reliant on glutamine quite possibly could be hobbled via dietary manipulations or novel pharmaceutical interventions stifling proliferation. Lipid metabolism alongside glucose metabolism and amino acid metabolism plays quite a prominently crucial role in manifesting Warburg effect. Cancer growth is potentially thwarted by diets heavy in omega-3 fatty acids or markedly low in saturated fats disrupting lipid metabolism pathways.

8. Harnessing Nutrients to Disrupt Tumour Bioenergetics for Cancer Therapy

Cancer cells display anomalous metabolic adaptability quite effectively through reprogramming biochemical mechanisms fostering swift proliferation and stubborn resistance to treatment. Cancer cells frequently switch over to aerobic glycolysis producing energy by fermenting glucose into lactate even amidst copious oxygen supply normally. Tumour cells derive multifaceted metabolic advantages quite liberally from Warburg effect a phenomenon mystifying many scientists for decades apparently. Glycolysis churns out ATP and various biosynthetic intermediates crucial for rapidly synthesizing nucleotides lipids and amino acids needed for cell division. Glycolysis quite frequently enables cancer cells thriving rather robustly in low oxygen environments a fairly typical hallmark of solid tumours (Liberti et al, 2016).

Glycolysis produces lactate which acidifies extracellular space thereby fostering a permissive environment for malignant cell growth and tumour metastasis quite readily. Rampant glycolytic activity and warped nutrient uptake largely manifest distinct metabolic traits in cancer cells providing fresh avenues for therapy. Dietary interventions have emerged rather promisingly as a potent strategy significantly influencing metabolic pathways and offering means for disrupting bioenergetics of malignant cells nowadays very effectively. Consuming copious refined sugars and simple carbs boosts glucose availability thereby fueling Warburg effect and accelerating proliferation of cancer cells very rapidly. Ketogenic diet drastically cuts glucose supply and fosters fatty acid utilization remarkably well as primary energy sources alongside ketone bodies (Liberti et al, 2016).

Malignant cells sloppily burn ketones for fuel and a drastic shift in metabolism may severely curb proliferation of tumours eventually. Amino acid metabolism plays a vital role in cancer cell growth curiously alongside glucose metabolism in some obscure manner. Glutamine fuels TCA cycle activity rather heavily and liberally supplies nitrogen for synthesis of various nucleic acids very extensively. Targeting glutamine metabolism through dietary restriction or potent pharmacological inhibition severely hampers proliferative ability of cancer cells quite greatly. Dietary tweaks that mess with availability of crucial metabolic players can revamp tumour energetics and make cancer cells sensitive to chemo and radiation thereby boosting outcomes.

8.1. The Role of Tumour Bioenergetics in Cancer Progression

Cancer cells exhibit metabolism profoundly altered under various physiological conditions rather differently from normal cells obviously. Tumour cells frequently hijack metabolic pathways towards aerobic glycolysis wherein glucose rapidly converts into lactate despite abundant nearby oxygen. Cancer cells satisfy skyrocketing energy needs via Warburg effect a peculiar metabolic shift woefully inefficient in producing ATP yet bizarrely effective anyway. Reprogramming occurs owing largely to complex interplay of critical oncogene mutations such as PIK3CA or KRAS alongside TP53 and dysregulation of key signaling pathways. Alterations facilitate swift biosynthesis of crucial cellular constituents necessary for cancer cells rapidly dividing and growing quite uncontrollably nowadays (Hammoudi et al, 2011).

Tumours derive several advantages from relying heavily on glycolysis for energy production, as it reaps myriad benefits by leaning very heavily on glycolytic pathways. Glycolysis generates biosynthetic intermediates like nucleotides and amino acids necessary for the synthesis of macromolecules that support rapid cell division. Metabolic intermediates such as α-ketoglutarate fuel tumour cell proliferation rapidly by being crucial for nucleotide synthesis and amino acid production. Lactate, a glycolytic byproduct, heavily accumulates in the tumour microenvironment, thoroughly acidifying surrounding tissues very rapidly. Acidification disrupts tissue architecture very significantly, thereby fostering a ripe environment for cell dissemination and boosting tumour invasion markedly (Hammoudi et al, 2011).

Glycolysis confers a survival advantage quite frequently in hypoxic conditions, fairly common inside most solid tumours, obviously very deep within tissue. Oxidative phosphorylation falters spectacularly in hypoxic environments, and glycolysis becomes a vital energy source, fueling the survival of tumour cells under severely harsh conditions. Tumour bioenergetics presents a highly promising cancer therapy strategy by targeting metabolic pathways crucial in cancer progression quite effectively nowadays. Manipulating nutrient availability drastically alters crucial metabolite concentrations like glucose and fatty acids, disrupting energy supply in tumour cells thereby (Zheng J, 2012).

Ketogenic diets or caloric restriction might strangely halt tumour cell proliferation rather quickly by depleting cells of vital nutrients needed for growth. Interventions like these might enhance conventional therapies such as chemotherapy by targeting metabolic vulnerabilities and enhancing effectiveness in cancer cells significantly. Tumour bioenergetics manipulation through dietary interventions or pharmacological agents may prove crucial in cancer treatment tailored very specifically.

8.2. Nutrient Modulation in Cancer Therapy

Cancer therapy now exploits nutrient manipulation as a potentially paradigm-shifting tactic derailing metabolic routes that turbocharge tumour growth extremely quickly. Cancer cells fuel proliferation rather haphazardly with quirky bioenergetics largely dependent on glucose and fatty acids or certain amino acids. Strategically manipulating crucial metabolic substrate availability impairs tumour cell function and potentially greatly enhances conventional therapy effectiveness, markedly under certain conditions. Glucose garners significant attention in cancer research nowadays as a nutrient of paramount importance, undergoing intense scrutiny in metabolic studies. Tumour cells rely heavily on glycolysis for energy production even when oxygen is present, largely due to some weird phenomenon known as Warburg effect (Hammoudi et al, 2011).

Aerobic glycolysis empowers cancer cells, generating ATP swiftly and crucial biosynthetic intermediates, fueling wildly unchecked proliferation quite effectively overall. Ketogenic diets and low-carbohydrate diets severely starve tumour cells by drastically limiting glucose intake, which serves as their primary energy source. Ketogenic diet radically shifts bodily functions towards fat metabolism, producing ketone bodies as an alternate energy source very rapidly in a peculiar manner. Cancer cells struggle to utilise ketones efficiently, thereby inducing stress metabolically that inhibits the growth of tumours, sparing fairly healthy cells adjacent. Fatty acids eerily assume a crucial role in cancer cells' metabolism alongside glucose in various obscure cellular processes, obviously. Malignant cells display unbridled synthesis of fatty acids essential for membrane production and store energy vigorously in abnormally large quantities (Hammoudi et al, 2011).

Diets rich in omega-3 fatty acids found mostly in fish oils and walnuts exert very potent anti-cancer effects through AMPK modulation pathways. Red meat and processed food rich in saturated fat have been strongly linked to inflammation and tumour progression that activates pro-survival pathways like PI3K/Akt/mTOR. Amino acids enhance the swift biosynthesis of proteins and lipids quite vigorously in diverse cancer cells under certain very pathological conditions. Glutamine fuels cellular growth substantially by feeding into the TCA cycle and providing nitrogen for nucleotide synthesis. Glutamine fuels cellular growth by catapulting into the TCA cycle vigorously and supplying nitrogen needed for synthesising nucleotides very energetically. Tweaking the diet extremely restricts glutamine and inhibiting glutaminase has shown quite promise in stifling tumour growth in several preclinical models (Hammoudi et al, 2011).

Glycine and serine substantially energise one-carbon metabolic pathways crucial for nucleotide synthesis in rapidly proliferating cell environments and cell division. Manipulation of dietary amino acid intake potentially curtails supply of crucial building blocks, thereby impairing tumour cell proliferation quite badly, really. Nutrient modulation offers a novel complementary cancer therapy approach effectively nowadays with tremendous potential, surprisingly under various circumstances. Dietary interventions disrupt tumour bioenergetics substantially by altering the availability of key metabolic substrates like glucose or fatty acids, thereby rapidly reducing tumour growth, and chemotherapy is enhanced. Modified nutrition strategies could play a vital role in developing highly effective personalised cancer therapies as correlations between diet and cancer metabolism become increasingly lucid.

8.2.1. Glucose Restriction and the Warburg Effect

Glucose fuels cellular energy production mechanisms extensively via glycolysis in various biological systems and plays a crucial role therein normally. Cancer cells weirdly display the Warburg effect, marked by reliance on glycolysis for energy production amidst plenty of oxygen being present. Metabolic reprogramming enables rapid ATP production, fuelling the biosynthesis of crucial macromolecules, crucial for unbridled cell growth and rampant proliferation. Tumour cells vigorously rely on glucose metabolism, thus creating an opportunity for therapeutic intervention by targeting glucose supply squarely. Glucose restriction appears rather promising as a cancer-fighting tactic through extremely low-carb diets or fairly ketogenic regimens, somewhat effectively (Liberti and Locasale, 2017).

Restrictive diets drastically cut glucose availability, thereby hobbling glycolysis and severely impairing the Warburg effect in cancer cells somewhat badly. Tumour cells heavily reliant on glycolysis for energy production become extremely vulnerable when glucose supply is abruptly withheld from them. Ketogenic diet triggers a profound metabolic shift characterised by extremely low carbohydrate intake and copious consumption of fats very rapidly. Under such conditions body enters a state of ketosis where cells obtain energy from ketone bodies formed by the conversion of fatty acids. Tumour cells typically display rather limited capacity for utilising ketone bodies efficiently, making them very susceptible to severe stress metabolically anyway. Normal cells adapt readily to utilising glucose or ketones and remain relatively unscathed by drastic dietary changes very much unharmed. Ketogenic diet remarkably reduces tumour growth fairly effectively in various cancers like gliomas, prostate cancer, and other such malignancies extremely well (Liberti and Locasale, 2017).

Depriving cancer cells of glucose and ramping up ketone body utilisation severely limits tumour growth and enhances traditional treatment efficacy very effectively. Ketogenic diet fosters oxidative stress very readily, inducing cell death or apoptosis in various quirky cancer cells, obviously nowadays. Glucose restriction holds promise therapeutically in cancer therapy and is now significantly amplified further, potentially yielding better outcomes. Glucose restriction presents a promising anticancer tactic largely via ketogenic diet regimen by preying on metabolic vulnerabilities inherent in cancer cells. Dietary interventions disrupt the Warburg effect and starve cancer cells of glucose while sparing normal cells in a hostile metabolic environment. Other strategies are markedly enhanced, and survival rates are boosted significantly by this approach in cancer treatment regimens quite nicely.

8.2.2. Amino Acid Modulation: Targeting Glutamine and Serine Metabolism

Amino acids rapidly fuel the growth of cells, providing vital precursors for protein synthesis and nucleotides or lipids necessary quickly for proliferating cancer cells. Cancerous cells often exhibit weird fluctuations in amino acid metabolic pathways, satisfying sudden surges in demand for sundry biosynthetic precursors. Glutamine and serine play pivotal roles in wildly altered cancer cell metabolism, presenting potential targets for some rather innovative therapeutic strategies. Cancer cells rely heavily on glutamine metabolism, and glutamine is one of the most abundant amino acids found in human body. It acts as crucial nitrogen and carbon donor, significantly contributing to the synthesis of α-ketoglutarate, a vital intermediate in the tricarboxylic acid cycle, fueling various cell processes (Endicott et al, 2021).

α-ketoglutarate not only fuels the TCA cycle, enabling ATP production, but also supports various biosynthetic pathways essential for cell growth, including nucleotide synthesis and amino acid production.

α-ketoglutarate fuels the TCA cycle, enabling ATP production and supports various biosynthetic pathways essential for cell growth, including the synthesis of nucleotides and amino acids. α-ketoglutarate fuels the TCA cycle, thereby enabling production of ATP and supporting various biosynthetic pathways crucial for cell growth via the synthesis of nucleotides and amino acids. Glioblastomas and some particularly vicious lung cancers display pronounced glutamine addiction relying heavily on exogenous sources for frenzied growth. Disrupting glutamine metabolism rampantly curtails energy production in such tumours with considerable efficacy, normally affecting various biosynthetic processes severely (Endicott et al, 2021).

Restricting glutamine through certain dietary manipulations or pharmaceutical interventions can very effectively starve cancer cells of this vital nutrient. Glutaminase inhibitors, blocking the conversion of glutamine into glutamate, show promising results in preclinical studies and are currently undergoing rigorous clinical trials nationwide. ASCT2 and similar glutamine transporters that enable cells to take up glutamine very effectively represent a novel potential therapeutic target. Inhibiting transporters quite effectively curtails glutamine supply in tumour cells, resulting in significant metabolic disruption and cell death eventually. Glutamine proves crucial for cancer cell metabolism alongside serine and one-carbon metabolism in a somewhat mystifying manner. Serine plays a crucial albeit largely underappreciated role in one-carbon metabolism, a vital biochemical pathway crucial for the synthesis of nucleotides. Serine significantly enhances the synthesis of glycine and methionine, which play crucial roles in sustaining various cellular functions especially inside rapidly proliferating cancer cells (Muranaka et al, 2024).

Cancer cells often display grossly upregulated serine biosynthesis pathways largely due to overexpression of the enzyme phosphoglycerate dehydrogenase, which catalyses the conversion of 3-phosphoglycerate into serine remarkably well. Tumours become heavily dependent on external serine sources due to metabolic adaptation that rapidly increases demand for serine supply. Inhibiting PHGDH or serine restriction disrupts one-carbon metabolism, impairing nucleotide synthesis, and tumour cell proliferation becomes significantly reduced suddenly. Targeting this metabolic pathway has shown considerable promise in preclinical research, particularly for certain malignancies like melanomas exhibiting rather high serine dependency. Glutamine and serine metabolic pathways represent tantalising targets for dietary tweaking as adjunct cancer treatment with considerable therapeutic promise, apparently. Restricting the consumption of specific amino acids or administering certain pharmaceuticals that impede their catabolism might potentially deprive tumour cells of essential nutrients (Muranaka et al, 2024). Adopting a plant-based diet or cutting back on glutamine-rich foods like meat and dairy yields surprisingly therapeutic benefits slowly. Dietary strategies limiting serine intake or shoring up metabolic pathways that reduce serine synthesis might be leveraged alongside traditional cancer therapies very effectively nowadays. Metabolic vulnerabilities tied up with serine metabolism and glutamine offer newfangled avenues for swift nutritional interventions disrupting the proliferation of cancerous cells.

8.2.3. Fatty Acid Metabolism: Targeting Lipid Synthesis in Cancer Cells

Fatty acids form crucial constituents of cell membranes and play a vital role in energy production remarkably well under normal conditions. Cancer cells undergo drastic reprogramming of lipid metabolism, rapidly supporting heightened demand for proliferation and abnormal cell division. Reprogramming entails upregulating lipogenesis, wherein fatty acid synthesis readily occurs, forming new membranes as tumour cells proliferate at an alarming rate. Fatty acid synthase FASN enzyme synthesises long-chain fatty acids and is frequently overexpressed in breast, prostate, and liver cancers nowadays. FASN overexpression manifests vigorously as a crucial aspect of tumour cell metabolism thriving under rapid division conditions very remarkably (Fu et al, 2020).

FASN catalyzes formation of palmitate, a long-chain saturated fatty acid vital for tumour lipid metabolic processes, from acetyl-CoA and malonyl-CoA. Palmitate serves as precursor for complex lipids like phospholipids and triglycerides crucial for maintaining the structural integrity of cell membranes. Cancer cells undergo rapid mitotic division, thereby boosting demand for energy and membrane components so lipid biosynthesis becomes crucial suddenly. FASN overexpression in cancer cells fuels rampant lipid production, enabling tumour cells sustain proliferative capacity and build new membranes rapidly. FASN activity inhibition very significantly hinders lipid biosynthesis, and tumour cell growth suffers badly as a direct consequence of this disruption (Fu et al, 2020).

Orlistat and other FASN inhibitors have shown considerable promise in preclinical studies and are being explored quite vigorously as cancer treatment options, potentially. FASN inhibitors severely disrupt lipid synthesis in tumour cells, leading to depletion of lipids and drastically impairing membrane production capability. FASN inhibition becomes an attractive therapeutic strategy in cancers exhibiting highly elevated FASN expression, particularly under certain conditions. Dietary modulation influences lipid metabolism very effectively under certain conditions, thereby impacting cancer progression with occasional pharmacological interventions. Consumption of various dietary fat types can significantly impact tumour growth and profoundly alter metabolism in cancerous cells. Omega-3 fatty acids found predominantly in fish oils and occasionally in flaxseeds or walnuts exhibit remarkably potent anti-cancer properties (Hao et al, 2023).

Polyunsaturated fatty acids have been shown to significantly reduce inflammation and suppress tumour metastasis in various cancer types including rather aggressive breast cancer. Omega-3 fatty acids exert effects via multiple quirky mechanisms including modulation of crucial metabolic pathways deeply entrenched in lipid metabolism . Crucial regulators AMPK and PPAR-α play somewhat mysterious significant roles in cellular metabolism governing fatty acid oxidation and lipid biosynthesis extensively. Omega-3 fatty acids rev up AMPK and PPAR-α resulting in notably diminished lipid synthesis and substantially elevated fatty acid oxidation rates suddenly thereafter. Changes foster prevention of excessive lipid buildup and spur oxidative stress damaging cancer cells thereby enhancing efficacy of chemotherapy and radiation therapy remarkably. Red meat and processed food rich in saturated fats have been linked rather strongly of late to fostering inflammation and tumour growth (Hao et al, 2023).

Diets rich in saturated fats trigger pathways such as PI3K/Akt/mTOR crucial for cell survival rewiring cancer cell metabolism radically further down the line. Targeting lipid metabolism in cancer cells represents a fresh remarkably promising strategy potentially treating various cancer forms quite effectively. FASN inhibitors coupled with dietary adjustments that significantly ramp up omega-3 intake and drastically slash saturated fat consumption vigorously hinder cancer cell growth. Omega-3 fatty acids possibly amplify efficacy of existing cancer treatments by starkly modulating metabolic pathways and profoundly reducing inflammation within the tumour microenvironment. Lipid metabolism plays a crucial role in cancer cell biology, with fatty acids deeply entrenched in membrane biosynthesis, generating energy prolifically. Tweaking diet or inhibiting FASN could potentially throw tumour cells' metabolism into disarray, stunting growth and hampering metastatic spread rapidly. Further research into lipid targeting therapies might uncover novel, potentially valuable adjuncts for traditional cancer treatments serving obscure ancillary roles effectively.

8.2.4. Micronutrients and Metabolic Regulation

Micronutrients play a vital role in tiny amounts, actually regulating energy production and maintaining proper cellular metabolic functions. Selenium and B vitamins play diverse roles supporting cellular functions, significantly influencing the progression of diseases like cancer under various physiological conditions. Micronutrients markedly enhance or thwart cancer cell proliferation depending on the metabolic requisites of tumours in diverse oncological settings, often quite radically. Vitamin D plays a crucial role within cells, sustaining mitochondrial function and regulating energy very effectively in various cellular contexts. Vitamin D profoundly affects mitochondrial biogenesis in healthy cells, optimising cellular energy production quite effectively at a very fundamental level. Vitamin D has been shown to modulate crucial pathways in cell cycle regulation, apoptosis, and immune surveillance very vigorously within various cancer cells (Gombart et al, 2020).

Vitamin D deficiency often correlates with an elevated risk of numerous malignancies, such as colon and breast cancer, very frequently nowadays. Vitamin D somewhat effectively reduces inflammatory cytokines in tumour microenvironments fraught with heightened oxidative stress and elevated inflammation. Vitamin D possibly helps disrupt the metabolic flexibility of cancer cells by promoting mitochondrial function and regulating sundry metabolic pathways for their ultimate downfall. Fruits and certain vitamins, like vitamin C, contain antioxidants that remarkably neutralise reactive oxygen species quite effectively in various physiological situations. ROS play crucial roles in cell signalling under normal physiological conditions, but excess production ravages cellular structures like DNA or proteins, thereby fueling tumourigenesis. ROS levels surge rather frequently in cancer cells owing largely to super rapid metabolic churn (Gombart et al, 2020).

Antioxidants very effectively maintain cellular integrity by mitigating oxidative stress and stifling mutations fueling cancerous growth beneath the cell surface. Antioxidant usage in cancer therapy settings must be meticulously regulated. Antioxidants shield normal tissues from oxidative stress and can curtail cell death, weirdly in tumour cells beset by oxidative damage. Antioxidants at high levels may unwittingly cloak cancer cells from treatments such as chemotherapy, inducing cell death via ROS-mediated pathways. Maximising therapeutic efficacy happens quite effectively while minimising damage to fairly healthy surrounding tissue with a balance between ROS and antioxidants. Selenium and B vitamins play a vital role in tumour metabolism alongside cellular antioxidant defence and DNA repair processes. Selenoproteins such as glutathione peroxidase utterly safeguard cells from oxidative stress, being a vital component crucial for cellular defence (Luo et al, 2022).

Selenium possibly possesses anti-cancer properties by modulating crucial signalling pathways deeply involved in cell proliferation and apoptosis irregularly. Selenium's impact on cancer progression fluctuates wildly depending on dosage, and excessive intake heightens the risk of some very nasty malignancies. B vitamins like B6, B12, folate and niacin play crucial roles in nucleotide synthesis and DNA methylation quite basically in cells. Folate and methionine cycles intertwine in one-carbon metabolism that fuels rapid cell division and growth remarkably well in diverse cancerous cells. Folate intake at elevated levels has been linked tenuously and somewhat controversially to progression of some cancers and implicated starkly in tumourigenesis. B6 plays a crucial role in sustaining immune function, while B12 regulates DNA synthesis, thereby helping prevent tumourigenesis by fostering cell cycle control mechanisms effectively (Luo et al, 2022).

Micronutrients subtly modulate tumour bioenergetics beneath surface-level observations in multifaceted ways that are surprisingly complex and deeply nuanced. Cancer cells frequently display peculiar nutrient dependencies stemming from utterly transformed cellular metabolic processes inside those abnormal cells. Dietary interventions potentially inhibit tumour growth quite effectively by influencing micronutrient availability and disrupting cancer cell metabolism, thereby. Tweaking antioxidant intake and boosting vitamin D levels really helps regulate mitochondrial activity, crucial for stifling the progression of tumours somewhat effectively. Balancing dietary intake of selenium and B vitamins modulates metabolic pathways in tumour cells, making them rather vulnerable to existing therapies very effectively.

9. Conclusion

Metabolic reprogramming emerges rather quickly as a hallmark of cancer, enabling tumour cells to adapt to bioenergetic needs sustaining tumultuous rapid growth. Cancer cells frequently skew markedly toward aerobic glycolysis with aberrant mitochondrial function and wonky glutaminolysis in a profoundly abnormal way. Metabolic adaptations fuel proliferation and foster stubborn resistance against therapy while contributing heavily, simultaneously to various immune evasion mechanisms. Tumour metabolism gets heavily swayed by dietary inputs, offering fresh prospects for therapeutic intervention in various cancer treatments effectively these days. Nutrients behave as signalling molecules fueling or thwarting cancer progression significantly by influencing myriad cellular processes in a rather complex manner (Navarro et al, 2022).

Diets severely restricted in certain amino acids or rich in healthy fats disrupt tumour bioenergetics and may effectively sensitise cancer cells to conventional therapies. Polyphenols and omega-3 fatty acids downregulate oxidative stress and epigenetically modulate genes related to metabolism quite remarkably. Deciphering complex interplays between eating habits and cancer cell metabolism reveals new avenues for therapeutic innovation through targeting metabolic pathways. Dietary modulation serves as a complementary non-invasive strategy rather haphazardly alongside pharmacological inhibitors of various enzymes involved in metabolism (Ruban et al, 2025). Ketogenic diets and intermittent fasting restrict nutrients very significantly and reduce insulin signaling thereby somewhat surprisingly enhancing chemotherapy efficacy in preclinical models. Translating such findings into clinical practice necessitates a nuanced understanding of tumour stage and patient metabolism, alongside overall nutritional status. Eventually, highly personalised dietary interventions will be developed with precision nutrition tailored somewhat by genetic background and metabolic profiling (Paoli et al, 2023).

Tumour bioenergetics can be significantly altered through dietary changes, representing a promising, largely untapped strategy in mainstream cancer treatment. Cancer cells' wonky metabolic processes can be targeted quite effectively, thereby thwarting tumour growth and boosting the efficacy of various treatment regimens very significantly. Metabolic insights deeply embedded in personalised oncology protocols, leveraging interdisciplinary collaboration, will profoundly transform cancer management strategies.

References

Aggarwal V, Tuli HS, Varol A, Thakral F, Yerer MB, Sak K, Varol M, Jain A, Khan MA, Sethi G. Role of Reactive Oxygen Species in Cancer Progression: Molecular Mechanisms and Recent Advancements. Biomolecules. 2019 Nov 13;9(11):735. doi: 10.3390/biom9110735. PMID: 31766246; PMCID: PMC6920770.

Alexandru I, Nistor D, Motofelea AC, Cadar Andone BA, Crintea A, Tatu C, Pop GN, Csep AN. Vitamins, Coenzyme Q10, and Antioxidant Strategies to Improve Oocyte Quality in Women with Gynaecological Cancers: A Comprehensive Review. Antioxidants (Basel). 2024 Dec 19;13(12):1567. doi: 10.3390/antiox13121567. PMID: 39765895; PMCID: PMC11672914.

Bader JE, Voss K, Rathmell JC. Targeting Metabolism to Improve the Tumour Microenvironment for Cancer Immunotherapy. Mol Cell. 2020 Jun 18;78(6):1019-1033. doi: 10.1016/j.molcel.2020.05.034. PMID: 32559423; PMCID: PMC7339967.

Caprara, G., Pallavi, R., Sanyal, S., & Pelicci, P. G. (2025). Dietary Restrictions and Cancer Prevention: State of the Art. Nutrients, 17(3), 503. https://doi.org/10.3390/nu17030503

Chen CI, Kuo DY, Chuang HY. FASN inhibition shows the potential for enhancing radiotherapy outcomes by targeting glycolysis, AKT, and ERK pathways in breast cancer. Int J Radiat Biol. 2025;101(3):292-303. doi: 10.1080/09553002.2024.2446585. Epub 2025 Jan 10. PMID: 39792986.

Cluntun AA, Lukey MJ, Cerione RA, Locasale JW. Glutamine Metabolism in Cancer: Understanding the Heterogeneity. Trends Cancer. 2017 Mar;3(3):169-180. doi: 10.1016/j.trecan.2017.01.005. PMID: 28393116; PMCID: PMC5383348.

Cunha A, Silva PMA, Sarmento B, Queirós O. Targeting Glucose Metabolism in Cancer Cells as an Approach to Overcoming Drug Resistance. Pharmaceutics. 2023 Nov 10;15(11):2610. doi: 10.3390/pharmaceutics15112610. PMID: 38004589; PMCID: PMC10675572.

Do LK, Lee HM, Ha YS, Lee CH, Kim J. Amino acids in cancer: Understanding metabolic plasticity and divergence for better therapeutic approaches. Cell Rep. 2025 Apr 22;44(4):115529. doi: 10.1016/j.celrep.2025.115529. Epub 2025 Apr 6. PMID: 40193251; PMCID: PMC12038367.

Doaei S, Gholamalizadeh M, Akbari ME, Akbari S, Feradova H, Rahimzadeh G, Mosavi Jarrahi A. Dietary Carbohydrate Promotes Cell Survival in Cancer Via the Up-Regulation of Fat Mass and Obesity-Associated Gene Expression Level. Malays J Med Sci. 2019 Mar;26(2):8-17. doi: 10.21315/mjms2019.26.2.2. Epub 2019 Apr 30. PMID: 31447604; PMCID: PMC6687223.

Du H, Xu T, Yu S, Wu S, Zhang J. Mitochondrial metabolism and cancer therapeutic innovation. Signal Transduct Target Ther. 2025 Aug 4;10(1):245. doi: 10.1038/s41392-025-02311-x. PMID: 40754534; PMCID: PMC12319113.

Endicott M, Jones M, Hull J. Amino acid metabolism as a therapeutic target in cancer: a review. Amino Acids. 2021 Aug;53(8):1169-1179. doi: 10.1007/s00726-021-03052-1. Epub 2021 Jul 22. PMID: 34292410; PMCID: PMC8325646.

Fu Y, Zou T, Shen X, Nelson PJ, Li J, Wu C, Yang J, Zheng Y, Bruns C, Zhao Y, Qin L, Dong Q. Lipid metabolism in cancer progression and therapeutic strategies. MedComm (2020). 2020 Dec 24;2(1):27-59. doi: 10.1002/mco2.27. PMID: 34766135; PMCID: PMC8491217.

Ge M, Xu Y, Cui L, Huang E, Liu Z, Yin K. Targeting amino acids in tumour therapy. Front Oncol. 2025 Jun 4;15:1582116. Doi: 10.3389/fonc.2025.1582116. PMID: 40535116; PMCID: PMC12174139.

Gombart AF, Pierre A, Maggini S. A Review of Micronutrients and the Immune System-Working in Harmony to Reduce the Risk of Infection. Nutrients. 2020 Jan 16;12(1):236. doi: 10.3390/nu12010236. PMID: 31963293; PMCID: PMC7019735.

Gupta D, Vashi PG, Trukova K, Lis CG, Lammersfeld CA. Prevalence of serum vitamin D deficiency and insufficiency in cancer: Review of the epidemiological literature. Exp Ther Med. 2011 Mar;2(2):181-193. doi: 10.3892/etm.2011.205. Epub 2011 Jan 20. PMID: 22977487; PMCID: PMC3440651.

Hammoudi N, Ahmed KB, Garcia-Prieto C, Huang P. Metabolic alterations in cancer cells and therapeutic implications. Chin J Cancer. 2011 Aug;30(8):508-25. doi: 10.5732/cjc.011.10267. PMID: 21801600; PMCID: PMC4013402.

Hao X, Zhu X, Tian H, Lai G, Zhang W, Zhou H, Liu S. Pharmacological effect and mechanism of orlistat in anti-tumour therapy: A review. Medicine (Baltimore). 2023 Sep 8;102(36):e34671. doi: 10.1097/MD.0000000000034671. PMID: 37682175; PMCID: PMC10489489.

Harachi M, Masui K, Okamura Y, Tsukui R, Mischel PS, Shibata N. mTOR Complexes as a Nutrient Sensor for Driving Cancer Progression. Int J Mol Sci. 2018 Oct 21;19(10):3267. doi: 10.3390/ijms19103267. PMID: 30347859; PMCID: PMC6214109.

Herst PM, Carson GM, Eccles DA, Berridge MV. Bioenergetic and Metabolic Adaptation in Tumour Progression and Metastasis. Front Oncol. 2022 Mar 17;12:857686. Doi: 10.3389/fonc.2022.857686. PMID: 35372069; PMCID: PMC8968714.

Huo M, Zhang J, Huang W, Wang Y. Interplay Among Metabolism, Epigenetic Modifications, and Gene Expression in Cancer. Front Cell Dev Biol. 2021 Dec 24;9:793428. Doi: 10.3389/fcell.2021.793428. PMID: 35004688; PMCID: PMC8740611.

Jiang J, Srivastava S, Zhang J. Starve Cancer Cells of Glutamine: Break the Spell or Make a Hungry Monster? Cancers (Basel). 2019 Jun 11;11(6):804. doi: 10.3390/cancers11060804. PMID: 31212591; PMCID: PMC6627209.

Jin J, Byun JK, Choi YK, Park KG. Targeting glutamine metabolism as a therapeutic strategy for cancer. Exp Mol Med. 2023 Apr;55(4):706-715. doi: 10.1038/s12276-023-00971-9. Epub 2023 Apr 3. PMID: 37009798; PMCID: PMC10167356.

Krzyszczyk P, Acevedo A, Davidoff EJ, Timmins LM, Marrero-Berrios I, Patel M, White C, Lowe C, Sherba JJ, Hartmanshenn C, O'Neill KM, Balter ML, Fritz ZR, Androulakis IP, Schloss RS, Yarmush ML. The growing role of precision and personalised medicine for cancer treatment. Technology (Singapore World Sci). 2018 Sep-Dec;6(3-4):79-100. doi: 10.1142/S2339547818300020. Epub 2019 Jan 11. PMID: 30713991; PMCID: PMC6352312.

Księżakowska-Łakoma K, Żyła M, Wilczyński JR. Mitochondrial dysfunction in cancer. Prz Menopauzalny. 2014 May;13(2):136-44. doi: 10.5114/pm.2014.42717. Epub 2014 May 21. PMID: 26327844; PMCID: PMC4520353.

Kumar R, Mishra A, Gautam P, Feroz Z, Vijayaraghavalu S, Likos EM, Shukla GC, Kumar M. Metabolic Pathways, Enzymes, and Metabolites: Opportunities in Cancer Therapy. Cancers (Basel). 2022 Oct 27;14(21):5268. doi: 10.3390/cancers14215268. PMID: 36358687; PMCID: PMC9656396.

Liberti MV, Locasale JW. The Warburg Effect: How Does it Benefit Cancer Cells? Trends Biochem Sci. 2016 Mar;41(3):211-218. doi: 10.1016/j.tibs.2015.12.001. Epub 2016 Jan 5. Erratum in: Trends Biochem Sci. 2016 Mar;41(3):287. Erratum in: Trends Biochem Sci. 2016 Mar;41(3):287. doi: 10.1016/j.tibs.2016.01.004. PMID: 26778478; PMCID: PMC4783224.

Liu X, Ren B, Ren J, Gu M, You L, Zhao Y. The significant role of amino acid metabolic reprogramming in cancer. Cell Commun Signal. 2024 Jul 29;22(1):380. Doi: 10.1186/s12964-024-01760-1. PMID: 39069612; PMCID: PMC11285422.

Longo VD, Fontana L. Calorie restriction and cancer prevention: metabolic and molecular mechanisms. Trends Pharmacol Sci. 2010 Feb;31(2):89-98. doi: 10.1016/j.tips.2009.11.004. Epub 2010 Jan 25. PMID: 20097433; PMCID: PMC2829867.

Luo M, Zhou L, Huang Z, Li B, Nice EC, Xu J, Huang C. Antioxidant Therapy in Cancer: Rationale and Progress. Antioxidants (Basel). 2022 Jun 8;11(6):1128. doi: 10.3390/antiox11061128. PMID: 35740025; PMCID: PMC9220137.

Menendez JA, Cuyàs E, Encinar JA, Vander Steen T, Verdura S, Llop-Hernández À, López J, Serrano-Hervás E, Osuna S, Martin-Castillo B, Lupu R. Fatty acid synthase (FASN) signalome: A molecular guide for precision oncology. Mol Oncol. 2024 Mar;18(3):479-516. doi: 10.1002/1878-0261.13582. Epub 2024 Jan 18. PMID: 38158755; PMCID: PMC10920094.

Mentella MC, Scaldaferri F, Ricci C, Gasbarrini A, Miggiano GAD. Cancer and Mediterranean Diet: A Review. Nutrients. 2019 Sep 2;11(9):2059. doi: 10.3390/nu11092059. PMID: 31480794; PMCID: PMC6770822.

Mitra S, Paul S, Roy S, Sutradhar H, Bin Emran T, Nainu F, Khandaker MU, Almalki M, Wilairatana P, Mubarak MS. Exploring the Immune-Boosting Functions of Vitamins and Minerals as Nutritional Food Bioactive Compounds: A Comprehensive Review. Molecules. 2022 Jan 16;27(2):555. doi: 10.3390/molecules27020555. PMID: 35056870; PMCID: PMC8779769.

Muranaka H, Akinsola R, Billet S, Pandol SJ, Hendifar AE, Bhowmick NA, Gong J. Glutamine Supplementation as an Anticancer Strategy: A Potential Therapeutic Alternative to the Conventional. Cancers (Basel). 2024 Mar 5;16(5):1057. doi: 10.3390/cancers16051057. PMID: 38473414; PMCID: PMC10930819.

Navarro C, Ortega Á, Santeliz R, Garrido B, Chacín M, Galban N, Vera I, De Sanctis JB, Bermúdez V. Metabolic Reprogramming in Cancer Cells: Emerging Molecular Mechanisms and Novel Therapeutic Approaches. Pharmaceutics. 2022 Jun 19;14(6):1303. doi: 10.3390/pharmaceutics14061303. PMID: 35745875; PMCID: PMC9227908.

Nong S, Han X, Xiang Y, Qian Y, Wei Y, Zhang T, Tian K, Shen K, Yang J, Ma X. Metabolic reprogramming in cancer: Mechanisms and therapeutics. MedComm (2020). 2023 Mar 27;4(2):e218. Doi: 10.1002/mco2.218. PMID: 36994237; PMCID: PMC10041388.

Paoli A, Bianco A, Moro T, Mota JF, Coelho-Ravagnani CF. The Effects of Ketogenic Diet on Insulin Sensitivity and Weight Loss, Which Came First: The Chicken or the Egg? Nutrients. 2023 Jul 12;15(14):3120. doi: 10.3390/nu15143120. PMID: 37513538; PMCID: PMC10385501.

Phan LM, Yeung SC, Lee MH. Cancer metabolic reprogramming: importance, main features, and potentials for precise targeted anti-cancer therapies. Cancer Biol Med. 2014 Mar;11(1):1-19. doi: 10.7497/j.issn.2095-3941.2014.01.001. PMID: 24738035; PMCID: PMC3969803.

Poff A, Koutnik AP, Egan KM, Sahebjam S, D'Agostino D, Kumar NB. Targeting the Warburg effect for cancer treatment: Ketogenic diets for management of glioma. Semin Cancer Biol. 2019 Jun;56:135-148. doi: 10.1016/j.semcancer.2017.12.011. Epub 2017 Dec 30. PMID: 29294371; PMCID: PMC6927557.

Qian L, Zhang F, Yin M, Lei Q. Cancer metabolism and dietary interventions. Cancer Biol Med. 2022 Dec 22;19(2):163–74. doi: 10.20892/j.issn.2095-3941.2021.0461. PMID: 34931768; PMCID: PMC8832959.

Rodriguez-Leyva D, Dupasquier CM, McCullough R, Pierce GN. The cardiovascular effects of flaxseed and its omega-3 fatty acid, alpha-linolenic acid. Can J Cardiol. 2010 Nov;26(9):489-96. doi: 10.1016/s0828-282x(10)70455-4. PMID: 21076723; PMCID: PMC2989356.

Ruban M, Pozhidaeva E, Bolotina L, Kaprin A. The Role of Diet and Nutrition in Cancer Development and Management: From Molecular Mechanisms to Personalised Interventions. Foods. 2025 May 18;14(10):1788. doi: 10.3390/foods14101788. PMID: 40428567; PMCID: PMC12110988.

Schiliro C, Firestein BL. Mechanisms of Metabolic Reprogramming in Cancer Cells Supporting Enhanced Growth and Proliferation. Cells. 2021 Apr 29;10(5):1056. doi: 10.3390/cells10051056. Erratum in: Cells. 2022 Nov 14;11(22):3593. doi: 10.3390/cells11223593. PMID: 33946927; PMCID: PMC8146072.

Sheeley MP, Andolino C, Kiesel VA, Teegarden D. Vitamin D regulation of energy metabolism in cancer. Br J Pharmacol. 2022 Jun;179(12):2890-2905. doi: 10.1111/bph.15424. Epub 2021 Apr 8. PMID: 33651382; PMCID: PMC9703876.

Stefanache A, Lungu II, Butnariu IA, Calin G, Gutu C, Marcu C, Grierosu C, Bogdan Goroftei ER, Duceac LD, Dabija MG, Popa F, Damir D. Understanding How Minerals Contribute to Optimal Immune Function. J Immunol Res. 2023 Nov 1;2023:3355733. Doi: 10.1155/2023/3355733. PMID: 37946846; PMCID: PMC10632063.

Talib WH, Mahmod AI, Kamal A, Rashid HM, Alashqar AMD, Khater S, Jamal D, Waly M. Ketogenic Diet in Cancer Prevention and Therapy: Molecular Targets and Therapeutic Opportunities. Curr Issues Mol Biol. 2021 Jul 3;43(2):558-589. doi: 10.3390/cimb43020042. PMID: 34287243; PMCID: PMC8928964.

Tan-Shalaby J. Ketogenic Diets and Cancer: Emerging Evidence. Fed Pract. 2017 Feb;34(Suppl 1):37S-42S. PMID: 30766299; PMCID: PMC6375425.

Tufail M, Jiang CH, Li N. Altered metabolism in cancer: insights into energy pathways and therapeutic targets. Mol Cancer. 2024 Sep 18;23(1):203. doi: 10.1186/s12943-024-02119-3. PMID: 39294640; PMCID: PMC11409553.

Wu W, Zhao S. Metabolic changes in cancer: beyond the Warburg effect. Acta Biochim Biophys Sin (Shanghai). 2013 Jan;45(1):18-26. doi: 10.1093/abbs/gms104. PMID: 23257292.

Yang K, Wang X, Song C, He Z, Wang R, Xu Y, Jiang G, Wan Y, Mei J, Mao W. The role of lipid metabolic reprogramming in the tumour microenvironment. Theranostics. 2023 Mar 13;13(6):1774-1808. doi: 10.7150/thno.82920. PMID: 37064872; PMCID: PMC10091885.

Yang WH, Qiu Y, Stamatatos O, Janowitz T, Lukey MJ. Enhancing the Efficacy of Glutamine Metabolism Inhibitors in Cancer Therapy. Trends Cancer. 2021 Aug;7(8):790-804. doi: 10.1016/j.trecan.2021.04.003. Epub 2021 May 18. PMID: 34020912; PMCID: PMC9064286.

Yu X, Pu H, Voss M. Overview of anti-inflammatory diets and their promising effects on non-communicable diseases. Br J Nutr. 2024 Oct 14;132(7):898-918. doi: 10.1017/S0007114524001405. Epub 2024 Oct 16. PMID: 39411832; PMCID: PMC11576095.

Zhang Y, Tang J, Jiang C, Yi H, Guang S, Yin G, Wang M. Metabolic reprogramming in cancer and senescence. MedComm (2020). 2025 Mar 4;6(3):e70055. Doi: 10.1002/mco2.70055. PMID: 40046406; PMCID: PMC11879902.

Zhao Y, Liu H, Riker AI, Fodstad O, Ledoux SP, Wilson GL, Tan M. Emerging metabolic targets in cancer therapy. Front Biosci (Landmark Ed). 2011 Jan 1;16(5):1844-60. doi: 10.2741/3826. PMID: 21196269; PMCID: PMC3117434.

Zhao Y, Ye X, Xiong Z, Ihsan A, Ares I, Martínez M, López-Torres B, Martínez-Larrañaga MR, Anadón A, Wang X, Martínez MA. Cancer Metabolism: The Role of ROS in DNA Damage and Induction of Apoptosis in Cancer Cells. Metabolites. 2023 Jun 27;13(7):796. doi: 10.3390/metabo13070796. PMID: 37512503; PMCID: PMC10383295.

Zheng J. Energy metabolism of cancer: Glycolysis versus oxidative phosphorylation (Review). Oncol Lett. 2012 Dec;4(6):1151-1157. doi: 10.3892/ol.2012.928. Epub 2012 Sep 20. PMID: 23226794; PMCID: PMC3506713.

Chapter 8

The Gut Microbiome-Host Axis: Dietary Determinants in Cancer Aetiology and Therapy Response

Ng. Joykumar Singh[1], Praneeth Juvvi[2], Sheetanshu Gupta[3*], Lokesh Kumar Mishra[4]

[1]Department of Food Process Engineering, College of Food Technology, Central Agricultural University (CAU), Imphal, Manipur, India

[2]Department of Food Processing Technology, College of Food Technology-Central Agricultural University, Imphal, Manipur, India

[3]Department of Food Safety and Quality Assurance, College of Food Technology, Central Agricultural University (CAU), Imphal, Manipur, India

[4]Department of BPME, College of Agriculture, Central Agricultural University (CAU), Imphal, Manipur, India

Abstract

The gut microbiome greatly influences host health facets like immune response and metabolism, alongside inflammation that plays a crucial role in cancer progression. Diet influences microbial composition profoundly, thereby affecting cancer progression substantially in intricate relationships with gut microbiome and treatment outcomes are altered. Diet-induced microbiome shifts drastically alter key processes like immune modulation and carcinogen metabolism, fueling inflammation deeply nested in cancer aetiology. Cancer therapies' efficacy and toxicity are partly mediated by gut microbiome activity, with treatments like chemotherapy being very heavily affected. Diet modulates microbial populations significantly and can boost therapy efficacy or mitigate the nasty side effects of various cancer treatments substantially. Folks who chow down on Western food loaded with processed edibles may face heightened cancer risk, whilst fibre intake nurtures gut health vigorously. Cutting-edge microbiome analysis technologies synergise rather effectively with preclinical models and clinical studies, furnishing insight into dietary regimens modulating gut microbiota, thwarting the onset of cancer. Diet modulates the gut microbiome-host axis fairly effectively in various cancer scenarios and potentially serves as a valuable therapeutic adjunct very often.

Keywords: Gut Microbiome, Cancer Aetiology, Therapy Response, Dysbiosis, Nutritional Modulation, Immune System

DOI: 10.1201/9781042010387-8

1. Introduction

Research into gut microbiome has surfaced as a vital field in cancer biology over the last ten years, uncovering myriad microorganisms lurking in the gut that play a crucial albeit obscure role in cancer development, progression and therapy. A diverse array of bacteria, fungi, viruses and sundry microbes inhabits the gut microbiome, intricately interfacing with host immune response and metabolic processes, quietly affecting overall wellbeing. Gut microbiota dynamically interacts with host physiological processes, influencing cancer aetiology remarkably and affecting response to cancer therapies nowadays quite significantly. Dietary factors profoundly influence microbiome composition, thereby impacting cancer initiation markedly in various cancerous states and altering treatment efficacy quite dramatically (Ağagündüz et al, 2023).

Cancer development unfurls as a gnarly, protracted process entailing lots of genetic mutations and exposures to environmental toxins very frequently. The gut microbiome acts remarkably as a key modulator of immune system inflammation and DNA repair mechanisms effectively at various crucial stages. Certain microbial communities either markedly enhance or utterly stifle tumour growth by modulating immune responses and producing metabolites that directly affect the tumour microenvironment greatly. Dysbiosis has been quite strongly linked with heightened risk of various cancers, including colorectal cancer, liver cancer and breast cancer too. Deciphering complex interactions between cancer pathogenesis and microbiome surprisingly yields novel recalibrations of microbial ecosystems for markedly better prognoses (Ağagündüz et al, 2023).

Diet hugely influences microbiome composition in a major way, really, for the overall well-being of humans and animals, apparently. Consumed food serves as the primary fuel for gut microbes, fueling fairly intricate metabolic processes remarkably and determining their overall composition suddenly. Diets rich in fibre foster the growth of beneficial gut bacteria fermenting dietary fibre into short-chain fatty acids such as butyrate with potent anti-inflammatory effects. Diets rich in processed food, red meat, and saturated fats prevalent in western cultures tenuously correlate with shifts in microbiome that curiously favour proliferation of pro-inflammatory microbial entities. Dietary patterns like these super inflammation in gut regions, known as a risk factor for various cancers, particularly colorectal tract cancers, which develop malignantly thereafter. Dietary patterns heavily sway the expression of oncogenes and tumour suppressor genes, partly by affecting various immune responses through microbiome-mediated modulation (Zhang P, 2022).

The connection between the gut and the immune system plays a crucial role in understanding the microbiome's profound influence on cancer development quite mysteriously. T lymphocytes and macrophages, along with dendritic cells, are besieged by signals originating from gut microbiota that modulate systemic responses very irregularly. Gut-associated lymphoid tissue crucially maintains immune homeostasis, and dysbiosis swiftly leads to immune dysfunction, thereby promoting chronic inflammatory responses. Microbial fermentation yields short-chain fatty acids crucial for upholding immune tolerance and encourages various peculiar immune responses quite effectively nowadays. They enhance regulatory T cells' function very effectively and thwart production of pro-inflammatory cytokines by various immune cells, thus mitigating systemic inflammation (Zhang P, 2022).

Pathogenic microbiota rather quickly spark inflammation through activation of toll-like receptors and sundry other weird immune pathways, promoting cancer progression vigorously. Cancer therapies' efficacy gets determined largely by the gut microbiome nowadays, and it influences overall cancer risk very significantly. Recent studies reveal microbiome profoundly impacts the effectiveness of chemotherapy alongside immunotherapy in diverse medical settings, particularly nowadays. Bacterial species peculiarly magnify anti-tumour effects of immune checkpoint inhibitors, which block proteins like PD-1, unleashing cancer-killing ability rather surreptitiously in some cases (Vivarelli et al, 2019).

Microbes alter the efficacy of immune responses by changing the composition and activity of sundry immune cells that heavily infiltrate tumourous tissue. Bacteroides fragilis remarkably boosts response vigorously to immune checkpoint inhibitors in preclinical models by activating CD8+ T cells very effectively. Conversely, some other bacteria may thwart the efficacy of treatment by fostering resistance in tumours or producing metabolites that drastically alter drug metabolic pathways (Pei et al, 2023).

Manipulating gut microbiota via targeted nutritional interventions presents a rather promising yet largely unexplored route for markedly improving cancer therapy results. Probiotics prebiotics and synbiotics a combo of both have been investigated rather thoroughly lately as potentially useful adjuncts in cancer therapy. Such interventions foster growth of beneficial microbes and restore microbial diversity thereby considerably improving immune function and enhancing therapeutic response greatly. Prebiotics such as dietary fibre stimulate growth of beneficial gut bacteria thereby promoting production of SCFAs and probiotics like Lactobacillus species heavily modulate various immune responses. Fruits and whole grains richly embedded in a plant-based diet markedly enhance microbiome composition and furnish bioactive polyphenols possessing markedly anti-cancerous properties (Roy and Dhaneshwar, 2023).

Integrating microbiome data into novel cancer therapy regimes effectively hinges on grasping highly variable individual microbiome composition intricately nowadays. Lifestyle alongside age and genetics significantly influences microbiome composition which affects individual responses to diet and therapies variably quite remarkably. Cancer treatment now encompasses a novel realm centered around highly personalized nutrition quite intricately linked with each person's distinct microbiome setup, offering diverse preventative measures. Microbiome profiling pinpoints unique microbial fingerprints that presage cancer susceptibility and forecast therapy response with fairly significant downstream ramifications very accurately. Merging cancer genomics with microbiome data enables creation of highly tailored interventions that optimize dietary regimens and enhance therapeutic efficacy remarkably well (Bhatt et al, 2017).

Gut microbiome and cancer have a fairly intricate relationship that will be explored somewhat extensively through various dietary habits in this chapter. Dietary factors profoundly shape microbiome composition and its functionality markedly impacting cancer risk downstream and modulating therapy response variably. Emerging research on microbiome-based therapies and dietary modulation that somewhat irregularly enhances conventional cancer treatment effectiveness will be explored deeply. Cancer care can be made rather more effective by leveraging gut microbiome knowledge and modulating diet very powerfully against tumours.

2. Exploring the Gut Microbiome's Role in Cancer Development and Progression

Myriad microorganisms like bacteria and archaea reside in human gut and facilitate overall bodily homeostasis extremely well. Microbes crucial for digestion significantly influence bodily functions like immune response and metabolism and also impact mental well-being, rather profoundly too. An increasing amount of research has rather quietly laid bare the profound effects of the gut microbiome on cancer biology in recent times. Evidence emerging rapidly indicates gut microbiome profoundly affects cancer initiation through complex mechanisms, thereby significantly influencing tumour development and metastasis. The microbiome residing beneath epithelial layers erratically modulates various immune responses quite heavily and significantly contributes to cancer development. Microbiota profoundly impacts the balance between pro-inflammatory immune cells and anti-inflammatory ones by interacting significantly with the host's immune system (Ogunrinola et al, 2020).

Immune surveillance plays a pivotal role in detecting nascent tumour cells effectively under normal physiological conditions, eliminating them very quickly. Microbial community imbalance severely impairs immune surveillance, thereby creating quite a favourable environment subsequently for tumourigenesis inside bodily tissues. Gut microbes enhance activation of regulatory T cells suppressing anti-tumour immune responses thereby quite vigorously promoting cancer growth. Microbiome influences cancer via metabolic pathways and modulates immune response through various obscure mechanisms quite effectively simultaneously. Gut bacteria facilitate breakdown of dietary constituents quite rapidly producing metabolites such as short-chain fatty acids that profoundly exert anti-inflammatory effects and vigorously suppress tumour growth (Ogunrinola et al, 2020).

Production of noxious metabolites like secondary bile acids can egregiously promote carcinogenesis particularly in gastrointestinal malignancies very frequently these days. Tumour microenvironment surrounding various cancerous tissues gets heavily influenced by the microbiome in a profoundly complex and often bewildering milieu. Tumour microenvironment gets modulated by microbial signals that influence angiogenesis or morph extracellular matrix, providing the structural support tumour cells need. Tumour microenvironment interactions with gut microbiome remarkably underscore the potential of probiotics nowadays in cancer treatment with microbiome-based therapies. Gut microbiome plays a somewhat obscurely a crucial role in cancer biology. Influence on immune function and tumour microenvironment rather effectively underscores nowadays potential as novel oncology therapies target quite remarkably.

2.1. Gut Microbiome and Immune Modulation in Cancer

Gut microbiome profoundly sculpts the immune system, influencing innate responses and modulating adaptive immunity with considerable impact on overall health, ostensibly. The gastrointestinal tract serves as the largest immune organ in the body, harbouring nearly 70 per cent of immune cells and facilitating the absorption of nutrients very effectively. Gut-dwelling microorganisms intricately interact with host immune cells, remarkably promoting immune system development and homeostasis maintenance therein very effectively. A balanced microbiome plays a crucial role in proper immune surveillance, detecting cancer cells quickly and eliminating them before rapid tumour establishment. A healthy gut microbiome enhances immune function somewhat mysteriously by vigorously modulating activation of various immune cells such as natural killer cells and T cells (Wiertsema et al, 2021).

Tumour cell identification and subsequent attacks are largely influenced by various microbial metabolites and mediated by crucial immune cell functions significantly. Gut bacteria churn out short-chain fatty acids very quickly during the fermentation of dietary fibre and these acids enhance immune responses quite significantly. Butyrate, propionate, and acetate exert profoundly anti-inflammatory effects inside tissues and rather slowly modulate T cell differentiation, fostering anti-tumour immunity. Dysbiosis manifests as severely compromised immune efficacy and fosters tumour progression effectively via stealthy mechanisms evading detection very quietly. Altered microbiome composition may thwart proper activation of immune responses, enabling cancer cells escape immune surveillance fairly unobtrusively in bodily tissues (Wiertsema et al, 2021).

Microbial communities weirdly influence the expression of immune checkpoint molecules such as PD-1 or CTLA-4, regulating T cell activation slowly in some instances. Cancer cells hijack such checkpoints very effectively, suppressing immune responses, thereby evading detection by almost every immune system quite often. Gut microbiome rather effectively modulates expression of checkpoint molecules, influencing the effectiveness of immunotherapy treatments targeting PD-1 in certain cases, while impacting CTLA-4.

Gut microbiome serves as a vital modulator significantly influencing the body's cancer-fighting prowess and response towards various immunotherapies, quite remarkably overall actually. Potentially novel avenues for augmenting anti-tumour immunity in cancer treatment emerge through probiotics or prebiotics and diet-based interventions restoring microbial balance. Gut microbiome exerts considerable influence on cancer biology through its ostensibly multifaceted functions and varied impact on immune response mechanisms. Novel therapeutic strategies for treating cancer now seem highly plausible as immune cell activation gets promoted (Cho et al, 2024). The microbiome plays a crucial role in immune checkpoint inhibitor therapy, fairly often these days, in various medical research studies, apparently. Patients with certain peculiar microbiome setups ostensibly respond remarkably well to ICIs in nasty malignancies like melanoma or lung cancer. Tumour immunotherapies enhance immune responses variably, but gut microbiome composition heavily influences their success in a rather unpredictable manner. *Akkermansia muciniphila* and *Bifidobacterium* apparently amplify therapy effectiveness, while other bacteria may disrupt immune response mechanisms.

2.2. Microbial Metabolites and Cancer Metabolism

Sundry microbial metabolites drastically alter tumour metabolism, and gut microbiome influences cancer development through quirky immune modulation very significantly. Fermentation byproducts originating from dietary constituents acted upon by gut microbes can either enhance or stifle cancer cell proliferation markedly. Microbial metabolites like butyrate, acetate, and propionate are heavily researched nowadays in various cancer studies involving short chain fatty acids. SCFAs emerge mainly from fermenting dietary fibres heavily in the colon and profoundly affect host physiology beyond just providing energy supply. Butyrate and other short-chain fatty acids crucially regulate epigenetics through histone deacetylation and DNA methylation, thereby maintaining cellular homeostasis. Butyrate has garnered attention lately owing largely to ostensibly potent anti-cancer properties in various significant research studies (Yang et al, 2023).

Researchers recently examined a process whereby cell differentiation is promoted, thereby halting the proliferation of cancerous cells uncontrollably. Butyrate markedly inhibits cancer cell proliferation and induces apoptosis or programmed death in tumour cells via microbiome activity quite effectively. Butyrate plays a protective role, maintaining gut epithelial barrier integrity beyond effects on various cancer cells, rather obviously in many respects. Nasty pathogens and toxic metabolites can seep very deeply into the bloodstream, triggering severe systemic inflammation from a compromised gut barrier. Cancer is driven notoriously driven by chronic inflammation, especially in some really nasty malignancies like colorectal cancer, very profoundly. Butyrate may mitigate tumourigenesis risk indirectly by fortifying gut barrier function, and it dampens local inflammatory responses very effectively. Production of SCFAs and maintenance of gut integrity extend protective effects remarkably beyond the gut into other organs very profoundly. Microbiome influence on systemic inflammation and localised immune responses intricately links gut health with broader cancer risk quite profoundly (Yang et al, 2023).

Microbial metabolites such as indole lactic acid and various short-chain fatty acids exhibit noteworthy effects on the biology of cancer cells. Gut bacteria produce indole, exerting profoundly anti-inflammatory effects deeply within tumour microenvironments by heavily modulating various immune system responses. Indole possibly fosters tumour suppressive immune responses while stifling pro-inflammatory pathways heavily contributing to various carcinogenic processes in a somewhat convoluted manner. Various lactic acid bacteria produce lactic acid that plays a somewhat convoluted role under certain peculiar conditions, on the other hand. It can foster an acidic environment somewhat thwarting tumour growth yet occasionally abetting proliferation of cancer cells in wildly disparate contextual scenarios.

Complex interaction between microbial metabolites and tumour biology is underscored by this dual role, with effects varying wildly across cancer types and local microenvironments. Butyrate and other SCFAs produced by the gut microbiome play crucial roles in regulating cancer metabolism extensively, and tumour progression happens rapidly. Metabolites maintain cellular homeostasis rather quietly and prevent cancer development vigorously inside gut epithelial cells by modulating gene expression and promoting apoptosis.

Metabolites like indole and lactic acid play crucial roles, underscoring a pressing need for a nuanced grasp of the microbiome's complex sway on cancer metabolism.

2.3. Gut Microbiome and Tumour Microenvironment (TME)

Tumour cells get enveloped by a dynamically shifting network replete with diverse cellular constituents like immune cells, stromal cells, non-cellular ECM proteins and blood vessels. Tumour development relies heavily on the environment playing a somewhat obscure, crucial role underground figuratively in a manner of speaking. Research increasingly shows gut microbiome profoundly impacts the tumour microenvironment via modulation of inflammation and various metabolic processes affecting tumour behaviour. Tumour microenvironment gets profoundly influenced by gut microbiome largely through its impact on inflammatory responses and various cellular processes modulation. Gut microbial community imbalance or dysbiosis has been linked tenuously quite often and fairly strongly with chronic inflammation fueling cancer progression. Signals from gut microbiome enter bloodstream and influence distant organs including tumours very effectively through some obscure mechanism (Anderson and Simon, 2020).

Several stages in colorectal cancer development have been tenuously linked to proliferation of nasty bacteria such as Fusobacterium nucleatum rather dubiously. Bacteria secrete various pro-inflammatory cytokines very heavily thereby creating a tumour-promoting microenvironment and tumour-associated macrophages infiltrate largely due to this. Tumour cells evade immune surveillance quite effectively with help from certain immune cells that ramp up metastasis by fostering ECM breakdown thereby facilitating migration. F stands out very starkly amidst surroundings. Fusobacterium nucleatum modulates immune responses within tumour microenvironments, subtly affecting activation of various T cells and surreptitiously promoting tolerance thereby further enhancing evasion of immune surveillance and facilitating rapid progression of tumours. Some gut bacteria produce carcinogenic metabolites such as secondary bile acids fairly readily in some cases from diverse dietary sources (Anderson and Simon, 2020).

Mutations emerge rapidly from reactive metabolites, damaging DNA in colon cells and driving tumourigenesis frequently in gastrointestinal tract cancers. Secondary bile acids accumulate very quickly, promoting genotoxicity, thereby heightening the likelihood of mutagenesis and DNA damage, accelerating tumour growth rapidly. A balanced gut microbiome exerts protective effects within TME by very effectively maintaining immune homeostasis under various circumstances. Species of Lactobacillus and Bifidobacterium produce metabolites that quite effectively encourage immune responses and thwart tumour escape mechanisms, rather ingeniously in various contexts. Beneficial microbes stimulate dendritic cells very vigorously, and these cells present tumour antigens sloppily to naive T cells encourage adaptive immunity effectively. Microbes facilitate activation of cytotoxic T lymphocytes, crucial for recognising tumour cells and killing them with considerable efficacy.

Bacteria surprisingly enhance anti-tumour immune response effectively amidst a balanced microbial makeup, preventing immune suppression typically seen in nasty tumours. Metabolites churned out by commensal bacteria in the gut tweak the tumour microenvironment significantly by influencing the formation of new blood vessels supplying oxygen. Tumour growth relies heavily on angiogenesis, and certain microbial metabolites either foster or thwart it depending on prevailing species. Butyrate and other short-chain fatty acids purportedly impede angiogenesis rather effectively by downregulating pro-angiogenic factors within tumour cells, restricting growth very significantly (Aghamajidi et al, 2022).

Tumour biology aspects, including immune regulation and inflammation, are influenced rather extensively by gut microbiome composition within TME alongside angiogenesis. Dysbiosis fuels chronic inflammation and carcinogenic compound production quite vigorously in various bodily contexts, facilitating tumour progression very relentlessly. A balanced microbiome fosters anti-tumour immunity, effectively reducing nasty inflammation, and potentially limiting the growth of tumours underneath epithelial layers. Interplay between gut microbiome and tumour microenvironment holds considerable promise, remarkably for the development of novel therapies encourage cancer treatment outcomes.

2.4. Microbiome-Targeted Therapies in Cancer

Novel cancer therapies have emerged recently targeting the gut microbiome with unusual fervor and they now leverage its influence very thoroughly. Researchers are fervently exploring sundry approaches nowadays modulate microbiome therapeutically via various unorthodox methods and obscure experimental techniques rapidly. Supplementing with beneficial microbes such as Lactobacillus or Bifidobacterium might vigorously promote anti-tumour immunity by restoring a healthy microbiome. Probiotics vigorously modulate immune responses and inhibit the growth of pathogenic bacteria linked with various cancer progression rather rapidly. Prebiotics rather quietly foster the growth of beneficial gut bacteria inside human intestines daily amidst a sea of other food components (Cho et al, 2024).

Diets rich in fibre and prebiotic-rich foods like fruits and whole grains markedly enhance production of SCFAs such as butyrate with protective anticancer effects. Faecal Microbiota Transplantation radically transfers gut microbiota from a healthy donor into cancer patients with considerable therapeutic intent. FMT profoundly reshapes the gut microbiome alongside immune checkpoint inhibitors and various cancer therapies, thereby promoting a very favourable immune response. Antibiotics traditionally kill harmful bacteria, but inappropriate use disrupts the gut microbiome, potentially impairing anti-tumour immunity significantly over time. Targeted antibiotic use might eradicate certain microbial species that contribute significantly to oncogenesis whilst preserving resilient beneficial microbes elsewhere in the body (Cho et al, 2024).

Cancer development is profoundly influenced by the gut microbiome through effects on the tumour microenvironment and microbial metabolism, essentially modulating immune responses. Dysbiosis fuels the progression of cancer rapidly by fostering chronic inflammation and enabling immune evasion in the gut microbiome quite precariously. Microbiome diversity markedly enhances anti-tumour immunity very effectively under certain conditions and fosters tumour growth inhibition rather noticeably. Dietary manipulation of gut microbiome using probiotics, prebiotics, and unorthodox therapies may enhance cancer treatment outcomes, significantly reducing cancer risk. Deeper probing into intricate mechanisms by which the microbiome profoundly influences oncogenesis will unlock novel therapeutic avenues tailored for cancer care specifically.

3. Diet-Microbiome Interactions: Implications for Cancer Aetiology

Gut microbiome interacts dynamically with diet in a complex manner, and recent research has vigorously explored cancer-causing implications. Trillions of microbes, like bacteria and weird fungi, vigorously regulate metabolism and immune response in the gut microbiome essentially playing a crucial role. Such processes play a crucial role very effectively in maintaining overall well-being and staving off maladies like rather nasty cancer. Consumption of certain foods drastically alters gut microbiota composition and overall function, with potentially dire implications for cancer development downstream. Fibre and sugar intake rapidly alters gut microbiota by fostering the growth of both beneficial and pathogenic microbial colonies very quickly. High-fibre diets enrich the gut microbiome with beneficial bacteria churning out short-chain fatty acids like butyrate having very potent anti-inflammatory effects. SCFAs ostensibly play protective roles in cancer pathogenesis by heavily modulating immune response and promoting apoptosis quite aggressively in malignant cells (Zhang P, 2022).

Microbes that promote healthier immune responses thrive on a high-fibre diet, reducing chronic inflammation markedly amidst various cancer risks, including colorectal cancer. Diets rich in fat and replete with heavily processed red meats have been tenuously linked with perturbations in the microbiome that heighten malignancy risk. Diets rich in specific nutrients can spur the growth of pathogenic bacteria that produce carcinogenic metabolites such as N-nitroso compounds, damaging cellular DNA. Fusobacterium nucleatum proliferation fuels colorectal cancer pathogenesis by inducing intense inflammation remarkably deep inside tumour microenvironments gradually. Gut microbiome plays a crucial albeit largely understated role in metabolising dietary components, fairly effectively modulating their sundry effects on various bodily systems dynamically. Polyphenols abundant in fruits and veggies get metabolised by gut bacteria into very potent bioactive compounds exhibiting rather interesting anti-cancer properties (Zhang P, 2022).

Metabolites modulate gene expression effectively and inhibit cancer cell growth by reducing oxidative stress somewhat in cells. Diets rich in antioxidants, fibre, and omega-3 fatty acids foster an anti-inflammatory state, altering microbiome composition significantly. Probiotics and prebiotics nowadays garner increasing attention for potential roles in rapidly treating various kinds of cancer effectively. Live beneficial microbes in probiotics enhance immune responses, thereby potentially mitigating cancer risk and inhibiting tumour growth in dysbiotic gut environments. Prebiotics stimulate the growth of beneficial microbes by fostering microbiota producing protective metabolites like SCFAs, which have remarkably analogous effects downstream. Pairing probiotics with prebiotics potentially offers a mighty strategy downstream for fostering a healthy gut microbiome and hindering cancer development (Berding et al, 2023).

Emerging evidence now suggests that diet microbiome interactions influence the efficacy of orally administered cancer treatments variably with considerable impact. Recent studies show chemotherapy effectiveness gets swayed very heavily by gut microbiome composition and gets altered drastically during certain immunotherapy treatments. Some microbiota may vigorously enhance immune response during cancer treatment, while others could possibly undermine treatment efficacy, leading to resistance. Modified cancer treatments leveraging immune system modulation, such as checkpoint inhibitors, necessitate consideration of microbiome variability, particularly nowadays. Cancer aetiology gets influenced rather intricately by gut microbiome and diet in a somewhat convoluted manner, obviously. Antioxidants and fibre-rich dietary regimens robustly foster immune function, supporting microbiomes that mitigate inflammation against various forms of cancer effectively. Consumption of garbage food laden with noxious lipids fuels the rampant growth of malignant microorganisms, thereby markedly elevating oncogenesis risk. Novel cancer research strategies hinge on grasping interactions between diet and microbiome, emphasising heavily diet as a modifiable risk factor (Berding et al, 2023).

3.1. Dietary Impact on the Gut Microbiome

Gut microbiome composition and its function are deeply influenced by dietary habits, with implications for health and disease prevention unfolding slowly. Trillions of microorganisms thrive remarkably well inside the gut microbiome, playing a vital role in digestion and significantly aiding various metabolic processes. Dietary patterns profoundly impact microbial ecosystems, nurturing healthy gut flora or precipitating dysbiosis with potentially grim health consequences, including oncogenesis. Diets heavy in processed food fuel the growth of nasty pathogenic bacteria like Fusobacterium nucleatum and suppress beneficial gut microbes quite effectively. Harmful microbes produce metabolites that very badly disrupt normal cellular functions and foster environments eerily conducive, rather rapidly, to cancer. Fusobacterium nucleatum rather haphazardly ramps up tumour progression in colorectal cancer by activating inflammatory pathways and very effectively fostering immune evasion (Hills et al, 2019).

Diets teeming with fibre from fruits and whole grains foster the growth of beneficial microbes such as Bifidobacteria that produce butyrate, namely short-chain fatty acids. SCFAs play a pivotal role in maintaining gut health, and their presence facilitates various protective functions therein quite effectively. Butyrate remarkably enhance gut epithelial cellular integrity significantly and safeguards vigorously against nasty inflammation, thereby preventing diseases like cancer very effectively. SCFAs profoundly modulate the activity of diverse immune cells, such as T cells and macrophages, in cancer surveillance and tumour cell destruction processes. A diet rich in fibre yet starved of processed food fosters a healthy microbiome, helping maintain optimal metabolic functions that support various physiological processes, including nutrient uptake, energy homeostasis and modulation of quirky immune responses. A balanced microbiome remarkably stymies the proliferation of pathogenic bacteria rather effectively thereby mitigating systemic inflammation that fuels cancerous tumour growth (Hills et al, 2019).

Obesity and insulin resistance frequently spawn low-grade inflammation fostering a pro-inflammatory tumour microenvironment that expedites cancer progression rapidly and metastasis occurs subsequently. Dysbiosis significantly influences various factors that alter immune function and metabolic processes linking it with several chronic diseases including cancer. Cancerous dysbiosis ramps up synthesis of nasty carcinogenic metabolites such as secondary bile acids and nitrate-derived stuff that nukes DNA fast. Altered microbiome drastically disrupts tumour microenvironment by fostering inflammation and suppressing immune responses thus cancer cells thrive fairly unnoticed. Fluctuations inside gut microbiota driven by diet erratically affect oncogenesis by encourage or thwarting progression of malignant tumours quite heavily sometimes (Iyengar et al, 2016).

Microbiome modulates TME's immune landscape significantly fostering cancerous immune evasion or somewhat effectively enhancing antitumour responses really quickly underground. Ramping up fibre intake or slashing processed foods loaded with fat may thwart cancer onset and fine-tune immune surroundings encourage treatments. Diets greatly impact gut flora, profoundly influencing overall well-being and various disease states in surprisingly complex, often quite unexpected ways, obviously. Diets rich in fibre foster the growth of beneficial microbes that produce anti-inflammatory metabolites, while food high in processed food promotes dysbiosis. A diverse gut microbiome plays a crucial role in preventing various chronic diseases, including cancer, by robustly supporting immune function. Dietary modulation enhances microbiome well-being and enhances immune efficacy, thereby unlocking fresh avenues for cancer therapy with massive prophylactic promise.

3.2. Gut Microbiome and Inflammation in Cancer Development

Chronic inflammation ominously fuels the development of various cancers, including colorectal cancer, liver cancer and pancreatic cancer, seemingly with some regularity. Gut microbiome quietly regulates inflammation centrally amidst a plethora of bodily functions and orchestrates various physiological processes very subtly. Gut microbes get severely skewed, and this spurs overproduction of heinous pro-inflammatory molecules like cytokines, sometimes inside human bodies rapidly. Fusobacterium nucleatum heavily promotes chronic inflammation by activating NF-κB signaling thereby fueling tumour growth very effectively, and metastasis occurs subsequently (Armstrong et al, 2018).

Dysbiosis, strongly linked to IBD, fosters colon cancer development rapidly in the gut microbiome's stark contribution to inflammatory maladies surfacing quite ominously. Microbiome interplay with inflammatory pathways underscores considerable potential for dietary interventions that modulate gut flora quite significantly, mitigating cancer risk. Diet profoundly influences inflammatory pathways through various recondite routes and sometimes triggers unexpected downstream biochemical cascades quite rapidly. Diets heavy in processed meats and red flesh often spur the growth of pro-inflammatory microbes, while fibre-rich plant-based regimens foster profoundly anti-inflammatory responses. Polyphenols found in fruits and veggies drastically reduce inflammatory markers and foster healthier gut microbiome composition very naturally in various studies.

3.3. Microbiome-Mediated Metabolism and Carcinogenesis

The gut microbiome plays a crucial roles in immune modulation and metabolic processes, directly impacting cancer risk through various convoluted biochemical routes. Microbiome interactions with dietary components, rather haphazardly sway various metabolic pathways and either thwart or foster cancer development somewhat unpredictably. Novel findings underscore microbial metabolites, notably short-chain fatty acids generated via dietary fibre fermentation, orchestrating pivotal shifts profoundly impacting tumourigenesis. Beneficial gut bacteria, such as Firmicutes, produce butyrate, a short-chain fatty acid, rather slowly during fermentation of various dietary fibres. Butyrate serves remarkably well as an energy source for colonocytes and exerts some very wild epigenetic effects, thwarting carcinogenesis in various cellular contexts. Butyrate specifically inhibits histone deacetylases or HDACs deeply, which regulate chromatin structure and gene expression quite significantly (Xu et al, 2025).

Butyrate induces histone acetylation rather slowly by inhibiting HDACs and leads curiously to changes in gene expression favouring tumour suppression. Butyrate helps maintain intestinal lining integrity, particularly within the colon and reduces colorectal cancer risk quite significantly over long periods of time. Butyrate very effectively fosters apoptosis in damaged cells, safeguarding against malignant transformations, rather sneakily down the line further. Consumption of copious saturated fats via a high-fat diet can bizarrely thwart microbiome health and considerably fuel carcinogenesis in various obscure ways. Diets heavy with saturated fats vigorously promote the growth of gut bacteria favoring production of secondary bile acids such as deoxycholic acid. Secondary bile acids brutally ravage intestinal cells, getting perilously linked to DNA damage that spawns heinous mutations, fueling colorectal cancer initiation very quickly. Bile acids induce genotoxicity quickly, leading rather profoundly to chromosomal instability, a hallmark often seen in various malignant cell types (Xu et al, 2025).

High-fat diets tweak gut microbiome severely, ramping up populations of bacteria that produce carcinogenic compounds rapidly inside the gut. Various metabolic pathways are influenced heavily by the gut microbiome, notably glucose metabolism frequently dysregulated rapidly in proliferating malignant cells within human tissues. Tumour cells favour glycolysis over oxidative phosphorylation eerily in energy generation via a phenomenon known as the Warburg effect, hallmarking various cancers. Gut microbiome modulates glucose metabolism effectively by producing metabolites that heavily influence insulin sensitivity and overall glucose utilisation in humans. Certain SCFAs, such as acetate, can influence insulin signalling quite profoundly, thereby enhancing insulin sensitivity and potentially reducing the risk of cancers like breast cancer, liver cancer and pancreatic cancer. Abnormal tumour cell survival gets fostered very readily by insulin resistance, which gets really bad due to poor dietary habits and dysbiosis occurring together, stimulating blood vessel growth under pro-inflammatory conditions (Murphy et al, 2015).

Microbiome alterations driven by dietary shifts heavily influence systemic metabolic processes by modulating lipid metabolism and tweaking inflammatory pathways concurrently. Gut microbiome modulates the balance between pro-inflammatory mediators and anti-inflammatory ones, rather slowly playing a critical role in tumour progression. Dysbiotic microbiome fuels chronic inflammation, driving cancer and forming a tumour-promoting microenvironment that greatly enhances the survival of tumour cells, metastasis and therapy resistance. Metabolic activities of the gut microbiome deeply impact the aetiology of cancer and progression within bodily systems fairly profoundly. Beneficial microbiota churns out SCFAs such as butyrate, thereby inducing far-reaching epigenetic changes and substantially encouraging immune responses very effectively. High-fat low-fibre diets fuel dysbiosis, fostering the production of carcinogenic metabolites such as secondary bile acids and promoting environments that initiate cancer (Murphy et al, 2015). The microbiome influences glucose metabolism profoundly, and insulin resistance is linked with dietary habits and various oncogenic risk factors simultaneously. Unlocking microbiome-mediated metabolic pathways reveals fresh cancer prevention avenues, mostly via dietary changes and therapy modulation, rather quietly.

3.4. Dietary Interventions and Microbiome-Modulated Cancer Prevention

Dietary interventions show considerable promise in cancer prevention given their profound impact on the microbiome and subsequent trajectories of cancer progression. High-fibre diets correlate with gut microbiome profiles remarkably more favorable alongside substantially reduced cancer risk. Whole grains, fruits, and veggies rich in fibre foster beneficial microbes that produce SCFAs, helping regulate inflammation and thwarting cancer cell growth rather effectively. Certain nutrients have shown considerable promise in significantly altering gut flora, thereby reducing the risk of specific cancers, rather surprisingly. Polyphenols present in various foods, such as berries or green tea, heavily modulate the microbiome and reduce tumourigenesis significantly in many cases naturally. Non-digestible food components fostering the growth of beneficial microbes have been shown to enhance gut microbiota fairly extensively. Fermented foods and probiotics are lately gaining traction quite rapidly as potentially efficacious tweakers of the microbiome that may confer anticancer benefits (Greathouse et al, 2022).

Lactobacillus species potentially enhance immune function vigorously and fend off nasty inflammation, thereby offering somewhat effective protection against cancer development. Interventions like these may prove rather salutary in folks harbouring a dysbiotic microbiome, thus furnishing a novel modus operandi for recalibrating microbial homeostasis. Dietary habits heavily influence the gut microbiome, which subsequently fuels cancer development through quirky immune responses and aberrant inflammation metabolism pathways. Unhealthy diets foster microbiome imbalance spurring cancer development, but remarkably, a balanced microbiome may thwart tumourigenesis very effectively in numerous cases. Cancer prevention strategies crucially rely on grasping fairly complex interactions between dietary habits and microbiota in the human gut quite accurately nowadays. People can effectively lower cancer risk by eating foods that support a healthy microbiome and subsequently enhance overall well-being quite remarkably. Research continually unearths intricate connections between diet and cancerous tumours, potentially rendering modified nutritional interventions pivotal for thwarting malignancies effectively nowadays (Greathouse et al, 2022).

4. The Gut Microbiome as a Modulator of Cancer Therapy Response

Remarkably swift progress in cancer therapy has been made in recent decades, owing largely to breakthroughs in chemotherapy and targeted therapy, yielding greatly improved survival rates. Response remains wildly inconsistent despite garnering successes from sundry unorthodox therapies and various other rather innovative treatment modalities lately. Some patients initially benefit quite significantly from treatment therapeutically but others develop resistance or experience recurrence of cancer despite its effectiveness. Research increasingly underscores a hitherto underappreciated yet pivotal factor in therapy results that vary wildly due to gut microbiome fluctuations erratically. Microorganisms like bacteria, fungi, and viruses thrive rather abundantly in the human gut amidst considerable complexity and highly varied microbial makeup. Microbial ecosystem regulates numerous physiological functions such as metabolism and immune response vigorously amidst intense inflammatory bouts fairly dynamically (Anand et al, 2022).

Fundamental processes crucial for maintaining health and amplifying cancer therapies exist ubiquitously and rather obviously within various medical treatment modalities. Evidence emerging rapidly from many recent studies suggests the gut microbiome profoundly influences response to various cancer treatments by modulating key factors deeply. Cancer therapy outcomes are influenced heavily by the microbiome that modulates the immune system rather effectively in sometimes surprisingly compelling, albeit unpredictable ways. Immunotherapy relies heavily on vigorously stimulating the body's immune response rather than haphazardly and eliminates malignant cells quite effectively sometimes. Gut microbiome exerts a somewhat nebulous influence nowadays on immune landscape thereby greatly shaping innate immune responses and adaptive ones too rather markedly. Certain microbial species amplify the efficacy of checkpoint inhibitors, which block immune checkpoints such as PD-1 or CTLA-4, enabling T cells to target tumours (Anand et al, 2022).

Bacteroides and Firmicutes are linked quite positively to immune checkpoint blockade therapy response, while the absence of beneficial microbes severely impairs the body's response, leading to therapy resistance. Surprisingly, drug metabolism gets heavily influenced by the microbiome under certain conditions fairly regularly in various bodily systems. Chemotherapy drugs often require liver enzymes rapidly metabolise them afterwards, rendering some fairly quickly inert or surprisingly activated. Gut microbiome alters activity of certain enzymes thereby impacting bioavailability and efficacy of various cancer drugs quite significantly nowadays is rephrased as: Nowadays various cancer drugs efficacy gets significantly altered by gut microbiome, modifying the activity of certain enzymes activity very drastically. Microbial metabolites such as short-chain fatty acids modulate the activity of certain cytochrome P450 enzymes quickly metabolise numerous chemotherapeutic agents in liver cells (Aggarwal et al, 2023).

Dysbiosis drastically alters drug metabolism thereby severely affecting pharmacokinetics and pharmacodynamics of cancer therapeutics potentially resulting in heightened toxicity or efficacy reduction greatly. Tumour microenvironment is crucially shaped by microbiome, a profound influence that determines cancer progression variably under specific treatments, obviously. TME comprises cancer cells and immune cells alongside stromal cells, blood vessels and various extracellular matrix components interacting rather intricately, regulating tumour growth. Research suggests gut microbiota heavily influences inflammatory responses within tumour microenvironment thereby significantly impacting tumour evasion and therapy resistance mechanisms. A balanced microbiome might help mitigate chronic inflammation and foster TME remarkably responsive naturally to therapies like radiation or very intense chemotherapy (Aggarwal et al, 2023).

Dysbiotic microbiome fosters inflammatory environments quite readily thereby supporting tumour progression and it enhance treatment resistance rather effectively. Microbiome somewhat significantly modulates response to radiation therapy in a fairly crucial manner under various circumstances. Radiation therapy efficacy gets somewhat haphazardly enhanceed or undermined in various ways by gut microbiome's highly irregular radiation-induced immune response. Germ-free mice lacking microbiome exhibit diminished tumour responses upon radiation and gut microbiome plays a crucial role in optimizing radiation treatment outcomes very effectively nowadays. Gut microbiome exerts profoundly significant influence on cancer treatment toxicity according to some very recent and unusually thorough studies. Aggressive treatment frequently induces very nasty side effects such as neutropenia or systemic inflammation in patients undergoing chemotherapy and radiotherapy. Gut microbiome crucially regulates immune system and epithelial integrity imbalances in microbial composition can severely exacerbate treatment related toxicity. Chemotherapy-induced mucositis drastically depletes gut microbiota linking such conditions very direly to outcomes while a healthy microbiome surprisingly may mitigate them.

4.1. The Microbiome's Role in Immunotherapy Response

Immunotherapy signifies a paradigm-shifting advancement in oncology largely through novel immune checkpoint inhibitors such as antibody therapies targeting PD-1 and CTLA-4 vigorously nowadays. Treatments for nasty cancers like melanoma and non-small-cell lung cancer have been upended quite remarkably by therapies these days. ICIs operate rather effectively nowadays by blocking certain inhibitory signals within immune system preventing T cells from annihilating malignant cells. Releasing this brake on immune system lets T cells recognize tumour cells more effectively and they get eliminated quite vigorously subsequently. Outcomes vary enormously among patients treated with ICIs which have succeeded rather remarkably in many instances despite being largely unpredictable normally. Some patients fare poorly with immunotherapy and develop nasty immune-related adverse events triggered essentially by a rogue immune system gone haywire. Newly excavated research surprisingly illuminates a previously underappreciated factor influencing immunotherapy efficacy profoundly through gut microbiome (Zhang et al, 2024).

Trillions of microorganisms residing in human gut impact various aspects of immune function rather profoundly including activation of inflammation and tolerance mechanisms. Nowadays studies imply gut microbiome hugely influences immunotherapy efficacy by significantly modulating immune system activity quite irregularly under various circumstances. Certain gut microbial species ostensibly enhance ICIs' efficacy while other species vitiate immune response thereby diminishing treatment effectiveness rather significantly. Beneficial bacteria such as Akkermansia muciniphila and Faecalibacterium prausnitzii frequently correlate with enhanced responses to ICIs these days fairly often. Dendritic cells get activated really strongly by microbes which greatly amplifies immune response against tumours and T cells respond vigorously (Zhang et al, 2024).

Akkermansia muciniphila has garnered considerable attention recently for potentially boosting PD-1 blockade effectiveness significantly in various murine tumour models effectively. CD8+ T cell activation surges remarkably around this bacterium proving crucial subsequently for eradication of tumour cells. Beneficial microbes presence has been rather strongly linked to increased anti-tumour immunity suggesting gut microbiome acts as very effective biological adjuvant enhancing response under immune checkpoint inhibitors. Pathogenic bacteria throng a dysbiotic microbiome which can drastically impair immune response and reduce immunotherapy effectiveness very significantly . Dysbiosis intricately links with suppressed immune function and fosters chronic inflammation which impairs T cell efficacy against tumours very effectively. Fusobacterium nucleatum bacterium very badly hinders response to ICIs in colorectal cancer patients under certain circumstances (Yan et al, 2021).

Fusobacterium nucleatum surreptitiously facilitates immune evasion through activation of specific checkpoint pathways and triggers release of various pro-inflammatory cytokines very effectively. Bacterium fosters profoundly immunosuppressive environments subduing cytotoxic T lymphocytes crucial for targeting tumour cells thereby largely inhibiting immunotherapy efficacy. Fusobacterium has been linked insidiously to tumour progression and fosters immune escape further muddling cancer treatment in cases thriving with this bacterium. Gut microbiome composition plays a crucial role in determining patient outcomes undergoing immunotherapy treatments influenced by immune checkpoint inhibitors fairly significantly. Beneficial bacteria thrive in diverse microbiomes greatly enhancing immunotherapy efficacy while dysbiosis festers with noxious microbes severely hindering treatment progress (Yan et al, 2021).

Microbiome's role in immunotherapy sprawls far beyond merely modulating immune cell activity and drastically reshapes tumour microenvironment surroundings very significantly. Novel strategies rooted deeply in microbiome research are being explored rather vigorously for optimizing cancer treatment amidst wildly varying immunotherapy responses. Restoring healthy microbial balance effectively might involve fecal microbiota transplants or probiotics alongside very drastic changes in diet quite radically. Early clinical studies rather surprisingly are exploring probiotics rapidly modulating gut microbiome and yielding promising results in certain cancers against ICIs.

4.2. Microbiome and Chemotherapy Efficacy

Chemotherapy remains crucial cancer treatment yet frequently entails numerous debilitating side effects like profound immune suppression and heightened risk of infection. Gut microbiome plays a peculiar dual role in chemotherapy influencing drug effectiveness and modulating toxicity rather significantly through various obscure mechanisms . Gut bacteria substantially influence pharmacokinetics and metabolism of some chemotherapy drugs under fairly specific physiological conditions sometimes. Microbiome rather quietly modulates activation of prodrugs inside human body where enzymatic conversion transforms compounds into their therapeutically active form. Cyclophosphamide effectiveness gets regulated by microbiome influencing its metabolic pathways in fairly complex unpredictable ways quite obviously underground (Li et al, 2023).

Gut microbes surprisingly activate certain cytochrome P450 enzymes involved in drug metabolism thereby remarkably altering each drug's overall pharmacological efficacy quite profoundly. Chemotherapy induced toxicity gets significantly impacted downstream by gut microbiome in a surprisingly major way often rather quietly. Dysbiosis correlates rather severely with heightened gastrointestinal toxicity manifesting as diarrhea or mucositis after chemotherapy and intestinal inflammation occurs. Chemotherapy-induced changes in microbiome result in drastic reduction of gut bacteria diversity depleting beneficial microbes such as Lactobacillus and Bifidobacterium very significantly. Disruption here severely impairs gut barrier function leading rapidly to heightened intestinal permeability and bacteria translocate into bloodstream exacerbating systemic inflammation (Li et al, 2023).

Research indicates prebiotics and probiotics may potentially restore balance somewhat in microbiome and mitigate bad side effects from harsh chemotherapy treatments. Lactobacillus or Bifidobacterium species drastically reduces intestinal damage obviously and remarkably enhances immune function under specific physiological conditions. Beneficial gut microbes thrive on certain fibres which shield against harsh chemotherapy toxicity and remarkably enhance recovery during grueling treatment.

4.3. Microbiome and Radiation Therapy Response

Radiation therapy plays a vital role in treatment of various malignancies effectively nowadays often used alongside surgery or chemotherapy. Radiation therapy has very nasty side effects eerily similar to chemo including major damage mostly in intestines and sometimes extremely painful mucosal inflammation. Recent studies imply gut microbiome mediates radiation therapy toxicity somewhat mystifyingly and modulates its effectiveness profoundly within varied clinical contexts. Radiation therapy targeting abdominal tumours induces drastic changes in gut microbiome composition very rapidly leading to dysbiosis full of radiation-induced maladies. Dysbiosis severely compromises intestinal barrier function allowing entry of harmful pathogens into bloodstream quite readily alongside nasty toxins normally kept out. Pathogenic bacteria and endotoxins proliferate wildly in gut after microbiome disruption and seep into bloodstream very badly exacerbating systemic inflammation (Majeed H, Gupta, 2023).

Radiation therapy precipitates gastrointestinal distress alongside diarrhea and fatigue resulting from this rather insidious phenomenon unfolding quite slowly. Dysbiosis caused by radiation has been tenuously linked through various obscure gastrointestinal effects locally to a severely weakened immune system. Immune cells responding cancerously function properly when gut microbiome teems with diverse microbiota ordinarily considered healthy in varying abundance . Radiation severely disrupts microbiome function thereby heightening risk of nasty systemic infections and inflammation remarkably across various bodily systems. Dysbiosis terribly exacerbates radiation therapy's nasty side effects but gut microbiome weirdly augments therapeutic effects of radiation under certain circumstances quite significantly. Radiation can heavily boost anti-tumour response in presence of diverse healthy microbiome by modulating functionality of immune system very significantly (Majeed H, Gupta, 2023).

Gut bacteria possibly promote activation of cytotoxic T lymphocytes crucial for destroying cancerous tumour cells with targeted precision effectively. CTLs function by pinpointing malignant cells displaying aberrant proteins and eliminating them quite effectively in a vital process for radiation therapy success. Microbial metabolites such as short-chain fatty acids produced during dietary fibre fermentation play quite a crucial role in significantly enhancing immune responses. Butyrate acetate and propionate remarkably support gut health exhibiting anti-inflammatory effects that enhance anti-tumour immune response fairly effectively. SCFAs foster T cell infiltration into tumours where cancer cells get attacked very vigorously with greatly heightened efficacy. Production of SCFAs helps regulate gene expression in immune cells thereby fostering a robust immune response that aids eradication of cancerous cells during radiotherapy (Vivarelli et al, 2019).

Microbiome and radiation therapy interactions underscore potential novel interventions that significantly improve cancer treatment outcomes under fairly specific conditions. Probiotics and prebiotics might mitigate radiation therapy toxicity significantly by fostering beneficial bacteria growth or restoring microbiome health thereby boosting its efficacy. Dietary interventions fostering SCFA-producing bacteria growth may remarkably optimize immune responses and improve overall therapeutic efficacy substantially in various ways. Fecal microbiota transplants being explored vigorously as potential therapy mitigating dysbiosis effects and encourage treatment outcomes fairly effectively in various medical contexts nowadays. FMT has shown considerable promise in restoring healthy microbiomes markedly during radiation therapy and enhance immune function (Vivarelli et al, 2019).

Gut microbiome plays a dual role in radiation therapy exacerbating toxicity rather alarmingly while enhancing treatment efficacy with remarkable unpredictability. Radiation-induced dysbiosis severely compromises gut barrier integrity fostering heightened systemic inflammation thereby contributing significantly to many debilitating side effects subsequently. Diverse microbiome robustly boosts immune response by promoting activation of cytotoxic T cells and production of metabolites like SCFAs very rapidly. Novel microbiome-based therapeutic strategies leveraging microbiome's role in radiation therapy could be integrated quite effectively into cancer care.

4.4. Harnessing the Microbiome to Improve Cancer Treatment

Gut microbiome has emerged as pivotal factor heavily influencing cancer treatment success through modulation of immune response and tumour microenvironment dynamics. Microbiome-based interventions are rapidly gaining traction as potential strategies for optimizing cancer therapy with minimized nasty side effects nowadays. Interventions like these might significantly enhance chemotherapy radiation therapy and immunotherapy efficacy while offering highly modified treatment opportunities rooted deeply in each person's unique gut microbiome. Crappy things occur very frequently nowadays. Fecal microbiota transplantation restores severely disrupted microbial ecosystems quickly by transferring fecal matter from a healthy donor into a patient. FMT has been utilized mainly for treating Clostridium difficile infections but cancer treatment potential sparks extremely fascinating research endeavors nowadays. Recent research indicates fecal microbiota transplantation can amplify responses to immunotherapy rather effectively by revitalizing gut flora and suppressing nasty inflammation quite (Kim et al, 2025).

FMT from patients responding remarkably well enhances anti-tumour immune response in recipients with gut microbiome directly influencing therapy efficacy variably. Patients beset by unrelenting toxicity from radiation therapy or experiencing severe chemo side effects may benefit hugely from this rather unorthodox new approach. Probiotics and prebiotics offer rather promising novel approach for modulating gut microbiome somewhat effectively in various fairly aggressive cancer treatments. Probiotics teeming with live beneficial microbes can rather effectively restore microbial balance by vigorously fostering growth of healthy gut bacteria. Prebiotics are non-digestible food bits like fibre that strangely foster growth of beneficial microbes deep within gut rather slowly. Supplementing with these remarkably boosts immune responses and improves overall microbiome health quite effectively during cancer treatment (Kim et al, 2025).

Probiotics might effectively mitigate chemotherapy-induced mucositis and reduce radiation-induced gastrointestinal tract damage allowing tolerable cancer treatment somewhat successfully. Diet profoundly impacts gut microbiome composition and influences response to cancer treatments quite dramatically in various therapeutic contexts effectively. Diets rich in fibre polyphenols and fermented foods promote growth of beneficial bacteria like Bifidobacterium and Lactobacillus producing short-chain fatty acids namely butyrate. SCFAs yield numerous perks encourage immune function rather quietly and diminish inflammatory responses inside gut lining supporting bodily tolerance of cancer therapies greatly. Polyphenols in various fruits and veggies have lately been shown to positively impact microbiome by fostering growth of certain anti-inflammatory gut bacterial strains. A fibre-rich diet markedly enhances immune response thereby substantially encourage treatment outcomes especially for therapies like immunotherapy in rather critical cases (Ciorba et al, 2015).

Cancer treatment frequently demands prudent antibiotic use with meticulous consideration during regimen planning and thorough patient monitoring afterwards every step. Misuse of antibiotics catastrophically leads to serious microbiome disruption in cancer patients with severely compromised immunity often under intense treatment. Antibiotics very quickly deplete beneficial gut flora leading rapidly to dysbiosis and impaired immune responses crucial for efficacy of cancer treatment. Evidence-based stewardship facilitates judicious antibiotic use minimizing profoundly negative impacts on gut microbiota extremely effectively over time naturally. Minimizing antibiotic use during cancer treatments may preserve microbiome's capacity very effectively thereby supporting immune system and potentially improving outcomes of chemotherapy radiation and immunotherapy substantially. Microbiome-based interventions might eventually become vital in personalized cancer treatment as research slowly untangles links between gut microbiome and cancer therapies. Oncologists might remarkably boost efficacy by tailoring treatments according to an individual's unique microbiome composition and significantly improve long-term outcomes. A drastic departure from traditional cancer treatments is signified by this novel approach focusing on tumour eradication and manipulating gut microbiota heavily.

5. Nutritional Influences on Microbial Composition and Tumourigenesis

Bacteria viruses and fungi forming complex diverse microbial communities inhabit human gut very quietly alongside trillions of other microbes. It plays a crucial part in sustaining overall well-being underground by governing quirky metabolic pathways and diverse physiological phenomena. Evidence highlights a substantial impact of nutrients on microbial makeup and tumour development haphazardly in various bodily contexts very irregularly. Nutrient intake influences gut microbiome composition variously thereby ratcheting up cancer risk substantially over time or mitigating it very significantly. Dietary effects are mediated by multiple key mechanisms mostly through vigorously altered carcinogen metabolism within highly inflammatory pathways and robust immune responses. Diet drastically reshapes microbial composition and functionality largely owing to its potent role as influencer of various microbiome formation environments naturally (Leonard and Toro, 2023).

Pernicious microbes proliferate rapidly in dysbiosis while salutary ones dwindle drastically and distinct eating habits can either foster robust microbiome or spiral into chaos. Diets rich in fibre polyphenols, and fermented foods foster the growth of beneficial microbes like Bifidobacterium and Lactobacillus associated with remarkably enhanced overall gut health. Beneficial microbes produce short-chain fatty acids like butyrate that play crucial roles in gut integrity maintenance and immune response regulation. Consumption of saturated fats and sugars fosters microbial dysbiosis rapidly, with subsequent heightened risk of various cancers ensuing very quickly thereafter. Diets rich in fat rather aggressively foster the proliferation of pathogenic bacteria like Fusobacterium nucleatum, tenuously linked to colorectal cancer development. Malignant microbes produce carcinogenic metabolites directly damaging DNA and sparking intense inflammation, which effectively fuels tumourigenesis in diverse cellular contexts. Gut microbiome influences inflammation fairly obscurely, playing a pivotal role in the regulation of cancer development, substantially fueled by chronic inflammation (Leonard and Toro, 2023).

Diet heavily influences downstream changes in the microbiome that modulate balance between pro-inflammatory microbes and ones exhibiting anti-inflammatory effects. Diets heavy in processed meats or saturated fats tend to correlate with overgrowth of pro-inflammatory gut bacteria secreting cytokines that fuel chronic inflammation. Inflammation can swiftly spark onset of various cancers especially colorectal cancer over a fairly short timespan. A fibre-rich diet fosters growth of beneficial gut bacteria that churn out SCFAs such as butyrate with profoundly anti-inflammatory effects downstream. Butyrate very effectively serves as energy source for colonic epithelial cells helping maintain gut lining integrity amidst diverse immune system reactions. Cancer risk somewhat abates very significantly with time as likelihood of inflammatory pathway dysregulation potentially leading cancer decreases markedly over prolonged periods. Balance of gut microbiome plays crucial role in detecting cancerous cells rapidly within human bodies and eradicating them effectively so. Tumours evade surveillance partly owing to severely impaired immune response under grossly compromised bodily defenses caused ordinarily by dysbiosis. Certain bacteria trigger immune checkpoint pathways that suppress T cell activation crucial for anti-cancer immunity very effectively in mysterious ways (Zhang P, 2022).

Microbiome dynamically modulates immune cell infiltration into tumours influencing tumour microenvironment quite significantly and altering its responsiveness therapeutically. Nutrition plays a pivotal role vigorously in shaping interactions between immune system and microbiome with increasingly crucial effects every single day. Oily fish harbour omega-3 fatty acids that very effectively modulate immune responses by fostering growth of certain gut microbes with anti-inflammatory properties. Diets heavy with refined sugars and trans fats readily foster inflammatory immune responses thereby facilitating cancer development and significantly promoting immune evasion. Dietary components very significantly alter carcinogen metabolism within gut flora in a manner that has profound impact (Zhang P, 2022). High-fat diets can strangely promote production of secondary bile acids that are weirdly churned out rapidly by gut bacteria in intestines. Deoxycholic acid profoundly exerts carcinogenic effects on colonocytes thereby heightening risk of colorectal cancer development significantly in certain obscure instances. Diets rich in fibre and polyphenols radically alter gut microbiome thereby lowering cancer risk significantly by hampering conversion of primary bile acids very effectively.

5.1. Diet as a Key Modulator of the Gut Microbiome

Diet profoundly impacts gut microbiome composition and its function being a potent environmental factor that significantly alters its delicate dynamics. Gut microbiome plays an essential role in maintaining gut health whilst modulating various physiological functions such as digestion and metabolism extremely effectively always. Daily consumption of various foods profoundly impacts gut microbiota diversity and its composition significantly influencing overall health and subsequent cancer risk development. A nutrient-rich diet fosters growth of beneficial gut bacteria while a diet high in fat and sugar strangely promotes gut dysbiosis very effectively. Fibre-rich diets hugely influence gut microbiome composition thereby playing quite a crucial role in shaping overall gut health obviously. Diets rich in fibre from whole grains legumes and various fruits support growth of beneficial gut bacteria like Bifidobacterium very effectively (Hills et al, 2019).

Beneficial microbes ferment fibre very slowly inside colon producing short-chain fatty acids like butyrate and sometimes propionate or acetate. SCFAs exert multifaceted beneficial influences profoundly on health very effectively within gut indeed. Butyrate serves as a primary energy source for colonocytes and plays a vital role in maintaining gut integrity rather obscurely. It robustly enhance gut epithelial barrier function thereby thwarting ingress of noxious pathogens into bloodstream and fosters tolerance within immune system very effectively. SCFAs display markedly potent anti-inflammatory effects helping regulate immune system function and thwarting chronic low-grade inflammation often accompanying cancer progression in diverse tissue types. SCFAs significantly protect against diseases like colorectal cancer by vigorously boosting immune responses and dampening inflammatory pathways effectively meanwhile. SCFAs modulate gene expression fairly significantly exerting wild epigenetic effects that influence cellular processes such as cell differentiation and apoptosis rather deeply. Diets heavy in saturated fats red meat and refined sugars drastically alter microbiome composition fostering growth of malign opportunistic bacteria (Hills et al, 2019).

Consumption of diets rich in saturated fats and red meat fosters proliferation of pathogenic microbes namely Fusobacterium nucleatum and Enterococcus faecalis alongside sundry Bacteroides species correlating with elevated oncological risk. Fusobacterium nucleatum has garnered significant attention lately owing largely to its strong link with colorectal cancer development recently. Bacterium spurs cancer progression by ratcheting up inflammatory pathways involving activation of NF-kB a crucial mediator downstream apparently. Tumour progression and immune evasion occur rapidly in many cases due largely to persistent stimulation of this pathway. Fusobacterium nucleatum significantly hampers immune surveillance by subtly altering dendritic cell function and T cell activity allowing tumour cells evade detection. Copious sugar and fat in Western diets fosters ambiance ripe for intestinal permeability and chronic inflammation thereby facilitating cancer initiation readily (Huang and Liu, 2019).

High-fat diets spur production of genotoxic secondary bile acids like deoxycholic acid which damages intestinal cells and fosters colorectal cancer development rather rapidly. Dietary components interacting with microbiome heavily influence inflammatory responses while playing a significant albeit rather obscure role metabolizing numerous carcinogens. Carcinogenic compounds lurk in alcoholic drinks and processed foods getting swiftly metabolized by gut bacteria into DNA-rattling mutagens that elevate cancer risk. Specific gut bacteria rapidly convert nitrates found in processed meats into highly carcinogenic nitrosamines under diverse physiological conditions quite frequently. Dietary factors substantially shape gut microbiome composition thereby possibly impacting various immune responses very significantly and altering overall health markedly. A diet rich in fibre and polyphenols substantially fosters growth of gut bacteria supporting immune function that naturally amplifies anti-tumour response. Diets rich in saturated fats and sugar shift gut microbiome towards rampant immune suppression rendering body unusually susceptible to marauding tumour cells (Huang and Liu, 2019).

5.2. Dietary Components and Their Effect on Tumourigenesis

Diet profoundly impacts gut microbiome constitution which can subsequently amplify cancer risk and gravely exacerbate disease progression very rapidly. Fibre polyphenols and fatty acids in diet profoundly impact microbial composition thereby influencing tumourigenesis intricately in various ways obviously. Diets rich in fibre comprising fruits and whole grains promote growth of beneficial bacteria like Bifidobacteria and Lactobacilli that produce short-chain fatty acids quite prolifically notably butyrate. SCFAs promote gut health remarkably while toning down inflammation very considerably and regulating diverse immune responses that protect against various cancers. Western diets rich in saturated fats and red meats strongly foster dysbiosis and enhance proliferation of malignant microbes like Fusobacterium nucleatum associated with colorectal cancer (Mansour et al, 2021).

Saturated fats spur production of secondary bile acids that damage gut cells frequently and contribute alarmingly to inflammation and cancer rather severely. Polyphenols in various fruits and tea act as remarkably potent antioxidants exhibiting anti-inflammatory properties against certain kinds of cancer very effectively. Beneficial microbial growth gets fostered very effectively and various metabolites are generated that enhance immune system responses significantly nowadays. Fatty acids particularly omega-3s derived from fish and olive oil display anti-inflammatory properties and are often linked with reduced cancer risk. Consumption of high-fat diets drastically alters microbial composition heightening risk of colorectal cancer in certain populations meanwhile (Mansour et al, 2021).

Protein sources manifest their influence haphazardly oftentimes in very peculiar ways across diverse contexts. Eating lots of red and processed meats fosters pathogenic microbe growth and generates very nasty carcinogenic compounds but plant-based proteins remarkably enhance gut health. Refined sugars heavily disrupt gut bacteria nowadays thereby significantly upping cancer risk and fostering insulin resistance and obesity very frequently. Diet profoundly affects gut microbiome composition and plays a crucial albeit sometimes counterintuitive role in either cancer prevention or fueling rapid progression.

5.2.1. Fibre and Microbial Metabolism

Profound implications for cancer prevention stem from dietary fibre found mainly in whole plant foods shaping gut microbiome composition significantly. Fermentation happens swiftly amidst gut microbiota upon consumption of fibre resulting in production of short-chain fatty acids namely butyrate and acetate. Butyrate stands out particularly for having potentially significant anti-cancer properties among them quite remarkably in various medical research studies. Cancer cell proliferation gets thwarted and apoptosis gets promoted rather vigorously meanwhile cell differentiation occurs very effectively under certain conditions. Butyrate influences carcinogenesis profoundly especially in colon where notably high levels naturally render its modulating effects crucial. Butyrate plays a crucial role somewhat underappreciated in gut epithelial barrier integrity preventing translocation of various pathogens into bloodstream very effectively. Pivotal barrier function significantly mitigates chronic inflammation reducing effectively a well-established risk factor for many cancer types (Fu et al, 2022).

Gut microbiota ferments fibre yielding lactic acid alongside butyrate and acetate thus lowering colon pH suppressing growth of some very nasty pathogenic bacteria. Acidic environments foster proliferation of beneficial microbes further promoting somewhat balanced microbiome thereby diminishing risk of oncogenesis-linked dysbiosis heavily. High-fibre diets correlate strongly with lowered colorectal cancer risk largely owing to beneficial effects on gut microbiota and increased SCFA production. Fermenting fibre's metabolic byproducts profoundly reconfigure microbial communities and vigorously regulate immune responses impeding tumour formation through various pathways. Dietary fibre plays a crucial role modulating microbial metabolic processes deeply inside gut thereby encourage overall gut health remarkably for cancer prophylaxis (Fu et al, 2022).

5.2.2. Polyphenols and Microbial Modulation

Polyphenols are a group of bioactive compounds found in various plant-based foods including fruits and vegetables and tea and whole grains. Compounds mitigate oxidative stress very effectively and alter gut microbiome composition in ways that lower cancer risk mostly. Polyphenols are known to promote the growth of beneficial gut bacteria such as Lactobacilli and Bifidobacteria, while suppressing the proliferation of pathogenic microbes. Microbial modulation plays crucial role in sustaining gut health and staving off cancer-predisposing conditions very effectively in individuals apparently. Upon reaching the colon, polyphenols undergo fermentation by gut microbiota, resulting in the production of bioactive metabolites like phenolic acids. Polyphenols apparently play a protective role in cancer prevention as metabolites exhibiting anti-inflammatory and anti-cancer effects strongly support this notion. In the case of colorectal cancer, specific polyphenols such as epigallocatechin gallate (EGCG) from green tea and ellagic acid from berries have been shown to inhibit cancer cell proliferation, reduce inflammation, and modulate microbial activity in the gut (Pandey and Rizvi, 2009).

Polyphenols can also reduce the production of carcinogenic compounds, including secondary bile acids and nitrosamines, which are often generated by microbial metabolism in the colon. Compounds implicated in tumourigenesis initiation cause DNA damage subsequently leading quite frequently to various nasty outcomes and awful health issues. By modulating the gut microbiome and reducing the formation of these harmful substances, polyphenols play a dual role in both reducing oxidative stress and promoting a gut environment that is less conducive to cancer development. Polyphenols ostensibly represent quite a promising dietary strategy modulating various microbial communities thereby somewhat reducing overall cancer risk.

5.2.3. Fatty Acids and Tumourigenesis

Type of dietary fat profoundly shapes composition of gut microbiome and markedly influences development of cancer in various contexts. Processed foods and animal products contain abundant saturated fats which have been strongly implicated in promoting severe gut dysbiosis rather frequently. High amounts of saturated fats spur growth of pro-inflammatory bacteria such as Fusobacterium nucleatum and Enterococcus faecalis fueling chronic inflammation heavily which is pivotal in tumourigenesis. Saturated fats ramp up secondary bile acid production including deoxycholic acid exhibiting carcinogenic properties in diverse bodily contexts fairly often apparently. Bile acids rapidly induce DNA damage and accelerate colorectal cancer development abnormally by disrupting cellular processes in colon tissues quite frequently. High-fat diets very conclusively suppress diversity of beneficial gut microbiota like Bifidobacteria and Lactobacilli which normally help fend off nasty inflammation (Conlon and Bird, 2014).

Microbial diversity reduction severely impairs gut protective mechanisms rendering body vulnerable extremely to tumourigenesis under pathological conditions subsequently. Omega-3 fatty acids found in fish oils flaxseeds and walnuts promote a significantly healthier microbiome quite remarkably in various bodily functions. Omega-3 fatty acids remarkably foster growth of beneficial anti-inflammatory microbes such as Lactobacillus and Bifidobacterium helping balance immune systems very effectively. Fats play a crucial role in regulating metabolic pathways remarkably affecting insulin sensitivity and oxidative stress vital for cancer prevention mechanisms . Omega-3 fatty acids exhibit markedly anti-cancer properties in breast cancer cases and fairly frequently in prostate and colon cancer nowadays. They act vigorously by encourage immune function and reducing chronic inflammation in support of microbial tumour suppression effectively (Conlon and Bird, 2014).

Omega-3 fatty acids help reduce pro-inflammatory cytokine expression fairly effectively and cytotoxic T cells ramp up tumour cell targeting activity vigorously. Consuming specific dietary fats drastically alters microbiome composition and functionality in various obscure ways rather significantly under certain conditions. Diets rich in saturated fats can foster pro-inflammatory tumour-promoting microbiome whereas those replete with omega-3 fatty acids strongly encourage protective anti-cancer microbes.

5.2.4. Protein and Cancer Risk

Consumption of protein from processed and red meats very frequently indeed correlates with heightened risk of certain cancers notably colorectal cancer. Eating lots of animal-based proteins from sources like beef or processed meats such as sausages drastically alters gut microbiome promoting carcinogenesis variously. High levels of animal protein intake facilitate rampant proliferation of pathogenic bacterial strains including Clostridia and Enterococcus producing carcinogenic N-nitroso compounds. Compounds inherently possess toxicity towards intestinal lining cells and induce DNA damage potentially leading to sporadic cancer development and freaky mutations. Microbes produce hydrogen sulfide tenuously linked lately to heightened inflammation a frequently cited risk factor in progression of various cancers. Colon inflammation chronically fosters an environment that promotes tumours accelerating tumourigenesis rapidly and boosts metastasis way downstream of initial lesion (Santarelli et al, 2008).

Proteins from legumes nuts and whole grains provide protection against various cancers very effectively these days in many different ways. Beneficial bacteria thrive quickly under plant-derived protein influence producing short-chain fatty acids and anti-inflammatory metabolites very abundantly. Butyrate and other short-chain fatty acids crucially preserve intestinal barrier function and thwart growth of cancer cells rather effectively. Plant-based proteins often arrive laden with fibre and polyphenols alongside antioxidants that synergistically cultivate a healthier gut environment reducing tumour risk. Abundance of noxious microbes may be curtailed and production of carcinogenic metabolites suppressed by swapping animal-based protein sources for plant-based ones lowering cancer risk. Plant-based proteins profoundly exert protective influence via microbial modulation significantly obscuring gut microbiome role in cancer prevention (Santarelli et al, 2008).

5.3. Nutritional Interventions for Cancer Prevention

Nutritional intake heavily influences gut microbiota and subsequent tumour development offering promising avenues for cancer prevention via modified dietary regimes. A diet rich in fibre alongside polyphenols remarkably fosters healthy gut microbiome which supports immune surveillance and curbs proliferation of cancer cells effectively. Fibre from plant-based foods fosters growth of beneficial microbes that produce short-chain fatty acids playing a critical role in cancer risk reduction by encourage gut integrity effectively and modulating various immune responses. Prebiotics and probiotics substantially optimize microbiome function remarkably enhancing cancer prevention effectively in many cases with quite dramatic results. Inulin and FOS aka fructooligosaccharides foster beneficial bacteria growth really deeply inside gut lining churning out SCFAs very effectively thereby quashing inflammation (Zhang P, 2022).

Probiotic supplementation with species like Lactobacillus helps restore microbial balance fairly effectively in people afflicted with dysbiosis, reducing potential cancer risk. Probiotics somewhat vigorously boost production of beneficial metabolites and help modulate various immune responses, thereby fostering a very reduced tumourigenic microenvironment rather quickly in various tissues. Cancer outcomes are profoundly swayed by nutritional choices, which substantially alter gut microbiome composition and influence risk in diverse populations. Polyphenols profoundly impact metabolic pathways and immune system regulation, thereby thwarting cancer prevention mechanisms effectively through various convoluted biochemical interactions (Zhang P, 2022).

Nutritional interventions strategically integrated furnish a potent tool for effectively preventing various cancers and treating them within the human body. Ongoing research into the diet microbiome cancer axis sheds new light on the potential for extremely targeted personalised therapies to be applied very effectively. Nutritional strategies aimed at optimising gut microbiota may become crucial in cancer care, offering fresh opportunities to reduce cancer risk very rapidly through dietary changes.

6. Gut Microbiota and Cancer

Trillions of microorganisms dwell deeply inside the human gut and form an intricate ecosystem supremely vital for bodily equilibrium while influencing digestion profoundly. Recently, scientific research has rather strikingly acknowledged a deep kinship between gut microbiota and cancer in fairly tumultuous times. Microbiota plays a crucial albeit somewhat obscure part in cancer progression, remarkably, while cancer itself drastically alters microbiota composition suddenly. Novel avenues have been opened up by dynamic interaction for comprehending the influence of gut health on cancer risk profoundly under various conditions. Diet plays a crucial role in substantially shaping the composition and function of gut microbiota within their convoluted symbiotic relationship quite dynamically. Consumed foods supply bodily nutrients and fuel festering gut microbes ordinarily serving as sustenance for flora in the gut (Thursby and Juge, 2017).

A diet rich in fibre polyphenols, and unsaturated fats fosters the growth of beneficial gut bacteria, helping maintain healthy gut barrier function vigorously. Western lifestyle diets loaded with sugar and fat, rather nastily, foster an imbalance of gut bacteria that promotes extensive inflammation. Emerging evidence strongly suggests that microbiota affects cancer risk via mechanisms including the production of short-chain fatty acids from fermenting fibre that have anti-inflammatory properties. Microbes ferociously metabolise dietary constituents into fiendishly toxic compounds like secondary bile acids or nitrosamines, damaging DNA grievously, fueling cancerous growth quite rapidly. Microbiota exerts considerable influence on immune function, thereby modulating tumour growth and shaping outcomes of novel immunotherapy approaches effectively nowadays. Cancer can drastically alter gut microbiota, on the other hand, quite remarkably within quite a short span of time, apparently (Thursby and Juge, 2017).

Tumour microenvironment releases inflammatory signals that disrupt microbial homeostasis, supporting a drastic shift in microbial populations, fueling quite aggressive tumour growth. Chemotherapy and radiation therapies perturb microbiota by fostering selective pressures that favour the growth of pathogenic bacteria, thus exacerbating treatment toxicity rapidly and cancer metastasis. Grasping the effects of diet on microbiota yields fresh avenues for broadly advancing cancer prevention and novel therapeutic strategies nowadays quite effectively. Dietary changes involving prebiotics and probiotics may markedly reduce inflammation and somewhat effectively boost cancer treatment efficacy by optimising the microbiome. Cancer research now takes a more nuanced view of gut microbiota, thereby providing a framework for personalised nutrition strategies aimed at modifying the microbiome effectively to prevent malignancies.

6.1. Gut Microbiota as a Driver of Cancer Development

Gut microbiota regulates various biological processes crucial for health, including immune function, metabolic pathways and inflammatory responses quite normally. Microbiota modulates tumourigenesis partly owing to intrinsic links with cancer development happening simultaneously beneath surface levels, rather quietly underground. Apparently, microbial composition sways tumour cell elimination prowess of the immune system, while dysbiosis fosters cancer-friendly environments via inflammatory routes and carcinogen metabolism alterations deeply. Gut microbiota fuels cancer development heavily through inflammation later inside human body. Chronic inflammation poses considerable risk for developing various cancers, and liver cancer occurs quite frequently alongside gastric cancer (Liu et al, 2024).

Dysbiosis mercilessly skews the balance toward inflammatory states by boosting the abundance of pro-inflammatory bacteria whilst depleting anti-inflammatory microbes rather significantly. Fusobacterium nucleatum and Enterococcus faecalis have lately been linked very insidiously with colorectal cancer onset and rapid progression. Microbes trigger inflammatory pathways that disrupt immune surveillance and impair bodily ability, inducing DNA damage and facilitating tumourous growth rapidly in colon cells. Microbial-derived metabolites heavily influence carcinogenesis via sundry mechanisms besides extensively modulating inflammation in a fairly haphazard manner. Gut bacteria transform primary bile acids into secondary bile acids, which are researched extensively as a peculiar class of metabolites (Liu et al, 2024).

Deoxycholic acid induces DNA damage quite rapidly in intestinal cells, thereby initiating colon cancer and promoting vigorous tumour growth. Microbial conversion of nitrates from processed meats forms very nasty compounds called nitrosamines, which strongly further implicate the microbiome in cancer risk. Mutagenic compounds wreak havoc on cellular DNA, rapidly fostering malignant transformations inside cells, thereby profoundly disrupting normal cellular function. Gut microbiota rapidly modulates inflammatory responses and deeply influences carcinogen metabolism, generating metabolites that very effectively foster tumourigenesis directly. Unravelling intricate microbial and cancer cell interplays rapidly yields novel strategies for cancer prevention and unorthodox therapeutic interventions simultaneously.

6.2. Cancer-Induced Alterations in Gut Microbiota

Malignant growths ravage bodily tissues and perturb gut microbiota concurrently fostering some curiously reciprocal bond between cancerous cells and diverse microbial communities. Tumours develop erratically, precipitating metabolic changes and aberrant immune responses that severely impact the composition of the gut microbiome locally. Alterations can foster peculiar environments conducive to the growth of microbial communities that further tumour progression very rapidly in some instances. Tumours in the colon drastically alter local gut microbiota quite remarkably in cases of colorectal cancer, for instance. Tumour growth drastically alters the environmental conditions surrounding it, like pH levels and oxygen availability, selecting for bacteria that thrive under harsh conditions (Ivleva and Grivennikov, 2022).

Malignant cells remarkably thrive inside a feedback loop created by dysregulated microbial flora that fuels virulent inflammation and cancer progression quite aggressively. Fusobacterium nucleatum grows rather prevalently and links quietly to cancer promotion via activation of inflammatory pathways, and immunity gets suppressed. Chemotherapy and radiation therapy can drastically alter gut microbiota over time, quite significantly, with treatments like these being rather harsh. Tumour-targeting therapies often wreak havoc on the microbiome, inadvertently causing dysbiosis and severely disrupting microbial community structures profoundly (Ivleva and Grivennikov, 2022).

Chemotherapy very rapidly depletes beneficial gut bacteria, weakening immune systems, and ratchets up side effects from cancer treatment like nasty intestinal inflammation. New findings suggest therapeutic benefits may emerge after cancer treatment from restoring balance in a deeply mystifying somewhat intriguingly helpful way. Probiotics and prebiotics interventions enhance beneficial microbes substantially thereby remarkably enhancing therapeutic outcomes and quite possibly improving immune function greatly. Microbiome alterations induced by cancer drastically affect disease progression and treatment responses opening up novel avenues for cancer therapy very rapidly.

6.3. The Role of Diet in Shaping the Gut Microbiome-Cancer Relationship

Diet drastically reshapes gut microbiome under various conditions with significant ramifications for cancer risk progressing at an alarming rapid rate. Consumed food types drastically alter gut microbiota composition and function because different dietary components directly impact microbial populations thereby modulating myriad biological processes influencing cancer development erratically. Fibre from veggies whole grains legumes plays a crucial role remarkably well in shaping microbiome health with considerable efficacy notably underground. Fibre serves as substrate for gut bacteria fermentation yielding short-chain fatty acids butyrate acetate and propionate at a remarkably rapid rate. SCFAs possess anti-inflammatory properties very effectively and help modulate immune function thereby mitigating cancer risk significantly downstream. A fibre rich diet has been consistently linked with a lower risk of colorectal cancer by fostering beneficial microbial profile and suppressing pro-inflammatory gut bacteria (Greathouse et al, 2022).

Diets high in saturated fats remarkably foster dysbiosis and energetically promote the growth of pro-inflammatory bacteria within various tissues, driving chronic inflammation. High-fat diets spur the production of secondary bile acids such as deoxycholic acid, which ravages DNA very quickly and fosters the development of colorectal cancer. Consuming protein mainly from red meats and highly processed products can profoundly alter the gut microbiome, thereby significantly ramping up cancer risk. Proteins facilitate the proliferation of pathogenic microbes like Clostridia and Enterococcus, which churn out carcinogenic metabolites such as N-nitroso compounds, rather vigorously damaging intestinal cells and fostering tumourigenesis. Polyphenols present in fruits and whole grains exhibit remarkably potent antioxidant effects and display fairly strong anti-inflammatory properties, rather mysteriously (Greathouse et al, 2022).

Oxidative stress gets significantly reduced, thereby promoting the growth of beneficial microbes such as Bifidobacteria and Lactobacilli, inhibiting growth of harmful bacteria. Bioactive compounds heavily modulate inflammatory responses, thereby possibly mitigating the production of carcinogenic metabolites and thwarting quirky immune reactions in cancer. Diet profoundly modulates microbial composition via various mechanisms, influencing interactions between microbiome and host immune systems with considerable potency.

6.3.1. Fibre and Gut Microbiota Composition

Dietary fibre modulates gut microbiota significantly over time and reduces the risk of various cancers naturally in humans very effectively. Gut bacteria ferment fibre into short-chain fatty acids like butyrate and propionate after slow ingestion occurs naturally in the digestive system. Short-chain fatty acids exert remarkably diverse beneficial effects on gut health but thwart cancer formation with considerable efficacy. Various research groups have studied butyrate vigorously for its anti-cancer properties, mostly within colon tissue, very extensively of late. It works by inhibiting histone deacetylases or HDACs, which are enzymes deeply involved in regulating gene expression, rather intricately. Inhibition spurs cell differentiation and apoptosis very effectively in cancerous cells, thereby diminishing tumour growth potential and suppressing unbridled cell proliferation (Cronin et al, 2021).

A diet rich in fibre from fruits and whole grains fosters the growth of beneficial gut microbes like Bifidobacteria and Lactobacilli key producers of SCFAs remarkably. Presence of such beneficial bacteria vigorously supports overall gut health by maintaining gut barrier integrity and helps reduce inflammation, a crucial factor in colorectal cancer development, rather insidiously. Butyrate and other SCFAs cultivate an acidic colon environment, heavily inhibiting the growth of pathogenic microbes, thereby thwarting production of potentially carcinogenic toxic metabolites. Diets rich in fibre particularly those loaded with soluble fibre have been consistently linked to significantly lower colorectal cancer risk. Production of SCFAs and their role in gut microbiota balance are heavily implicated in this phenomenon, fairly obviously down the line. Eating foods rich in fibre quite effectively supports microbiome health and prevents cancer development, particularly in the colon areas (Cronin et al, 2021).

6.3.2. Fat and Microbial Dysbiosis

Various fats exhibit wildly different effects on overall health, partly influencing cancer risk, as dietary fats significantly shape the gut microbiome. Red meats and processed foods contain saturated fats strongly linked to microbial dysbiosis, essentially an imbalance within gut microbiota populations. Dysbiosis heavily fuels chronic inflammation, particularly during colon cancer development and acts as a key driver in this pathological process. High-fat diets ramp up production of secondary bile acids like deoxycholic acid, which apparently possess very nasty carcinogenic properties. Bile acids wreak havoc on the DNA of colon cells rather aggressively, thereby fueling the initiation and progression of colorectal cancer downstream. Omega-3 fatty acids found in fatty fish-like salmon, possess potent anti-inflammatory properties and support a balanced microbiome, somewhat generally, through various mechanisms. Omega-3 fatty acids foster the growth of beneficial microbes like Bifidobacteria and boost the production of short chain fatty acids, such as butyrate having protective anticancer effects (Zhang P, 2022).

Fats deemed healthy have a profound impact on sundry metabolic pathways, thereby substantially ameliorating sensitivity to insulin and downregulating oxidative stress rampant in oncogenic processes. Omega-3 fatty acids modulate inflammation very effectively and support various beneficial microbial communities, thereby potentially mitigating the risk of colorectal cancer markedly. Certain fat types consumed sway microbial makeup and crucial immune function pathways quite directly for thwarting processes that are cancerous in nature. Replacing saturated fats with unsaturated ones, especially omega-3 fatty acids, may offer a dietary strategy for mitigating microbial dysbiosis and significantly lowering inflammatory responses (Zhang P, 2022).

6.3.3. Polyphenols and Cancer Prevention

Polyphenols, a diverse group of bioactive compounds found in plant-based foods like berries and green tea, have garnered significant attention quite recently for cancer prevention. Compounds exhibit potent antioxidant properties and anti-inflammatory effects, mitigating oxidative stress somewhat slowly while thwarting cancer development quite rapidly. Polyphenols are rapidly broken down by gut microbiota into bioactive metabolites such as phenolic acids after oral ingestion. Polyphenols fairly effectively foster the growth of beneficial microbes such as Lactobacillus and Bifidobacterium within gut microbiota whilst hindering pathogenic bacterial colonies. Alteration in microbial composition facilitates reestablishment of gut equilibrium very significantly over time and supports largely diminished inflammatory reactions (Ciupei et al, 2024).

Polyphenols may help maintain gut barrier function, thereby forestalling the influx of noxious metabolites and toxins readily contributing to carcinogenesis. Polyphenols very effectively curb the formation of carcinogenic compounds under specific obscure conditions, rather mysteriously. Polyphenols found in green tea, such as epigallocatechin gallate EGCG heavily curb the production of carcinogenic secondary bile acids and nitrosamines through various microbial metabolic pathways. Polyphenols greatly lower the risk of various cancers, including colorectal and breast cancer, by reducing DNA damage and suppressing the formation of aberrant compounds heavily. Polyphenols crucially curb cancer naturally, owing largely to antioxidant properties and effects modulating microbiome (Ciupei et al, 2024).

6.4. Strategies to Modulate the Microbiome for Cancer Prevention

Innovative cancer treatment approaches emerge slowly as intricate relationships between gut microbiome and cancer become increasingly recognised as key prevention factors. Trillions of microorganisms swarm the gut microbiome, forming a complex ecosystem with profoundly impactful effects on physiological processes such as immune modulation and metabolism. Tweaking diet modulates gut microbiome presenting exciting strategy for cancer prevention and enhance treatment efficacy while substantially mitigating the risk of recurrence. Diet profoundly shapes gut microbiome composition, influencing overall functionality greatly through multifaceted pathways and various obscure mechanisms simultaneously. Remarkably effective dietary approaches fostering a healthy microbiome reduce the risk of various cancers significantly, thereby promoting overall well-being quietly (Maddern et al, 2023).

High-fibre diets very rapidly influence the microbiome by vigorously promoting the growth of beneficial bacteria that produce short-chain fatty acids like butyrate. SCFAs crucially maintain gut barrier integrity and effectively downregulate inflammatory processes whilst orchestrating diverse immune responses fairly effectively under varied circumstances. Fruits, vegetables, whole grains and legumes in the diet foster SCFA-producing bacteria growth and link quite strongly with lowered colorectal cancer incidence. Diets rich in polyphenols from plant-based foods like berries possess strong antioxidant properties and exert profoundly anti-inflammatory effects. Gut bacteria catabolize polyphenols into myriad bioactive metabolites such as phenolic acids that stifle cancer cell proliferation and mitigate oxidative stress significantly (Maddern et al, 2023).

Compounds help reduce cancer cell growth by promoting beneficial bacteria like Lactobacillus, which further enhance protection and support microbial diversity greatly. Probiotics and prebiotics offer another very promising intervention alongside rather innovative therapeutic strategies being explored fairly recently, apparently. Live beneficial microbes in probiotics somewhat restore balance during or after harsh cancer treatments like intense radiation therapy or chemotherapy. Prebiotics, on other hand, foster the growth of beneficial microbes like inulin and fructooligosaccharides FOS rather effectively in a normal human gut. Collectively, such interventions very significantly improve overall therapeutic outcome by restoring the diversity of gut microbiota and boosting immune responses (Sankarapandian et al, 2022).

Reducing consumption of processed meats remarkably lowers cancer risk every single day as an effective critical dietary strategy very effectively. Red meats and processed meats spur the formation of carcinogenic metabolites like N-nitroso compounds, fueling inflammation and damaging DNA very badly. Drastically reducing the consumption of certain foods effectively helps prevent dysbiosis and mitigates the risk of colorectal cancer and various other tumour types. People can cultivate cancer-resistant microbial environments rather effectively by consuming probiotics alongside fibre-rich food and polyphenol supplements very slowly. Further research into microbiome-cancer connections will yield glimpses of novel cancer prevention methods and spawn surprisingly efficacious interventions ultimately.

7. Dietary Factors that Shape the Gut Microbiome in Cancer Prevention and Treatment

Diverse microbial communities form the gut microbiome, playing a crucial role modulating bodily functions like digestion and various metabolic processes extremely effectively. Cancer development progression and response to treatments have been starkly influenced by microbiome remarkably across several decades recently. Gut microbiome composition influences immune responses profoundly, alongside inflammatory pathways crucial for cancer initiation and carcinogen metabolism gets altered subsequently. Diet profoundly reshapes the gut microbiome, and grasping influence of sundry dietary elements on microbial composition proves crucial for devising cancer prevention strategies. Fibre supports growth of beneficial gut bacteria extensively producing short-chain fatty acids like butyrate and acetate, profoundly altering microbiome dynamics. SCFAs exert potent anticancer effects mainly in the colon by inhibiting tumour cell proliferation and, rather slowly, fostering differentiation of cells (Bhatt et al, 2017).

Fibre-rich diets loaded with fruits, veggies, legumes and whole grains remarkably foster a microbiome that mitigates the risk of colorectal cancer and boosts immunity. Fibre reinforces gut barrier integrity by boosting production of SCFAs, thereby preventing harmful pathogens from seeping into the bloodstream and sparking nasty inflammation. Fruits and veggies and tea and whole grains typically teem with polyphenols that freely exert antioxidant properties and somewhat crudely modulate microbiome. Polyphenols somewhat vigorously alter microbial composition by promoting the growth of beneficial microbes like Lactobacillus and inhibiting pathogenic bacteria proliferation rather effectively. Phenolic acids produced from polyphenols by gut bacteria suppress cancer cell growth and reduce inflammation, thus lowering the risk of cancer significantly (Bhatt et al, 2017).

Unsaturated fats play a very crucial role in cancer prevention by significantly influencing the gut microbiome, or so researchers vaguely suggest. Omega-3 fatty acids found in fatty fish and plant oils like flaxseed substantially foster anti-inflammatory bacteria growth, promoting a healthy microbiome. Healthy fats remarkably boost gut health and modulate various metabolic pathways linked with insulin sensitivity or oxidative stress, crucial for preventing cancer. Abundant consumption of saturated fats presents in red meat and processed food fosters pro-inflammatory bacterial growth, producing carcinogenic metabolites. Protein intake from animal sources substantially heightens the risk of cancer, evidently. Diets heavy with red and processed meats spur overgrowth of harmful microbes that produce carcinogenic compounds like N-nitroso compounds, damaging intestinal cell DNA (Costantini et al, 2017).

Proteins from plants found in legumes, nuts and seeds maintain a fairly healthy microbial balance and reduce cancer risk noticeably. Probiotics and prebiotics modulate gut microbiota composition effectively, offering a strategy for balancing the microbiome harshly during cancer treatments like chemotherapy. Probiotics harbour live microbes that revive beneficial gut bacteria, while prebiotics are non-digestible fibres nourishing those microbes fairly heavily. They can very effectively alleviate treatment-induced dysbiosis and boost immune responses, thereby potentially enhancing therapy outcomes greatly in many cases. Polyphenol-rich fibres and healthy fats found in probiotic-rich plant-based foods can effectively influence the microbiome, thus reducing cancer risk and encouraging treatment responses. Investigating microbiome-cancer interplay might propel scientists toward vastly tailored dietary regimens relatively successfully in oncology therapeutics nowadays.

7.1. Dietary Fibre

Profoundly influencing gut microbiome composition, dietary fibre remains a crucial element in foods like whole grains and various fruits naturally. Gut bacteria fervently ferment fibre as primary substrate, producing short-chain fatty acids like butyrate and propionate in copious amounts. SCFAs vitally maintain gut health while providing somewhat effective protection against cancer development inside human bodies under normal circumstances. Butyrate stands out amongst short-chain fatty acids owing largely to fairly potent anti-cancer properties in various cellular contexts. Butyrate very effectively inhibits histone deacetylase activity, thereby promoting epigenetic changes beneficial in cells very rapidly. Malignant cells undergoing programmed death experience apoptosis precipitously as changes quell rampant proliferation and spur cellular differentiation very rapidly (Fu et al, 2022). Butyrate's ability to maintain gut barrier integrity rather crucially in colorectal cancer by helping prevent deeply penetrating harmful pathogens in the intestinal lining. Mitigating chronic inflammation risk happens quite obviously because it drives cancer development very significantly in most bodily systems. Butyrate significantly mitigates inflammation within intestinal tissues often very frequently linked nowadays with various carcinogenic processes. A high-fibre diet somewhat effectively promotes beneficial gut microbes like Bifidobacteria under various physiological conditions, and Lactobacilli too. Bacteria enhance immune function significantly, thereby fostering balance in the gut ecosystem and vigorously suppressing nasty microbes that cause inflammation (Fu et al, 2022).

Eating plenty of fibre-rich food fosters beneficial microbial species growth thereby encourage diversity crucial for gut well-being and potentially mitigating cancer risk. Research evidence plentifully indicates diets high in fibre correlate with markedly reduced risk of colorectal cancer development overall. SCFAs produced from fibre fermentation rather effectively modulate immune responses and enhance gut barrier function remarkably preventing cancer. Eating loads of fibre-rich plant-based foods can remarkably enhance gut well-being and thwart cancer development very effectively over time.

7.2. Polyphenols: Antioxidants that Modulate the Microbiome

Polyphenols comprise a vast array of bioactive compounds mostly inhabiting fruits vegetables whole grains tea and surprisingly dark chocolate rich in antioxidants. Polyphenols exert a profound impact on gut microbiome dynamics vital for thwarting cancer while very effectively neutralizing free radicals amidst heightened oxidative stress. Polyphenols get broken down rather quickly by gut microbes into quite bioactive compounds like phenolic acids or various lignans. Such metabolites very significantly exhibit anticancer properties and directly influence microbial composition in gut with marked anti-inflammatory effects downstream. Polyphenols curiously foster proliferation of beneficial microbes such as Lactobacillus and Bifidobacterium renowned for safeguarding gut health remarkably (Wang et al, 2022).

Beneficial bacteria churn out metabolites supporting immune function and thwart pro-inflammatory Enterococcus faecalis very frequently in cancerous developments . Epigallocatechin gallate predominantly found in green tea has garnered considerable attention for exhibiting numerous health benefits as a polyphenol exemplar. EGCG remarkably modulates gut microbiota diversity thereby fostering an environment that is conducive very much for protective microbial species proliferation. EGCG very conclusively reduces production of carcinogenic metabolites like secondary bile acids and nitrosamines in gut flora heavily infested with pathogenic bacteria often tied to colorectal cancer. Polyphenols are very much everywhere and significantly modulate inflammatory pathways heavily implicated in the development of cancerous tumours within various bodily tissues (Wang et al, 2022).

Berries, tea and nuts rich in polyphenol have been shown quite effectively slashing pro-inflammatory cytokine levels somewhat in cancerous bodily tissues. Polyphenols notoriously lower nitrosamine levels deep within colon tissues quite effectively and are known for thwarting carcinogenesis rather successfully. Consuming polyphenol-rich foods offers protective effects by mitigating oxidative stress fairly and promoting a somewhat balanced gut microbiome naturally. Polyphenols act crucially as antioxidants influencing gut health profoundly and aid cancer prevention significantly in various bodily processes naturally.

7.3. Fatty Acids: The Role of Fats in Cancer Risk and Microbial Balance

Gut microbiome gets heavily influenced by type and quality of dietary fats eaten with sudden implications for risks of certain cancers emerging. Red meats and processed foods contain saturated fats that can cause microbial dysbiosis disrupting gut microbiota and leading to severe imbalance heavily. High intake of saturated fats tends to promote growth of pro-inflammatory gut bacteria like Clostridia and Enterococcus while diminishing beneficial Bifidobacterium populations rather significantly. Dysbiosis cultivates inflammatory milieu within gut fostering development of various malignancies especially colorectal cancer with ferocity that can be downright considerable (Zhang P, 2022).

Omega-3 fatty acids found in fish oils and flaxseeds promote a remarkably healthier gut microbiome quite naturally alongside walnuts. Omega-3 fatty acids enhance Faecalibacterium prausnitzii growth remarkably and modulate systemic inflammation deeply beneath gut barrier integrity very effectively. Omega-3s exhibit profoundly anti-inflammatory properties crucial for preventing cancer as tumourigenesis frequently involves unbridled chronic inflammation rampantly. Omega-3 fatty acids tenuously correlate with modulated gut microbial composition and vigorous support of various immune functions reducing breast prostate and colorectal cancer risks vigorously. Omega-3 fatty acids intricately modulate metabolic pathways heavily implicated in insulin sensitivity under oxidative stress and erratic lipid metabolism (Zhang P, 2022).

Crucial factors help maintain metabolic homeostasis thereby reducing cellular damage associated with oncogenesis very effectively during prevention efforts obviously. Omega-3s heavily influence various signaling pathways controlling cell growth and apoptosis essentially preventing cancerous tissue from undergoing wildly uncontrolled cell division. Unsaturated fats from fatty fish and nuts profoundly enhance immune function and mitigate cancer risk by regulating various metabolic processes at a glacial pace. Dietary fats play a somewhat enigmatic dual role nowadays in shaping gut microbiome and modulating cancer risk quite effectively in prevention strategies.

7.4. Protein: The Impact of Animal vs. Plant-Based Proteins on the Microbiome

Dietary protein source plays a crucial albeit oft overlooked role in shaping gut microbiome and significantly influences risk of some very nasty cancers. Proteins from animal sources especially red and processed meats have been fairly consistently linked nowadays with heightened risk of colorectal cancer. Meats contain heme iron and nitrates alongside saturated fats promoting Clostridia and Enterococcus growth readily within gut flora very quickly. Bacteria fairly frequently churn out nasty metabolites such as N-nitroso compounds and hydrogen sulfide in various environments exhibiting notoriously carcinogenic properties. N-nitroso compounds ravage intestinal cell DNA quite severely and disrupt normal cellular processes entirely while hydrogen sulfide impairs gut barrier functionality badly (Wu et al, 2022).

DNA damage heavily fosters tumourigenesis in colon regions under conditions of chronic inflammation particularly. Plant-based proteins found abundantly in legumes nuts and whole grains rather quietly foster gut microbiomes that are surprisingly healthier. Proteins like these often pair with polyphenols and healthy fats in fibre-rich diets that strangely foster Bifidobacteria growth quite vigorously. Beneficial microbes produce short-chain fatty acids like butyrate that help maintain gut barrier integrity and reduce inflammation encourage cancer prevention significantly. Plant-based proteins tend curiously enough to diminish pro-inflammatory bacteria ostensibly linked to cancer promotion in murky biological contexts. Diets rich in plant proteins foster a relatively benign microbial environment offering cancer-protective benefits alongside various other substantial health advantages (Wu et al, 2022).

Plant-based diets substantially reduce risk of metabolic syndrome and lower cholesterol levels thereby encourage cardiovascular health which curtails cancer risk very significantly further. Plant proteins naturally contain less saturated fat which reduces inflammation linked with cancer development significantly over prolonged periods. Embracing plant-based proteins fosters a robust microbiome and provides extensive cancer protection thereby significantly lowering overall cancer risk.

7.5. Probiotics and Prebiotics: Enhancing Microbial Diversity for Cancer Protection

Probiotics and prebiotics provide targeted strategies for modulating gut microbiome thereby reducing cancer risk effectively and encourage various treatment outcomes quite remarkably. Ingesting sufficient amounts of live microorganisms remarkably confers various health benefits normally on people earnestly seeking overall wellness and optimal bodily function. Beneficial bacteria flourish in fermented foods like yogurt and kimchi and in rather exotic sauerkraut alongside some varieties of kefir. Probiotics restore microbial balance fairly effectively in folks beset by dysbiosis largely stemming from antibiotic use or woefully inadequate nutrition. Probiotics effectively restore balanced gut flora supporting immune function and inhibiting cancer-promoting bacteria growth thereby reducing inflammation quite substantially. Probiotics enhance gut resilience very effectively against nasty pathogens and foster robust intestinal barriers crucial for mitigating cancers driven by inflammation (Cho et al, 2024).

Probiotic strains such as Lactobacillus churn out metabolites that directly impede cancerous cell growth thereby underscoring their role in cancer prevention. Probiotics modulate production of carcinogenic secondary bile acids rather tenuously linked to colorectal cancer development quite frequently in gut flora. Prebiotics foster growth of beneficial gut microbes selectively and significantly boost their activity in quite unusual ways. Garlic and onions and leeks are chock-full of prebiotics and asparagus and bananas contain them rather surprisingly too. Foods abundant in oligosaccharides and inulin nurture a multitude of bacteria like Lactobacilli and Bifidobacteria which feed on fibrous nutrients quite vigorously. Prebiotics somewhat effectively balance gut microbiome by stimulating production of short-chain fatty acids like butyrate with extensively anti-inflammatory properties. Prebiotics foster diverse microbial communities quite effectively, thereby markedly encourage gut health and immune function while aiding efforts against cancer somewhat (Cho et al, 2024).

Probiotics and prebiotics yield a remarkably synergistic effect dubbed synbiotics holding promise in cancer prevention and recovery remarkably well nowadays. Prebiotics furnish nutrients necessary for sustaining beneficial bacteria whereas probiotics ordinarily restore fairly healthy microbial composition somewhat effectively. They optimize gut health synergistically and enhance immune responses while mitigating chronic inflammation rapidly from grueling cancer treatments such as chemo. Research unfolds slowly revealing intricate links between diet microbiome and cancer and probiotics alongside prebiotics emerges quite unexpectedly as rather quirky complementary cancer fighting strategy. Fostering a very balanced diverse microbiome these strategies may offer a mighty tool for speedy recovery and cancer prevention treatment.

8. Microbial Ecosystems in Cancer: Bridging Nutrition and Therapeutic Outcomes

Human gut harbors a complex microbial ecosystem remarkably well playing a fundamental role in maintaining health and preventing various diseases normally. Recently scientific research has profoundly illuminated gut microbiota's mystifying influence on cancer development and response to various treatments vigorously. Gut microbiome modulates immune function significantly impacting therapeutic outcomes profoundly in cancer care while affecting various metabolic processes vigorously. Crucially nowadays understanding microbial ecosystems' role in cancer biology underpins development of innovative treatment strategies and optimizing patient outcomes effectively. Gut microbiome influences cancer therapy profoundly through myriad complex mechanisms affecting treatment outcomes quite significantly every time. Cancer cells behave unpredictably under chemotherapy and radiation therapy paired with immunotherapy mostly due to its mystifying deep-seated somewhat inexplicable impact (Bull and Plummer, 2014).

Microbial species sporadically churn out metabolites which haphazardly augment or debilitate efficacy of chemotherapy drugs within diverse bodily tissues and fluids. Certain microbes sabotage cancer treatment efficacy rather quickly by messing with drug metabolism and conjuring resistance mechanisms in very sneaky ways. Microbiome mediates cancer treatment side effects fairly effectively alongside numerous other bodily functions very normally under various circumstances. Chemotherapy ravages gut microbiota very badly fostering dysbiosis rapidly and amplifying ghastly side effects like gastrointestinal toxicity and suppression of immune function. Microbiome markedly influences therapeutic response and its capacity either mitigates or exacerbates treatment side effects thereby underscoring its importance as intermediary between nutrition and therapeutic success. Dietary interventions have emerged rather promisingly as a strategy for modulating gut microbiome thereby significantly enhancing effectiveness of cancer treatment (Bull and Plummer, 2014).

Diets rich in fibre polyphenols and healthy fats very positively influence microbial composition by fostering beneficial bacteria growth supporting robust immune function. Dietary factors effectively maintain gut barrier integrity and enhance metabolic pathways crucial for optimizing cancer treatment outcomes remarkably well. Probiotics and prebiotics have gained considerable attention lately as potentially beneficial adjuncts for restoring microbial balance during various cancer treatments. Probiotics teeming with live beneficial microbes can help replenish gut flora ravaged by aggressive cancer treatments administered extremely quickly. Prebiotics being non-digestible fibres can rather vigorously promote growth of microbes somewhat significantly enhancing their metabolic activity under specific gut conditions (Kumar et al, 2019).

Probiotics coupled with prebiotics very markedly amplify immune responses and prevent nasty side effects from treatment thereby fairly significantly improving overall efficacy of therapy. Microbiome nutrition and cancer therapy form a gnarly axis beset with intricate nonlinear dynamics and subtle unforeseen interactions beneath surface. Scientists investigating microbial impacts on oncological treatments might stumble upon novel modified therapies shaped partly by intestinal microbiota and eating habits. Microbiome-targeted interventions remarkably boost treatment efficacy and substantially improve quality of life for cancer patients notably nowadays.

8.1. The Role of the Gut Microbiome in Cancer Development and Progression

Trillions of microorganisms including archaea fungi bacteria and viruses residing roughly inside human gut microbiome play quite a fundamental role maintaining overall health. Onset and progression of various diseases including some cancers are markedly impacted by this microbiome very significantly in many cases. Microbial imbalance inside gut has been tenuously linked somewhat mysteriously to elevated cancer risk largely through immune modulation and deep inflammation. Microbiome influences cancer progression via silent interaction with immune system undermining bodily defenses effectively over prolonged periods very quietly. Gut-associated lymphoid tissue exists mainly within gut acting as a somewhat quirky interface between immune system and myriad microbial populations rather abundantly. Beneficial microbes like Lactobacillus vigorously boost immune responses by fostering T cell activation and differentiation that swiftly recognize tumour cells (Pickard et al, 2017).

Fusobacterium nucleatum kinda breeds chronic inflammation very effectively fostering immune tolerance and suppressing activity of immune cells in colorectal cancer. Dysbiosis fosters tumour growth and metastasis by creating an immunosuppressive microenvironment thereby highlighting a potentially pernicious role in cancer progression rapidly. Microbiome profoundly influences cancer development via production of sundry microbial metabolites like butyrate and acetate which are short-chain fatty acids. Beneficial gut bacteria produce SCFAs mainly during fermentation of dietary fibre in a very intricate biochemical rigmarole apparently. SCFAs very effectively exert salubrious multifaceted effects on human health via anti-inflammatory properties and often thwart cancer development remarkably. Butyrate acts very much ubiquitously as histone deacetylase inhibitor leading thereby epigenetic modifications that promote cell differentiation or slowly induce apoptosis (Pickard et al, 2017).

Butyrate significantly enhance gut barrier integrity and shields intestinal regions from colorectal cancer development while remarkably dampening inflammation. SCFAs partly regulate tumour microenvironment by modulating immune system effectively and reduce oxidative stress while promoting DNA damage repair. Such properties underscore significance of microbiome replete with SCFA-producing bacteria in providing protection against cancer particularly colon cancer development. Tweaking diet or popping probiotic supplements can potentially enhance production of protective metabolites and ramp up immune responses hugely for cancer prevention. Gut microbiome plays a multifaceted role rather intricately in cancer development and its further progression. Beneficial metabolites like SCFAs modulate immune responses really deeply and directly impact tumour microenvironment thereby altering overall cancer risk significantly. Tweaking lifestyle habits and making informed dietary choices can somewhat mitigate cancer risk and enhance efficacy of treatment very effectively.

8.2. Microbiome and Cancer Treatment: The Influence of Diet

Mounting evidence suggests gut microbiome heavily influences cancer risk as research into links between nutrition and cancer treatment outcomes evolves rapidly nowadays. Gut microbiota can either enhance or undermine chemotherapy efficacy and spawn nasty side effects while immunotherapy and radiotherapy treatments unfold simultaneously. Tumour response to treatment gets heavily influenced by microbiome necessitating a thoroughly integrative cancer therapy approach within patients and their gut ecosystem. Chemotherapy savagely targets rapidly dividing cancer cells but very badly harms healthy cells residing in gastrointestinal tract or other sensitive areas. Chemotherapy related side effects such as gastrointestinal toxicity and mucositis are modulated quite effectively by gut microbiome in cancer patients. Microbial imbalance manifests severely in chemotherapy patients and has been tenuously linked to increased incidence of adverse effects subsequently (Vivarelli et al, 2019).

Gut bacteria rather curiously crank up metabolism of specific chemo agents thereby substantially altering toxic effects and overall efficacy in a big way. Microbes strangely flip chemotherapy drugs on or off thereby altering efficacy very dramatically in rather obscure ways under various circumstances obviously. Research indicates very strongly diverse microbial ecosystems somewhat alleviate negative impacts under specific circumstances occurring very naturally in various environments. Certain probiotics and prebiotics may deeply restore gut microbial balance and enhance gut barrier integrity ultimately improving outcomes somewhat effectively. Bifidobacterium and Lactobacillus species ramp up production of short-chain fatty acids thereby boosting chemotherapy efficacy with markedly anti-inflammatory effects. Immunotherapy supercharges body's immune response against cancer cells very effectively in specific malignancies nowadays showing considerable promise (Vivarelli et al, 2019).

Gut microbiome factors wildly sway immunotherapy efficacy and its success varies greatly from one patient to another rather unpredictably. Specific microbial communities encourage T cell activation crucial for effective cancer surveillance influence immunotherapy response very significantly under varying conditions. Firmicutes and Bacteroidetes bacterial species have been strongly linked recently to enhanced responses to immune checkpoint inhibitors greatly revolutionizing treatment of cancer. Microbial dysbiosis can conversely impair immune system functionality potentially reducing effectiveness of immunotherapy quite drastically in certain weird conditions. Altered microbiota may precipitously lead to a surge in immune-suppressive cells thereby diminishing immune system's ability to target tumour cells quite effectively. Tweaking gut microbiota with diet or probiotics may possibly enhance immunotherapy response thereby rendering this research area very vital these days (Zhang et al, 2023).

High-energy radiation therapy annihilates malignant cells and significantly perturbs gut flora by ravaging healthy cells within gastrointestinal tract simultaneously. Radiotherapy drastically alters microbiome composition leading quite significantly and exacerbating side effects like rather severe gastrointestinal issues and inflammation sometimes very badly. A disrupted microbiome alters radiotherapy drug metabolism significantly much like it does chemotherapy thereby impacting effectiveness of these treatments. Various studies suggest maintaining balanced gut flora during radiation therapy quite possibly mitigates nasty reactions and enhance efficacy significantly in patients. Restoration of gut microbiota diversity potentially via prebiotics or probiotics or a fibre-rich diet has been proposed as therapeutic strategy mitigating dire effects of radiotherapy (Zhang et al, 2023).

Beneficial microbes produce SCFAs which markedly improve patients' overall quality of life during treatment by protecting gut from radiation-induced damage and inflammation. Dietary interventions play a crucial role in shaping gut microbiome thereby profoundly influencing effectiveness of various cancer therapies these days significantly. Diets rich in fibre polyphenols and healthy fats very effectively foster growth of beneficial microbes subsequently encourage immune function and reducing inflammation. A high-fibre diet boosts production of SCFAs with anti-inflammatory and anticancer effects and helps restore microbial diversity in cancer patients undergoing therapy.

8.2.1. Nutrition and Immunotherapy Response

Immunotherapy has emerged as a promising cancer treatment advancement particularly in melanoma and non-small cell lung cancer malignancies where chemotherapy falters badly. Immunotherapy vigorously stimulates body's immune response recognizing cancer cells via immune checkpoint inhibitors such as anti-PD-1/PD-L1 antibodies rather effectively. Considerable success notwithstanding ICIs don't work equally well for all patients and underlying reasons remain largely shrouded in obscurity still. Fresh perspectives on treatment efficacy emerge as research intimates gut microbiome profoundly influences immune system response under immunotherapy. Gut microbiome swarming with archaea and fungi and viruses plus various bacteria has a profound impact on body's immune system obviously nowadays. Research uncovered specific advantageous gut microbes such as Akkermansia muciniphila and Faecalibacterium prausnitzii linked with remarkably enhanced immunotherapy responses (Garg et al, 2024).

Bacteria remarkably boost immune function by promoting activation of T cells crucial for recognizing tumour cells and vigorously attacking them subsequently. Akkermansia muciniphila has been linked strongly to enhanced anti-tumour immunity by vigorously boosting activation of CD8+ T cells and their proliferation. Malignant microorganisms festering in a dysbiotic gut microbiome can utterly debilitate immunotherapy effectiveness and severely cripple immune function rather quickly. Pathogenic bacteria can weirdly fuel inflammation and immune suppression hindering ability of immune system to mount effective cancer response very badly. Crucially a healthy microbiome might significantly improve outcomes for patients undergoing immunotherapy in some manner rather effectively it seems. Gut microbiome plays crucial role modulating immune responses under immunotherapy and dietary interventions offer rather promising optimization strategy quite effectively meanwhile (Garg et al, 2024).

High-fibre diets foster proliferation of beneficial gut flora producing short-chain fatty acids such as butyrate very effectively amidst bacterial colonies. SCFAs exhibit anti-inflammatory properties very effectively and enhance immune system's cancer response mechanisms fairly significantly in gut. Microbial metabolites may help mitigate systemic inflammation that frequently sabotages efficacy of immunotherapy markedly in diverse clinical contexts. Foods rich in polyphenol are garnering considerable attention lately alongside fibre for encourage immunotherapy responses somewhat effectively. Berries teem with polyphenols and dark chocolate boasts very potent antioxidant properties alongside considerable anti-inflammatory effects in green tea. Epigallocatechin gallate EGCG profoundly affects gut microbiome by fostering growth of beneficial microbes and amplifying various immune responses substantially in the body. Research indicates EGCG could possibly augment immune checkpoint blockade therapy rendering it a fairly valuable addition in treating various cancers including melanoma (Xiong et al, 2022).

Cruciferous veggies like broccoli and kale turmeric citrus fruits rich in polyphenol can further enhance immune function and microbial health remarkably. Incorporating such edibles might enhance microbiome diversity and mitigate inflammation stemming from certain immunotherapies very effectively in some cases. Gut microbiome crucially modulates immune responses within certain cancer immunotherapy contexts and does so rather significantly under specific conditions . Dietary interventions potentially enhance immunotherapy efficacy quite significantly and nasty side effects dwindle thereby yielding much better outcomes overall for cancer patients. A diet rich in fibre polyphenols and sundry nutrients supporting microbiome health might enhance conventional cancer treatments by greatly enhancing therapeutic efficacy and vigorously revving up immune function. Growing evidence underscores importance of diet and microbiome health in future cancer treatment yet further exploration of these complex relationships is sorely needed.

8.2.2. Nutrition and Chemotherapy Efficacy

Chemotherapy plays a crucial role in cancer treatment but often induces heinous side effects like gastrointestinal toxicity with severe nausea vomiting and mucositis. Side effects can drastically impair patient well-being and muddy treatment compliance very badly in some instances naturally occurring very frequently. Trillions of microorganisms residing in gut play a critical role in chemotherapy efficacy and its often debilitating side effects recently. Chemotherapy-induced dysbiosis gravely hampers gut recovery exacerbating inflammation rather badly thereby limiting efficacy of treatment and further compromising weakened immune function. Chemotherapy brutally depletes beneficial gut microbes such as Lactobacillus or Bifidobacterium crucial for maintaining gut integrity and supporting immune system function properly nowadays. Microbes remarkably produce short-chain fatty acids such as butyrate having anti-inflammatory properties and they strengthen gut barrier very well (Li et al, 2024).

Depletion of beneficial gut flora can exacerbate intestinal inflammation precipitating nasty GI symptoms such as diarrhea and mucositis affecting treatment outcomes very badly. Microbial dysbiosis drastically alters drug metabolism thereby influencing efficacy of chemotherapy significantly by modifying bodily processes responding to cancer drugs. Novel eating plans present an untested method for rejuvenating gut flora amidst grueling chemo treatments with somewhat unpredictable outcomes. A fibre-rich diet acts as substrate for beneficial microbes and rather slowly enhances gut health by promoting growth of SCFA-producing bacteria. Fermentation of fibre produces butyrate which rather effectively mitigates damage and inflammation in gut induced by chemotherapy. Garlic and onions and bananas rich in prebiotics rapidly foster beneficial bacteria growth thereby improving immune function and facilitating swift gut recovery. Probiotics being beneficial bacteria restore balance of microbes rather effectively in a very significant manner obviously (Li et al, 2024).

Saccharomyces boulardii strains rather effectively stabilize gut microbiome thereby mitigating chemotherapy-related diarrhea and mucositis alongside Lactobacillus rhamnosus very helpfully. Probiotics significantly enhance immune function thereby remarkably boosting tolerance during treatment and potentially lowering risk of infection quite effectively overall. Fibre prebiotics and probiotics remarkably improve chemotherapy outcomes significantly by supporting a healthy gut microbiome very effectively nowadays. Novel cancer therapies surprisingly enough benefit from such interventions which enhance immune response and mitigate pernicious side effects thereby optimizing treatment efficacy greatly. Insights into microbiome's role in cancer treatment accumulate steadily and nutrition-based approaches play a pivotal role in personalized cancer care.

8.2.3. Diet and Radiation Therapy

Radiation therapy aimed at pelvis for rectal cancer treatment ravages gut microbiome quite horribly resulting in various nasty gastrointestinal maladies. Radiation directly ravages intestinal cells sparking dysbiosis or a nasty imbalance in microbial populations that severely heightens inflammation and gut permeability disrupting normal gut function badly. Alterations may severely exacerbate side effects like nausea and diarrhea thereby badly hindering efficacy of radiation treatment for patients terribly. Radiation therapy brutally decimates microbial diversity mostly in gut's beneficial bacteria namely Lactobacillus and Bifidobacterium often with gravely unforeseen calamitous consequences. Gut barrier integrity relies heavily on microbes churning out beneficial metabolites like short-chain fatty acids possessing markedly anti-inflammatory properties. Radiation therapy brutally ravages microbial colonies leading heavily compromised gut health and greatly diminished gut repair capacity resulting in ghastly aftereffects (Oh et al, 2021).

Dietary interventions show considerable promise in alleviating such side effects by restoring balance somewhat to gut bacteria and supporting recovery vigorously of gut health. Prebiotics such as inulin and fructooligosaccharides or FOS help stimulate growth of beneficial microbes crucial for maintaining gut health naturally. Prebiotics can markedly enhance gut barrier function whilst encourage production of SCFAs and reducing radiation-induced inflammatory damage significantly. Prebiotics foster growth of Lactobacillus and Bifidobacterium thereby helping maintain microbial equilibrium very effectively encourage gut's reparative capacity. Berries and grapes loaded with polyphenols exhibit radioprotective properties fairly obviously in various studies alongside green tea extracts. Radiation exposure generates free radicals that cause oxidative stress which antioxidant-rich foods can very effectively mitigate in many instances. Polyphenols in certain foods may enhance growth of beneficial microbes further enhancing microbiome resilience against disruption caused by radiation (Oh et al, 2021).

Polyphenol-rich dietary intake remarkably modulates immune response and offers quite significant protection against radiation-induced DNA damage during therapy sessions. Polyphenol-rich foods and prebiotics might somewhat effectively counteract ghastly radiation therapy side effects on gut flora rather surprisingly. Enhancing microbial diversity and reducing inflammation alleviates severe treatment-related side effects and potentially amplifies overall therapeutic response significantly under radiation therapy. Nutritional strategies will play an essential role slowly in optimizing radiation therapy outcomes and improving patient well-being as microbiome's role becomes clearer.

8.3. Bridging Nutrition, Microbial Ecosystems, and Cancer Therapy

Gut microbiome plays a crucial albeit largely unexplored role slowly in oncology outcomes for cancer treatment presenting novel possibilities very quietly underground. Microbiome impact manifests variably across diverse therapeutic regimens like immunotherapy or chemotherapy and radiotherapy affecting treatment outcomes significantly . Nutritional interventions aimed at modulating microbiome garner considerable attention as potential tools remarkably for improving cancer therapy outcomes and enhancing patient life quality. Nutrition intricately links with microbiome offering cancer therapy a potentially groundbreaking novel approach that transforms treatment modalities rather remarkably. Probiotics and fibre-rich foods potentially alter gut microbial ecosystem significantly with polyphenol-rich diets very effectively under certain circumstances. Changes remarkably improve treatment outcomes and quite effectively mitigate side effects like fatigue or gastrointestinal distress suppressing immune problems effectively (Kim et al, 2025).

Probiotics rather effectively reinstate beneficial gut flora after nasty disruptions brought about harshly by chemotherapy or very strong antibiotic medications. Prebiotics nurture beneficial microbes quite vigorously by furnishing requisite nutrients for flourishing abundantly in environs surrounding them. Fibre-rich food especially stuff containing soluble fibres like inulin fuels fermentation which produces short-chain fatty acids really encourage gut health very effectively. Berries and dark chocolate rich in polyphenol offer antioxidant benefits that deeply support microbial health within cellular protection mechanisms overall. Integration of microbiome-based nutritional strategies into clinical oncology nowadays signifies a major stride toward rather precise medicine suddenly. Modified dietary interventions crafted according to individual microbial profiles can markedly optimize cancer treatment responses in patients remarkably well nowadays (Kim et al, 2025).

Evidence suggests a balanced microbiome boosts immunotherapy effects vigorously by modulating immune checkpoint activity and enhancing body's natural defense mechanisms. Dietary changes can profoundly impact chemotherapy's effects on various microbial populations thereby helping preserve gut health and mitigate nasty side effects. Fostering a gut environment conducive tissue repair and diminishing inflammation effectively yields markedly better long-term outcomes and heightened treatment responses in patients. Dietary strategies appear remarkably effective overall in encourage resilience of patients navigating complexities of cancer therapy with considerable success. Bodies of research connecting nutrition intricately to cancer treatment strangely open fresh avenues for markedly better outcomes silently in various clinical settings. Targeted dietary tweaks may recalibrate microbiome profoundly bridging nutrition and therapeutic triumph quite effectively in oncology yielding super personalized treatments.

9. Conclusion

Gut microbiome has emerged as pivotal player in human health exerting a rather profound influence on host metabolism and immunity intimately connected with various cancers. Diet drastically shapes microbial makeup nowadays as increasing knowledge of gut microbiome-host dynamics unfolds rapidly under intense scrutiny. Nutrition influences microbial ecology deeply thereby shaping local environments and encourage bodily defenses or occasionally fuelling erratic carcinogenic processes haphazardly within bodily systems. Certain nutrients and dietary patterns greatly influence production of metabolites and microbial diversity thereby affecting cancer risk significantly altering therapeutic outcomes. Diets rich in fibre and fermented products tend to foster diverse anti-inflammatory gut microbiota producing beneficial metabolites like short-chain fatty acids rapidly (Hills et al, 2019).

Consumption of processed foods and red meats fosters a pro-inflammatory gut microbiome thereby vigorously amplifying production of genotoxic compounds substantially in body. Gut microbiome modulates response rather effectively to some cancer therapies especially immunotherapies and chemotherapeutics with varying degrees of success apparently. Specific microbial taxa correlate strongly with improved outcomes whereas dysbiosis and severe microbial imbalances often precipitate heightened toxicity and reduced responsiveness. Rapidly unfolding dynamic interactions offer novel therapeutic opportunities through modified dietary interventions and prebiotics targeting gut microbiome effectively nowadays. Microbiome science merging with nutritional oncology slowly holds rather obscure promise for personalized medicine ahead in very novel ways (Lee et al, 2023).

Challenges persist obstinately in standardization of microbiome analysis and identification of causal relationships yet slowly emerging clinical practices prove somewhat actionable. Rabidly interdisciplinary collaboration and gnarly longitudinal studies hugely refining understanding of cancer trajectories alongside wonky multi-omics integration deeply influence diet microbiome host triad. Gut microbiome acts as a crucial mediator between diet and cancer biology rather subtly ultimately influencing overall tumour dynamics. Nutritional choices informed by this axis offer a novel cancer prevention approach and optimize treatment fairly effectively these days rather quietly. Advances in research will likely render microbiome science and dietary intervention synergistic and foundational in precision oncology and maybe even integrative cancer therapeutics.

References

Ağagündüz D, Cocozza E, Cemali Ö, Bayazıt AD, Nanì MF, Cerqua I, Morgillo F, Saygılı SK, Berni Canani R, Amero P, Capasso R. Understanding the role of the gut microbiome in gastrointestinal cancer: A review. Front Pharmacol. 2023 Jan 24;14:1130562. doi: 10.3389/fphar.2023.1130562. Erratum in: Front Pharmacol. 2025 Jul 30;16:1662597. doi: 10.3389/fphar.2025.1662597. PMID: 36762108; PMCID: PMC9903080.

Aggarwal N, Kitano S, Puah GRY, Kittelmann S, Hwang IY, Chang MW. Microbiome and Human Health: Current Understanding, Engineering, and Enabling Technologies. Chem Rev. 2023 Jan 11;123(1):31-72. doi: 10.1021/acs.chemrev.2c00431. Epub 2022 Nov 1. PMID: 36317983; PMCID: PMC9837825.

Aghamajidi A, Maleki Vareki S. The Effect of the Gut Microbiota on Systemic and Anti-Tumour Immunity and Response to Systemic Therapy against Cancer. Cancers (Basel). 2022 Jul 22;14(15):3563. doi: 10.3390/cancers14153563. PMID: 35892821; PMCID: PMC9330582.

Anand U, Dey A, Chandel AKS, Sanyal R, Mishra A, Pandey DK, De Falco V, Upadhyay A, Kandimalla R, Chaudhary A, Dhanjal JK, Dewanjee S, Vallamkondu J, Pérez de la Lastra JM. Cancer chemotherapy and beyond: Current status, drug candidates, associated risks and progress in targeted therapeutics. Genes Dis. 2022 Mar 18;10(4):1367-1401. doi: 10.1016/j.gendis.2022.02.007. Erratum in: Genes Dis. 2024 Jan 20;11(4):101211. doi: 10.1016/j.gendis.2024.101211. PMID: 37397557; PMCID: PMC10310991.

Anderson NM, Simon MC. The tumour microenvironment. Curr Biol. 2020 Aug 17;30(16):R921-R925. doi: 10.1016/j.cub.2020.06.081. PMID: 32810447; PMCID: PMC8194051.

Armstrong H, Bording-Jorgensen M, Dijk S, Wine E. The Complex Interplay between Chronic Inflammation, the Microbiome, and Cancer: Understanding Disease Progression and What We Can Do to Prevent It. Cancers (Basel). 2018 Mar 20;10(3):83. doi: 10.3390/cancers10030083. PMID: 29558443; PMCID: PMC5876658.

Berding K, Vlckova K, Marx W, Schellekens H, Stanton C, Clarke G, Jacka F, Dinan TG, Cryan JF. Diet and the Microbiota-Gut-Brain Axis: Sowing the Seeds of Good Mental Health. Adv Nutr. 2021 Jul 30;12(4):1239-1285. doi: 10.1093/advances/nmaa181. PMID: 33693453; PMCID: PMC8321864.

Bhatt AP, Redinbo MR, Bultman SJ. The role of the microbiome in cancer development and therapy. CA Cancer J Clin. 2017 Jul 8;67(4):326-344. doi: 10.3322/caac.21398. Epub 2017 May 8. PMID: 28481406; PMCID: PMC5530583.

Bull MJ, Plummer NT. Part 1: The Human Gut Microbiome in Health and Disease. Integr Med (Encinitas). 2014 Dec;13(6):17-22. PMID: 26770121; PMCID: PMC4566439.

Cho YS, Han K, Xu J, Moon JJ. Novel strategies for modulating the gut microbiome for cancer therapy. Adv Drug Deliv Rev. 2024 Jul;210:115332. doi: 10.1016/j.addr.2024.115332. Epub 2024 May 15. PMID: 38759702; PMCID: PMC11268941.

Ciorba MA, Hallemeier CL, Stenson WF, Parikh PJ. Probiotics to prevent gastrointestinal toxicity from cancer therapy: an interpretive review and call to action. Curr Opin Support Palliat Care. 2015 Jun;9(2):157-62. doi: 10.1097/SPC.0000000000000134. PMID: 25872116; PMCID: PMC4852157.

Ciupei D, Colişar A, Leopold L, Stănilă A, Diaconeasa ZM. Polyphenols: From Classification to Therapeutic Potential and Bioavailability. Foods. 2024 Dec 20;13(24):4131. doi: 10.3390/foods13244131. PMID: 39767073; PMCID: PMC11675957.

Conlon MA, Bird AR. The impact of diet and lifestyle on gut microbiota and human health. Nutrients. 2014 Dec 24;7(1):17-44. doi: 10.3390/nu7010017. PMID: 25545101; PMCID: PMC4303825.

Costantini L, Molinari R, Farinon B, Merendino N. Impact of Omega-3 Fatty Acids on the Gut Microbiota. Int J Mol Sci. 2017 Dec 7;18(12):2645. doi: 10.3390/ijms18122645. PMID: 29215589; PMCID: PMC5751248.

Cronin P, Joyce SA, O'Toole PW, O'Connor EM. Dietary Fibre Modulates the Gut Microbiota. Nutrients. 2021 May 13;13(5):1655. doi: 10.3390/nu13051655. PMID: 34068353; PMCID: PMC8153313.

Garg P, Pareek S, Kulkarni P, Horne D, Salgia R, Singhal SS. Next-Generation Immunotherapy: Advancing Clinical Applications in Cancer Treatment. J Clin Med. 2024 Oct 30;13(21):6537. doi: 10.3390/jcm13216537. PMID: 39518676; PMCID: PMC11546714.

Greathouse KL, Wyatt M, Johnson AJ, Toy EP, Khan JM, Dunn K, Clegg DJ, Reddy S. Diet-microbiome interactions in cancer treatment: Opportunities and challenges for precision nutrition in cancer. Neoplasia. 2022 Jul;29:100800. doi: 10.1016/j.neo.2022.100800. Epub 2022 Apr 29. PMID: 35500546; PMCID: PMC9065883.

Hills RD Jr, Pontefract BA, Mishcon HR, Black CA, Sutton SC, Theberge CR. Gut Microbiome: Profound Implications for Diet and Disease. Nutrients. 2019 Jul 16;11(7):1613. doi: 10.3390/nu11071613. PMID: 31315227; PMCID: PMC6682904.

Huang P, Liu Y. A Reasonable Diet Promotes Balance of Intestinal Microbiota: Prevention of Precolorectal Cancer. Biomed Res Int. 2019 Jul 25;2019:3405278. doi: 10.1155/2019/3405278. PMID: 31428633; PMCID: PMC6683831.

Ivleva EA, Grivennikov SI. Microbiota-driven mechanisms at different stages of cancer development. Neoplasia. 2022 Oct;32:100829. doi: 10.1016/j.neo.2022.100829. Epub 2022 Aug 4. PMID: 35933824; PMCID: PMC9364013.

Iyengar NM, Gucalp A, Dannenberg AJ, Hudis CA. Obesity and Cancer Mechanisms: Tumour Microenvironment and Inflammation. J Clin Oncol. 2016 Dec 10;34(35):4270-4276. doi: 10.1200/JCO.2016.67.4283. Epub 2016 Nov 7. PMID: 27903155; PMCID: PMC5562428.

Kim K, Lee M, Shin Y, Lee Y, Kim TJ. Optimizing Cancer Treatment Through Gut Microbiome Modulation. Cancers (Basel). 2025 Apr 7;17(7):1252. doi: 10.3390/cancers17071252. PMID: 40227841; PMCID: PMC11988035.

Kumar Singh A, Cabral C, Kumar R, Ganguly R, Kumar Rana H, Gupta A, Rosaria Lauro M, Carbone C, Reis F, Pandey AK. Beneficial Effects of Dietary Polyphenols on Gut Microbiota and Strategies to Improve Delivery Efficiency. Nutrients. 2019 Sep 13;11(9):2216. doi: 10.3390/nu11092216. PMID: 31540270; PMCID: PMC6770155.

Lee C, Lee J, Eor JY, Kwak MJ, Huh CS, Kim Y. Effect of Consumption of Animal Products on the Gut Microbiome Composition and Gut Health. Food Sci Anim Resour. 2023 Sep;43(5):723-750. doi: 10.5851/kosfa.2023.e44. Epub 2023 Sep 1. PMID: 37701742; PMCID: PMC10493557.

Leonard JM, Toro DD. Defining the Microbiome Components (Bacteria, Viruses, Fungi) and Microbiome Geodiversity. Surg Infect (Larchmt). 2023 Apr;24(3):208-212. doi: 10.1089/sur.2023.014. PMID: 37010972; PMCID: PMC10061322.

Li S, Zhu S, Yu J. The role of gut microbiota and metabolites in cancer chemotherapy. J Adv Res. 2024 Oct;64:223-235. doi: 10.1016/j.jare.2023.11.027. Epub 2023 Nov 26. PMID: 38013112; PMCID: PMC11464465.

Liu Q, Yang Y, Pan M, Yang F, Yu Y, Qian Z. Role of the gut microbiota in tumourigenesis and treatment. Theranostics. 2024 Mar 17;14(6):2304-2328. doi: 10.7150/thno.91700. PMID: 38646653; PMCID: PMC11024857.

Maddern AS, Coller JK, Bowen JM, Gibson RJ. The Association between the Gut Microbiome and Development and Progression of Cancer Treatment Adverse Effects. Cancers (Basel). 2023 Aug 28;15(17):4301. doi: 10.3390/cancers15174301. PMID: 37686576; PMCID: PMC10487104.

Majeed H, Gupta V. Adverse Effects of Radiation Therapy. [Updated 2023 Aug 14]. In: StatPearls [Internet]. Treasure Island (FL): StatPearls Publishing; 2025 Jan-. Available from: https://www.ncbi.nlm.nih.gov/books/NBK563259/

Mansour SR, Moustafa MAA, Saad BM, Hamed R, Moustafa AA. Impact of diet on human gut microbiome and disease risk. New Microbes New Infect. 2021 Feb 2;41:100845. doi: 10.1016/j.nmni.2021.100845. PMID: 34035924; PMCID: PMC8138677.

Murphy EA, Velazquez KT, Herbert KM. Influence of high-fat diet on gut microbiota: a driving force for chronic disease risk. Curr Opin Clin Nutr Metab Care. 2015 Sep;18(5):515-20. doi: 10.1097/MCO.0000000000000209. PMID: 26154278; PMCID: PMC4578152.

Ogunrinola GA, Oyewale JO, Oshamika OO, Olasehinde GI. The Human Microbiome and Its Impacts on Health. Int J Microbiol. 2020 Jun 12;2020:8045646. doi: 10.1155/2020/8045646. PMID: 32612660; PMCID: PMC7306068.

Oh B, Eade T, Lamoury G, Carroll S, Morgia M, Kneebone A, Hruby G, Stevens M, Boyle F, Clarke S, Corless B, Molloy M, Rosenthal D, Back M. The Gut Microbiome and Gastrointestinal Toxicities in Pelvic Radiation Therapy: A Clinical Review. Cancers (Basel). 2021 May 13;13(10):2353. doi: 10.3390/cancers13102353. PMID: 34068216; PMCID: PMC8153110.

Pandey KB, Rizvi SI. Plant polyphenols as dietary antioxidants in human health and disease. Oxid Med Cell Longev. 2009 Nov-Dec;2(5):270-8. doi: 10.4161/oxim.2.5.9498. PMID: 20716914; PMCID: PMC2835915.

Pei B, Ma X, Wu N, Wang C, Yang W. Effect of microbiome group on immune checkpoint inhibitors in treatment of gastrointestinal tumours. Chin J Cancer Res. 2023 Jun 30;35(3):252-265. doi: 10.21147/j.issn.1000-9604.2023.03.05. PMID: 37440825; PMCID: PMC10334499.

Pickard JM, Zeng MY, Caruso R, Núñez G. Gut microbiota: Role in pathogen colonization, immune responses, and inflammatory disease. Immunol Rev. 2017 Sep;279(1):70-89. doi: 10.1111/imr.12567. PMID: 28856738; PMCID: PMC5657496.

Roy S, Dhaneshwar S. Role of prebiotics, probiotics, and synbiotics in management of inflammatory bowel disease: Current perspectives. World J Gastroenterol. 2023 Apr 14;29(14):2078-2100. doi: 10.3748/wjg.v29.i14.2078. Erratum in: World J Gastroenterol. 2023 Sep 21;29(35):5178-5179. doi: 10.3748/wjg.v29.i35.5178. PMID: 37122604; PMCID: PMC10130969.

Sankarapandian V, Venmathi Maran BA, Rajendran RL, Jogalekar MP, Gurunagarajan S, Krishnamoorthy R, Gangadaran P, Ahn BC. An Update on the Effectiveness of Probiotics in the Prevention and Treatment of Cancer. Life (Basel). 2022 Jan 2;12(1):59. doi: 10.3390/life12010059. PMID: 35054452; PMCID: PMC8779143.

Santarelli RL, Pierre F, Corpet DE. Processed meat and colorectal cancer: a review of epidemiologic and experimental evidence. Nutr Cancer. 2008;60(2):131-44. doi: 10.1080/01635580701684872. PMID: 18444144; PMCID: PMC2661797.

Thursby E, Juge N. Introduction to the human gut microbiota. Biochem J. 2017 May 16;474(11):1823-1836. doi: 10.1042/BCJ20160510. PMID: 28512250; PMCID: PMC5433529.

Vivarelli S, Salemi R, Candido S, Falzone L, Santagati M, Stefani S, Torino F, Banna GL, Tonini G, Libra M. Gut Microbiota and Cancer: From Pathogenesis to Therapy. Cancers (Basel). 2019 Jan 3;11(1):38. doi: 10.3390/cancers11010038. PMID: 30609850; PMCID: PMC6356461.

Wang X, Qi Y, Zheng H. Dietary Polyphenol, Gut Microbiota, and Health Benefits. Antioxidants (Basel). 2022 Jun 20;11(6):1212. doi: 10.3390/antiox11061212. PMID: 35740109; PMCID: PMC9220293.

Wiertsema SP, van Bergenhenegouwen J, Garssen J, Knippels LMJ. The Interplay between the Gut Microbiome and the Immune System in the Context of Infectious Diseases throughout Life and the Role of Nutrition in Optimizing Treatment Strategies. Nutrients. 2021 Mar 9;13(3):886. doi: 10.3390/nu13030886. PMID: 33803407; PMCID: PMC8001875.

Wu S, Bhat ZF, Gounder RS, Mohamed Ahmed IA, Al-Juhaimi FY, Ding Y, Bekhit AEA. Effect of Dietary Protein and Processing on Gut Microbiota-A Systematic Review. Nutrients. 2022 Jan 20;14(3):453. doi: 10.3390/nu14030453. PMID: 35276812; PMCID: PMC8840478.

Xiong RG, Zhou DD, Wu SX, Huang SY, Saimaiti A, Yang ZJ, Shang A, Zhao CN, Gan RY, Li HB. Health Benefits and Side Effects of Short-Chain Fatty Acids. Foods. 2022 Sep 15;11(18):2863. doi: 10.3390/foods11182863. PMID: 36140990; PMCID: PMC9498509.

Xu K, Motiwala Z, Corona-Avila I, Makhanasa D, Alkahalifeh L, Khan MW. The Gut Microbiome and Its Multifaceted Role in Cancer Metabolism, Initiation, and Progression: Insights and Therapeutic Implications. Technol Cancer

Res Treat. 2025 Jan-Dec;24:15330338251331960. doi: 10.1177/15330338251331960. Epub 2025 Apr 10. PMID: 40208053; PMCID: PMC12032467.

Yan J, Sheng L, Li H. Akkermansia muciniphila: is it the Holy Grail for ameliorating metabolic diseases? Gut Microbes. 2021 Jan-Dec;13(1):1984104. doi: 10.1080/19490976.2021.1984104. PMID: 34674606; PMCID: PMC8726741.

Yang Q, Wang B, Zheng Q, Li H, Meng X, Zhou F, Zhang L. A Review of Gut Microbiota-Derived Metabolites in Tumour Progression and Cancer Therapy. Adv Sci (Weinh). 2023 May;10(15):e2207366. doi: 10.1002/advs.202207366. Epub 2023 Mar 23. PMID: 36951547; PMCID: PMC10214247.

Zhang D, Zhao J, Zhang Y, Jiang H, Liu D. Revisiting immune checkpoint inhibitors: new strategies to enhance efficacy and reduce toxicity. Front Immunol. 2024 Dec 10;15:1490129. doi: 10.3389/fimmu.2024.1490129. PMID: 39720720; PMCID: PMC11666512.

Zhang M, Liu J, Xia Q. Role of gut microbiome in cancer immunotherapy: from predictive biomarker to therapeutic target. Exp Hematol Oncol. 2023 Sep 28;12(1):84. doi: 10.1186/s40164-023-00442-x. PMID: 37770953; PMCID: PMC10537950.

Zhang P. Influence of Foods and Nutrition on the Gut Microbiome and Implications for Intestinal Health. Int J Mol Sci. 2022 Aug 24;23(17):9588. doi: 10.3390/ijms23179588. PMID: 36076980; PMCID: PMC9455721.

Chapter 9

Ultra-Processed Foods and Cancer Risk: Mechanistic Insights and Public Health Implications

Sheetanshu Gupta[1], Praneeth Juvvi[2*], Sarfraj Ahmad Siddiqui[3], and Ng. Joykumar Singh[4]

[1]Department of Food Safety and Quality Assurance, College of Food Technology, Central Agricultural University (CAU), Imphal, Manipur, India

[2]Department of Food Processing Technology, College of Food Technology-Central Agricultural University, Imphal, Manipur, India

[3]Department of Biochemistry, King George's Medical University, U.P., India

[4]Department of Food Process Engineering, College of Food Technology, Central Agricultural University (CAU), Imphal, Manipur, India

Abstract

Ultra-processed foods have been increasingly linked with the elevated risk of diseases such as cancer and other chronic diseases quite frequently nowadays. UPFs may rapidly exacerbate cancer development through complex and largely obscure mechanisms quietly over time in various bodily systems. Dubious fats and copious added sugars in ultraprocessed foods severely disrupt cellular functions, thereby fueling carcinogenesis at an alarmingly rapid rate. Bizarre eating habits enormously heighten the risk of cancer, worryingly by dysregulating the gut microbiome and fostering insulin resistance quite alarmingly. Tumour-promoting environments heavily fostered in genotoxicity induction involve acrylamide, trans fats, and high-fructose corn syrup playing crucial roles. Globally, UPF consumption persists with an outsized impact on impoverished demographics and sparks trepidation about glaring health inequities manifesting starkly across them. Nationwide epidemiological evidence and mechanistic studies in animal models vigorously underscores necessity for public health interventions curbing ultra-processed food consumption. Ridiculously stringent food labelling and hefty taxation of junk food products are recommended for mitigating the growing global cancer burden significantly worldwide.

Keywords: Ultra-Processed Foods, Carcinogenesis, Metabolic Disruption, Inflammation, Epidemiology, Public Health

DOI: 10.1201/9781042010387-9

1. Introduction

Rampant global consumption of ultra-processed foods has bizarrely synchronized with the skyrocketing incidence of various non-communicable diseases like cancer in recent decades. Ultra-processed foods constitute a sizeable portion of contemporary diets, mostly in wealthy countries, drastically altered with artificial additives and preservatives. Growing unease surrounds a potential nexus between the consumption of processed edibles and increasing global cancer rates in many parts of the world. Epidemiological studies and mechanistic research evidence suggest UPFs might significantly heighten various cancer risks while underlying biological pathways stay woefully complex (Kliemann et al, 2022).

Nowadays, research focuses on how ultra-processing drastically alters nutritional profiles of foods in ways that may substantially heighten cancer risk. Processed meats and refined sugars harbour carcinogenic constituents that largely elevate cancer risk somewhat ominously in certain dietary contexts. UPFs have peculiar traits largely owing to the presence of artificial additives, flavour enhancers, and various emulsifiers, sparking concerns about links to carcinogenesis potentially. Refined carbs and copious added sugars teem in ultra-processed foods and fuel obesity, notoriously risking various cancers like breast and colorectal cancer. Gobbling loads of hyper-processed food such as saccharine beverages and munchies heightens risk of metabolic mayhem and insulin dysfunction fueling cancerous terrain. Overproduction of growth factors such as insulin-like growth factor 1 occurs in various bodily processes due largely to dysregulation of insulin metabolism (Kliemann et al, 2022).

Ultra-processed foods contain weird preservatives and dodgy colorants alongside flavor enhancers and emulsifiers that seem very fishy most likely. Emerging evidence suggests some food additives might trigger cancerous growth with prolonged exposure although deemed safe by regulatory agencies. Concerns are raised by certain studies regarding nitrates and nitrites present in processed meats forming carcinogenic nitrosamines quite rapidly upon metabolism. Aspartame and saccharin kindle controversy surrounding potentially fuelling cancerous cells rampantly with evidence remaining woefully inconclusive still. Certain additives like polysorbates and carboxymethylcellulose present in ultra processed foods tweak gut microbiota very frequently sparking inflammation and thereby fostering tumourigenesis (Kliemann et al, 2022).

UPFs eaten regularly profoundly alter gut microbiota playing a pivotal role downstream in mediating carcinogenic effects fairly significantly within bodily systems. Emerging evidence increasingly implicates gut microbial community dysbiosis in various chronic diseases including myriad forms of cancer rather slowly nowadays. UPFs highly refined nature completely devoid of fibre and essential prebiotics drastically shifts microbiome toward a decidedly pro-inflammatory profile in gut. Certain additives found in ultraprocessed foods namely emulsifiers and artificial sweeteners severely disrupt gut microbiota promoting inflammatory responses which contribute significantly to development of colorectal cancer. Dysbiosis spawns chronic low-grade inflammation vigorously fueling tumour initiation and metastasis very intensely in certain cancer cases anyway (Rondinella et al, 2025).

Production of reactive oxygen species or ROS and oxidative stress significantly ups cancer risk via numerous twisted biochemical routes . Consumption of trans fats rampant in processed baked items and deep-fried comestibles boosts ROS generation precipitating DNA lesions and oncogenic mutations alongside inflammatory cascade activation pivotal in tumourigenesis. Artificial additives break down frenetically during digestion possibly generating rogue free radicals that exacerbate oxidative damage and spark carcinogenic processes rapidly. Recent cancer research scrutinizes dietary influences on treatment efficacy with intake of ultra-processed foods playing a crucial albeit murky role . Cancer treatments such as chemotherapy trigger severely suppressed immunity and gut dysbiosis thereby increasing oxidative stress that hampers patient recovery badly (Waris and Ahsan, 2006).

Evidence emerging rapidly now suggests diets heavy in ultraprocessed food might amplify nasty side effects of therapy and hamper some treatments' efficacy badly. Dietary habits potentially modulate immune function by heavily influencing gut microbiome thereby altering response to immunotherapy and fostering gradual development of treatment resistance. Growing evidence quite alarmingly links UPF consumption cancer risk and treatment outcomes for public health with stark worrying efficacy implications. Carefully designing public health policies around potential risks of ultra-processed foods fosters encouragingly healthier dietary choices very effectively nowadays. Nationwide initiatives targeting low-income populations alongside dietary guidelines and opaque food labeling may be implemented unevenly with varying degrees of success (Rondinella et al, 2025).

Nationwide public health initiatives might very effectively promote consumption of fruits and whole grains linked overall with significantly lower cancer risk. Cancer risk may be fueled by UPFs through obscure pathways warranting in-depth exploration here. Evidence linking ultra-processed foods to various cancer types will be scrutinized particularly in relation to their impact on metabolic health and inflammation. Emerging roles of dietary interventions in cancer risk reduction will be deliberated upon quite thoroughly now including efforts replacing UPFs with nutrient-dense alternatives. Rising intake of ultra-processed edibles has dire consequences for public health and sundry tactics can be wielded somewhat mitigating cancer risk. Elucidating underlying mechanisms by which UPFs affect cancer risk and societal ramifications of dietary habits informs public health policy and fosters healthier eating.

2. The Rise of Ultra-Processed Foods

Ultra-processed foods have reconfigured global food systems very quietly over past few decades with striking rapidity and alarming stealthiness. Massively industrialized manufacturing processes churn out heaps of ultra-processed foods riddled with copious artificial ingredients and buckets of refined sugar nowadays. Ultra-processed foods now pervade global diets mainly because of their handy availability and suspiciously lengthy storage duration at cheap rates. Public health experts are getting mighty concerned nowadays about ultra-processed foods fuelling rising tide of diet-related illnesses very rapidly. Ultra-processed foods pack plenty of vacuous calories and surprisingly little nutritional oomph fuelling stark deficiencies in fibre and sundry vital nutrients. Consuming foods loaded with copious sugar and dubious fats can really mess with metabolic health and catastrophically fuel development of obesity type 2 diabetes and heart disease (Leite et al, 2022).

Recently consumption of ultra processed foods has been tied loosely to increased body fat and higher rates of metabolic issues. Surging obesity rates globally heighten unease over UPFs' ties with chronic ailments that frequently give rise to nasty cancers subsequently. Ultra-processed foods catastrophically ravage public health systems and severely damaged individual health outcomes result from such destructive dietary habits . Global populations increasingly adopt diets laden with UPF and healthcare systems get heavily burdened over time in many geographical areas. Enormous resources are squandered on treating diet-related maladies that severely strain healthcare coffers and sap productivity nationwide due to morbidity. A public health crisis erupts suddenly nationwide demanding extremely urgent attention alongside drastic swift intervention from various authorities very quickly (Leite et al, 2022).

Ultra-processed foods mayhem ravages gut microorganisms lurking stealthily in digestive tracts and possibly trigger nasty unforeseen health debacles down line . Studies suggest consumption of ultra-processed foods likely disrupts gut bacteria fairly profoundly thereby fostering chronic inflammation and aberrant immune system reactions. Ultra-processed foods drastically need reduction for yielding long-term health benefits as gut microbiome composition gets severely altered by such diets. Nationwide a drastic overhaul of public health policies is imperative amidst a surging tide of diet-related health issues caused by ultra-processed food consumption. Tactics like ultra-transparent nutritional labeling and heavily subsidized public education initiatives promote wholesome eating habits while stringent regulations stifle egregious marketing gimmicks preying on youngsters. Fostering food systems that privilege whole unadulterated food can nudge dietary equipoise back on track and cultivate salubrious global futures rather quietly (Rondinella et al, 2025).

2.1. What Are Ultra-Processed Foods?

Ultra-processed foods get heavily manipulated industrially turning raw materials into ridiculously convenient products with lots of obscure additives inside. Ultra-processed foods frequently contain artificial ingredients alongside synthetic additives and preservatives devoid of natural nutrients nearly always entirely. Engineered foods become ridiculously palatable making them staple fare in most diets and fairly visually appealing to consumers nowadays. Extensive processing exacts a steep toll on nutritional value frequently anyway. Ultra-processed foods bear lengthy ingredient lists containing obscure unpronounceable substances seldom found in average household pantries or on grocery shelves. Some additives might be weird artificial flavorings or colorings and sweeteners alongside emulsifiers that stabilize foods with really obscure textural effects (Monteiro et al, 2019).

Processed foods frequently harbor hydrogenated oils and preservatives like BHT alongside artificial sweeteners such as aspartame and high-fructose corn syrup. Processed foods contain additives boosting flavor remarkably and prolong shelf life yet typically lack vital nutrients such as fibre and assorted vitamins. Ultra-processed foods tend to be ridiculously energy-dense and very lacking in essential micronutrients overall. Ultra-processed foods are loaded with copious amounts of added sugars and copious unhealthy fats and salt yielding ridiculously addictive flavor and remarkably long shelf life. Undesirably strong flavors get masked quite effectively with certain ingredients used sporadically in lots of disparate food products very successfully. Ultra-processed food often teems with energy yet yields paltry nutritional value resulting in dietary distress when it monopolizes daily eats (Monteiro et al, 2019).

Sugary soft drinks and chips alongside packaged baked goods and processed meats like hot dogs get classified as ultra-processed foods nearly everywhere. Busy people and families grasping for ease gobble down these food options needing minimal prep or zero fuss altogether. Heavily marketed via ad blitzes they're peddled as ridiculously quick dirt cheap food that's sort of tasty alternative to your own sloppy cooking. Growing consumption of ultra-processed foods has raised significant concerns regarding public health recently in many countries somewhat surprisingly. Diets heavy in UPFs have lately been tied quite strongly to myriad health issues including obesity and type 2 diabetes rather frequently. UPFs devoid of essential nutrients and fibre spur proliferation of detrimental bacteria within gut microbiome thus fostering rather poor gastrointestinal well-being significantly. Ultra-processed foods spark vociferous demands for greater awareness and novel public health strategies fostering whole foods consumption for markedly better health outcomes.

2.2. Health Implications of Ultra-Processed Foods

Globally ultra-processed foods intake has skyrocketed nowadays fueling a rather rapid surge in obesity type 2 diabetes and heart ailments. Foods loaded with added sugars and unhealthy fats are very much nutritionally vacuous posing significant risks to public health nowadays quite frequently. Eating ultra-processed foods raises eyebrows largely because of glaringly poor nutritional value and some very inferior overall dietary quality. Such foods frequently pack plenty calories yet fall remarkably short on fibre vitamins and various micronutrients essentially lacking in crucial antioxidants normally. People stuck on ultra processed foods frequently endure nasty deficiencies precipitating health calamities like crappy immune responses and very severe metabolic syndrome issues suddenly. UPFs lacking fibre severely impair digestive health and play a somewhat crucial role in overall health by contributing to poor gut microbiome diversity (Valicente et al, 2023).

Ultra-processed foods get engineered rather cleverly with added sugars or unhealthy fats and salt making them basically super addictive. Overeating occurs rather frequently and trouble controlling daily calorie consumption subsequently happens with significant regularity very often in many cases. Ultra-processed foods are formulated with cunning precision to fuel excessive consumption but whole foods typically satiate hunger very effectively. High energy density fuels overeating very readily and over time weight gain manifests eventually culminating in frank obesity. Obesity markedly elevates risk of chronic diseases like type 2 diabetes and certain cancers or heart disease suddenly over time. Eating ultra-processed foods regularly has been tenuously linked to insulin resistance a harbinger of nasty metabolic syndrome quite notoriously (Valicente et al, 2023).

Consuming lots of refined sugars and trans fats commonly present in ultra-processed foods badly disrupts bodily functions that regulate blood sugar levels thereby heightening type 2 diabetes risk. Insulin resistance chronically precipitates inflammation and increased fat accumulates haphazardly around vital organs sparking sudden dysfunction in key metabolic pathways. People ingesting huge quantities of heavily processed edibles nowadays might be quite possibly rather more prone to cardiovascular disease and metabolic dysregulation. Ultra-processed foods detrimentally affect bodily functions and foster low-grade chronic inflammation negatively impacting weight and metabolic health very badly. Artificial additives and preservatives hiding in ultraprocessed foods may foster imbalance in gut microbiome thereby precipitating a weird condition called dysbiosis (Almarshad et al, 2022).

Dysbiosis signifies a drastically altered gut microbial ecosystem linked rather tenuously to nasty afflictions like obesity and various carcinomas. Consuming copious amounts of salt sugar and fat fuels inflammation that merges with a wonky gut microbiome rampantly exacerbating chronic health risks. Studies reveal people gorging on heavily processed food often have diets sorely deficient in vital nutrients and bereft of fresh fruit. Unhealthy eating habits spirally downwards very quickly resulting in woefully poor health outcomes over time and perpetuate themselves vigorously . Ultra-processed foods grievously exacerbate health inequities worldwide amongst lower-income populations rather badly these days. People struggling financially bear a greater load of non-communicable diseases largely due to their significant contributing factors (Almarshad et al, 2022).

Convenience comes at a steep price now and detrimental effects on health are glaringly obvious. Their association with obesity type 2 diabetes cardiovascular disease and cancer highlights need for swift nationwide action and greater awareness rapidly everywhere. Nationwide diet-related disease epidemics can be reversed through policy reforms alongside dietary education that severely limit availability of ultra-processed foods.

2.2.1. Obesity and Metabolic Disorders

Obesity gets fueled fairly significantly by ultra-processed food consumption amidst growing concerns over their rather detrimental impact on overall wellbeing. Ultra-processed foods get formulated with intense flavor profiles exceptionally tasty and ridiculously crave-worthy by clever design nearly every time. Combining copious sugars unhealthy fats and salt results in highly addictive foods triggering brain pleasure centers very effectively in some obscure manner. Such foods frequently render moderation quite elusive leading rapidly to gluttony and excessive calorie intake. Over time quite drastically excessive intake fosters a very stark imbalance between bodily energy expenditure and overall caloric consumption normally. Ultra-processed foods crammed with calories and devoid of nutrients offer minimal satiety thus people often wolf down extra food far beyond daily energy needs. Such egregious behavior fosters weight gain and precipitously contributes enormously to onset of obesity globally in alarming proportions eventually (Dicken and Batterham, 2024).

Obesity gets driven substantially by eating energy-dense junk foods like UPFs due largely to various underlying complex health factors. Obesity links rather alarmingly nowadays with various nasty metabolic disorders including type 2 diabetes and hypertension alongside dyslipidemia very tightly. Visceral fat around vital organs swells precipitously fostering systemic inflammation and insulin resistance with lipid metabolism going haywire rapidly. Type 2 diabetes manifests with marked insulin resistance whereby cells curiously stop responding effectively and blood sugar levels surge precipitously. Metabolic issues erupt rapidly further worsening obesity and formation of other vile chronic ailments down line very darn quickly. Research shows folks wolfing down heaps of highly processed junk food frequently display weird metabolic markers such as rapidly rising blood glucose and sketchy lipid profiles (Dicken and Batterham, 2024).

Metabolic disturbances significantly ramp up risk of cardiovascular diseases and diabetes which are major global killers causing substantial disability worldwide. Pernicious vicious cycles erupt rapidly when coalescing conditions spiral out of control with alarming ferocity in decidedly dire poor health circumstances. Ultra-processed foods consumption fuels global obesity epidemic heavily and spawns various nasty metabolic disorders worldwide nowadays with alarming frequency. Addictive qualities of these foods and poor nutritional content hugely facilitate overeating and subsequent weight gain putting people at greatly heightened risk of contracting life-threatening chronic ailments such as diabetes. Nationwide initiatives coupled with rigorous education effectively curb consumption of ultra-processed foods thereby markedly improving public health outcomes over time.

2.2.2. Cardiovascular Disease

Rising global prevalence of cardiovascular disease correlates strongly with consumption of ultra-processed foods and it remains a prominent mortality cause worldwide. Ultra-processed foods laden with trans fats sodium and added sugars play a significant role in development of nasty cardiovascular maladies. Trans fats constitute a rather disconcerting component lurking within many ultra processed food products nowadays. Packaged treats and processed baked goods frequently harbor them mainly to very substantially tweak texture and boost shelf life. Trans fats very conclusively raise levels of low-density lipoprotein cholesterol deemed bad by most medical professionals nowadays in many countries. Elevated LDL cholesterol levels spur formation of arterial plaques subsequently leading atherosclerosis a condition marked by narrowed arteries hardening and impairing blood flow greatly (Juul et al, 2021).

Older adults nowadays face terribly heightened risk of heart attacks and strokes or peripheral artery disease quite significantly often. Ultra-processed food loaded with sodium contributes substantially to cardiovascular disease risk alongside trans fats very significantly in most cases. Sodium abounds very heavily in processed meats and snack foods but surprisingly canned soups contain rather alarmingly high amounts too. A high-sodium diet precipitates hypertension quite suddenly a major risk factor for stroke and myocardial infarction. Elevated blood pressure puts strain squarely on heart and blood vessels thereby heightening likelihood of damage rapidly fostering various cardiovascular events. Frequent consumption nowadays of ultra-processed foods heightens risk of coronary artery disease significantly and puts people at risk of heart failure. UPFs vigorously fuel fat buildup and sodium retention within bloodstream and foster inflammation very intensely throughout various bodily tissues (Juul et al, 2021).

Chronic inflammation severely hampers vascular integrity triggering endothelial dysfunction which significantly impairs dilatory capacities of blood vessel lining rather properly. Nationwide systemic inflammation may be severely exacerbated by disruption of beneficial gut microbiota caused by consumption of ultra-processed foods. UPFs unleash profound inflammatory effects deeply within cardiovascular system rendering arteries highly susceptible to maladies such as heart failure quite suddenly. Ultra-processed foods drastically affect cardiovascular disease by badly impacting cholesterol blood pressure and overall vascular health severely nowadays. Consumption of such foods often entails trans fats excessive sodium and added sugars accelerating atherosclerosis development boosting hypertension risk and fuelling systemic inflammation crucial in cardiovascular disease pathogenesis. Fostering relatively healthier eating habits and curbing consumption of ultra-processed foods greatly enhance overall heart health and prevents cardiovascular disease.

2.2.3. Cancer

Higher risk of certain cancers notably breast and prostate cancer increasingly links to a rise in consumption of ultra-processed foods. Studies reveal certain ingredients in ultra-processed edible products namely copious added sugars and highly refined carbs fuel cancerous tumour development rampantly. Factors conducive to tumour growth exist ubiquitously nowadays under specific conditions and environments are virtually everywhere fostering such development. Ultra-processed foods foster cancer risk significantly by promoting insulin resistance gradually in human bodies over an extended period. Diets rich in refined sugars and carbs cause wildly fluctuating blood glucose levels resulting in elevated insulin levels over a protracted period. Elevated insulin levels and quirky insulin-like growth factors spur cell proliferation and stifle apoptosis very profoundly during cancerous tumour development (Isaksen and Dankel, 2023).

Insulin resistance plays a crucial role rather frequently in tumourigenesis of cancers such as breast and prostate cancer. Chronic inflammation factors significantly into cancer risk rather frequently amidst many diet-related diseases being marked by such persistent inflammation. Ultra-processed foods teem with trans fats and added sugars that very frequently trigger low-grade systemic inflammation throughout one's body. Inflammation fuels cellular damage and oxidative stress spurring DNA mutations rapidly within cells leading to cancerous tumour formation very quickly. UPFs foster a profoundly inflammatory milieu crucial for tumourigenesis and cancer progression as TNF-alpha heavily influences neoplastic cell survival amidst metastasis (Isaksen and Dankel, 2023).

Quite often nowadays health risks arise from carcinogenic compounds that form during storage of ultra-processed edibles in sundry processing facilities. International Agency for Research on Cancer has recently deemed acrylamide a probable human carcinogen found prevalently in oily fried foods. Processed meats like bacon contain nitrates and nitrites which get converted into carcinogenic nitrosamines during gastrointestinal digestion thereby potentially heightening colorectal cancer risk greatly. Studies show consumption of copious amounts of ultra processed foods correlates with elevated risk of gastrointestinal malignancies notably colorectal and breast cancers. Insulin resistance and inflammation linked to obesity greatly heighten cancer development susceptibility in such individuals fairly substantially over time naturally.

Ultra-processed foods teeming with unhealthy fats badly alter fat metabolism potentially fueling progression of hormone-sensitive cancers such as breast cancer vigorously. Ultra-processed foods remarkably often pose significant risk for development of various cancer types in disparate demographic groups frequently nowadays. Certain dietary components trigger inflammation and altered fat metabolism alongside carcinogenic chemicals thereby significantly boosting likelihood of cancer development remarkably. Drastically cutting consumption of ultra-processed foods slowly could be crucial in cancer prevention and improving health outcomes by shifting towards whole foods (Kliemann et al, 2022).

2.3. Ultra-Processed Foods and the Global Obesity Epidemic

Ultra-processed foods consumption surged rapidly becoming a key driver of obesity epidemic globally across various nations these days. Foods riddled with artificial additives and loaded with copious amounts of saturated fats and added sugars have proliferated worldwide very rapidly. UPFs have become ridiculously appealing especially in low-income nations where traditional food gets swiftly supplanted by hyperpalatable calorie-dense food often. Food tech breakthroughs drastically altered eating habits worldwide and now super processed food pervades every corner of the globe essentially nowadays. Global urbanization accelerates rapidly making sugary drinks and packaged edibles ubiquitous nowadays for masses of people in sprawling metropolises everywhere. Super cheap foodby eats frequently supplant home-cooked meals in global metropolises particularly within some developing nations around our planet usually (Poti et al, 2017).

Processed snacks supplant whole foods like fruits and legumes rather alarmingly in this societal context nowadays with rapidity. Ultra-processed edibles touted as quick panaceas for frenzied lifestyles harbour negligible nourishment and loads of calories fuelling obesity rates surging nationwide rapidly. Such trends appear very disconcerting nowadays when musing over its far-reaching effects very rapidly on youngsters and teenagers these days. Rates of childhood obesity surge alarmingly worldwide largely owing to eating ultra-processed foods and sending alarm bells ringing among health experts suddenly. Childhood obesity portends adult obesity and signals future health calamities like type 2 diabetes amidst diverse metabolic maladies unfolding slowly. Youngsters wolfing down heavily processed junk food are very apt to cultivate dodgy munching habits and possibly turn into obese adults down line (Poti et al, 2017).

Nutritional patterns drastically impact scholastic achievement and psychological wellbeing rather badly on the whole in most cases apparently. Public health authorities must intervene swiftly nowadays because obesity strongly correlates with consumption of ultra-processed food items very frequently. Tackling such gnarly issues necessitates a very diverse approach starting with nutrition ed aimed squarely at heightening risk awareness linked with dodgy processed foodstuffs. Nutritional content of packaged food could be highlighted effectively through stringent labeling regulations thereby somewhat empowering consumers very much for making fairly healthy choices. Policymakers and public health organizations should vigorously champion radical overhauls in food production targeting youngsters with junk food ubiquitously available.

Prevalence of ultra-processed foods correlates heavily with global obesity epidemic nowadays almost invariably across diverse strata worldwide socioeconomically. Younger populations eating such foods at a rather alarming rate these days suffer profoundly grave long-term health consequences fairly frequently nowadays. Tackling obesity worldwide requires a ridiculously complex response involving extensive education and somewhat radical reform of food production for better health outcomes.

2.4. Public Health Strategies to Address Ultra-Processed Food Consumption

Nowadays globally obesity epidemic worsens rapidly fuelled by a surge in consumption of ultra-processed food and soaring rates of nasty cancers. A garrulous multifaceted strategy is needed nowadays very slowly to tackle negative health impacts of ridiculously affordable widely accessible foods. Sweeping policy reforms alongside stringent regulatory oversight of food production and individual behavioral modifications become necessary public health strategies quite often. Obscurity emanates erratically from numeral one with fervent ranting bursting forth in a plethora of obtuse utterances rather suddenly. Nutritional education serves crucially as tactic heightening awareness about risks linked with daily consumption of ultra-processed foods in modern diets. Public health initiatives vigorously promote healthier food choices emphasizing whole grains legumes and fairly minimally processed fruits and various vegetables (Beal et al, 2024).

Nutrient-dense foods stave off diet-related maladies fairly effectively overall and benefit health in myriad subtle yet profoundly impactful ways. Educating folks about perks of wholesome food inspires radically healthier lifestyle choices and slashes intake of junk eats drastically every year. Food marketing towards kids nowadays plays a significant albeit oft-maligned role in rapidly shaping dubious dietary habits in sundry ways. Slick ads peddle ultra-processed foods very effectively nowadays globally fueling rampant overconsumption in diverse regions (Beal et al, 2024).

Regulating food marketing vehemently appears critical nowadays in combating rather egregious issues somewhat effectively across various demographics globally. Rules restricting junk food ads mainly on TV and online could somewhat effectively reduce kids intake of sugary nutrient poor stuff. Nationwide regulations could greatly spur promotion of fruits and whole grains among children thereby significantly diminishing obesity rates in various environments. Sugary food and processed edibles taxation has very successfully diminished nationwide purchase of such junk over fairly significant periods lately (Beal et al, 2024).

Imposing a levy on sweetened beverages remarkably curbs overeating and fosters healthy dietary habits among populations with excessive junk food consumption. Revenue generated from such taxes might be funneled back into quirky public health programs or subsidies for unusually effective health education nationwide. This approach proves effective mainly within poor demographics that lack access to decent nutrition for various deeply ingrained socioeconomic reasons. Clear labeling on food products enables consumers rather easily making informed decisions daily with a substantial degree of regularity every day.

Nutritional labels highlighting calories and added sugars enable consumers very easily to identify fairly unhealthy food these days. Labeling that signifies processing level of edibles informs consumers about refinement degree in bought food prompting healthier eating habits and diminishing dependency on overly processed food. Nationwide drastic measures addressing health crises spawned by gobbling ultra-processed food must be swiftly taken very effectively right now. Quirky nutritional education tactics and wacky food marketing regs alongside taxation can very significantly improve global public health outcomes worldwide.

3. Mechanisms of Carcinogenesis

Consumption of ultra-processed foods has skyrocketed lately spawning significant public health concerns across many nations worldwide over recent decades rapidly. Diets riddled with copious added sugars unhealthy fats and dubious preservatives contribute heavily to obesity and spur cancer development rather alarmingly nowadays. Myriad genetic and environmental factors swirl together with dubious lifestyle choices in a maddening complex dance fueling carcinogenesis very slowly. Evidence piles up rather quickly suggesting ultra-processed foods play a crucial role in global obesity development these days very much everywhere. Biological mechanisms underlying UPFs' role in cancer are meticulously examined here with differing levels of empirical evidence and nuanced analysis. A solitary numeral exists quietly in obscurity with stupid mundanity (Poti el al, 2017).

Ultra-processed foods significantly ramp up cancer risk mostly through chronic inflammation which festers stealthily deep within bodily tissues very quietly. Consuming large amounts of refined carbohydrates and unhealthy fats found alongside various additives in ultra processed foods rapidly activates inflammatory pathways deeply within bodily tissues. Chronic low-grade inflammation very badly damages DNA and thereby fosters mutations creating a super favorable environment for uncontrollably thriving cancer cells. Ultra-processed foods loaded with trans fats and refined sugars trigger pro-inflammatory cytokines and aggressive immune responses which can heighten cancer risk over time in tissues such as colon and breast tissue. Oxidative stress embodies a crucial carcinogenic pathway rather intriguingly tied with intake of ultra processed edibles in sundry fairly alarming research lately (Poti el al, 2017).

Refined sugars fats and preservatives abundant in UPFs notably accelerate free radical production bodily within humans under certain conditions naturally. Unstable molecules rapidly wreak havoc on cellular components like DNA proteins and lipids leading to mutations and swift cancer initiation. Processed meats contain nitrates and artificial sweeteners that foster oxidative stress and promote malignancy development in stomach and liver quite readily. Consumption of ultra-processed foods strongly correlates with insulin resistance a condition characterized by bodily cells becoming less responsive rather rapidly to insulin. Persistently elevated blood glucose levels foster cancer cell growth and insulin surges facilitate rapid proliferation of malignant cells very effectively. Elevated insulin levels rampantly stimulate overproduction of various growth factors like insulin-like growth factor which rapidly accelerates development of certain nasty cancers especially breast cancer and prostate cancer (Poti el al, 2017).

Insulin resistance ramps up fat storage remarkably fostering inflammation thereby furthering a cancer-promoting microenvironment in bodily tissues with aggressive rapidity. Ultra-processed foods significantly disrupt gut microbiome crucial for modulating severe inflammatory responses and supporting overall immune function . High sugar and fat content in ultraprocessed foods drastically alters balance of beneficial gut bacteria thereby promoting growth of rather pathogenic microbes fueling chronic inflammation. Research indicates a diet rife with ultra-processed edibles can precipitate rampant proliferation of Fusobacterium nucleatum bacteria linked to colorectal cancer onset. A disrupted microbiome may severely impair bodily ability to detoxify nasty carcinogens and DNA damage gets repaired poorly ratcheting up cancer risk further.

Ultra-processed foods harbour potentially carcinogenic compounds formed during processing or storage in fairly dodgy conditions and packaging is often lacklustre. Blistering heat during frying procedures unleashes ominously acrylamide a known potent carcinogen in starchy foods often subjected to such treatments. Nitrates and nitrites present in processed meat products such as bacon or sausages readily form carcinogenic compounds called nitrosamines inside human body. Compounds brutally ravage DNA fostering heinous mutations deep within stomach tissues or colon where cancerous transformations get triggered rather quickly. Eating ultra-processed foods triggers obscure biological responses that greatly amplify risk of developing certain cancers rather quietly over time (Kliemann et al, 2022).

Oxidative stress and insulin resistance conspire with gut microbiome disruption rapidly increasing cancer risk exposure to various carcinogenic compounds heightens this danger. Research slowly uncovers influence of ultra-processed foods on carcinogenesis and lowering their consumption significantly improves overall health markedly. Global cancer incidence could drastically decline with public health initiatives vigorously promoting consumption of whole foods processed barely at all industrially.

3.1. Inflammation and Cancer

Ultra-processed foods play significant role driving systemic inflammation within various bodily systems and chronic inflammation markedly fuels cancer progression. Consuming food rich in saturated fats refined carbs and sketchy additives tends to ignite pro-inflammatory pathways very deep inside human anatomy. Western diet loaded with ultra-processed food substantially boosts release of pro-inflammatory molecules like TNF-α and IL-6 alongside C-reactive protein promoting cancer. Ultra-processed foods trigger low-grade systemic inflammation directly impacting immune function badly through some dodgy mechanisms probably involving heaps of nasty biochemicals. Refined sugars and unhealthy fats lurking in ultra processed foods trigger immune cells recklessly producing pro-inflammatory cytokines (Tristan et al, 2023).

Cytokines wreak havoc on normal cellular function fairly aggressively thereby fueling tumour initiation and metastasis quite rapidly in some nasty cases. Foodby comestibles spawn low-level inflammation fostering milieu unusually conducive to proliferation of cancer cells and boosting odds of tumour cells evading immune surveillance. Ultra-processed foods trigger a substantial spike in reactive oxygen species nasty molecules that ravage cellular structures and DNA fairly badly. Reactive oxygen species wreak havoc on cellular genetic stuff thereby precipitating heinous mutations that massively amplify oncogenic potential suddenly. ROS accelerates cancer cell proliferation with high levels of pro-inflammatory cytokines by spurring angiogenesis which entails forming new blood vessels rapidly (Tristan et al, 2023).

Tumour growth accelerates rapidly getting blood supply that enables metastasis freely in other body parts with alarming swiftness. Ultra-processed foods severely hamper bodily immune response and foster inflammation rendering immune cells less adept at obliterating malignant cells rapidly. Mechanisms of the immune system usually lurk stealthily in background awaiting suspicious activity ruthlessly detecting and eliminating rogue cellular entities very swiftly. Frequent intake of ultraprocessed foods fuels inflammatory responses that drastically impair immune response weakening bodily defenses against cancerous tumour formation rather significantly. Pre-cancerous cells flourish rapidly while abnormal cells that would have normally been eliminated manage to survive under peculiar circumstances. Research robustly backs a linkage between ultra-processed food consumption and heightened inflammation risk and cancer development significantly nowadays.

Eating ultra-processed foods rampantly fosters DNA damage and fuels cellular proliferation thereby creating an environment eerily conducive to tumour growth. Ultra-processed foods consumption reduction could remarkably lower cancer risk worldwide and improve public health significantly in diverse populations.

3.2. Oxidative Stress and DNA Damage

Ultra-processed foods spawn cancer risk by triggering oxidative stress that fosters formation of free radicals and reactive oxygen species rather readily. Ultra-processed foods bursting with copious refined sugars and dodgy trans fats boost production of highly reactive free radicals ravaging cellular components mercilessly. Oxidative stress ravages cells very badly causing genomic instability a hallmark of cancerous cells and significantly fuels cancer progression. Metabolizing ultra-processed foods in body tissues quite rapidly spawns hordes of free radicals and reactive oxygen species fostering genomic instability. Reactive molecules ravage cell nuclei very badly and trigger mutations in genes that regulate vital processes such as cell growth and apoptosis. Genetic mutations spawned by oxidative damage impair cellular function rather haphazardly and unbridled cell proliferation eventually forms tumours fairly quickly (Sainz et al, 2012).

Free radicals and ROS are particularly pernicious because they ravage genetic material within cells resulting in mutations in tumour suppressor genes that drive cancer. Abnormal cells circumvent growth regulation haphazardly under disrupted genetic control becoming crucial very quickly in carcinogenic processes rather mysteriously. Oxidative stress may severely debilitate DNA repair mechanisms over time when damage persists extensively and becomes quite problematic . Prolonged consumption of ultra-processed foods induces oxidative stress that overwhelms body repair systems which normally fix damaged DNA eventually. DNA damage inflicted by UPFs may spiral out of control and mutated cells survive proliferating haphazardly beneath radar largely unnoticed subsequently. Mutation accumulation over time substantially contributes to genomic instability a hallmark feature typically found in various kinds of cancerous cells (Sainz et al, 2012).

Ultra-processed foods harbor numerous additives alongside sugars and fats that very significantly fuel oxidative stress in myriad bodily processes rather stealthily. Aspartame and other artificial sweeteners found in diet sodas and sugar-free products generate free radicals rapidly during metabolic breakdown apparently.

Preservatives and colorings in UPFs can rather quickly induce oxidative stress within diverse cellular milieus under very specific conditions. Additives may directly inflict DNA damage and rather quietly interact with bodily compounds exacerbating oxidative stress and surreptitiously promoting carcinogenesis. Eating ultra-processed foods rampantly fosters oxidative stress that substantially fuels cancer development in humans relatively quickly nowadays.

UPFs intensify free radical production thereby severely damaging DNA and fostering an environment of genomic instability that spurs rather anarchic tumour formation and cell proliferation. Additives sneaking into foods can crank oxidative stress way up thereby significantly escalating cancer risk down line very badly. Reducing consumption of highly processed foodstuffs very significantly curtails oxidative stress thereby furnishing a potent stratagem for lessening cancer risk and generally encourage overall wellbeing.

3.3. Insulin Resistance and Cancer Progression

Ultra-processed foods rather insidiously foster insulin resistance a very gnarly metabolic state deeply implicated in cancer's somewhat sinister progression. Ultra-processed foods are typically replete with refined sugars and rather low in fibre and loaded with very dodgy fats that spark rapid surges in blood glucose. Spikes trigger overproduction of insulin a hormone that helps regulate blood sugar and insulin-like growth factor 1 remarkably deep within various cellular structures. Elevated insulin and IGF-1 levels have been rather closely associated with heightened risk of various cancer types including breast prostate and some colorectal cancers. Diets comprising heavily processed foods mercilessly foster insulin resistance in most people over an extended period of time gradually (Nijenhuis-Noort et al, 2024).

Cells in body grow sluggishly responsive to insulin forcing pancreas and liver to release copious insulin frantically amidst chaotic glucose regulation efforts. Insulin levels surge and IGF-1 levels subsequently swell further vividly stimulating cell growth heavily while inhibiting apoptosis very thoroughly. Rampant cell proliferation alongside failure of damaged cell elimination typically occurs during tumour formation and growth in cancer progression stages. Insulin-driven signaling pathway fosters wildly proliferating cellular environments heavily promoting tumourigenesis in diverse bodily contexts. Excessive insulin saturates bloodstream precipitating chronic hyperinsulinemia and subsequently boosts bioavailability of IGF-1 very significantly almost always. Cell division accelerates rapidly in this cycle and damaged cells evade natural elimination normally staving off cancer progression further downstream (Nijenhuis-Noort et al, 2024).

Gorging daily on copious amounts of ultra processed junk foods greatly exacerbates insulin resistance wherein obesity plays a crucial underlying role. Obesity fosters chronic low-grade inflammation thereby exacerbating insulin resistance very badly over time in lots of people. Insulin resistance ramps up insulin production in body further hiking IGF-1 levels and speeding tumour progression at an alarming rate over time. Lackluster eating habits characterized by ultra processed victuals foster insulin resistance which ostensibly ups cancer risk markedly downstream. Tumour growth and metastasis get fueled largely through insulin resistance a mechanism underlying cancer progression from ultra-processed foods very frequently (Nijenhuis-Noort et al, 2024). Elevated insulin levels drastically stimulate cell growth and inhibit apoptosis in tumour development fairly significantly alongside surging IGF-1 levels. Consuming ultra-processed foods fosters obesity which markedly exacerbates insulin resistance fueling a vicious cycle that greatly heightens risk of cancer. Eating fewer ultra-processed foods remarkably improves public health outcomes and plays a crucial role in thwarting cancer development nationwide slowly.

3.4. Disruption of the Gut Microbiome

Human gut microbiome teems with bacteria and viruses and fungi and other microorganisms playing a very critical role in regulating immune responses vigorously. Heightened risk of various extremely heinous cancers occurs very frequently worldwide due to tenuous links with gut microbiome disruptions. Ultra-processed foods teeming with refined sugars and saturated fats drastically disrupt gut microbiota balance resulting in dysbiosis rather mysteriously. Dysbiosis denotes microbial community imbalance marked by proliferation of noxious bacteria and diminution of beneficial microbes remarkably quickly. Consumption of ultra-processed foods significantly disrupts gut microbiome thereby precipitating development of cancer particularly aggressive forms of colorectal cancer. Risk of cancer goes up very significantly with frequent intake of these kinds of foods. Malignancy emerges rather insidiously within a milieu of thoroughly dysregulated microbiome (Ogunrinola et al, 2020).

Colorectal cancer surfaces quite frequently under such harsh conditions often found in certain populations worldwide apparently every year. Disturbance within microbiome culpably occurs quite frequently under certain conditions and with noticeable consequences thereafter in many instances. Disrupted microbiome can spur production of really nasty compounds like bile acids and nitrosamines which are very carcinogenic stuff basically. Specific gut microbes degrade dietary compounds rapidly into toxic substances that ravage DNA and trigger oncogenic mutations with alarming swiftness. Dysbiosis severely impairs gut function in detoxifying nasty compounds and heightens overall cancer risk significantly over time in a rather insidious manner. Gut microbiome connects intricately with immune system and microbial population imbalance severely impairs body's ability to fight tumour cells very effectively (Ogunrinola et al, 2020).

Beneficial gut bacteria like Lactobacillus trigger activation of immune cells very rapidly which helps detect and eliminate cancerous cells fairly quickly. Fusobacterium nucleatum interacts very aggressively with tumour cells and fosters inflammation fueling rather cancerous growth quite directly in many cases. Dysbiosis-induced inflammation furthers cancer progression by heavily promoting tumour growth and metastasis and fostering formation of new blood vessels vigorously. Chronic inflammation often manifests in dysbiosis states creating tumour-friendly microenvironments that foster cancer cells thriving under fuzzy immune surveillance. Profoundly immune-modulatory properties of a healthy microbiome remarkably enhance cancer cell detection ability of immune system in this context. Disruptions can weaken immune responses significantly allowing tumours progress quickly unchecked in some very bad cases essentially without much resistance suddenly.

Interesting research findings suggest dietary tweaks may help recalibrate gut flora substantially lowering oncogenic risk according to some experts. Increasing fibre intake can support growth of beneficial bacteria producing short-chain fatty acids like butyrate which have anti-inflammatory properties quite effectively. Reducing consumption of heavily processed foods linked heavily to gut dysbiosis fosters a relatively healthier gut microbiome thereby significantly lowering risk of cancer. Ultra-processed foods brutally ravage gut flora and grossly debilitate immune response thereby fostering inflammation that turbocharges oncogenesis at an alarming rate. Consuming copious amounts of fibre while eschewing heavily processed garbage may substantially mitigate cancer risk stemming from gut bacteria imbalance.

3.5. Carcinogenic Compounds in Ultra-Processed Foods

Ultra-processed foods harbor a slew of pernicious compounds that very rapidly jack up risk of contracting certain very nasty cancers. Dubious compounds frequently emerge during food processing while others stealthily lurk within ingredients used in ultra-processed foods festering quietly. Research highlights key carcinogenic substances in ultra-processed foods which increase cancer likelihood very significantly through murky mechanisms often involving nasty free radicals. Processed meats such as sausages and bacon rank among rather perturbing examples frequently cited these days with unsettling regularity nowadays. Products contain nitrates or nitrite preservatives weirdly used rather effectively in some processing plants enhancing color noticeably. Very potent carcinogens form essentially during digestion as these compounds get converted into nitrosamines rather quickly. Nitrosamines have been linked tenuously rather alarmingly to heightened gastric cancer risk and occurrence of colorectal cancer in many cases (Kliemann et al, 2022).

Studies reveal a robust association exists between consuming processed meat products rapidly and markedly increased risk of developing specific notoriously pernicious cancers. Ultra-processed foods often harbour acrylamide a potentially deadly compound frequently lurking in fried snacks and rather dubious baked goods. Starchy foods like potatoes rapidly form this substance when cooked at scorching temperatures during deep frying or intense baking sessions. International Agency for Research on Cancer has deemed acrylamide possibly carcinogenic and it has been loosely associated with bladder and kidney cancers. Scorching temperatures trigger Maillard reaction in food producing acrylamide a rather insidious compound very harmfully thereby damaging bodily functions quite severely. Food packaging amplifies carcinogenic risks lurking ominously in ultra-processed food alongside dubious ingredients riddled heavily with nasty toxins (Kliemann et al, 2022).

Phthalates and bisphenol A seep into food from plastic wrapping slowly when subjected intensely to heat over time. Phthalates and BPA notoriously disrupt endocrine function wreaking havoc very badly on hormone regulation within bodily systems. Numerous studies have linked certain chemicals to increased risk of hormonally associated cancers such as prostate and breast cancer. Chemicals in packaging seep unobtrusively into bodily systems posing a stealthy menace silently over prolonged periods of exposure. Carcinogenic effects of ultra-processed foods stem partly from weird interactions not solely attributed to presence of nitrates or nasty chemicals like BPA. Rapid consumption of ultraprocessed foods markedly hastens cancer development through numerous convoluted pathological mechanisms underlying tumourigenesis (Bleak TC, Calaf et al, 2021).

Carcinogenesis thrives on oxidative stress and insulin resistance fuelled by chronic inflammation often greatly worsened by consuming ultra processed foods devoid of nutrients. Diets laden with ultra processed foods starkly exacerbate gut microbiome disruption thereby facilitating rapid development of cancer with alarming swiftness. Ultra-processed foods contribute cancer risk through multifaceted mechanisms intricately interconnected with sundry physiological processes rather insidiously within human bodies. Carcinogenic compounds like nitrosamines and acrylamide spark major concern and broader impact on inflammation heavily influences cancer progression gradually (Bleak TC, Calaf et al, 2021). Curbing consumption of ultra-processed foods effectively and promoting whole-food-based dietary habits rigorously mitigates cancer risk substantially in people generally. Mitigating cancer's public health burden substantially over a long period enhances health outcomes markedly thereby improving overall wellbeing significantly.

4. Dietary Patterns and Cancer

Diet plays a crucial role in prevention of various diseases and cancer progression stands out starkly as quite a prominent glaring example. Dietary patterns have shifted considerably over past few decades and a worrying trend manifests itself in widespread consumption of ultra-processed foods nowadays. Artificially concocted ultra-processed foods saturated with dodgy preservatives have remarkably surged in prevalence within modern eating habits nowadays globally. Rampant consumption of ultra processed edibles has precipitated alarm owing largely to dubious links with development of several chronic health issues including carcinoma. Ultra-processed foods tend be very nutritionally bankrupt harboring copious amounts of refined sugars and unhealthy fats alongside excessive sodium (Mittelman SD, 2020).

Conveniently packaged foods frequently lack beneficial compounds like antioxidants and phytochemicals present in whole foods that fiercely combat oxidative stress naturally. Engineered foods harbour cancer risk through various shady mechanisms owing largely to mass production and unnecessarily prolonged shelf life. Ultra-processed food consumption gets linked heavily to carcinogenesis and obesity via insulin resistance and chronic inflammation rather increasingly. Diseases frequently foreshadow cancer and foster an environment that readily allows tumour growth and metastasis deeply within bodily tissues (Mittelman SD, 2020).

Eating copious ultra-processed foods high in calories exacerbates obesity rather quickly and triggers overproduction of insulin and other crucial hormones. Refined sugars and saturated fats in ultra-processed foods foster systemic inflammation thereby accelerating various cancer initiations and progression very rapidly. Tissues get badly ravaged in environments fostering unbridled growth of cancer cells which evade immune surveillance and proliferate freely. Nitrates lingering ominously in cured meats and acrylamide fester quietly beneath surface of starchy foods crisped black by intense heat elevate cancer risk appreciably.

Regular consumption of certain compounds has been linked to DNA damage and promotion of mutations that heavily contribute to cancer development. Consumption of ultra-processed foods rises alarmingly nowadays sparking concerns over cancer risk and other far-reaching consequences on public health dramatically. Drastic dietary interventions promoting whole-food-based diets very strongly get underscored by evidence tenuously linking various cancers to ultra-processed foods. Understanding cancer-fueling mechanisms of UPFs effectively tackles global cancer burden and heightens health outcomes worldwide for numerous individuals substantially.

4.1. The Link Between Ultra-Processed Foods and Cancer Risk

Ultra-processed foods are surging in modern diets constituting a seismic shift in 21st century eating habits with far-reaching repercussions worldwide presently. Processed meats and packaged baked goods alongside sugar sweetened beverages have become daily staples particularly in industrialized nations with many instant meals readily available too. Processed foods abound rapidly in relatively impoverished regions and diet-related cancers surge there and in affluent nations simultaneously now. Numerous confounding mechanisms inside human bodies rapidly fuel carcinogenesis linking ultra-processed foods quite strongly with heightened cancer risk. Ultra-processed foods are remarkably low in vital nutrients like fibre and essential vitamins and minerals being very calorie-dense overall naturally. Nutrient imbalance fuels obesity becoming a well-established risk factor for various cancers including colorectal breast and endometrial cancer quite obviously (Elizabeth et al, 2020).

Obesity fuels chronic inflammation and insulin resistance thereby accelerating tumourigenesis substantially through some very significant alterations in various hormone levels. Ultra-processed foods are remarkably bereft of fibre a vital component quite crucial for promoting health of gut microbiome and gastrointestinal well-being. A fibre-rich diet shields against various cancers including colon and rectum cancers by fostering beneficial gut bacteria very effectively. Ultra-processed foods lacking sufficient fibre can instigate dysbiosis in gut very badly disrupting balance among microbes and fostering chronic inflammatory responses. Dubious artificial additives and wonky preservatives lurking in some ultra-processed foods apparently remain a pressing concern these days (Elizabeth et al, 2020).

Processed meats such as bacon harbour nitrates that transmogrify into very potent carcinogens dubbed nitrosamines upon digestion and strongly correlate with colorectal cancer. Compounds like acrylamide form rapidly when starchy foods are scorched at sizzling temperatures and they've been pegged as probable carcinogens by some researchers lately. Global consumption of ultra-processed foods rises steadily worldwide and obesity prevalence swells markedly with attendant dire metabolic disruptions heightening cancer risk.

Evidence suggests reliance on edibles fuels global cancer rates prompting calls for interventions that foster somewhat healthier eating habits urgently nowadays.

4.2. Dietary Patterns and Cancer Development: Obesity and Metabolic Syndrome

Ultra-processed foods heavily fuel cancer development through highly abnormal biochemical pathways largely by fostering obesity and metabolic syndrome. Rare cancers like endometrial cancer and breast cancer have long been associated with obesity which poses a major risk factor. Consumption of ultra-processed foods ridiculously high in calories and refined sugars yet woefully low in fibre significantly fosters weight gain and insulin resistance fueling cancer onset rather ominously. Obesity fuels cancer growth in myriad mysterious ways often through insidious mechanisms deeply rooted within various bodily systems and physiological processes. Adipose tissue releases pro-inflammatory cytokines like TNF-α and IL-6 functioning somewhat mysteriously as an endocrine organ rather than just storing energy. Molecules with inflammatory properties fuel cancer growth quite markedly by fostering low-grade inflammation that persists chronically (Anastasiou et al, 2025).

Cancer cells proliferate rapidly under these circumstances and tumour growth is fostered in inflammatory conditions that facilitate metastasis quite freely. Chronic inflammation fosters an environment teeming with genomic mutations that accumulate rapidly and fuel cancer development further downstream. Insulin resistance plays a critical role in cancer progression and manifests fairly often amidst obesity-related pathological transformations nowadays under various conditions. Body stubbornly resists insulin and compensates by excessively ramping up insulin production leading rapidly to hyperinsulinemia. Elevated IGF-1 levels frequently manifest in obese individuals and get linked with rampant cell proliferation and rather suppressed apoptosis. Cancer cells proliferate frenetically surviving remarkably longer than anticipated owing largely to aberrant changes facilitating evasion of normative apoptotic pathways (Anastasiou et al, 2025).

Obesity triggers chronic inflammation that disrupts normal immune response quite insidiously and rather frequently in bodily systems. Molecules causing inflammation often severely cripple cancer cell detection ability of immune system rather rapidly in numerous cases. Malignant cells swiftly evade immune detection and proliferate into sizable tumours at an alarmingly fast rate under various circumstances. Obesity triggers inflammatory pathways heavily implicated in development of several cancers including colorectal cancer and surprisingly pancreatic cancer rather mysteriously. Ultra-processed foods foster pro-inflammatory environments rather heavily in bodily systems ultimately contributing to nasty cancer development over time. Consumption of such foods precipitates metabolic turmoil thereby increasing risk of obesity-linked cancers and undermining innate mechanisms for tumour suppression quite vigorously.

4.3. The Gut Microbiome

Trillions of microorganisms including bacteria and fungi reside in gut microbiome playing a pivotal role in overall health maintenance silently. Microbes effectively facilitate regulation of immune response and absorb nutrients fairly well maintaining integrity of intestinal lining very simultaneously. A diverse microbiome protects surprisingly effectively against various cancers including colorectal cancer and gastric cancer in many instances quite remarkably. Growing consumption of ultra-processed foodstuffs loaded with weird additives and saturated fats royally messes up that delicate bodily ecosystem quite thoroughly. Dysbiosis emerges from disruption wherein balance between beneficial microbes and harmful ones gets severely disturbed under fairly calamitous conditions. Dysbiosis emerges with pathogenic bacteria proliferating rapidly alongside a sharp drop in beneficial microbes crucial for maintaining gut health (Colella et al, 2023).

Dysregulation of gut microbiota profoundly unsettlingly affects cancer risk alarmingly downstream amid complex physiological processes rather insidiously. Bacterial overgrowth spawns nasty inflammation in gut lining and leaky gut syndrome enabling very noxious substances surreptitiously into bloodstream through permeable gut walls. Gut integrity disruptions spur production of carcinogenic metabolites like bile acids and nitrosamines fueling cancer development particularly in colon cancer. Ultra-processed foods contain staggeringly high amounts of sugar and fat nowadays which greatly exacerbates problems. Such diets cultivate an environment rife with inflammatory bacteria that release toxins and sundry noxious metabolic byproducts that rather severely damage intestinal lining (Colella et al, 2023).

Damage fosters development of DNA mutations rapidly in intestinal tract cells potentially leading to fairly quick cancerous growth afterwards. Tumour cells evade detection rather easily when bodily immune surveillance gets severely impaired by an imbalanced microbiome remarkably. Consumption of ultra-processed foods drastically alters gut microbiome nowadays fostering production of carcinogenic compounds and ramping up inflammation significantly in various ways. Sizable changes foster development of gastrointestinal cancers and greatly impair bodily ability against various tumours rather effectively nowadays in some cases. Consuming copious amounts of whole foods rich in nutrients fosters robust gut flora thereby lowering cancer risk very significantly over time.

4.4. Carcinogenic Compounds in Ultra-Processed Foods

Ultra-processed foods harbour myriad carcinogenic compounds that foster cancer development directly in many unsuspecting individuals very insidiously over time. Dubious chemicals and nasty toxins lurk frequently in processed foods posing significant risks nearly always for human well-being. Processed meats such as bacon sausages and hot dogs often contain rather alarming quantities of nitrates and nitrites very frequently. Compounds get converted into nitrosamines deep inside human bodies subsequently morphing into extremely potent carcinogens over time rather slowly. Nitrosamines aggressively foster cancerous cell formation in colon thereby heightening colorectal cancer risk by damaging DNA quite rapidly. Acrylamide forms in starchy foods like potatoes and cereals when cooked at scorching temperatures typically by deep frying or radiant baking (Isaksen IM, Dankel, 2023).

International Agency for Research on Cancer deemed acrylamide a probable human carcinogen in some rather alarming research findings very recently. It often lurks in food like crunchy potato chips and sweet baked goodies beneath layers of salty flavorful toppings. Research suggests acrylamide quite readily sparks DNA damage and mainly fosters cancerous growth inside gastrointestinal tract and various digestive organs. Ultra-processed foods packaging frequently involves chemicals such as bisphenol A that can leach into food under certain conditions quite readily. BPA acts very erratically as an endocrine disruptor severely messing with hormonal systems in various physiological processes very badly nowadays. Prolonged exposure linking BPA has been observed quite alarmingly in hormone-related cancers including breast cancer risk and prostate cancer risk very significantly (Isaksen IM, Dankel, 2023).

Pervasive BPA use in plastic packaging poses significant concern as tiny amounts accumulate slowly inside human bodies over surprisingly lengthy periods. Rising incidence of diet-related cancers correlates very strongly with growing global consumption of ultra-processed foods in diverse populations rapidly nowadays. Obesity promotion and introduction of carcinogenic compounds into diet suddenly facilitate cancer development from certain foods and nasty culinary habits. Consumption of ultra-processed foods frequently results in drastic weight gain and obesity remains a prominent risk factor for various cancer types. Eating whole nutrient-dense foods like fruits substantially reduces cancer risk while minimizing ultra-processed foods greatly benefits overall health. Nutritional education initiatives significantly heighten awareness about detrimental dietary habits and foster relatively healthier eating patterns by revamping food labels effectively nationwide. Public health gets a substantial boost from slashing intake of heavily processed edibles thereby gradually gathering steam in cancer prevention endeavors nationwide.

5. Chemical Additives and Cancer

Ultra-processed foods and processed food now rule global markets affordably largely owing to remarkable convenience and very long shelf lives. Extensive use of chemical additives like preservatives and colorants has become an integral part of food production globally nowadays. Concerns emerge rapidly about their potential role in cancer development and other chronic diseases owing largely to various dubious additives. Regulatory bodies such as FDA and European Food Safety Authority deem chemical additives like artificial sweeteners and synthetic colors sufficiently safe. Organizations nowadays approve substances based on brief somewhat rigorous studies evaluating direct health impacts of additives on humans fairly regularly. A plethora of scientific evidence now indicates regularly consuming highly processed foods laced with such additives can have very detrimental long-term health effects. Biological mechanisms underlying cancer development from certain substances remain somewhat opaque but research indicates additives could drastically disrupt normal cellular functions quietly (Adams et al, 2020).

Aspartame and saccharin these artificial sweeteners fall under a category of additives scrutinized intensely lately by various health experts. Research on animal subjects links sugar-free products with heightened cancer risk especially in brain and bladder tissues somewhat surprisingly. Human studies haven't definitively confirmed these findings yet controversy persists owing largely to their presence in myriad modern consumer goods. Sodium nitrite and potassium nitrate frequently used in processed meats have been linked rather mysteriously to elevated cancer risk. Consumption of such additives can lead formation of nitrosamines potent carcinogens associated with elevated risk of various cancers including gastric cancer. Nitrosamines form under acidic conditions like during digestion or cooking at scorching temperatures and accumulate in bodily tissues quite slowly (Adams et al, 2020).

Preservatives interact haphazardly with human biology nowadays posing a growing public health concern rather alarmingly in various unexpected ways. Artificial food colorants like Red 40 and Yellow 5 are used frequently nowadays in candies baked goods and many soft drinks. Studies indicate certain artificial colourings may damage DNA fairly significantly and disrupt normal cell functions thereby heightening risk of cancer over time substantially. Numerous studies vociferously demand stricter regulations on levels presently used in sundry foodstuffs and fairly thorough safety assessments are being called for. Processed foods nowadays frequently utilize emulsifiers like carboxymethylcellulose or polysorbate 80 for enhancing overall consistency and texture quite remarkably.

Emerging research has linked long-term exposure quite alarmingly with inflammation fueling development of colorectal cancer and gut microbiome disturbances. Heightened public awareness of risks associated with consuming processed foods containing chemical additives desperately needs reevaluation of current food safety regulations now. Extensive research focusing on cumulative effects of multiple additives in cancer development sorely needs clearer insights very quickly these days. Consumers should prioritize whole foods that are largely unprocessed and stay very vigilant about lurking risks in their daily diets..

5.1. Chemical Additives in Processed Foods

Chemical additives crucially enable modern food production yielding enhanced shelf life and rather obscurely improved flavor profiles very naturally. Sneaky additives lurk in a vast array of food including fizzy drinks and snacks and tinned foods and baked goods and dairy products. These substances render food remarkably palatable and sufficiently stable for human consumption very darn effectively under various environmental conditions. Stringent safety evaluations by bodies such as Food and Drug Administration and European Food Safety Authority utterly fail to mitigate escalating apprehensions regarding protracted health impacts upon excessive consumption. Sundry additives stealthily present in processed edibles get slotted into diverse categories fulfilling some mystifying role and enormously boosting food product . Preservatives are basically weird chemicals that stifle microbial growth within packaged edibles and prolong shelf life of various food products dramatically.

Preservatives like sodium nitrate benzoates and sulfites are commonly found nowadays in many products especially some quite obscure food items. Additives help stave off spoilage from bacteria mold and yeast thus keeping food remarkably fresh for fairly long odd durations subsequently. Preservatives like nitrates and nitrites react vigorously with various stomach compounds forming potentially carcinogenic nitrosamines linked heavily to colorectal cancer risk. Very much sugar-free sweetness lurks in various products thanks largely to chemicals such as sucralose and saccharin and aspartame. Sugar-free beverages and candies typically contain sweeteners often used nowadays in various processed food products generally found everywhere. High levels of long-term exposure remain rather contentious despite plethora of studies suggesting such sweeteners are ostensibly safe in ordinarily consumed food products daily. Artificial sweeteners possibly linked ominously to various cancers, notably malignancies rather rampantly affecting bladder in some animal studies (Sambu et al, 2022).

Synthetic dyes like Red 40 and Yellow 5 get added liberally to processed foods making them look rather visually appealing very much instantly. Additives frequently replicate vibrant unnatural hues found in processed snacks and sweet treats normally occurring rather infrequently in nature. Daily consumption of dubious coloring agents sparks growing unease about potential allergic reactions and weird behavioral changes in kids very sensitive. Certain dyes such as Red 40 or Yellow 5 have been dubbed putative carcinogens in murine studies highlighting heightened oncogenic potential. Monosodium glutamate or MSG rather effectively heightens savory flavors in processed foods and remains a notoriously well-known flavor enhancer. MSG often gets slipped into frozen dinners and savory snacks very frequently nowadays in many different products. Excessive MSG consumption possibly precipitates nasty health issues like headaches and obesity thereby potentially inducing neurotoxicity with utterly baffling consequences. Scientific research hasn't conclusively proven a direct link between MSG and cancer yet findings on the matter remain fairly inconclusive still (Sambu et al, 2022).

Lecithin and polysorbates are emulsifiers that maintain texture somewhat erratically in processed foods by halting separation of water and fat. Margarine and baked goods frequently contain them alongside salad dressings these days in many different products very regularly. Evidence emerging slowly suggests certain emulsifiers disrupt gut health over time leading inexorably to chronic inflammation a risk factor notoriously for colorectal cancer. Research increasing nowadays scrutinizes lingering effects of such additives in comestibles raising alarm about their deleterious aggregate impact on human well-being significantly. Chemicals get ingested together frequently over fairly long periods with collective effects not being entirely understood by researchers these days often . Studying long-term implications of chemical additives in diet remains vital for protecting public health amidst a rising tide of chronic diseases. Consumers are urged meanwhile be super mindful of processed food they eat opting for whole foods barely tampered with daily.

5.2. Preservatives and Their Potential Carcinogenic Effects

Preservatives play crucial roles rather safely in extending shelf life of processed foods by effectively thwarting microbial growth and maintaining product quality. Chemicals pop up fairly regularly in various food including bizarre meat snacks and some rather delectable baked goods nowadays. Growing concern surrounds potentially carcinogenic risks associated with preservative substances used markedly to reduce spoilage and foodborne illness. Several preservatives have been researched thoroughly in relation to cancer showing evidence of carcinogenic effects under fairly unusual experimental conditions. Sodium nitrate and sodium nitrite frequently preserve processed meats such as bacon sausages hot dogs and many deli meats very effectively nowadays. Compounds get added haphazardly to maintain vibrant color and boost flavor while thwarting nasty bacterial growth such as Clostridium botulinum that causes debilitating botulism. Searing heat during grilling or frying can very rapidly morph nitrates and nitrites into rather carcinogenic nitrosamines under some wonky conditions (Teshome et al, 2022).

Nitrosamines represent an extremely carcinogenic category of compounds notoriously exhibiting significant health hazards in diverse animal studies obviously. Studies show consuming nitrite-preserved meats greatly heightens risk of various gastrointestinal malignancies including colorectal cancer and stomach cancer rather alarmingly. Processed meats laced with nitrates and nitrites were classified as Group 1 carcinogens by International Agency for Research on Cancer under WHO umbrella. Evidence conclusively links specific substances quite ominously to human cancer thereby warranting such a dire classification mercifully. Risk arises ostensibly from nitrosamines muddling normal cellular activity thereby inducing freaky mutations in DNA that foster cancer development subsequently in affected tissues (Teshome et al, 2022).

Risk associated with sodium nitrate and nitrites is especially perturbing because these preservatives saturate commonly eaten chow and their cumulative exposure over time rather alarmingly exacerbates long-term health issues. People looking for lower cancer risk nowadays are advised reducing intake of processed red meats or opting for nitrate-free alternatives very much entirely. Butylated hydroxyanisole aka BHA and butylated hydroxytoluene or BHT are synthetic antioxidants frequently added in processed foods preventing fat oxidation rapidly. Preservatives lurk surreptitiously in processed edibles like baked goods or salty snacks and meats served at breakfast gatherings frequently. They effectively prevent rancidity thereby ensuring freshness and maintaining flavor of food products with varying texture very successfully. Safety concerns surrounding BHA and BHT have sporadically emerged largely due to potentially nasty carcinogenic effects ominously lurking in dark shadows.

High doses of such compounds can induce tumour formation mostly in liver and lungs of previously studied animal models under various conditions. Evidence ominously suggests BHA disrupts endocrine systems rather alarmingly leading to hormonal imbalances and heightened risk of hormone-related cancers such as prostate cancer. Human studies have raised alarm about potentially pernicious long-term sequelae of ingesting sizable amounts of BHA and BHT on a fairly regular basis. U rather quietly existed beneath layers of obscurity. S sounds very sketchy. National Toxicology Program lists BHA as possible human carcinogen whereas IARC categorizes it as Group 2B carcinogen possibly causing cancer in humans. BHT has relatively lower carcinogenic risk compared to BHA yet both are often used together in various processed foods heightening potential risk over time. Nowadays consumers might think twice about ditching products containing BHA and BHT which are rife in all sorts of processed food (Teshome et al, 2022).

Choosing products with natural preservatives such as vitamin E or ascorbic acid may provide somewhat safer alternatives very naturally. Preservatives such as sodium nitrate or BHT serve crucial functions in food industry by preventing spoilage yet potential carcinogenic effects loom large ominously. A plethora of emerging evidence links certain additives rather alarmingly significantly and disturbingly with various forms of cancer raising sundry health concerns. Consumers must be informed about dubious additives stealthily lurking in processed food products and make consciously healthy decisions rather haphazardly. Eating nutrient-rich whole foods and cutting back on heavily processed meats remarkably boosts overall well-being and significantly lowers risk of cancer.

5.3. Artificial Sweeteners and Their Controversial Role in Cancer

Artificial sweeteners are utilized copiously in processed comestibles and potables as sugar substitute proffering sweetness with negligible caloric accretion. Folks keen on slimming down or regulating blood sugar levels have rapidly taken to drastically cutting down on sugar consumption. Such sugar substitutes remain swathed in controversy largely due fairly recently alleged potentially carcinogenic effects on humans. Many studies now indicate potentially dire long-term health consequences from ingesting artificial sweeteners especially with respect to cancer development possibility. Aspartame lingers ubiquitously in sundry sugar-free treats such as diet sodas and artificially sweetened desserts remarkably often these days. Much sweeter than sugar roughly 200 times it gets used extremely sparingly in ridiculously minute quantities with tremendous efficacy often. Aspartame has been subject of intense scrutiny quietly over many years (Sharma et al, 2016).

Regulatory bodies like FDA and World Health Organization have concluded after reviewing extensive studies on aspartame's safety that it remains safe for human consumption. Fears linger regarding carcinogenic potential amidst much fanfare from high-profile backers lately. Several animal studies hint at a possible connection between prolonged aspartame intake and onset of lymphomas leukemia and assorted brain tumours fairly surreptitiously. Research settings often involve unusually high aspartame dosages that greatly surpass typical human intake levels in myriad experimental configurations. Some very compelling findings have emerged yet results in humans remain rather inconclusive with big epidemiological studies failing utterly to show a definitive link between aspartame and various cancers. National Cancer Institute claims available human studies have failed utterly to yield convincing evidence linking aspartame directly to cancer formation (Sharma et al, 2016).

Mixed results have sparked fervent controversy among experts urgently calling for further investigations into potentially deleterious effects of aspartame on human health longterm. Saccharin has had a checkered past being one old artificial sweetener with controversy swirling around it quite vigorously indeed nowadays. Studies highly publicized ominously linked saccharin with bladder cancer in 1970s sparking rather vociferous alarms involving rats raised under various conditions. Large amounts of saccharin fed mostly to rats resulted in bladder tumours forming and subsequently got banned temporarily in several nations. Further studies revealed saccharin causes cancer in rats through a mechanism oddly entangled with rodent physiology irrelevant very much entirely for humans. Saccharin got reclassified as a Group 2B carcinogen by IARC around same time FDA lifted its ban in 2000 on fairly scant evidence. Saccharin remains embroiled in controversy still years after its ban was lifted amidst considerable fanfare and vociferous public outcry (Doueihy et al, 2025).

Long-term saccharin consumption may potentially disrupt endocrine function somewhat despite humans showing fairly weak evidence of being carcinogenic. Such effects may wildly disrupt hormone balance spiraling into severe metabolic problems or other egregious maladies down line very badly. Saccharin remains somewhat dubious regarding long-term health impact especially when consumed recklessly in bucketloads over ridiculously prolonged durations. Sucralose and acesulfame potassium face intense scrutiny over potentially carcinogenic effects despite scant research having been conducted on these substances. Safety concerns surrounding such substances stem largely from animal studies where doses administered far exceed typical human consumption levels greatly (Doueihy et al, 2025).

Artificial sweeteners remain a confounding factor in cancer risk assessments nowadays yielding largely inconclusive results across various human population studies still. Profoundly more rigorous investigation into potentially pernicious health impacts of artificial sweeteners becomes necessary due to growing concerns fueled by disparate findings. Research investigating cumulative impacts of sweeteners on populations heavily reliant on them battling obesity or managing conditions such as diabetes is urgently needed. Rigorous studies are necessary rather urgently for thoroughly comprehending risks posed by such substances on human health particularly regarding cancerous developments.

5.4. Coloring Agents and Their Carcinogenic Potential

Artificial colouring agents curiously enhance visual appeal in processed foods and beverages thereby attracting consumers very effectively nowadays. Vibrant hues get liberally sprinkled onto diverse edibles including candies sodas baked goods and dairy products echoing tints of freshly prepared fare. Concerns about safety of food additives have emerged sporadically over years mainly regarding potential links to increased cancer risk in humans. Some synthetic chemicals and coal tar derivatives suspected of being very toxic are possibly quite carcinogenic in nature nowadays. Red 40 and Caramel Color have faced intense scrutiny in numerous studies for possibly being carcinogenic with some alarming results surfacing recently. Red 40 and Yellow 5 are found alongside Blue 1 in myriad candies beverages processed snacks and some pharmaceuticals quite ubiquitously. Experts at various regulatory agencies worldwide hotly debate potential health risks linked to such dyes particularly with respect to cancer (Varghese and Ramamoorthy, 2023).

Red 40 also known as Allura Red has undergone quite extensive research recently for sundry potential health risks apparently in humans. Some animal studies murkily suggest links between Red 40 and cancers like brain tumours and leukemia popping up fairly frequently in test subjects. Evidence suggests Red 40 may be culpable in hyperactivity and behavioral changes in kids particularly sensitive ones under some very specific circumstances. Concerns persist about cumulative effects of Red 40 when consumed regularly over quite a long period particularly alongside other artificial food additives. Tartrazine or Yellow 5 has sparked controversy very much everywhere surrounding several knotty issues for quite some considerable time now. Research sparks worries regarding possible hyperactivity links and kids' behavioral issues especially at dosages commonly found in edibles nowadays. Evidence exists suggesting long-term exposure has very bad carcinogenic effects on colorectal cancer from ingesting Yellow 5 dye (Varghese and Ramamoorthy, 2023).

High doses of Tartrazine probably induce tumours in certain animal studies but mechanisms behind these occurrences remain rather inexplicably shrouded in deep mystery. Yellow 5 gets a nod of safety generally but murky potential long-term repercussions on human health linger ominously with copious consumption. Blue 1 another oft utilized artificial dye has been incriminated very thoroughly overseas in various animal studies probing potentially carcinogenic effects. Certain studies imply Blue 1 potentially worsens leukemia risk and spawns brain tumours in lab animals under extremely high dosage regimens. Human studies have failed miserably to provide definitive evidence of a direct link with cancer but results remain largely inconclusive still. Blue 1 stays allowed in food at controlled amounts with very much no proof it poses huge cancer risk ordinarily (Varghese and Ramamoorthy, 2023).

Artificial colorings accumulating over time pose questions regarding lengthy impact on human well-being particularly amongst youngsters gorging heavily on daily processed foods. Scientists vehemently call for rigorous studies probing putative connections between synthetic dyes and malignancies under lengthy low-level exposure scenarios. Caramel color stays hugely popular nowadays in sodas and baked goods and boozy beverages and sauces fairly frequently. Heating sugar with alkaline chemicals spawns various compounds like 4-Methylimidazole via a multifaceted reaction process under certain conditions naturally. Caramel color is generally regarded safe yet 4-MEI formation raises concerns due to potential carcinogenic effects in various food products nowadays. California Environmental Protection Agency labels 4-MEI a known carcinogen and sets limits on its presence in foodstuffs. Dark beverages like colas often contain this chemical that gets brown color from caramel coloring primarily in most formulations nowadays.

5.5. Emulsifiers and Their Role in Cancer Development

Emulsifiers frequently pop up in processed nosh augmenting texture and staving off segregation of oil and H2O thereby ensuring a consistent appearance throughout shelf life. Polysorbates and lecithin show up heavily in baked goods and very frequently in processed snacks or occasionally in ice cream. Research lately raised red flags about impact of certain emulsifiers on human health particularly in relation to various nasty forms of cancer. Evidence mounting rapidly suggests certain emulsifiers disrupt gut microbiome very badly leading inflammation in intestines and heightening risk of developing colorectal cancer. Polysorbates like Polysorbate 80 and carboxymethylcellulose or CMC are commonly found in processed foods consumed daily by many people. Additives like these very effectively help stave off separation of ingredients in products such as dodgy salad dressings and fancy ice cream sauces (Partridge et al, 2019).

Studies reveal specific emulsifiers drastically alter microbial environment in gut resulting in condition known as gut dysbiosis fairly recently. Gut dysbiosis fosters precariously skewed microbiota wherein malignant microbes proliferate rapidly whilst beneficial microbial entities dwindle markedly within. Disruption quite frequently triggers inflammation in intestines a risk factor for various nasty diseases including IBD and colorectal cancer. Polysorbate 80 and CMC promote intestinal inflammation significantly by drastically altering gut bacteria composition in various animal studies apparently. Toxins seep rather suddenly into bloodstream from badly compromised intestinal barrier triggering a fierce inflammatory response deep inside quietly. Colorectal cancer emerges slowly from chronic inflammation often over rather lengthy periods. Research indicates emulsifiers trigger gut inflammation thereby markedly boosting reactive oxygen species production and oxidative stress that severely damages DNA (Partridge et al, 2019).

Oxidative stress coupled with gut dysbiosis rather quickly fosters growth of cancerous cells in rectum and colon through some obscure indirect pathway. Ulcerative colitis and Crohn's disease which are types of inflammatory bowel diseases significantly boost risk of colorectal cancer due largely to chronic intestinal inflammation. Certain emulsifiers like polysorbates or CMC potentially exacerbate inflammation very significantly thereby accelerating progression of intestinal bowel disease fairly rapidly. Emulsifier consumption might worsen disease severity substantially over time in individuals predisposed to gastrointestinal maladies heightening cancer risk very significantly. Research indicates gut microbiota plays a crucial role in modulating various immune responses quite heavily alongside levels of inflammation fairly significantly. A balanced microbiome remarkably enhance resistance against various pathogens and fosters intestinal barrier integrity quite effectively inside human hosts (Pratt et al, 2021).

Emulsifiers may undermine bodily ability to regulate inflammation and foster cancerous cell growth remarkably well in quite a favorable environment. Evidence sporadically mounting implicates certain emulsifiers in development of colorectal cancer underscoring need for scrutiny of various chemical additives in processed food products. Preservatives and artificial sweeteners play crucial roles nowadays in greatly enhancing taste appearance and shelf life of processed foods very significantly. Long-term consumption of such substances especially in vast amounts may quietly exert detrimental effects on human health gradually over prolonged periods. Gut dysbiosis and chronic inflammation triggered by food additives ostensibly facilitate carcinogenesis via mechanisms involving DNA damage and heightened oxidative stress. Cancer prevalence surges globally with colorectal cancer reaching epidemic proportions so consumers and regulatory bodies must heed findings with utmost gravity (Pratt et al, 2021).

Regulatory agencies like FDA and EFSA often deem food additives safe at approved consumption levels but cumulative effects remain woefully under-studied over surprisingly long periods. Further investigation now appears utterly necessary for grasping long-term hazards linked with myriad chemical additives and deciphering their obscure role in fostering maladies like cancer. Mounting research on cumulative effects of various food additives vehemently calls for re-evaluation of current food safety standards nowadays very extensively. Food additives must undergo very stringent safety testing assessing their potentially deleterious impact on human health quite significantly over long periods.

6. Nutritional Consequences of Ultra-Processed Diets

Ultra-processed foods consumption surges rapidly nowadays raising huge public health concerns amidst stark changes in modern dietary habits very quickly. Ultra-processed foods made with industrial techniques frequently harbour copious refined sugars unhealthy fats dubious protein sources and heaps of artificial additives. Nutritional consequences can significantly impair health and elevate cancer risk very readily despite convenience and fairly tasty offerings. Ultra-processed foods frequently pack ridiculously high calorie counts but often remain shockingly low in essential nutrients altogether surprisingly. Foods plentiful in calories abound copiously supplying energy yet lacking vital nutrients and fibre substantially in most such edible items. Nutrient deficiencies and poor metabolic health often stem from such an imbalance fostering chronic diseases like cancer rather frequently these days (Shim JS, 2025).

Diets high in refined sugars and unhealthy fats including trans and saturated fats are alarmingly concerning these days very much everywhere nowadays. Obesity and insulin resistance alongside chronic inflammation are known risk factors that cause breast cancer and colorectal cancer quite frequently. Low-quality proteins prevalent in UPFs alongside woefully inadequate dietary fibre badly compromise gut health thereby markedly heightening risk of colorectal cancer. Ultra processed foods ravage metabolic wellbeing rather catastrophically fostering nasty conditions like metabolic syndrome manifested as obesity high blood pressure and dyslipidemia. Various physiological conditions normally heighten risk of liver and breast cancers significantly and endometrial cancer under abnormal bodily states (Shim JS, 2025).

Ultra-processed foods harbour endocrine disruptors such as phthalates and bisphenol-A often lurking in packaging that messes with hormone regulation thereby significantly raising cancer risk. Ultra-processed foods are rather strongly linked with chronic inflammation and oxidative stress both of which play a critical role in cancer development . Many UPFs contain heinous artificial additives or dubious preservatives that spark intense inflammation deep in bodily tissues rather suddenly. Oxidative stress triggers DNA damage crucial for cancer initiation while inflammation fuels tumour growth and metastasis with alarming rapidity. Mounting evidence rather alarmingly links consumption of ultraprocessed foods quite directly to various kinds of cancer prompting drastic changes in dietary habits nowadays. Focusing on whole grains lean proteins and plenty of fruits and vegetables rather than UPF remarkably lowers cancer risk improving metabolic health significantly. Consuming predominantly plant-based food packed with antioxidant and anti-inflammatory properties can very effectively shield against cancer these days. People ditch ultra-processed food entirely for stellar nutrition and drastically lower cancer risk thereby boosting overall health remarkably.

6.1. The Nutritional Profile of Ultra-Processed Foods

Ultra-processed foods dominate modern diets harbouring a glaringly poor nutritional profile that royally messes with overall bodily functions so badly. Foods like these often lack vital nutrients such as fibre and antioxidants needed for maintaining cellular health and preventing cancer rather naturally nowadays. Ultra-processed foods are rife with copious amounts of refined sugars and trans fats and saturated fats alongside sodium fuelling metabolic maladies namely obesity and type 2 diabetes. A single assertion merely exists quietly underneath. Refined sugars and carbohydrates are liberally sprinkled in UPFs severely skewing nutritional profile with odious additions like saccharine high-fructose corn syrup. Sugars quickly spike blood glucose levels thereby vigorously promoting insulin production and fairly rapid release of IGF-1 in response. Hormones very vigorously stimulate cellular proliferation and stifle cell death thereby potentially leading unchecked cell division and tumour progression both hallmarks of cancer (Elizabeth et al, 2020).

Frequent ingestion of sucrose fosters insulin resistance intricately tied obesity and emergence of sundry metabolic disorders heightening risk of contracting various neoplasms especially colorectal carcinoma and breast cancer. Ultra-processed foods frequently harbour artificially created trans fats during processing which have chronic links to obesity and various cardiovascular maladies. Trans fats sabotage cell signaling rather aggressively fostering tumourigenic microenvironments inside bodily tissues and promote cancer cell proliferation quite energetically. Saturated fats abundant in numerous ultra-processed foods disrupt lipid metabolism very severely thereby heightening risk of various cancers of digestive system. Fats link strongly with metabolic diseases that worsen cancer risk via inflammation and develop strong insulin resistance gradually over long periods (Elizabeth et al, 2020).

Fibre crucially regulates various metabolic processes very effectively thwarting gastrointestinal malignancies including rather nasty colorectal cancer in gut health . Ultra-processed foods typically contain little fibre naturally or virtually none at all in most cases obviously. Inside intestines very intensely inflammation gets triggered largely due to absence of sufficient fibre negatively affecting gut microbiome badly. Chronic inflammation silently ravages gastrointestinal tracts nowadays fostering a milieu ostensibly very ripe for development of colorectal cancer fairly quickly. Fibre binds carcinogenic compounds remarkably tightly and fosters regular bowel movements subsequently underscoring its importance in cancer prevention very effectively. Ultra-processed foods harbor dubious chemical additives like saccharin and tartrazine that augment flavor rather prolifically and protract shelf life somewhat.

Additives like these may somewhat disrupt normal cellular functions while rather quietly helping with convenience in various everyday situations. Processed meats containing nitrates and nitrites very readily morph into carcinogenic nitrosamines when seared at extremely high temperatures fueling cancer growth vigorously. Artificial sweeteners such as aspartame have been tied up with endocrine disruption and Red 40 allegedly heightens leukemia risk in animal test subjects. Ultra-processed foods harbour nasty stuff like refined sugars and unhealthy fats alongside bogus additives rather surprisingly lacking essential nutrients. Certain dietary constituents markedly exacerbate obesity and insulin resistance thereby significantly heightening inflammation and metabolic derangement which elevates cancer risk substantially. Radical dietary overhauls focused on wholesome nutrient-dense comestibles are necessitated by chronic ailments exacerbated substantially by ultra-processed edibles.

6.2. Obesity and Cancer Risk: The Role of Ultra-Processed Diets

Eating ultra-processed foods correlates strongly with obesity becoming major risk factor for several cancer types rather alarmingly nowadays. People often wolf down heaps of vacuous calories because ultra-processed foods are frequently obscenely high in energy yet weirdly bereft of nutrients. Excessive weight gain occurs due to caloric imbalance thereby heightening cancer risk through multiple convoluted pathways involving various serious physiological derangements subsequently. One appears first very much always. Obesity very much everywhere in body induces state of chronic low-grade inflammation with seriously debilitating consequences often manifesting quite severely. Hormones secreted copiously by fat cells namely adipokines and pro-inflammatory cytokines surge markedly in this quite unusual pathological state. Ravaging brutally healthy tissues fosters cancer development quietly in a decidedly conducive environment. TNF-α and IL-6 inflammatory markers play crucial roles in rapidly forming new blood vessels essential for tumour growth underneath tissues (Poti et al, 2017).

Chronic inflammation fosters an environment that quite aggressively supports initiation and progression of various cancers including colorectal breast and liver cancer.. Visceral fat accumulates haphazardly around vital organs and fosters chaos hormonally thereby significantly amplifying cancer development risk very drastically. Adipose tissue releases estrogens and heightened estrogen levels are linked with increased risk of ovarian endometrial and several breast cancers. Estrogen originates predominantly from adipose tissue in postmenopausal women who exhibit this phenomenon quite markedly under such circumstances. Obesity ramps up production of insulin and insulin-like growth factor 1 IGF-1 rather substantially in many instances very frequently. Elevated hormone levels spur cell proliferation vigorously and inhibit apoptosis enhancing tumour progression substantially upping cancer risk in prostate colorectal and pancreatic cancers (Poti et al, 2017).

Obesity nowadays tends to deteriorate rapidly from eating copious amounts of ultra-processed foods and subsequently breeds insulin resistance very quickly. Body becomes unresponsive remarkably slowly resulting in chronically high insulin levels mostly in this condition under various physiological circumstances. IGF-1 levels surge subsequently playing a crucial role very significantly in fostering cancer cell proliferation and survival quite vigorously afterwards. Elevated insulin levels and IGF-1 have been rather strongly linked to heightened risk of various cancers including breast prostate and some colorectal cancers. Insulin resistance fosters accumulation of fat particularly around abdominal areas thereby further heightening risk factors for several nasty cancers very significantly. Ultra-processed diets fuel obesity very significantly thereby heightening risk of cancer via chronic inflammation hormonal imbalances and insulin resistance. Energy-dense and nutrient-poor diets promote weight gain readily enough fostering an environment conducive very much entirely to cancer development. Radically healthier diets are adopted and consumption of ultra-processed edibles curbed very effectively mitigating risk of obesity-linked cancer.

6.3. The Gut Microbiome and Cancer Prevention

Fungi and viruses and bacteria thrive very cryptically deep inside human guts forming intricate microbiota in various bodily regions oddly enough. It remarkably plays a crucial part deep within bodily processes and enhance immune function gradually alongside cancer prevention somewhat. A diverse healthy microbiome vigorously facilitates degradation of numerous nutrients producing vitamins crucial for human health extremely effectively against pathogens. It aids regulation of immune system somewhat effectively by detecting abnormal cells and destroying rather cancerous ones very frequently. Eating loads of vibrant fruits and cruciferous veggies fosters very diverse gut flora crucial for overall bodily function almost invariably. Beneficial gut bacteria thrive remarkably inside human digestive tracts when consumed foods are richly endowed with fibre and various antioxidants (Leonard and Toro, 2023).

Diets ridiculously high in ultra-processed junk teeming with artificial crap and loads of bad fats severely disrupt gut microbiome causing nasty dysbiosis. Disruption sometimes triggers severely detrimental effects on digestive health and utterly thwarts cancer prevention measures with potentially calamitous outcomes quite drastically. Ultra-processed foods vigorously foster gut bacteria imbalance linked with intestinal inflammation a significant risk factor for colorectal cancer development . Gut inflammation fosters intestinal permeability often dubbed leaky gut wherein noxious substances seep surreptitiously into bloodstream through intestinal lining remarkably porous from inflammation. Inflammation can be triggered thereby damaging DNA of cells inside intestinal tissues promoting fairly rapid cancerous growth within body. Heinously nasty metabolites like nitrosamines and secondary bile acids are churned out by unhealthy microbiomes and sometimes shown downright carcinogenic (Leonard and Toro, 2023).

Gut microbiome exerts a vital role in regulating body's immune responses dynamically amidst various physiological processes and erratic cancer progression . A healthy microbiome trains immune systems fairly effectively distinguishing normal cells from cancerous ones amidst considerable turmoil within cellular environments. Ultra-processed foods savagely disrupt microbiome balance thereby very effectively impairing immune function and fostering cancerous tumour growth with alarming rapidity. Cancer cells thrive in such impairment fostering an environment that facilitates evading immune surveillance and progression happens rapidly uncontrollably thereby. Prevention of cancer depends quite heavily on gut microbiome particularly in context of colorectal cancer developing rapidly and often fatally. Gut inflammation and formation of carcinogenic substances occur rapidly inside intestinal tract due to excessive consumption of ultra-processed foods fairly quickly. Profoundly debilitated immune response renders quashing malignant cells remarkably arduous in a severely perturbed physiological milieu. Consuming nutrient-dense foods enhance bodily defenses naturally helping maintain a fairly healthy gut microbiome somewhat resistant to cancer development.

6.4. Implications for Cancer Prevention

Vigorously adopting whole food-based diets and slashing ultra-processed food intake should be prioritized nowadays by cancer prevention strategies very effectively. Diets rich in veggies whole grains lean proteins and good fats found in Mediterranean style eating patterns offer numerous benefits for overall cellular health. Bioactive compounds found in foods replete with fibre and phytochemicals very effectively counter damage and negate nasty effects of ultra-processed food. Nutrient-dense whole foods play a crucial role remarkably in prevention of various cancers very effectively on daily basis. High-fibre foods deeply nurture gut health preventing colon cancer by encourage a healthy microbiome which reduces inflammation inside digestive tracts. Antioxidants lurking in sundry fruits and veggies somewhat help neutralize errant free radicals that spark DNA damage and lead cancer (Esquivel MK, 2022).

Phytochemicals such as flavonoids possess potent anti-cancer properties blocking cancer cell growth very rapidly and promoting their destruction very effectively. Focusing on nutrient-dense foods enables individuals quite effectively fight cancerous cellular changes thereby lowering risk of tumour development overall. Nationwide policy changes and individual dietary tweaks play crucial roles in cancer prevention fairly remarkably effectively across various demographics. Promoting nutritional literacy and curbing marketing of ultra-processed foods that target kids greatly cuts down formation of unhealthy eating habits. Fostering consumption of whole foods and informing people about health risks associated with ultra-processed food can ultimately slash cancer burdens related to diet. Ultra-processed foods harbor egregious nutritional flaws which rather alarmingly contribute significantly towards cancer development owing partly to seeming convenience (Esquivel MK, 2022). Consuming edibles packed with copious refined sugars and dubious artificial additives can potentially trigger obesity and inflammation strongly tied to elevated cancer risk. People nowadays can very significantly mitigate risk of cancer fairly regularly by eating whole foods rich in nutrients overall. Fostering healthier eating habits globally relies heavily on public health interventions which effectively mitigate worldwide cancer burden in some manner.

7. Public Health Strategies to Mitigate Cancer Risk from Ultra-Processed Foods

Consumption of ultra-processed foods rises sparking significant public health concern largely due to links with chronic diseases like cancer. Ultra-processed foods harbour copious artificial additives dubiously alongside unhealthy fats and pack a very high caloric punch basically. Cancer development mechanisms are very strongly linked to foods that foster obesity and gut microbiome disruption via insulin resistance and inflammation. Nationwide multifaceted health initiatives must be undertaken rather vigorously to curb intake of ultra-processed foods and foster relatively healthier eating habits. Many evidence-based approaches for mitigating risk of cancer are presented below rather succinctly. Clearer labeling on food products nowadays significantly aids consumers in making informed choices generally with somewhat crucial information being provided. Indicating processing level clearly on product packaging helps individuals spot relatively healthy options quickly online or in most retail stores (Kliemann et al, 2022).

Nationwide campaigns promoting nutritional literacy ought rapidly educate public about risks of ultra-processed edibles and benefits of whole unadulterated food. Empowering consumers happens very quietly with rather obscure dietary tips and fairly actionable advice on generally healthier eating habits. Government regulation plays a pivotal role curbing consumption of ultra-processed foods especially among kids and other very susceptible demographics nationwide. Limiting ads for ultra-processed food on television and online can significantly curb kids' exposure somewhat to very unhealthy food options daily. Nationwide regulations get enacted swiftly limiting availability of unhealthy processed food in schools and public institutions thereby fostering healthier environs rather effectively (Kliemann et al, 2022).

Boosting availability of whole unprocessed foods nationwide reduces reliance on ultra-processed edibles significantly for many folks every day. Subsidizing wholesome food like fruits whole grains makes adopting relatively healthy diets ridiculously easier for folks living deep in underserved areas. Public health campaigns nowadays help individuals access fresh produce effectively and learn preparing meals quite nutritiously at community gardens and farmers markets. Taxes on sugary drinks and junk food have been touted nationwide as potent strategy for suddenly curbing ultra-processed food consumption. Taxation drastically curbs consumption of unhealthy food generating revenue quietly reinvested in nationwide public health initiatives funding quirky nutrition awareness schemes.

Public health bodies ought vigorously promote national dietary guidelines which emphasize consumption of fairly unprocessed foods and thoroughly discourage ultra-processed options. Initiatives promoting dietary regimens somewhat akin to Mediterranean diet heavily emphasizing copious fruits vegetables whole grains lean proteins and copious healthy fats may mitigate cancer risk. Promoting fairly healthy eating habits among large populaces may potentially stave off rising obesity rates and related metabolic issues that exacerbate cancerous tumour formation. Initiatives grounded deeply in local communities can play a crucial role promoting radical nationwide change in people's dietary habits very effectively. Such programs offer support locally through nutrition counseling and cooking classes. Forming alliances with diverse community organizations very much guarantees people access to info and tools for embracing super healthy lifestyles (van Tulleken C, 2025). Social support networks facilitate long-term adherence quite effectively and promote relatively healthier environments thereby spreading awareness fairly ubiquitously. Heightened consumption of ultra-processed comestibles poses a plethora of significant health concerns owing largely risk of sundry neoplasms. Regulatory measures curbing adverts aimed squarely at youngsters and subsidies for wholesome food can mitigate cancer rates very effectively alongside public health education. Public health authorities can effectively mitigate cancer burden by heavily promoting whole nutrient-dense foods and fostering somewhat healthier diets overall.

7.1. Strengthening Nutritional Education and Public Awareness

Promoting balanced nutrient-dense diets greatly reduces cancer risk nowadays effectively among public largely unaware of ultra-processed foods detrimental health impacts. Consumers remain astonishingly oblivious to potential health hazards linked with eating ultra-processed foods often marketed deceitfully as wholesome nutritional options. Public health initiatives play crucial roles empowering individuals making savvy dietary decisions effectively preventing myriad forms of cancer under various circumstances. Nutritional education requires facilitating comprehension among people about foods deemed ultra-processed very frequently nowadays for various obvious reasons. Many people oblivious remain of differences between entire insect snacks and highly processed rubbish riddled with dubious ingredients and extraneous sugar heaps (Cotter et al, 2021).

Public health initiatives ought to rather loosely define food highlighting very serious risks alarmingly associated with consumption somewhat ominously in certain contexts. Consumers can make very savvy decisions dining out or eating fast at various eateries by grasping perils associated with such food. Public health initiatives ought to very much always vigorously promote people ditching highly processed food for relatively healthier food options over time. Eating plenty of veggies whole grains lean meats and good fats naturally enhance prevention of cancer with key nutrients fairly effectively. Foods rich in fibre and phytochemicals promote overall cellular health very effectively by reducing inflammation and shielding cells against oxidative damage. Healthy eating becomes very achievable for people of all ages with quirky recipe books and detailed nutrition guides readily available online daily (Cotter et al, 2021).

Regularly cooking meals at home can quietly diminish reliance on heavily processed foods and foster somewhat healthier dietary habits over time. Home-cooked meals typically turn out very healthy and remarkably affordable allowing greater control over ingredients used quite freely nowadays. Public health initiatives offer resources such as ridiculously simple recipes and rigorously tested meal plans making home cooking significantly more accessible nowadays. This approach promotes healthier eating habits rather vigorously and fosters deep connection with food amidst various nutritional underpinnings simultaneously. Public health authorities must fairly regularly forge alliances with schools workplaces and various media outlets nationwide to maximize educational efforts impact. Schools vigorously infuse curricula with nutrition education while workplaces offer healthier meal options and conduct intensive workshops side by side nationwide and media outlets sporadically raise awareness through targeted campaigns. Social media television and print are potent tools for disseminating evidence-based info on risks of ultra-processed food and benefits of relatively healthier dietary choices obviously. Nutritional education significantly empowers individuals making relatively healthier food choices nowadays thus reducing cancer risk very effectively across the population.

7.2. Regulation of Food Labeling and Marketing

Food labeling plays a vital albeit oft overlooked role in furnishing fairly transparent info about contents of packaged foods thereby very significantly empowering consumers. Ultra-processed foods masquerade as healthy fare replete with refined sugars loads of saturated fats and dubious artificial additives quite deceptively. Strengthening food labeling regulations very quickly empowers consumers grasp nutritional quality of foods they purchase and make savvy decisions subsequently. Simplistic nutrition labels plastered on packaging constitute a vital step forwards almost magically within a surprisingly short span. Labelling schemes like Nutri-Score or Traffic Light System might aid consumers somewhat rapidly in evaluating nutritional worth of product offerings very effectively. Labels furnish very clear color-coded info about added sugars and unhealthy fats plus calories enabling shoppers make fairly healthy purchasing decisions (Shangguan et al, 2019).

Consumers make super healthy choices by opting for products bearing very clear labels thus avoiding food loaded with toxic substances. Regulatory bodies should really crack down on shonky health claims like sugar-free or all-natural slapped on heaps of ultra-processed junk food. Such assertions frequently obscure unhealthy additives and preservatives lurking beneath ostensibly wholesome foods rendering them very darn detrimental overall. Crucial regulation curbs dubious marketing tactics masquerading as wholesome options targeting youngsters with unhealthy food promotion very effectively nowadays. Regulatory bodies can sternly curb dubious assertions thereby ensuring food marketing reflects true nutritional value of products on shelves accurately nowadays (Shangguan et al, 2019).

Displaying calorie counts and basic nutrition info on menus at eateries proves very effective these days at curbing unhealthy eating somewhat. Awareness gets raised rapidly about calories sneaking into dishes made with ultra-processed foods and dubious ingredients at various eateries nationwide suddenly. Eating out smartly nowadays enables diners very effectively manage overall caloric intake and dodge unhealthy food outside their own kitchens. Fairly effectively nowadays public health policies help consumers navigate complexities of food choices by cracking down on misleading marketing very vigorously. Measures will ostensibly guide people toward healthier purchasing decisions ultimately reducing risks associated with ultra-processed foods and encourage public health across America suddenly.

7.3. Taxation and Subsidies on Foods

Taxation on junk food and subsidies for nutritious eats remarkably curb consumption of ultra-processed edibles nowadays very effectively. Several nations overseas have employed this approach very effectively reducing consumption of sugar-sweetened drinks and other fairly unhealthy food. Policy initiatives might encompass sugar taxes which Mexico Hungary and parts of United Kingdom have enacted very vigorously across entire nation. Manufacturers tweak product formulas under sugar taxes and consumers get nudged towards picking rather healthier alternatives quietly instead. Governments can shell out financial incentives to make whole grains and veggies super affordable (Tamir et al, 2018).

Governments can offer financial incentives or subsidies making fruits and whole grains rather more affordable for people down the line. Taxation on ultra-processed meats contains harmful preservatives like nitrates and nitrites classified as Group 1 carcinogens by International Agency for Research on Cancer. Mitigating stark price differences between ultra processed junk food and wholesome edibles may coax poorer folks into choosing healthier eats thus preventing diet related cancers. Ultra-processed meats containing dodgy preservatives like nitrates or nitrites attract taxation and are deemed Group 1 carcinogens by International Agency for Research on Cancer.

7.4. Promoting Healthy Environments in Schools and Workplaces

Public health policies ought focus heavily on crafting surroundings that foster relatively healthy eating habits mostly within schools and various community centers nationwide. Ultra-processed foods exert peculiarly deleterious long-term effects on certain groups making timely interventions crucial for cancer prevention and overall health. Schools play a pivotal role in shaping eating habits of kids significantly through various means very deeply inside their young lives. Restricting sugary junk food in cafeterias rather slowly over quite some time can help kids develop very healthy eating habits. Schools oughta embed nutrition ed into curricula kinda thoroughly teaching youngsters about significance of balanced food and perks of unprocessed eats for averting cancer. Instilling sound gastronomical habits in youngsters right from square one can have a profoundly lasting impact on their eating proclivities well into old age. Workplaces nowadays remain profoundly influential settings for very effective promotion of healthy eating habits (Gorski and Roberto, 2015).

Employers cultivate a nutritious environment by offering staff wholesome snacks and guidance on dietary habits through very unconventional means normally. Such initiatives enhance health significantly and can remarkably boost overall workplace productivity and staff morale extremely well too. Employers prioritize healthy eating in a markedly supportive environment thereby fostering lowered cancer risk amongst employees and encouraging remarkably ecofriendly habits. Nationwide community programs play crucial roles quietly making healthy eating a somewhat realistic option for people from very diverse socioeconomic walks. Super cool initiatives such as wacky gardening projects and ridiculously fun cooking classes equip people with skills needed for nutritious meals at home quickly (Gorski and Roberto, 2015). Such initiatives foster robust social support systems that enhance wholesome behaviors and nudge people towards informed eating decisions very effectively nowadays. Profoundly impactful public health efforts fostering deeply rooted nutrition environments yield far-reaching changes across diverse demographics nationwide over time slowly. Embedding healthy eating habits into daily life necessitates freakishly supportive environments very much everywhere in schools workplaces and various communal settings. Heavily promoting nutrition education and healthier food options fosters long-term public health improvements by reducing ultra-processed food consumption greatly. Sustained dietary changes on societal scale foster remarkably healthier populations and lower cancer risk significantly over time eventually.

7.5. Reformulating Ultra-Processed Foods

Food reformulation remains crucial nowadays for improving public health significantly alongside strategies altering consumer behavior quite remarkably. Reformulating ultra-processed edibles by drastically cutting sodium and dodgy additives can notably enhance nutritional worth and lessen grave health hazards such as cancer. Governments and public health organizations can implement key initiatives very quietly nationwide by collaborating with food manufacturers. Rigorous reformulation standards get established thereby fostering a healthier food environment all of a sudden very markedly. Governments work very intimately with behemoth food corporations establishing fairly stringent targets rapidly for truncating sodium content in sundry processed food. Manufacturers would get guided by such standards reducing very harmful stuff fairly gradually while mostly keeping products quite safe. Specific goals like slashing sugar content or ridding products of quite pernicious additives effectively mitigate health risks for consumers seeking fairly healthier options (Onyeaka et al, 2023). Promoting natural preservatives rapidly becomes crucial in reformulation efforts replacing nasty chemicals like nitrates or nitrites very effectively nowadays. Processed meats often harbor dubious chemicals which morph into carcinogenic stuff when blasted with searing heat whilst being cooked very vigorously. Governments can help curb cancer risks associated with processed foods by pushing manufacturers towards adopting alternatives such as rosemary extract or ascorbic acid. Shift toward relatively safer preservatives might drastically lower levels of potentially carcinogenic substances in food supply contributing significantly to better public health outcomes. Governments public health organizations and food industry must work together quite critically nowadays for success of reformulation efforts effectively (Onyeaka et al, 2023).

Engaging with food manufacturers and setting incentives fosters innovation in creating ridiculously healthy products extremely low in sodium or sugar. Regulatory policies cleverly embed reformulation incentives that cultivate surprisingly healthier eating environments and permit consumers loads of choice. Multifaceted public health strategies involving radical food reformulation are desperately needed nowadays to mitigate cancer risk linked with ultra-processed food consumption. Governments can back a swing towards healthier food by setting reformulation targets and pushing food makers towards using fairly innocuous ingredients swiftly. Efforts alongside education and stringent labeling regulations might considerably mitigate cancer burden and vigorously promote nutrient rich whole food diets.

8. From Consumption to Carcinogenesis

Lately concerns have been raised significantly about consumption of ultra-processed foods largely due to links with various chronic diseases including cancer. Ultra-processed foods teem with refined sugars galore and unhealthy fats aplenty alongside heaps of artificial additives and preservatives in most modern diets. Such foods are often remarkably dense in energy and surprisingly lacking in nutrients making them somewhat risky for developing certain cancers. Processed foods contribute quite profoundly to carcinogenesis via bodily inflammation and genomic metabolic dysregulation in deep underlying biological mechanisms sometimes.

One begins ostensibly by altering things quite erratically in a rather haphazard manner with some frequency (Kliemann et al, 2022).

Ultra-processed foods surprisingly effectively foster cancer development largely through various complex biochemical pathways inducing chronic low-grade inflammation. Consuming food chock-full of trans fats and refined sugars rather quickly triggers release of pro-inflammatory molecules such as cytokines and adipokines. Rampant cellular proliferation and aberrant angiogenesis are fueled deeply within bodily tissues spawning a milieu prone to cancer. Malignant transformations unfold very haphazardly in various tissues ravaged by inflammatory environments that mutate cellular DNA fairly extensively over time (Kliemann et al, 2022).

Metabolic dysregulation and insulin resistance form a major pathway linking ultra-processed foods quite directly with development of various cancerous malignancies. Ultra-processed foods teeming with copious refined sugars and dubious fats frequently precipitate insulin resistance wherein bodily responsiveness diminishes alarmingly fast. Insulin resistance triggers elevated insulin and insulin-like growth factor 1 levels rather vigorously promoting abnormal cell growth and inhibiting apoptosis very effectively. Insulin resistance frequently manifests alongside obesity fostering an environment ripe for tumour initiation and progression in cancers such as breast cancer or liver cancer. Foods laced with artificial preservatives and flavor enhancers can very rapidly induce genomic instability a major factor in malignancy development. Processed meats contain chemicals like nitrates and nitrites which form nasty carcinogenic nitrosamines when cooked at extremely high temperatures (Kliemann et al, 2022).

Mutations and DNA damage stem largely from such reactive compounds resulting in chromosomal abnormalities that typically foster cancerous cellular proliferation quite uncontrollably. Ultra-processed foods severely disrupt gut microbiome an essential part of human health regulating digestion and encourage immune function quite vigorously. Diets comprising heavily processed foods loaded with artificial additives and remarkably low in fibre promote dysbiosis an imbalance festers in gut microbiota. Dysbiosis fosters chronic inflammation inside bodily tissues quite deeply and produces carcinogenic byproducts thereby heightening risk of colorectal cancer significantly.

Microbiome disruption hampers immune system's ability severely detecting cancerous cells becomes arduous and destruction of them gets impeded furthering rapid cancer progression. Ultra-processed foods and cancer are linked through a frequently occurring complex interplay of inflammation metabolic disruption and genomic instability in gut microbiome. Public health officials and researchers can tackle cancer prevention more effectively by grasping crucial dietary pathways for their overall efforts. Shifting towards a whole food diet rich in fibre and natural antioxidants remarkably reduces cancer risk and improves health outcomes significantly.

8.1. Inflammation: A Crucial Link between Processed Foods and Cancer

Ultra-processed foods contribute significantly to cancer risk through chronic inflammation that acts as a crucial underlying factor largely. Eating copious amounts of ultraprocessed food loaded with refined carbs sugars and noxious fats cultivates chronic low-grade systemic inflammation fostering a tumour-friendly environment. Inflammation driven mainly by UPFs plays a pivotal role in propelling cancer forward at a rather disconcertingly rapid pace inexplicably. Obesity correlates fairly strongly with consumption of ultra-processed comestibles that fuel inflammation extensively throughout various bodily tissues and systems rather pervasively. Excessive body fat secretes pro-inflammatory cytokines like IL-6 and TNF-α alongside C-reactive protein fairly often around various internal organs (Anastasiou et al, 2025).

Tumour cells rapidly hijack host immune systems and swiftly unleash various pro-inflammatory molecules that foster chronic inflammation evading detection mechanisms entirely. Excess body fat fosters profoundly inflammatory environments that alter cellular processes quite radically encourage survival of cancer cells very effectively . Adipokines like leptin secreted by fat cells stimulate cancer cells to proliferate very vigorously further exacerbating inflammation effects that promote cancer. Refined sugars trans fats and unhealthy fats in ultra-processed foods very quickly fuel key inflammatory pathways deep within human bodies. Nuclear factor kappa-light-chain-enhancer of activated B cells, namely NF-kB pathway constitutes a crucial signalling mechanism very apparently in cells (Anastasiou et al, 2025).

Diet-induced inflammatory responses chronically activate this pathway resulting in haphazard production of pro-inflammatory molecules fairly irregularly over time. Molecules wield multifaceted effects that markedly enhance tumour proliferation via augmented angiogenesis and heightened survival prospects of rather malignant cells. UPFs fuel vicious cycles fostering environments conducive cancer thrives and metastasizes rapidly within bodily tissues very quickly most everywhere. Ultra-processed foods spur chronic inflammation largely via obesity and inflammatory pathways tied heavily to diet that foster cancerous environments. UPFs substantially foster tumour development by radically altering key cellular processes and promoting secretion of inflammatory molecules quite vigorously. Mitigating cancer risk entails drastically cutting consumption of ultra-processed edibles and adopting whole food diets possessing markedly anti-inflammatory properties.

8.2. Insulin Resistance and Metabolic Dysregulation

Consumption of ultra-processed foods fuels cancer development through pathways involving insulin resistance and metabolic dysregulation very basically. Ultra-processed foods packed with sugar and dubious fats trigger huge spikes in insulin levels fostering insulin resistance quite rapidly. Metabolic disruption plays a crucial role in onset of various cancers quickly under certain gnarly conditions fairly remarkably. Bodily resistance surges and pancreas boosts insulin and IGF-1 production rapidly lowering glucose levels somewhat sluggishly in a rather ineffective manner. Elevated insulin levels vigorously stimulate secretion of IGF-1 a protein crucial for cell growth survival and numerous other cellular functions obviously. High levels of IGF-1 quite vigorously promote cancerous growth by stimulating cell proliferation and inhibiting apoptosis or programmed death of cells (Almarshad et al, 2022).

IGF-1 overexpression has ostensibly been linked rather strongly to development of various malignancies including breast and prostate cancers very frequently nowadays. Ultra-processed foods foster hyper-proliferation by sustaining high IGF-1 levels thereby encouraging cancer cells grow uncontrollably and divide rather rapidly. Eating ultra-processed foods frequently triggers insulin resistance and obesity subsequently worsening metabolic dysfunction severity very markedly in many individuals. Excess fat especially visceral fat markedly enhance production of pro-inflammatory cytokines further debilitating insulin sensitivity very severely in many instances. Obesity paired with insulin resistance rapidly fosters in most people a metabolic environment remarkably conducive to swift cancer development. Insulin resistance and inflammation spark pro-carcinogenic pathways involved deeply in cell cycle regulation fostering mutations and tumour formation quite rapidly (Almarshad et al, 2022). Metabolic disruption heavily contributes quite frequently to type 2 diabetes and cardiovascular disease alongside cancer in many chronic conditions. Tumours emerge partly from severely dysregulated cellular metabolism and insulin insensitivity triggered by eating copious amounts of highly processed edibles. Elevating insulin levels and IGF-1 quite substantially fosters inflammation and metabolic dysfunction thereby creating an environment ripe for rapid cell proliferation. Pivotal biological processes remarkably drive cancer pathogenesis highlighting significance of nutrient-dense diet in reducing cancer risk substantially with varied outcomes.

8.3. Genomic Instability and DNA Damage

Consuming processed foods laced with artificial additives and dubious preservatives can precipitously induce genomic instability characteristic of cancerous cells in some instances. Some ultra-processed foods contain mutagenic chemicals that directly damage DNA thereby sometimes suddenly leading to cancer development rapidly in certain cases. Processed meats such as bacon or sausages frequently harbour nitrites and nitrates serving as preservatives thereby fuelling significant health anxieties among consumers these days. Nitrates morph into potent carcinogenic nitrosamines at scorching cooking temperatures wreaking havoc on DNA with reckless abandon slowly (Kliemann et al, 2022).

Nitrosamines disrupt DNA replication very badly causing eerily subtle point mutations in genetic code that can activate oncogenes or knock out tumour suppressors. DNA damage rampantly heightens risk of gastric cancer and sundry other cancer types linked obscurely to consumption of notoriously processed meat. Processed foods yield acrylamide quite rapidly a noxious compound generated during intense heat treatment of starchy edibles like burnt potato chips. Acrylamide rather insidiously forms DNA adducts through attachments of chemical moieties onto fragile genetic material in a decidedly pernicious manner. Such adducts severely disrupt DNA structure thereby leading chromosomal abnormalities fairly frequently in complex biological processes unfolding rapidly (Kliemann et al, 2022).

Acrylamide very fundamentally induces mutations and DNA strand breaks in cancer initiation and progression apparently too under various cellular conditions. Eating processed foods containing nitrates or acrylamide substantially amplifies risk of genomic instability a key factor underlying development of various cancers rapidly. Chemicals directly damage DNA resulting in mutations that spur formation of tumours and very rapid progression occurs afterwards very quickly. Eating fewer processed meats and starchy foods cooked in oil or baked remarkably helps reduce exposure to carcinogenic compounds lowering cancer risk dramatically.

8.4. Disruption of the Gut Microbiome and Cancer Risk

Human gut microbiome plays a vital role deeply in maintaining immune function and overall gut health intricately links with metabolic processes . Consuming copious amounts of ultra-processed foods rife with sugars and dubious fats utterly ravages gut microbiota precipitating dysbiosis rather quickly. Dysbiosis stealthily contributes significantly to elevated risks of nasty cancers in humans very frequently under certain rather abnormal physiological conditions. Dysregulated microbiome precipitates leaky gut syndrome thereby facilitating ingress of deleterious substances through intestinal lining fairly readily into bloodstream. This process triggers chronic low-grade inflammation which serves as precursor mostly to colorectal cancer and various other cancer types. Molecules possessing inflammatory properties get produced in response to gut dysbiosis thereby damaging intestinal cells and fostering tumour formation vigorously inside (Rondinella et al, 2025).

A microbiome gone haywire churns out carcinogenic metabolites such as secondary bile acids and nitrosamines fueling DNA damage and tumourigenesis quite rampantly. Gut microbiome plays a crucial role very effectively in maintaining body's immune surveillance under fairly normal circumstances. Beneficial gut bacteria help regulate immune system function very vigorously including T-cells and other cells crucial for detecting cancer cells and annihilating them swiftly. Microbiome dysbiosis severely hampers immune response rather mysteriously often in various ways beneath surface of seemingly healthy individuals (Rondinella et al, 2025). Tumour cells proliferate unabated in people beset by weakened immunity thereby significantly upping likelihood of cancer progression drastically. Ultra-processed foods wreak havoc on gut microbiome thereby fuelling increased inflammation and substantially compromising immune function alongside production of carcinogenic metabolites. Changes foster environments rife with cancer development very rapidly nowadays particularly in colorectal regions. Eating copious amounts of fibre rich edibles and fermented fare may effectively lower cancer risk in people very generally or so it seems.

8.5. The Role of Food Additives in Carcinogenesis

Ultra-processed foods containing artificial colorants and flavor enhancers have sparked quite alarming concerns over cancer links nowadays. These additives may leverage various biological mechanisms like genotoxicity and tumour promotion rather significantly contributing to carcinogenesis through DNA damage. Numerous murky investigations surrounding artificial sweeteners lately have extensively studied aspartame and saccharin for potential links to cancer. Certain animal studies hazily imply a tenuous connection between bladder cancer and degenerate products of sweeteners that rather severely disrupt cellular processes or harm DNA. Evidence remains curiously mixed and further research seems desperately needed nowadays apparently to confirm risk in humans. Red 40 and Yellow 5 potentially damage DNA and spur tumour growth ominously heightening cancer risk somewhat in humans (Kliemann et al, 2022).

Studies in animals have shown certain colorants bind erratically with cellular DNA resulting in mutations or chromosomal damage that increases cancer risk significantly. Obscure channels operating simultaneously nowadays involve intricate mechanisms underlying ultra-processed foods' contribution to various cancer risks multifacetedly. Genomic instability and microbiome imbalances alongside chronic inflammation deeply entwine with various pathological processes very disruptively in metabolic contexts. Factors conspire rather surreptitiously fostering an environment rife with cancerous potential by ratcheting up inflammation and abetting proliferation of malignant cells vigorously. Nowadays grasping role of food additives in carcinogenesis becomes crucial very quickly and reduction in consumption of ultra-processed foods gains importance rapidly. Additives heighten cancer risk rapidly by inducing DNA damage and altering metabolic functions through swift promotion of inflammation chronically. Stricter regulation and better food labeling education backed by public health initiatives can slash cancer burden linked heavily to artificial additives in modern diets (Kliemann et al, 2022).

9. Conclusion

Globally consumption of ultra-processed foods poses significant concern for public health regarding chronic diseases like cancer these days. Evidence links UPF consumption quite alarmingly and strongly to elevated risk of various cancers including colorectal malignancies and postmenopausal breast cancer. Mechanistic insights emerging somewhat rapidly validate these associations by revealing disruption of physiological homeostasis and rampant promotion of carcinogenesis by foods processing badly. Ultra-processed foods contain copious refined sugars and unhealthy fats and sundry food additives but lack essential nutrients entirely and dietary fibre. UPFs notoriously foster chronic low-grade inflammation and insulin resistance alongside oxidative stress and gut microbiota dysbiosis facilitating tumour development substantially.

Novel compounds like acrylamides and nitrosamines formed during processing may exert direct genotoxic effects rather frequently under certain conditions . UPFs are deeply entrenched in modern diets and rather peculiar lifestyle choices beyond obvious physiological health factors nowadays apparently. Extremely palatable foods get consumed very extensively largely driven by super aggressive marketing and great convenience among very vulnerable demographic groups. Ultra-processed foods displace nutrient-dense options in ones diet and rather alarmingly contribute to obesity nasty metabolic issues linked to various cancers. Urgently needed now are multifaceted strategies for mitigating risks amidst a plethora of mounting uncertainties and severely unstable situations.

Public health interventions ought to largely focus on nutrition education and policies that promote access fairly readily to minimally processed healthful foods. Long-term studies incorporating both experimental methodologies and epidemiological analyses are sorely needed to investigate UPFs and associated cancer risk very thoroughly. Consumption of ultra-processed food rather strikingly correlates with heightened cancer risk according largely to both epidemiological trends and mechanistic insight. Cancer prevention efforts should prioritize curbing rampant ultra processed foods presence in global food systems amidst a rising tide of diet-related maladies. Public health systems play a pivotal role in mitigating cancer risk by empowering individuals with knowledge of healthier lifestyle options fairly effectively nowadays.

References

Adams J, Hofman K, Moubarac JC, Thow AM. Public health response to ultra-processed food and drinks. BMJ. 2020 Jun 26;369:m2391. doi: 10.1136/bmj.m2391. PMID: 32591348; PMCID: PMC7318879.

Almarshad MI, Algonaiman R, Alharbi HF, Almujaydil MS, Barakat H. Relationship between Ultra-Processed Food Consumption and Risk of Diabetes Mellitus: A Mini-Review. Nutrients. 2022 Jun 7;14(12):2366. doi: 10.3390/nu14122366. PMID: 35745095; PMCID: PMC9228591.

Anastasiou IA, Kounatidis D, Vallianou NG, Skourtis A, Dimitriou K, Tzivaki I, Tsioulos G, Rigatou A, Karampela I, Dalamaga M. Beneath the Surface: The Emerging Role of Ultra-Processed Foods in Obesity-Related Cancer. Curr Oncol Rep. 2025 Apr;27(4):390-414. doi: 10.1007/s11912-025-01654-6. Epub 2025 Feb 27. PMID: 40014232; PMCID: PMC11976848.

Beal T, Manohar S, Miachon L, Fanzo J. Nutrient-dense foods and diverse diets are important for ensuring adequate nutrition across the life course. Proc Natl Acad Sci U S A. 2024 Dec 10;121(50):e2319007121. doi: 10.1073/pnas.2319007121. Epub 2024 Dec 2. Erratum in: Proc Natl Acad Sci U S A. 2025 Jul 22;122(29):e2516301122. doi: 10.1073/pnas.2516301122. PMID: 39621916; PMCID: PMC11648672.

Bleak TC, Calaf GM. Breast and prostate glands affected by environmental substances (Review). Oncol Rep. 2021 Apr;45(4):20. doi: 10.3892/or.2021.7971. Epub 2021 Mar 2. PMID: 33649835; PMCID: PMC7879422.

Colella M, Charitos IA, Ballini A, Cafiero C, Topi S, Palmirotta R, Santacroce L. Microbiota revolution: How gut microbes regulate our lives. World J Gastroenterol. 2023 Jul 28;29(28):4368-4383. doi: 10.3748/wjg.v29.i28.4368. PMID: 37576701; PMCID: PMC10415973.

Cotter T, Kotov A, Wang S, Murukutla N. 'Warning: ultra-processed' - A call for warnings on foods that aren't really foods. BMJ Glob Health. 2021 Dec;6(12):e007240. doi: 10.1136/bmjgh-2021-007240. PMID: 34933866; PMCID: PMC8666852.

Dicken SJ, Batterham RL. Ultra-processed Food and Obesity: What Is the Evidence? Curr Nutr Rep. 2024 Mar;13(1):23-38. doi: 10.1007/s13668-024-00517-z. Epub 2024 Jan 31. PMID: 38294671; PMCID: PMC10924027.

Doueihy NE, Ghaleb J, Kfoury K, Khouzami KK, Nassif N, Attieh P, Ghadieh HE, Azar S, Kanaan A, Harb F. Aspartame and Human Health: A Mini-Review of Carcinogenic and Systemic Effects. J Xenobiot. 2025 Jul 7;15(4):114. doi: 10.3390/jox15040114. PMID: 40700161; PMCID: PMC12286081.

Elizabeth L, Machado P, Zinöcker M, Baker P, Lawrence M. Ultra-Processed Foods and Health Outcomes: A Narrative Review. Nutrients. 2020 Jun 30;12(7):1955. doi: 10.3390/nu12071955. PMID: 32630022; PMCID: PMC7399967.

Esquivel MK. Nutrition Benefits and Considerations for Whole Foods Plant-Based Eating Patterns. Am J Lifestyle Med. 2022 Apr 22;16(3):284-290. doi: 10.1177/15598276221075992. PMID: 35706588; PMCID: PMC9189583.

Gorski MT, Roberto CA. Public health policies to encourage healthy eating habits: recent perspectives. J Healthc Leadersh. 2015 Sep 23;7:81-90. doi: 10.2147/JHL.S69188. PMID: 29355201; PMCID: PMC5740998.

Isaksen IM, Dankel SN. Ultra-processed food consumption and cancer risk: A systematic review and meta-analysis. Clin Nutr. 2023 Jun;42(6):919-928. doi: 10.1016/j.clnu.2023.03.018. Epub 2023 Mar 30. PMID: 37087831.

Juul F, Vaidean G, Parekh N. Ultra-processed Foods and Cardiovascular Diseases: Potential Mechanisms of Action. Adv Nutr. 2021 Oct 1;12(5):1673-1680. doi: 10.1093/advances/nmab049. PMID: 33942057; PMCID: PMC8483964.

Kliemann N, Al Nahas A, Vamos EP, Touvier M, Kesse-Guyot E, Gunter MJ, Millett C, Huybrechts I. Ultra-processed foods and cancer risk: from global food systems to individual exposures and mechanisms. Br J Cancer. 2022 Jul;127(1):14-20. doi: 10.1038/s41416-022-01749-y. Epub 2022 Mar 2. PMID: 35236935; PMCID: PMC9276654.

Leite FHM, Khandpur N, Andrade GC, Anastasiou K, Baker P, Lawrence M, Monteiro CA. Ultra-processed foods should be central to global food systems dialogue and action on biodiversity. BMJ Glob Health. 2022 Mar;7(3):e008269. doi: 10.1136/bmjgh-2021-008269. PMID: 35346976; PMCID: PMC8895941.

Leonard JM, Toro DD. Defining the Microbiome Components (Bacteria, Viruses, Fungi) and Microbiome Geodiversity. Surg Infect (Larchmt). 2023 Apr;24(3):208-212. doi: 10.1089/sur.2023.014. PMID: 37010972; PMCID: PMC10061322.

Mittelman SD. The Role of Diet in Cancer Prevention and Chemotherapy Efficacy. Annu Rev Nutr. 2020 Sep 23;40:273-297. doi: 10.1146/annurev-nutr-013120-041149. Epub 2020 Jun 16. PMID: 32543948; PMCID: PMC8546934.

Monteiro CA, Cannon G, Levy RB, Moubarac JC, Louzada ML, Rauber F, Khandpur N, Cediel G, Neri D, Martinez-Steele E, Baraldi LG, Jaime PC. Ultra-processed foods: what they are and how to identify them. Public Health Nutr. 2019 Apr;22(5):936-941. doi: 10.1017/S1368980018003762. Epub 2019 Feb 12. PMID: 30744710; PMCID: PMC10260459.

Nijenhuis-Noort EC, Berk KA, Neggers SJCMM, Lely AJV. The Fascinating Interplay between Growth Hormone, Insulin-Like Growth Factor-1, and Insulin. Endocrinol Metab (Seoul). 2024 Feb;39(1):83-89. doi: 10.3803/EnM.2024.101. Epub 2024 Jan 9. PMID: 38192102; PMCID: PMC10901670.

Ogunrinola GA, Oyewale JO, Oshamika OO, Olasehinde GI. The Human Microbiome and Its Impacts on Health. Int J Microbiol. 2020 Jun 12;2020:8045646. doi: 10.1155/2020/8045646. PMID: 32612660; PMCID: PMC7306068.

Onyeaka H, Nwaiwu O, Obileke K, Miri T, Al-Sharify ZT. Global nutritional challenges of reformulated food: A review. Food Sci Nutr. 2023 Mar 6;11(6):2483-2499. doi: 10.1002/fsn3.3286. PMID: 37324840; PMCID: PMC10261815.

Partridge D, Lloyd KA, Rhodes JM, Walker AW, Johnstone AM, Campbell BJ. Food additives: Assessing the impact of exposure to permitted emulsifiers on bowel and metabolic health - introducing the FADiets study. Nutr Bull. 2019 Dec;44(4):329-349. doi: 10.1111/nbu.12408. Epub 2019 Nov 25. PMID: 31866761; PMCID: PMC6899614.

Poti JM, Braga B, Qin B. Ultra-processed Food Intake and Obesity: What Really Matters for Health-Processing or Nutrient Content? Curr Obes Rep. 2017 Dec;6(4):420-431. doi: 10.1007/s13679-017-0285-4. PMID: 29071481; PMCID: PMC5787353.

Pratt M, Forbes JD, Knox NC, Bernstein CN, Van Domselaar G. Microbiome-Mediated Immune Signaling in Inflammatory Bowel Disease and Colorectal Cancer: Support From Meta-omics Data. Front Cell Dev Biol. 2021 Nov 16;9:716604. doi: 10.3389/fcell.2021.716604. PMID: 34869308; PMCID: PMC8635193.

Rondinella D, Raoul PC, Valeriani E, Venturini I, Cintoni M, Severino A, Galli FS, Mora V, Mele MC, Cammarota G, Gasbarrini A, Rinninella E, Ianiro G. The Detrimental Impact of Ultra-Processed Foods on the Human Gut Microbiome and Gut Barrier. Nutrients. 2025 Feb 28;17(5):859. doi: 10.3390/nu17050859. PMID: 40077728; PMCID: PMC11901572.

Sainz RM, Lombo F, Mayo JC. Radical decisions in cancer: redox control of cell growth and death. Cancers (Basel). 2012 Apr 25;4(2):442-74. doi: 10.3390/cancers4020442. PMID: 24213319; PMCID: PMC3712695.

Sambu S, Hemaram U, Murugan R, Alsofi AA. Toxicological and Teratogenic Effect of Various Food Additives: An Updated Review. Biomed Res Int. 2022 Jun 24;2022:6829409. doi: 10.1155/2022/6829409. Retraction in: Biomed

Res Int. 2024 Jan 9;2024:9792751. doi: 10.1155/2024/9792751. PMID: 35782077; PMCID: PMC9249520.

Shangguan S, Afshin A, Shulkin M, Ma W, Marsden D, Smith J, Saheb-Kashaf M, Shi P, Micha R, Imamura F, Mozaffarian D; Food PRICE (Policy Review and Intervention Cost-Effectiveness) Project. A Meta-Analysis of Food Labeling Effects on Consumer Diet Behaviors and Industry Practices. Am J Prev Med. 2019 Feb;56(2):300-314. doi: 10.1016/j.amepre.2018.09.024. Epub 2018 Dec 17. PMID: 30573335; PMCID: PMC6340779.

Sharma A, Amarnath S, Thulasimani M, Ramaswamy S. Artificial sweeteners as a sugar substitute: Are they really safe? Indian J Pharmacol. 2016 May-Jun;48(3):237-40. doi: 10.4103/0253-7613.182888. PMID: 27298490; PMCID: PMC4899993.

Shim JS. Ultra-Processed Food Consumption and Obesity: A Narrative Review of Their Association and Potential Mechanisms. J Obes Metab Syndr. 2025 Jan 30;34(1):27-40. doi: 10.7570/jomes24045. Epub 2025 Jan 17. PMID: 39820152; PMCID: PMC11799601.

Tamir O, Cohen-Yogev T, Furman-Assaf S, Endevelt R. Taxation of sugar sweetened beverages and unhealthy foods: a qualitative study of key opinion leaders' views. Isr J Health Policy Res. 2018 Jul 31;7(1):43. doi: 10.1186/s13584-018-0240-1. PMID: 30064503; PMCID: PMC6069556.

Teshome E, Forsido SF, Rupasinghe HPV, Olika Keyata E. Potentials of Natural Preservatives to Enhance Food Safety and Shelf Life: A Review. ScientificWorldJournal. 2022 Sep 23;2022:9901018. doi: 10.1155/2022/9901018. PMID: 36193042; PMCID: PMC9525789.

Tristan Asensi M, Napoletano A, Sofi F, Dinu M. Low-Grade Inflammation and Ultra-Processed Foods Consumption: A Review. Nutrients. 2023 Mar 22;15(6):1546. doi: 10.3390/nu15061546. PMID: 36986276; PMCID: PMC10058108.

Valicente VM, Peng CH, Pacheco KN, Lin L, Kielb EI, Dawoodani E, Abdollahi A, Mattes RD. Ultraprocessed Foods and Obesity Risk: A Critical Review of Reported Mechanisms. Adv Nutr. 2023 Jul;14(4):718-738. doi: 10.1016/j.advnut.2023.04.006. Epub 2023 Apr 18. PMID: 37080461; PMCID: PMC10334162.

van Tulleken C. Ultra-processed foods and public health: Evidence of harm and of conflicts of interest in the food industry to evade regulation. Future Healthc J. 2025 Jun 30;12(2):100263. doi: 10.1016/j.fhj.2025.100263. PMID: 40692632; PMCID: PMC12277474.

Varghese R, Ramamoorthy S. Status of food colorants in India: conflicts and prospects. J Verbrauch Lebensm. 2023;18(2):107-118. doi: 10.1007/s00003-023-01427-y. Epub 2023 Mar 13. PMID: 37265594; PMCID: PMC10009361.

Waris G, Ahsan H. Reactive oxygen species: role in the development of cancer and various chronic conditions. J Carcinog. 2006 May 11;5:14. doi: 10.1186/1477-3163-5-14. PMID: 16689993; PMCID: PMC1479806.

Chapter 10

Phytochemicals as Chemopreventive Agents: Mechanisms of Action

Lokesh Kumar Mishra[1], Sheetanshu Gupta[2], Praneeth Juvvi[3*], and Sarfraj Ahmad Siddiqui[4]

[1]Department of BPME, College of Agriculture, Central Agricultural University (CAU), Imphal, Manipur, India
[2]Department of Food Safety and Quality Assurance, College of Food Technology, Central Agricultural University (CAU), Imphal, Manipur, India
[3]Department of Food Processing Technology, College of Food Technology-Central Agricultural University, Imphal, Manipur, India
[4]Department of Biochemistry, King George's Medical University, U.P., India

Abstract

Phytochemicals have recently garnered considerable attention as potentially bioactive compounds found inside various plants, playing crucial roles in many cancer prevention mechanisms. Phytochemicals exert profoundly protective effects against carcinogenesis slowly through myriad mechanisms thoroughly reviewed here. Terpenoids and carotenoids, alongside glucosinolates, modulate molecular pathways deeply entwined in cancer initiation naturally, while flavonoids play a big role too. Phytochemicals remarkably influence various cellular processes like apoptosis and cell cycle regulation, with antioxidant defence mechanisms under inflammatory responses being heavily. Special focus rests heavily on proteins interacting with transcription factors like p53, regulating genes deeply involved in stress responses cellularly. Phytochemicals modulate gene expression profoundly inside cells, heavily inhibiting oncogenic signalling pathways during DNA repair processes with considerable irregularity. Phytochemicals modulate the tumour microenvironment, effectively impacting immune function heavily and influencing angiogenesis suddenly in a very intricate manner. Certain phytochemicals, such as curcumin and sulforaphane, display pronounced anticancer properties heavily in preclinical research and some shaky human trials.

Keywords: Phytochemicals, Chemoprevention, Antioxidants, Apoptosis, Signal Transduction, Carcinogenesis

DOI: 10.1201/9781042010387-10

1. Introduction

Cancer remains a leading cause of mortality worldwide notwithstanding tremendous strides in diagnostic techniques and sundry prophylactic measures. Many patients have benefited from conventional therapies like chemotherapy but such treatments frequently result in nasty side effects and dubious efficacy especially in latter disease stages. Rapid growth in chemoprevention research involves employing a vast array of natural and synthetic substances that somewhat effectively inhibit carcinogenic processes. Bioactive compounds possessing antioxidant properties and anticarcinogenic effects are deemed promising chemopreventive agents found abundantly in various plant species (Zafar et al, 2025).

Naturally occurring substances have shown considerable promise in preclinical studies and some clinical trials as preventive agents for sundry aggressive cancers. Phytochemicals comprise diverse bioactive compounds such as polyphenols and flavonoids found abundantly in fruits and many whole grains typically. Diets rich in phytochemicals ostensibly lower cancer risk significantly and myriad health benefits are found in largely plant-based eating habits. Consumption of phytochemically rich foods inversely correlates with incidence of various cancer types notably breast and prostate cancers in numerous epidemiological studies. Effects of these compounds mediate multiple molecular pathways that regulate key processes in carcinogenesis including cell proliferation and apoptosis heavily (Zafar et al, 2025).

Phytochemical mechanisms underlying action are badly needed nowadays for effective application in cancer therapy quite crucially. Phytochemicals exert chemopreventive effects very effectively inside cells over time by modulating various quirky cellular signaling pathways. Phytochemicals haphazardly disrupt signaling of various growth factors crucial for survival and proliferation of certain malignant cells quite evidently. Compounds like curcumin present in turmeric resveratrol sourced from grapes and epigallocatechin gallate found abundantly in green tea suppress PI3K/Akt pathway remarkably dysregulated in several cancer types. Phytochemicals effectively modulate certain cellular pathways thereby arresting cycle progression and inducing apoptosis preventing uncontrolled proliferation in cancer (Rudzińska et al, 2023).

Phytochemicals fiercely combat oxidative stress marked by accumulation of reactive oxygen species and serve as potent antioxidants regulating cell survival pathways deeply. Oxidative stress precipitates carcinogenesis by inducing DNA damage and mutagenesis whilst activating signaling pathways that drive tumour progression very relentlessly. Quercetin and catechins scavenge free radicals thereby neutralizing reactive oxygen species and preventing mutations that spur cancerous cell growth rapidly. Phytochemicals markedly boost antioxidant enzyme activity including superoxide dismutase very effectively fortifying bodily defense against oxidative stress in various ways. Phytochemicals play a somewhat nebulous yet crucial role modulating inflammatory responses that become key in promoting cancer progression rather haphazardly (Rudzińska et al, 2023). Carcinogenesis gets driven substantially by chronic inflammation and many cancers result from prolonged inflammatory responses especially in liver and colorectal tissues. Sulforaphane derived from cruciferous veggies and curcumin and resveratrol vigorously suppress pro-inflammatory cytokines and enzymes such as COX-2. Compounds can naturally curb cancer initiation and progression quite significantly by reducing inflammation deeply inside various bodily tissues.

Phytochemicals profoundly influence epigenetic mechanisms by regulating gene expression subtly without altering DNA sequence itself in a very nuanced manner. DNA methylation and histone modification tweak epigenetic machinery heavily silencing tumour suppressors and ramping up oncogene activation in cancer onset scenarios. Phytochemicals like curcumin and genistein from soy modulate epigenetic marks quite effectively restoring normal gene function involved in cell cycle control apoptosis and DNA repair mechanisms. Phytochemicals emerge as riveting candidates for chemoprevention because epigenetic influences possibly provide avenues to counteract or entirely overturn cancerous cell transformations. Phytochemicals profoundly impact cancer progression by heavily influencing angiogenesis and metastasis while also affecting cell proliferation inflammation and oxidative stress variably (Shankar et al, 2013).

Tumour growth relies rather heavily on angiogenesis forming new blood vessels so cancer cells get oxygen and nutrients necessary for their survival. Resveratrol and curcumin very effectively inhibit angiogenesis by blocking vascular endothelial growth factor action rather thoroughly in various studies. Phytochemicals sabotage cancer cells' ability to invade surrounding tissues rather vigorously and exhibit profoundly anti-metastatic properties in various ways. Recently EGCG has been shown remarkably effectively inhibiting epithelial-mesenchymal transition a key process related to metastasis in various cancer studies. Phytochemicals' effectiveness as chemopreventive agents depends heavily on bioavailability namely how thoroughly they are absorbed and utilized by human body utterly. Phytochemicals typically display somewhat limited bioavailability thus curtailing therapeutic efficacy rather significantly in many cases (Shankar et al, 2013).

Research endeavours scrutinize bioavailability and delivery systems of such compounds vigorously in experimental settings nowadays with varying degrees of intensity. Nanotechnology has been very extensively explored as a means to enhance delivery of various phytochemicals in cancer prevention therapy remarkably. Preclinical studies show phytochemicals hold considerable promise in cancer prevention but human clinical trials remain very scarce somewhat surprisingly. Phytochemicals show promise in cancer treatment yielding fairly encouraging results and greatly enhancing various therapeutic outcomes very effectively in numerous clinical studies. Phytochemicals will likely wield considerable influence in cancer chemoprevention via modified approaches slowly tailored for individual genetic profiles and diverse malignancies (Chavda et al, 2022).

Phytochemicals serve as potent chemopreventive agents via multitudinous mechanisms which this chapter outlines with exhaustive thoroughness in significant depth. Bioactive compounds effectively exert protective effects against cancer through various molecular pathways including epigenetic regulation and cell cycle arrest. Delving deeply into complexities surrounding bioavailability of phytochemicals and their tricky delivery we examine possible integration into various cancer prevention tactics nowadays. Nowadays cancer prevention therapy approaches incorporating phytochemicals will be scrutinized very thoroughly against a backdrop of clinical evidence. Phytochemicals play a crucial role nowadays in remarkably mitigating burdens of cancer and encourage health outcomes through fairly vigorous exploration.

2. Phytochemicals in Cancer Prevention

Cancer remains a gargantuan global health threat culpable for astronomical mortality rates annually worldwide with fatalities mounting steadily each passing year. Extensive research quietly underscored importance of prevention through rather quirky dietary adjustments and other lifestyle modifications over many years. Phytochemicals found naturally in various plants have rather promisingly emerged as effective agents in cancer prevention nowadays. Naturally occurring substances are found in diets globally being primarily derived from plant-based foods like fruits legumes whole grains and various herbs. Phytochemicals like flavonoids possess anticancer properties that remarkably interfere with cancer progression at multiple stages fairly effectively in various ways (Kamaraju et al, 2020).

Crucial molecular mechanisms underlying their action fight cancer effectively nowadays with emerging significant therapeutic potential rather slowly. Phytochemicals act stealthily as sly modulators of vital cell processes underlying cancer initiation and swift uncontrolled tumour growth mechanisms. Cell cycle regulation serves as primary mechanism whereby compounds exert effects heavily through various downstream signaling pathways quite naturally underground. Cell division runs amok in cancerous tumours that exhibit wildly aberrant growth and frequently spawn potentially ruinous physiological effects downstream. Phytochemicals including flavonoids effectively modulate cyclin-dependent kinases and cyclins critical for cell cycle progression apparently quite rapidly (Kamaraju et al, 2020).

Phytochemicals effectively stunt cancerous cell growth at multiple stages by inhibiting crucial regulators and preventing further proliferation rather rapidly. Programmed cell death plays a crucial role rather effectively in cancer prevention within bodily tissues and bodily functions deteriorate subsequently. Cancer cells survive proliferation wildly in irregular cellular contexts where extensively disrupted apoptotic pathways no longer function properly . Phytochemicals such as curcumin from turmeric and resveratrol abundant in grapes trigger pro-apoptotic proteins like p53 and suppress anti-apoptotic Bcl-2 proteins. Cancerous cells die quite selectively whereas normal cells remain utterly unscathed beneath layers of therapeutic potency surprisingly still. Certain phytochemicals rev up DNA repair enzymes quite vigorously thereby precluding accumulation of genetic mutations that could potentially spawn cancer very slowly.

Angiogenesis spawns new blood vessels fairly rapidly through a mechanism rather crucial in progression of cancer relentlessly. Tumours require a steady blood supply subsequently growing quite rapidly and metastasizing elsewhere in body with alarming speed. Flavonoids and sulforaphane present in cruciferous veggies very effectively downregulate pro-angiogenic factors like vascular endothelial growth factor inhibiting angiogenesis thereby. Disruption hinders tumour growth very rapidly by severing supply lines of necessary nutrients and oxygen inside surrounding tissue. Inflammation plays quite a pivotal role rather centrally in cancer development. Chronic inflammation fosters a milieu ripe for tumourigenesis very readily within bodily tissues surrounding vital organs and other structures. Phytochemicals exhibit anti-inflammatory properties very effectively by modulating cytokines and signaling pathways like NF-κB in various cellular contexts or through COX-2 inhibition sometimes (Lugano et al, 2020). Polyphenols present in green tea or certain berries rather significantly mitigate oxidative stress and inflammatory responses thus reducing cancer risk fairly. Phytochemicals profoundly impact cell cycle regulation and apoptosis quite significantly while also affecting angiogenesis DNA repair very markedly and inflammation. Phytochemicals present a tantalizing prospect for thwarting cancer and intervening therapeutically by targeting various molecular pathways essential in oncology research.

2.1. Phytochemicals and Cell Cycle Regulation

Phytochemicals significantly curb cancer onset by modulating cell cycle a rigorously controlled mechanism governing growth and precipitating cell death suddenly. Cells divide under precise regulation only when necessary and undergo programmed death when severely damaged utterly or quite dysfunctional apparently. Cell proliferation runs amok fairly often in cancer largely due to aberrant regulation of cell cycles manifesting with ominous portentousness. Unchecked cell division precipitates genetic mutations accumulating rapidly inside bodily tissues and formation of malignant tumours occurs fairly quickly. Restoring proper cell cycle control becomes critical in cancer therapy and phytochemicals emerge as potent modulators of cell cycle progression rather effectively. Phytochemicals induce cell cycle arrest halting cancer cells from proliferating uncontrollably in various phases of their division cycle quite rapidly (Rahman et al, 2021).

Flavonoids a diverse group of polyphenolic compounds derived from plants are known for influencing cell cycle regulation very effectively nowadays. Quercetin a flavonoid found in various berries and onions and apples has recently been shown to induce G1/S phase arrest. Cells get snagged at some super crucial point between G1 phase where they sorta vet readiness for division and S phase where DNA replication happens subsequently. Quercetin effectively halts proliferation of cancer cells stalling progression from G1 phase and subsequently reduces tumour growth rapidly and metastasis. Kaempferol another flavonoid abundant in fruits and some veggies has shown an ability interfering with cell cycle at G1/S boundary thus inhibiting cancer cells proliferating rapidly. Blockage of DNA synthesis occurs thereby halting further cell division and promoting death of abnormal cells very quickly underground basically (Rahman et al, 2021).

Curcumin a polyphenolic compound present abundantly in turmeric spice has garnered extensive attention recently for its anticancer properties. Curcumin modulates activity of crucial cyclin-dependent kinases fairly effectively in regulation of cell cycle and impacts various cellular processes. CDK4 and CDK6 drive cell cycle progression from G1 phase into S phase rapidly alongside CDK2 in fairly quick succession. Curcumin effectively inhibits kinase activity thereby blocking G1 phase transition and subsequently halting progression of cell cycle quite remarkably. Inhibition of CDKs precipitates cell cycle arrest and sensitizes cancer cells to chemotherapy thereby markedly enhancing efficacy of treatments overall (Rahman et al, 2021).

Curcumin remarkably reduces tumour cell proliferation by targeting key cell cycle regulators and boosts likelihood of therapeutic intervention successfully. Phytochemicals play a crucial role naturally regulating cell cycles fundamental in cancer prevention. Phytochemicals like flavonoids and curcumin modulate crucial cell cycle checkpoints remarkably slowing proliferation of cancer cells and making them promising chemoprevention candidates. Cancer prevention strategies can be developed rather effectively by researchers grasping underlying molecular mechanisms of various compounds very quickly.

2.2. Induction of Apoptosis: Phytochemicals as Pro-apoptotic Agents

Apoptosis or programmed cell death enables body elimination of damaged mutated cells quite effectively every day with utter ruthless efficiency. Cells turning malignant are effectively removed by this mechanism acting as a robust safeguard against various cancers in numerous instances. Apoptosis happens fairly regularly in healthy bodily systems ensuring damaged cells succumb rather quietly in this peculiar form of cellular self-destruction. Dysregulation of apoptotic pathways occurs frequently in cancerous tissues inexorably fuelling survival of cells harbouring many mutations thereby driving tumour growth and metastasis. Apoptotic pathways restoration selectively triggers death in cancerous cells thwarting tumour growth effectively under some rather specific physiological conditions (Elmore S, 2007).

Phytochemicals occurring naturally in certain plants show significant promise in activating apoptotic pathways namely mitochondrial pathways and death receptor mediated ones. Sulforaphane a rather bioactive compound abundant in cruciferous veggies like broccoli exhibits remarkably pro-apoptotic effects having been quite thoroughly researched already in kale. Sulforaphane activates p53 tumour suppressor protein playing a crucial role in regulating apoptosis effectively under various cellular conditions (Elmore S, 2007).

p53 induces cell cycle arrest normally but initiates apoptosis vigorously if damage appears irreparable utterly. Function of p53 in cancer cells frequently undergoes mutation or inactivation allowing damaged cells with dire consequences downstream to survive unabated. Sulforaphane restores apoptosis very effectively by activating p53 and triggering death of malignant cells through complex cellular mechanisms. Sulforaphane inhibits NF-κB signaling pathway a crucial regulator of cell survival and inflammation rather separately from its effect on p53. NF-κB surges uncontrollably in malignant cells quite often fostering stubborn resistance against programmed cell death nourishing tumour-friendly inflammation around rapid growth. Sulforaphane suppresses NF-κB thereby reducing survival signals in cancer cells further encourage apoptotic response very significantly inside malignant tissues (Chen J, 2016).

Sulforaphane activates caspases crucial very much downstream of various cell signaling pathways during execution phase of apoptosis obviously. Caspases cleave various cellular substrates very rapidly and dismantle cell structures ensuring its death rather orderly in a swift manner. Resveratrol a polyphenolic compound found in foods like grapes and peanuts has garnered attention for inducing apoptosis effectively in various cancerous cells. Resveratrol somewhat intricately activates Bax/Bcl-2 pathway from within cellular environments regulating mitochondrial membrane integrity very delicately. Delicate balance of pro-apoptotic proteins like Bax and anti-apoptotic proteins such as Bcl-2 determines mitochondrial membrane permeability rather precisely ordinarily. Bax activation spurs release of pro-apoptotic factors like cytochrome c from mitochondria into cytoplasm triggering caspase activation and subsequent cell death. Bcl-2 overexpression prevents mitochondrial disruption effectively and inhibits apoptosis rather aggressively in various cancer cells with high malignancy. Resveratrol very effectively fosters mitochondrial dysfunction by significantly tilting Bax/Bcl-2 ratio heavily towards apoptosis and subsequent eradication of cancer cells (Parrish et al, 2013).

Resveratrol's effects on apoptosis aren't confined merely to mitochondria and it very effectively sensitizes cancer cells to various pro-apoptotic signals thereby boosting potential therapeutic outcomes further. Sulforaphane and resveratrol exhibit phytochemical ability targeting key apoptotic pathways that trigger selective death of cancer cells rather effectively. Molecular mechanisms underlying their action underscore huge potential of phytochemicals in cancer prevention and innovative treatment strategies are being developed rapidly nowadays. Phytochemicals trigger apoptosis through tumour suppressor activation like p53 and pro-apoptotic proteins such as Bax and concurrently inhibit cell survival pathways.

Restoring natural programmed cell death these compounds offer a promising new approach for reducing tumour growth quite effectively and metastasis. Nowadays a wealth of evidence underscores importance of various phytochemicals in cancer chemoprevention strategies remarkably through apoptotic effects very effectively. Modulating crucial apoptotic pathways naturally presents a less toxic alternative cancer treatment making them ridiculously exciting avenues for very future therapeutic development.

2.3. Inhibition of Angiogenesis: Phytochemicals and Tumour Vascularization

Tumour growth relies heavily on angiogenesis a vital process that spawns new blood vessels rapidly from pre-existing ones. Tumours expanding rapidly necessitate sufficient blood flow fueling proliferation of cells quickly within tumour mass for oxygen supply and nutrients. Tumours stay severely stunted in growth largely due to insufficient oxygen and simultaneous severe nutrient deprivation without angiogenesis being present. Angiogenesis inhibition has emerged as a pivotal tactic nowadays in cancer prevention therapy very aggressively these days worldwide. Phytochemicals show great promise inhibiting angiogenesis effectively by targeting critical molecules in various signaling pathways during blood vessel formation (Lugano et al, 2020).

Epigallocatechin gallate a catechin found predominantly in green tea has been studied extensively for various anti-angiogenic properties recently. EGCG throttles angiogenesis very effectively by messing with vascular endothelial growth factor signaling a crucial player in neovascularization processes. VEGF binds fairly potently to VEGFR2 receptor on endothelial cells lining interior surfaces of blood vessels and promotes cellular proliferation and migration. EGCG blocks crucial angiogenic processes very thoroughly by downregulating VEGF expression and inhibiting its interaction with VEGFR2 rather effectively downstream. Tumour growth potential dwindles as severely curtailed blood vessel formation falters within malignant tissue masses and metastatic ability gets hampered greatly. EGCG very effectively inhibits various pro-angiogenic factors and signaling pathways like matrix metalloproteinases involved in extracellular matrix remodeling and facilitating endothelial cell migration (Lugano et al, 2020).

Lycopene a very potent carotenoid in tomatoes and other orange fruits exhibits markedly anti-angiogenic properties under various circumstances. Lycopene quite effectively suppresses expression of MMPs a group of enzymes playing crucial roles in extracellular matrix breakdown mechanisms normally. Degradation of ECM components enables endothelial cells migrating invasively into surrounding tissues forming new blood vessels fairly rapidly. Lycopene hinders angiogenic process rather effectively by suppressing MMP activity thus diminishing endothelial cell migration very markedly in various cellular contexts. Tumour growth gets thwarted not just by prevention of angiogenesis within neoplastic masses but also by hindering cancer cells' invasive capabilities in surrounding tissues facilitating metastasis. Lycopene remarkably reduces secretion of various factors involved in angiogenesis including VEGF thereby further enhancing anti-angiogenic effects under diverse physiological conditions.

EGCG and lycopene vigorously exhibit antioxidant properties markedly reducing oxidative stress associated with cancer progression by affecting various angiogenic factors indirectly. Oxidative stress activates signaling pathways that support angiogenesis including NF-κB and HIF-1α pathways under diverse physiological and sometimes pathological states. Phytochemicals neutralize reactive oxygen species thus reducing pro-angiogenic pathway activation and significantly contributing to tumour blood vessel formation inhibition. Phytochemicals such as EGCG and lycopene very effectively offer multifaceted approaches nowadays for inhibiting angiogenesis in various cancer cells (Lugano et al, 2020). Compounds targeting key molecules like VEGF and enzymes such as MMPs disrupt establishment of tumour vascular networks involved heavily in angiogenesis through VEGFR2. Tumour growth gets stunted very quickly and metastasis of cancer cells in distant organs is significantly reduced obviously under certain conditions. Naturally occurring compounds heavily inhibit angiogenesis making them stellar prospects for cancer prevention offering potential alternatives rather quietly alongside conventional vascularization targeting treatments.

2.4. DNA Repair and Genomic Stability

Genomic stability maintains genetic material integrity within cells crucially and its disruption plays a key somewhat insidious role in cancer development. Oxidative stress sparks DNA damage which rapidly breeds mutations over time thus transforming normal cells into malignant ones very quickly. Repairing DNA damage effectively plays a crucial role in preventing cancer inside human bodies owing largely genetic integrity being maintained. Phytochemicals somewhat enhance genomic stability by facilitating DNA repair and very significantly diminishing mutation accumulation in various plant species. Phytochemicals confer protection against carcinogenesis very effectively by modulating cellular DNA repair mechanisms and exhibiting remarkably high antioxidant activity (Yao and Dai, 2014).

Phytochemicals foiling DNA damage mostly happen through strong antioxidant properties inside cells. Beta-carotene abounds in vibrant orange veggies such as carrots and sweet potatoes and acts as a very potent natural antioxidant. Beta-carotene neutralizes reactive oxygen species harbouring unstable molecules extremely adept at wreaking havoc on various cellular components notably DNA. Reactive oxygen species emerge from normal cellular processes but significantly spike in cancerous tissues owing largely to inflammation and grave mitochondrial dysfunction. ROS interacting with DNA can spur very severe oxidative damage leading rapidly to mutations and genomic instability occurs subsequently (Yao and Dai, 2014). Beta-carotene very effectively neutralizes ROS thereby significantly reducing risk of carcinogenic mutations by mitigating oxidative DNA damage. Beta-carotene markedly boosts expression of DNA repair genes and tumour suppressor genes thereby enhancing genomic stability through fairly potent antioxidant effects. Beta-carotene substantially boosts activity of tumour suppressor protein p53 which regulates cell cycle and induces apoptosis rapidly after DNA damage occurs. p53 plays crucial role in activating various mechanisms very swiftly under certain conditions to facilitate DNA repair rather effectively. Beta-carotene very effectively mitigates oxidative DNA damage and enhance genome repair thereby staving off mutagenic transformations that spark cancerous cellular changes. Berberine a bioactive compound extracted from roots of various Berberis plant species profoundly affects genomic stability and boosts DNA repair mechanisms remarkably (Didier et al, 2023).

Berberine has been shown rather convincingly boosting homologous recombination repair a crucial pathway involved deeply in mending DNA double-strand breaks very effectively. DSBs rank amongst most lethal forms of DNA damage leading rapidly to catastrophic chromosomal fragmentation and loss of vital genetic information suddenly. Genotoxic agents or radiation therapy can fairly readily induce this damage under certain circumstances owing to oxidative stress. Berberine boosts genome integrity rather effectively by ramping up homologous recombination thereby repairing DSBs and it staves off potentially carcinogenic mutations effectively downstream. Homologous recombination uses a sister chromatid as template rather accurately repairing damaged DNA very much error-free (Didier et al, 2023).

Berberine boosts DNA repair pathways quite accurately thereby mitigating risk of nasty chromosomal mutations and instability rather effectively. Berberine manifests as a potent guardian against genetic harm and potentially useful addition in oncology treatments entailing DNA-disrupting modalities such as chemo and radiotherapy. Berberine's effects on DNA repair heavily influence regulation of checkpoint kinases and other proteins sensing damage and coordinating various cellular responses. Damaged DNA gets mended rapidly under genotoxic duress thereby encourage cellular responsiveness and precluding really deleterious mutations from cropping up subsequently. Phytochemicals like beta-carotene enhance genomic stability remarkably by supercharging DNA repair mechanisms effectively amidst significant DNA damage mitigation efforts. Beta-carotene effectively counteracts ROS via antioxidant activity and prevents oxidative DNA damage while spurring activation of genes that repair DNA. Berberine rather curiously boosts repair of DNA double-strand breaks improving genomic integrity meanwhile significantly reducing risk of nasty genetic mutations. Phytochemicals emerge as valuable allies in cancer prevention by fiercely maintaining genomic integrity and thwarting accumulation of various carcinogenic mutations. Phytochemicals hold tremendous promise in preventing cancer and serve as adjuncts in existing therapies offering rather natural genomic stability thereby greatly reducing mutagenesis (van Helden et al, 2009).

2.5. Modulation of Inflammation: Phytochemicals as Anti-inflammatory Agents

Chronic inflammation fosters development of various cancer types rapidly over quite an extended period of time very much everywhere. Genetic damage thrives in such a microenvironment fostering survival and metastasis quintessential traits associated with cancerous cells proliferating rapidly. Prolonged inflammatory responses intensely fuel activation of various oncogenic pathways making inflammation very much a crucial target for multifaceted cancer prevention. Phytochemicals have demonstrated significant anti-inflammatory properties naturally rendering them very valuable candidates in fight against various nasty cancers. Compounds modulate inflammatory pathways thereby reducing chronic inflammation significantly mitigating associated cancer risk very effectively in various bodily systems. Gingerol a very potent anti-inflammatory phytochemical is found rather deeply within ginger and acts as active compound (Singh et al, 2019).

Gingerol exhibits numerous bioactivities and its anti-inflammatory action is remarkably prominent amidst these diverse physiological effects notably. It exerts effects mainly by inhibiting COX-2 enzyme which produces pro-inflammatory prostaglandins fairly quickly within bodily tissues rather deeply. COX-2 gets overexpressed frequently in various cancer cells fostering an inflammatory microenvironment promoting tumourigenesis significantly and vigorously encouraging metastasis. Gingerol inhibits COX-2 very significantly thereby reducing production of inflammatory molecules and effectively diminishing inflammatory response within tumour cells variously. Gingerol very significantly suppresses production of pro-inflammatory cytokines like TNF-α and IL-6 alongside IL-1β affecting COX-2 expression substantially (Singh et al, 2019).

Cytokines surge frequently in cancer patients and play crucial roles in various cancer progression stages including tumour initiation and rampant metastasis downstream. TNF-α sparks signaling pathways fostering cell survival and apoptosis resistance while IL-6 fuels epithelial-mesenchymal transition boosting cancer cell invasiveness with heightened metastatic potential. Gingerol quite effectively suppresses inflammatory signaling in various cellular contexts by downregulating key mediators that fuel cancer progression. Curcumin a vibrant yellow compound deeply embedded in turmeric possesses potent anti-inflammatory properties somewhat akin very much to various other obscure phytochemicals found elsewhere. Curcumin has been studied extensively modulating various signaling pathways inside cells particularly NF-κB pathway deeply during inflammatory responses (Lan et al, 2021).

NF-κB acts as crucial regulator of myriad immune responses and inflammatory processes frequently getting tangled up in development of nasty chronic maladies like cancer. NF-κB stays bound up very tightly in cytoplasm normally owing largely to association with inhibitory protein IκBα. Inflammatory signals trigger phosphorylation of IκBα leading swiftly to NF-κB activation which then translocates into nucleus inducing expression of genes that promote inflammation rapidly and cell survival. Curcumin effectively inhibits IκBα phosphorylation thereby preventing NF-κB activation in diverse cellular settings with considerable efficacy. Curcumin diminishes expression of pro-inflammatory genes encoding cytokines such as TNF-α or IL-6 and chemokines thereby slowly driving cancer progression (Lan et al, 2021).

Curcumin's suppression of NF-κB activity profoundly impacts various cellular processes deeply involved in apoptosis and cell cycle regulation alongside angiogenesis crucial for tumour growth control. Gingerol and curcumin are very potent phytochemicals regulating molecular inflammation effectively thereby reducing chronic inflammation often accompanying cancer development slowly. Compounds heavily target COX-2 enzyme and NF-κB signaling pathways thereby preventing microenvironment that supports initiation and progression of cancer inflammatorily. Their ability markedly reduces inflammation not only lessening risk of cancer but also encourage efficacy of conventional therapies otherwise badly compromised by inflammatory responses raging uncontrollably (Wang et al, 2012).

Phytochemicals like gingerol exhibit deeply anti-inflammatory effects crucial for cancer prevention nowadays effectively in many bodily processes. Certain compounds mitigate chronic inflammation contributing significantly to tumour growth and metastasis by modulating key inflammatory pathways effectively. Phytochemicals offer promising complementary cancer prevention emphasizing importance of diet rich in various obscure plant-based foods for overall drastic health improvement.

2.6. Phytochemicals in Synergy

Phytochemicals occur naturally in sundry plants and have garnered considerable scientific attention owing largely to their ostensible role in thwarting cancer. Research emerging strongly from various studies indicates true power rests in quirky combinations of phytochemicals fighting cancer via numerous molecular pathways. Multiple plant-derived compounds consumed together yield a significantly greater cancer prevention effect than sum of their individual actions possibly due to phytochemical synergy. Abundant evidence compellingly surrounds curcumin a principal curcuminoid found in turmeric and epigallocatechin gallate EGCG a major catechin abundant in green tea. Co-administration of both compounds in various cancer models has revealed remarkably enhanced ability to inhibit angiogenesis and cell proliferation significantly in many studies (Choudhari et al, 2020). Tumour growth relies heavily on angiogenesis supplying oxygen rapidly to cancer cells dividing uncontrollably and metastasis occurs with abundant nutrient availability. Curcumin and EGCG exert a very potent anti-angiogenic effect by modulating various signaling pathways like JAK/STAT3/IL-8 pathway crucial for new blood vessel formation rather quietly. Aberrant signaling cascades drive unchecked cellular division wildly through intricate interplay with various cell cycle regulators under their combined influence . Frenetic cellular growth and blood supply undergo synergistic inhibition launching a potent dual-pronged attack on tumour progression quite effectively (Choudhari et al, 2020).

Resveratrol present abundantly in red grapes combines quite potently with sulforaphane found in cruciferous veggies like broccoli showcasing enormous synergistic potential elsewhere effectively. Both compounds induce apoptosis or programmed cell death individually in various cancer cell lines very effectively. Their capacity triggers apoptosis significantly when administered together quite rapidly and it gets amplified via a fairly complex cascade. Enhanced apoptotic induction arises simultaneously from complementary actions on diverse cellular pathways within various cells rather quietly and unpredictably. Resveratrol fairly significantly influences p53 a critical tumour suppressor protein and other cell survival pathways inside cells under normal conditions. Sulforaphane potently induces phase II detoxification enzymes in cancerous cells and inhibits histone deacetylases ultimately leading down a path of apoptosis. Phytochemicals dismantle cancer cells' survival mechanisms very effectively through obscure biochemical routes and rather simultaneously in multifaceted convoluted ways (Jiang et al, 2010).

Phytochemicals exhibit remarkable chemopreventive actions by modulating molecular pathways linked intricately with initiation of cancer and subsequent deep progression. Crucial roles exist in cell cycle regulation maintaining orderly cell division heavily and preventing wildly uncontrolled growth rather haphazardly in various cellular contexts. Apoptosis gets induced quite readily eliminating grossly damaged or budding pre-cancerous cells with remarkable frequency in various cellular contexts (Jiang et al, 2010). Angiogenesis gets strongly inhibited thereby starving increasing tumours of necessary blood supply very effectively in a rather peculiar manner. DNA repair mechanisms get markedly enhanceed thereby affording protection against freaky genetic mutations possibly inciting onset of various cancers down line.

Chronic inflammation undergoes significant dampening being a driver of carcinogenesis widely recognized nowadays apparently. Bioactive compounds from plants exert a profoundly protective effect against cancer onset via multifaceted machinations and progression quite significantly. A diverse dietary regime rich in fruits whole grains legumes and veggies thwarts cancer remarkably well effectively very much across the board. Such diet furnishes elaborate mesh of protective compounds backing primary cancer prevention tactics and secondary prevention entailing swift detection or hindering disease progression rapidly (Jiang et al, 2010). Further scientific exploration unequivocally probing intricate molecular underpinnings of phytochemical synergy profoundly refines understanding of dietary patterns impacting cancer risk significantly nowadays. Sophisticated dietary-based therapeutic strategies will emerge ultimately from enhanced knowledge offering powerful new avenues in ongoing fight against cancer.

3. Mechanisms of Action

Phytochemicals a diverse assortment of bioactive compounds synthesized by plants have garnered considerable attention largely owing to their chemopreventive properties. Compounds found abundantly in fruits whole grains and various herbs offer natural multifaceted cancer prevention therapy rather effectively. Malignant cells emerge through a wonky multistep process of carcinogenesis involving initiation and very drastic subsequent molecular changes altering normal cell function drastically. Phytochemicals remarkably intervene at multiple stages influencing key cellular events such as DNA damage repair and apoptosis under diverse conditions very effectively (Hossain et al, 2025).

Phytochemicals wield anticancer effects predominantly via modulation of sundry metabolic enzymes deeply implicated in carcinogen bioactivation and subsequent detoxification pathways. Sulforaphane and isothiocyanates present in cruciferous veggies markedly upregulate phase II detoxifying enzymes such as glutathione S-transferases and NADPH quinone oxidoreductase enzymes rapidly. Enzymes very effectively facilitate excretion of carcinogens and curtail their propensity for binding DNA thereby hindering tumour initiation downstream significantly. Phytochemicals act as mighty antioxidants vigorously neutralizing reactive oxygen species thereby contributing heavily to prevention of resultant genomic instability. Quercetin and resveratrol enhance cellular antioxidant defenses remarkably mitigating oxidative stress closely linked with various cancerous developments in human bodies (Hossain et al, 2025).

Phytochemicals induce apoptosis crucially in damaged abnormal cells through a naturally programmed death process basically of cells. Curcumin genistein and apigenin trigger cell death pathways vigorously by altering mitochondrial membrane potential and upregulating pro-apoptotic proteins like Bax. Cells harbouring oncogenic mutations get eradicated very effectively thereby. Cell cycle progression gets arrested suddenly at crucial checkpoints by these compounds effectively inhibiting cell proliferation in a rather aberrant manner. Flavonoids downregulate cyclins and cyclin-dependent kinases whilst upregulating CDK inhibitors which leads quite effectively to suppression of tumour growth. Phytochemicals target chronic inflammation and tumour-promoting immune signaling effectively sometimes in various contexts biologically quite often underground.

Anti-inflammatory effects emerge very quickly by dialing down pro-inflammatory transcription factors such as NF-κB and stifling cytokine production including IL-6 or TNF-α. Phytochemicals thwart tumour expansion effectively by inhibiting metastasis and angiogenesis vital processes for cancer cell invasion very quickly underground. They effectively downregulate VEGF and matrix metalloproteinases thereby hindering formation of new blood vessels quite substantially and extracellular matrix barrier breakdown. Phytochemicals impact diverse molecular targets therapeutically offering promising avenues for cancer prevention via various dietary regimens with some success evidently.

3.1. Inhibition of Cell Cycle Progression

Precise regulation of cell cycle progression under normal physiological conditions essentially supports genomic integrity and cellular homeostasis heavily. Disruption of tightly controlled cellular mechanisms becomes characteristic of cancer allowing aberrant cells with damaged DNA to evade various checkpoints slowly. Phytochemicals exert anti-cancer effects quite effectively in various complex manners largely through modulation of cell cycle progression obviously. Bioactive plant compounds induce cell cycle arrest halting proliferation of malignant cells thereby facilitating apoptosis or repair mechanisms quite effectively inside tumour cells. Multiple phases like G1 gap 1 and S DNA synthesis and G2 gap 2 and M mitosis are encompassed by cell cycle under various checkpoints monitoring DNA integrity (Ma and Gurkan-Cavusoglu, 2024).

Cyclins and cyclin-dependent kinases governed by complex mechanisms rapidly transition cells through various phases under fairly normal physiological conditions. Aberrant activation of CDKs in cancer cells frequently triggers rampant cell proliferation and loss of checkpoint control ensuing uncontrollably. Flavonoids remarkably regulate cell cycles with considerable efficacy being present in numerous fruits and veggies as diverse polyphenolic compounds. Quercetin and kaempferol induce cell cycle arrest effectively at key transition points such as G1/S checkpoint very much every time normally. Flavonoids very effectively downregulate cyclin D1 and inhibit CDK4/6 activity thereby preventing retinoblastoma protein phosphorylation and blocking progression of S phase. Interruption inhibits proliferation enabling potential DNA repair or apoptotic pathways activation fairly readily in somewhat abnormal cells. Curcumin a principal curcuminoid derived from Curcuma longa rhizome or turmeric has been extensively studied for cell cycle modulation. It exerts effects by inhibiting key regulators like CDK2 and CDK4 alongside corresponding cyclins namely Cyclin E and D1 rather effectively (Ma and Gurkan-Cavusoglu, 2024).

Curcumin-mediated arrest typically transpires at G1 phase in various cancer models such as breast prostate and rather ferocious colorectal cancer cells. Curcumin upregulates CDK inhibitors like p21^Cip1 and p27^Kip1 thereby reinforcing a block in cell cycle progression markedly beyond mere CDK inhibition. Phytochemicals like flavonoids and curcumin suppress tumour growth quite effectively by restoring regulatory control over cell cycle rather rapidly. Them selectively arrest rapidly dividing cancer cells without severely affecting normal cells thus highlighting potential as cancer therapy adjuncts.

3.2. Induction of Apoptosis: Programmed Cell Death

Damaged cells harbouring latent danger deep within bodily tissues are quietly eliminated through apoptosis or programmed cell death surprisingly effectively. Cells harbouring genomic instability or oncogenic mutations get eliminated rapidly thereby serving as vital bulwark against cancer progression inside body. Malignant cells proliferate uncontrollably in dire cancers with severely impaired apoptosis regulation and evade death rather quietly always. Phytochemicals lately garnered considerable attention for restoring apoptotic pathways in cancer cells thereby suppressing tumour growth quite vigorously. Phytochemicals target two primary apoptotic pathways namely intrinsic pathway mediated heavily by mitochondria and extrinsic pathway triggered rather haphazardly through death receptors. Mitochondrial membrane integrity plays crucial role in intrinsic pathway regulation with Bcl-2 family proteins exercising tight control over it through pro-apoptotic Bax and anti-apoptotic members like Bcl-xL (Chen et al, 2022).

Pro-apoptotic signaling predominates releasing cytochrome c into cytosol subsequently triggering caspase activation as mitochondrial outer membrane permeabilization occurs freely. Sulforaphane triggers intrinsic apoptotic pathway via several mystifying cellular mechanisms found in cruciferous veggies like broccoli rather extensively. Tumour suppressor protein p53 activity gets enhanced quite effectively playing a crucial role in apoptosis by upregulating pro-apoptotic genes like Bax. Sulforaphane vigorously boosts expression of caspase-3 and caspase-9 and promotes destruction of cancer cells quietly without much inflammation. Resveratrol very clearly exerts pro-apoptotic effects through intrinsic pathways and extrinsic ones in red grapes and peanuts rather obviously. It modulates expression of Bcl-2 family proteins rather substantially boosting Bax/Bcl-2 ratio and promotes permeabilization of mitochondrial membrane effectively (Chen et al, 2022).

Cytochrome c release occurs swiftly and apoptosome formation happens subsequently activating caspase cascade extremely quickly downstream in cells undergoing apoptosis. Resveratrol stimulates extrinsic pathway fairly significantly by upregulating death receptors expression like Fas and TRAIL receptors on cell surfaces variously. Sulforaphane reasserts apoptotic control in cancer cells through molecular mechanisms erratically while resveratrol does so diversely with some overlap. Malignant cells undergo programmed cell death sparking interest as novel agents in oncology research effectively targeting tumours while sparing normal tissue.

3.3. Modulation of Oxidative Stress and Antioxidant Activity

Oxidative stress plays a crucial albeit oft underappreciated role rapidly initiating carcinogenesis under certain conditions during cancer progression. Reactive oxygen species production rapidly outpaces neutralizing capacity of bodily antioxidant defenses under fairly unusual stress conditions surprisingly. Free radicals such as superoxide anions wreak havoc on cells alongside non-radical molecules like hydrogen peroxide and highly reactive hydroxyl radicals. Oxidative modification of DNA bases happens simultaneously with lipid peroxidation fostering mutagenesis and genomic instability that fuels slow malignant cellular transformation. Mitigating oxidative stress effectively nowadays plays a crucial role in cancer prevention strategies under fairly normal bodily conditions (Li et al, 2023).

Phytochemicals possess remarkably potent antioxidative properties counteracting reactive oxygen species and encourage endogenous defenses extremely effectively safeguarding cellular wholeness meanwhile. Compounds act via two primary mechanisms namely direct scavenging of free radicals and modulation of cellular antioxidant enzyme systems rather effectively. Beta-carotene exhibits potent free radical scavenging activity ordinarily in rather vibrant orange vegetables like rather large spoonsful of cooked pumpkin. It stabilizes ROS very effectively by donating electrons thus mostly preventing oxidative damage to fragile DNA strands in cells. Beta-carotene substantially enhances endogenous enzymes like superoxide dismutase which converts superoxide radicals into hydrogen peroxide rapidly and glutathione peroxidase detoxifies it quickly (Li et al, 2023).

Enzymatic support diminishes oxidative stress within cells quite effectively and contributes significantly to genomic stability maintenance under fairly normal physiological conditions. EGCG and other green tea polyphenols have garnered rather considerable attention lately exhibiting potent antioxidant properties very remarkably in various studies. EGCG very effectively nowadays acts as direct antioxidant neutralizing various ROS and induces expression of phase II detoxifying enzymes like glutathione-S-transferase. Dual mechanisms amplify cellular resistance against oxidative stress significantly within cells ravaged by harsh environmental conditions very badly (Randisi et al, 2025). EGCG inhibits ROS-generating enzymes like NADPH oxidase quite significantly contributing rather broadly to reduction in cellular oxidative stress states. Phytochemicals maintain redox homeostasis fairly effectively and rapidly interrupt various cancer development stages through obscure biochemical mechanisms. Antioxidant activity manifests peculiarly toward cancer cells enduring heightened oxidative stress relative somewhat to normal cells under apparently differing circumstances. Selectivity enhance potential of these agents as safe cancer chemoprevention options and highlights value of phytochemical rich diets mitigating overall cancer risk .

3.4. Inhibition of Angiogenesis

Angiogenesis is a physiological process where new blood vessels burst forth from pre-existing vasculature playing a vital albeit oft-maligned role in tissue repair and cancer progression. Angiogenesis plays crucial role in furnishing oxygen and nutrients rapidly for cancerous tissue proliferation during tumourigenesis. Tumour cells spread very quickly through bloodstream thereby heavily contributing to metastasis. Tumour growth heavily relies on activation of angiogenic switch which has surfaced as plausible target in novel cancer prevention strategies effectively nowadays. Phytochemicals very evidently possess anti-angiogenic properties as bioactive compounds naturally present in various foods derived from plants mostly. Compounds mainly disrupt key signaling pathways in neovascularization mediated by vascular endothelial growth factor its receptor VEGFR and various matrix metalloproteinases (Saman et al, 2020).

Epigallocatechin gallate a major catechin found abundantly in green tea demonstrated remarkably potent anti-angiogenic activity in various in vitro models and in some in vivo studies subsequently. EGCG exerts its effects very effectively nowadays mainly by downregulating VEGF a major driver of angiogenesis in various tumour microenvironments. VEGF vigorously promotes endothelial cell proliferation and spawns new capillary formation frenetically inside tumour microenvironment rather haphazardly. EGCG inhibits VEGF/VEGFR2 signaling thereby reducing angiogenic markers expression and decreasing microvessel density ultimately impairing tumour vascularization significantly in various tumours. EGCG reportedly messes with various other angiogenic mediators such as platelet-derived growth factor and basic fibroblast growth factor very significantly amplifying its anti-angiogenic potential (Saman et al, 2020).

Lycopene quite remarkably exhibits significant anti-angiogenic effects in tomatoes and watermelon and pink grapefruit very frequently indeed. Lycopene markedly suppresses activity of matrix metalloproteinases particularly MMP-2 and MMP-9 enzymes that degrade extracellular matrix components rapidly. Degradation occurs beforehand facilitating endothelial cell migration and capillary sprouting extensively within various angiogenic processes fairly rapidly. Lycopene thwarts angiogenic restructuring somewhat by heavily suppressing MMP expression and activity and curtails tumour cell invasive potential very effectively. Phytochemicals foster an anti-angiogenic microenvironment starving tumours of oxygen and nutrients effectively reducing metastatic spread somewhat irregularly overall. Diet-derived agents like EGCG and lycopene thwart angiogenesis strongly underscoring promise in cancer prevention and encourage dietary strategies rich with phytochemicals.

3.5. Anti-inflammatory Effects: Modulating Inflammation in Cancer

Carcinogenesis gets fueled largely by chronic inflammation nowadays almost everywhere rather quietly and its recognition is increasingly pervasive. Chronic inflammation spawns tenacious immune hyperactivity that subtly cultivates fertile soil for cancerous cells with extreme prejudice very quietly underground. Prolonged production of inflammatory mediators such as cytokines and prostaglandins promotes genetic instability haphazardly and supports metastasis quite vigorously sometimes. Cancer prevention involves vigorously targeting inflammation crucially and many complex biological processes are naturally implicated in treatment. Phytochemicals from plant-based foods exhibit potent anti-inflammatory activities by regulating key signaling pathways associated with inflammation very effectively downstream (Fishbein et al, 2021).

Compounds can very effectively attenuate chronic inflammation underlying tumour development by modulating expression of various transcription factors and cytokines. Curcumin a principal curcuminoid present in turmeric spice Curcuma longa exhibits significant anti-inflammatory properties among highly studied phytochemicals quite ordinarily. Nuclear factor-kappa B, a central transcription factor in inflammatory responses gets inhibited quite frequently via one primary mechanism. NF-κB gets constitutively activated in many cancers leading upregulation of pro-inflammatory cytokines like tumour necrosis factor-alpha and sundry interleukins fairly often nowadays. Cytokines vigorously promote tumour cell survival and metastasis while stimulating proliferation fairly extensively in certain cases (Fishbein et al, 2021).

Curcumin hinders activation of NF-κB by thwarting degradation of inhibitor IκBα thereby blocking its translocation very deeply into nucleus. Markedly diminished expression of downstream inflammatory mediators results and tumour-promoting inflammation gets suppressed significantly under certain peculiar conditions basically. Gingerol a pungent bioactive compound in ginger Zingiber officinale fairly remarkably exhibits notable anti-inflammatory effects with great efficacy suddenly. Gingerol effectively inhibits expression of cyclooxygenase-2 or COX-2 an inducible enzyme that catalyzes formation of pro-inflammatory prostaglandins rapidly from arachidonic acid. COX-2 overexpression manifests rather frequently in diverse malignancies especially virulent forms of colorectal cancer and correlates with markedly enhanced tumourigenesis (Olivera et al, 2012). Gingerol quite effectively diminishes prostaglandin production by downregulating COX-2 expression thereby dampening inflammatory microenvironment that supports cancer development. Curcumin and gingerol together rather effectively exemplify how certain phytochemicals present in diet intervene in oncogenesis driven heavily by inflammation. Modulating inflammatory signaling pathways makes them very promising candidates in cancer prevention strategies employed nowadays with considerable integrative efficacy apparently. Adjunctive therapies and dietary interventions might effectively target inflammatory roots of tumour biology thus mitigating cancer risk quite significantly.

3.6. Epigenetic Modulation: Phytochemicals and Gene Expression

Gene expression undergoes heritable yet reversible epigenetic modifications fairly often sans alterations of underlying DNA sequence whatsoever normally. Silencing tumour suppressor genes and activating oncogenes rapidly fuels cancer initiation and metastasis via aberrant regulatory processes. Phosphorylation of non-coding RNAs like microRNAs and DNA methylation histone acetylation play quite a crucial albeit largely underappreciated role obviously. Epigenetic alterations are potentially reversible unlike genetic mutations making them rather attractive targets for cancer therapy quite possibly today. Phytochemicals have surfaced rather promisingly as epigenetic modulators influencing gene expression deeply within cellular phenotype under diverse physiological conditions. Certain natural compounds reactivate genes that halt cell cycle progression and stimulate DNA repair mechanisms alongside cellular detoxification processes effectively (Gu et al, 2024).

Sulforaphane a rather well-studied isothiocyanate derived from cruciferous veggies like broccoli exhibits strong epigenetic activity in various cells very effectively. Histone deacetylases are very strongly inhibited by it leading rather quickly to chromatin condensation and gene silencing ultimately occurs. Sulforaphane fosters relatively open chromatin structure by heavily inhibiting various HDACs and thereby facilitates transcription of some tumour suppressor genes like p21 or BAX. Sulforaphane modulates DNA methyltransferases somewhat effectively by inhibiting enzymes that rapidly add methyl groups to cytosine residues in CpG islands often leading gene silencing. Sulforaphane very effectively reactivates silenced tumour suppressor genes through various epigenetic actions and represses oncogenes aberrantly expressed inside cancerous cells (Gu et al, 2024).

Resveratrol heavily influences epigenetic regulation naturally in various organisms found predominantly in red grapes and berries or peanuts. DNA methylation patterns get modulated particularly in genes heavily involved in cancer progression nowadays very frequently and quite robustly. Resveratrol effectively inhibits DNMTs leading to demethylation and re-expression of silenced tumour suppressor genes like p16INK4a and RASSF1A in various cancer cells. Resveratrol markedly influences activity of sirtuins a disparate family of histone deacetylases reliant on NAD+ that play crucial roles in chromatin remodeling during intense cellular stress conditions. Phytochemical action prevents cancer fairly effectively nowadays by epigenetic means collectively underscoring various intriguing aspects of this complex phenomenon. Sulforaphane and resveratrol somewhat restore normal gene expression profiles in cancerous cells by modulating epigenetic regulators very effectively. Phytochemicals irregularly exhibit broad therapeutic potential due to epigenetic effects that couple with influence over cell cycle apoptosis oxidative stress and angiogenesis. Diets heavy with plant-based food naturally offer multi-pronged cancer prevention and substantial long-term wellness benefits quite effectively overall.

4. Bioactive Plant Compounds

Cancer remains a major cause of morbidity globally exhibiting complex pathophysiology characterized by genetic mutations and aberrant cellular signaling remarkably downstream. Conventional therapies such as chemotherapy have significantly improved outcomes in various cancer types but toxicity and resistance often crop up. Growing scientific interest fuels exploration of bioactive plant compounds as complementary agents for cancer prevention alongside conventional treatments. Phytochemicals occur rather abundantly in fruits and medicinal herbs and whole grains and vegetables naturally.

Various compounds are found naturally including flavonoids and carotenoids alongside alkaloids glucosinolates phenolic acids terpenoids polyphenols and many other such substances. They've demonstrated considerable aptitude in interacting with molecular targets deeply entwined in carcinogenesis and modulating signalling pathways governing cell proliferation and apoptosis significantly downstream. Phytochemicals exhibit remarkably diverse actions on numerous cellular processes with considerable potency in various contexts simultaneously and with great efficacy. Turmeric's curcumin suppresses inflammatory signalling remarkably by inhibiting the NF-κB pathway and induces apoptosis largely through activation of caspase enzymes (Tungmunnithum et al, 2018).

Epigallocatechin gallate abundant in green tea potently inhibits angiogenesis by blocking VEGF signaling and reduces oxidative stress significantly. Phytochemicals profoundly impact cell cycle regulation a crucial process severely dysregulated in malignant cancer cells very often fortunately. Quercetin and genistein very effectively induce cell cycle arrest at various checkpoints thwarting proliferation rather unchecked in a multitude of cancerous cells. Bioactive plant compounds modulate tumour microenvironment rather effectively by reducing inflammation and oxidative stress which heavily contribute to tumour progression obviously. Phytochemicals crucially exhibit selective toxicity toward cancer cells and spare relatively normal tissues remarkably in a healthy state. Such property makes them tantalizing candidates for chemopreventive and therapeutic applications either alone or paired with conventional therapies enhancing efficacy remarkably (Tungmunnithum et al, 2018). Bioactive plant compounds exert anti-cancer effects through intricate molecular machinations unfolding sluggishly within harsh cellular environments under various conditions. They heavily regulate cell cycle control and programmed cell death and angiogenesis underscoring their potential as mighty agents in managing cancer effectively.

4.1. Modulation of the Cell Cycle: Regulating Cancer Cell Proliferation

Cell cycle regulation maintains normal cellular function and genomic integrity deeply within tissues that are undergoing rapid homeostasis basically. Cell cycle entails several tightly regulated phases G1 S G2 and M with intricate molecular checkpoints vigilantly assessing DNA integrity and replication fidelity. Cancer arises partly from breakdowns in cellular regulation allowing cells circumventing vital checkpoints and proliferating wildly with DNA lesions and aberrant molecular cues. Restoring control over cell cycle progression becomes quite an effectively promising strategy in cancer prevention and therapy somewhat obviously. Bioactive plant compounds particularly flavonoids exert strong anti-proliferative effects very effectively by messing with cell cycle machinery (Barnum and O'Connell, 2014).

Cancer cells get arrested very selectively at specific phases namely G1/S transition which is crucial for commitment to DNA synthesis and subsequent cell division. Quercetin and catechins are remarkably well known in apples onions and green tea for arresting cell cycles in cancer cells variously. Quercetin heavily suppresses expression and activity of cyclin-dependent kinases CDK2 and CDK4 alongside their regulatory partners cyclin D and E. Kinases crucially enable phosphorylation of retinoblastoma protein a step that necessitates G1 progression fairly rapidly into S phase now. Quercetin effectively halts cell cycle progression by maintaining Rb in hypophosphorylated active form and suppresses tumour cell proliferation quite vigorously. Epigallocatechin gallate EGCG profoundly stalls G1 phase by downregulating cyclin D1 and boosting expression of CDK inhibitors p21 and p27 rather effectively (Barnum and O'Connell, 2014). Curcumin quite vividly exhibits potent properties modulating cell cycle being a yellow polyphenol derived from turmeric spice Curcuma longa. Inhibition of CDK4/6 and cyclin D1 expression occurs frequently in various cancer cell lines such as breast cancer cells and prostate cancer cells. Curcumin modulates crucial G1/S regulators thereby halting cells from entering DNA synthesis phase and restricting expansion of malignant cell populations heavily. Bioactive plant compounds offer a promising approach controlling cancer cell proliferation by targeting multiple molecular regulators deeply within cell cycle processes. Tumour cells undergo selective induction of cell cycle arrest whereas normal cells remain unaffected thus encourage their potential as cancer chemoprevention agents.

4.2. Induction of Apoptosis: Promoting Programmed Cell Death

Programmed cell death entails intricate cellular processes vital for tissue homeostasis and eliminates genetically unstable cells rather swiftly. Malignant cells flagrantly evade apoptosis with unrelenting persistence under most circumstances, displaying anomalous resilience in various cancer contexts very frequently. Cancer cells harbour accrued mutations and proliferate very unabatedly under complex circumstances resisting various therapies with enabled disruption. Bioactive plant compounds show significant therapeutic promise as effective treatment often necessitates reinstatement of apoptotic machinery in cancer cells. Phytochemicals trigger apoptosis fairly selectively in cancer cells through intrinsic mitochondrial pathways and death receptor mediated extrinsic routes quite simultaneously (Elmore S, 2007).

Pro-apoptotic signals get amplified usually in malignant tissues and anti-apoptotic mechanisms get inhibited thereby shifting balance decisively toward cell death. Sulforaphane potently induces apoptosis in various cancer cells being a sulfur-containing compound abundant mostly in cruciferous veggies like broccoli kale. Tumour suppressor protein p53 gets activated via one primary mechanism and serves as critical regulator of various stress responses cellularly. Sulforaphane riles up p53 very vigorously inducing expression of pro-apoptotic proteins like Bax and PUMA thus facilitating mitochondrial outer membrane permeabilization rather extensively. Cytochrome c release into cytoplasm triggers initiator caspases such as caspase-9 which subsequently activates downstream executioner caspases like caspase-3 (Elmore S, 2007). Cancer cell death ultimately results from systematic degradation of various cellular components occurring randomly over a fairly prolonged period. Notably effects manifest predominantly in models relating to lung cancer and prostate cancer under various experimental conditions. Resveratrol exhibits remarkably strong pro-apoptotic effects in cancer cells found mainly in red grapes and also in peanuts occasionally. It heavily modulates expression of Bcl-2 family proteins tipping balance toward apoptosis. Resveratrol strongly upregulates pro-apoptotic Bax while downregulating anti-apoptotic Bcl-2 thus fostering mitochondrial outer membrane permeabilization and liberation of cytochrome c subsequently (Selvaraj et al, 2015).

Caspase activation subsequently unfolds resulting in cell death under tightly regulated conditions ensuing ordinarily from such a catastrophic molecular cascade. Resveratrol has shown remarkable efficacy inducing apoptosis effectively in various cancer types including colon breast and pancreatic cancer cells. Sulforaphane and resveratrol target regulatory proteins and enzymes representing promising agents for cancer therapy notably downstream and quite upstream effectively. Phytochemicals show rather considerable promise somewhat surprisingly in less toxic cancer treatments and more integrative strategies overall apparently.

4.3. Inhibition of Angiogenesis: Preventing Tumour Blood Supply

Angiogenesis involves new blood vessels bursting forth rapidly from existing vasculature underlying embryonic development wound healing and tissue regeneration remarkably. Angiogenesis plays a pathological role facilitating cancer progression as tumours grow beyond a critical size and metastasize quite rapidly distantly. Tumours stimulate angiogenesis by secreting various pro-angiogenic factors, most notably vascular endothelial growth factor, which binds endothelial receptors vigorously, promoting endothelial cell proliferation and migration. Tumour starvation via angiogenesis inhibition has emerged slowly as a potent therapy strategy aiming stealthily at cutting off the blood supply. Bioactive plant compounds possessing anti-angiogenic properties offer promising natural agents complementing existing cancer-fighting strategies fairly effectively these days.

Epigallocatechin gallate, a major catechin found abundantly in green tea, Camellia sinensis has been studied very extensively for various anti-angiogenic effects lately. EGCG suppresses expression and signaling of VEGF a potent angiogenic cytokine secreted copiously by tumour cells under extremely hypoxic stressful conditions. EGCG very effectively thwarts endothelial cell proliferation migration and tube formation by disrupting VEGF/VEGFR signaling pathway somewhat irregularly it appears. Suppression severely disrupts vascular networks tumours rely on effectively limiting tumour growth and metastatic potential over a fairly long period of time. EGCG exerts antioxidant effects very significantly and anti-inflammatory effects, further reducing the pro-angiogenic microenvironment surrounding tumours rather effectively (Singh et al, 2011).

Lycopene very abundantly displays strong anti-angiogenic activity in tomatoes watermelon and pink grapefruit being basically a lipophilic carotenoid. Lycopene effectively inhibits expression and activity of matrix metalloproteinases particularly MMP-2 and MMP-9 downstream in various cells very potently. Enzymes facilitate degradation of extracellular matrix rapidly enabling endothelial cells to migrate and new capillaries sprout during various angiogenic processes. Lycopene very effectively stabilizes extracellular environment and suppresses neovascularization by toning down MMP expression thereby halting endothelial cell remodeling entirely. Lycopene has been shown very effectively under certain conditions to downregulate inflammatory cytokines and oxidative stress markers stimulating angiogenesis.

Lycopene's anti-angiogenic effects very remarkably enhance its chemopreventive properties in stomach cancers and various prostate cancer cells effectively. Bioactive plant compounds thwart angiogenesis via diverse molecular mechanisms thus presenting a strong rationale for therapeutic inclusion in cancer prevention protocols. Tumour growth sustainment gets impaired by natural agents and they hinder capacity for invasion and metastasis making them very valuable tools comprehensively in cancer control.

4.4. Anti-inflammatory Effects

Chronic inflammation plays a rather pivotal albeit oft overlooked role in cancer initiation and metastasis fuelling progression somewhat rapidly nowadays. Tumour microenvironment abounds with inflammatory signals harboring cytokines alongside prostaglandins and reactive oxygen species interacting with oncogenic pathways facilitating transformation into malignant phenotypes rather rapidly. Inflammation fosters DNA damage rapidly stimulating angiogenesis fairly quickly thereby facilitating immune evasion and creating fertile ground for cancerous growth (Nishida and Andoh, 2025). Focusing on inflammation appears remarkably promising overall for cancer prevention strategies and devising new treatment approaches effectively nowadays.

Bioactive compounds from plant sources exhibit multifaceted anti-inflammatory properties quite effectively mitigating chronic inflammation linked with various cancer types. Extensively studied phytochemical properties in curcumin a principal curcuminoid of turmeric remarkably exhibit anti-inflammatory and anti-cancer effects very thoroughly. Nuclear factor-kappa B signaling pathway gets inhibited mainly via some crucial mechanism very effectively underneath various biological contexts. NF-κB regulates expression of pro-inflammatory genes like tumour necrosis factor-alpha and interleukin-6, quite frequently acting downstream of various stimuli. NF-κB activation happens perpetually in cancers such as breast cancer and pancreatic cancer, fuelling inflammation and tumourigenesis (El-Saadony et al, 2023).

Curcumin inhibits NF-κB translocation into the nucleus thereby suppressing expression of downstream pro-inflammatory mediators and disrupting inflammatory milieu fostering cancer cell survival extensively; 6-gingerol a pungent constituent present in Zingiber officinale is renowned for multifaceted chemopreventive attributes and anti-inflammatory effects (El-Saadony et al, 2023). Gingerol quite rapidly suppresses COX-2 expression a crucial enzyme catalyzing prostaglandin production from arachidonic acid with significant efficacy. PGE2 and similar prostaglandins play a vital role in fostering tumour growth effectively alongside suppressing immune response quite vigorously and resisting apoptosis. Gingerol very effectively diminishes pro-tumourigenic inflammatory response by downregulating COX-2 and curbing synthesis of prostaglandin in a fairly significant manner. Gingerol exhibits potent anticancer effects in gastric and liver malignancies via modulation of various inflammation-related signalling cascades like PI3K/Akt pathways. Bioactive plant compounds such as curcumin and gingerol modulate key inflammatory pathways driving tumourigenesis effectively in diverse oncological contexts. Interfering with oncogenic signaling and diminishing expression of inflammatory mediators makes them very valuable nowadays in cancer prevention strategies. Integrating natural agents into dietary regimens or therapy may somewhat mitigate carcinogenesis driven largely by inflammatory responses reducing reliance heavily on pharmaceuticals.

4.5. Inhibition of Metastasis

Metastasis remains a predominant factor globally in deaths related very closely with various nasty forms of cancer nowadays, obviously. Cancer cells set off on a tortuous journey, detaching from primary tumours and invading surrounding tissues very readily into bloodstream or lymphatic vessels. Multiple molecular events converge rather haphazardly, driving changes in cellular adhesion and degradation of matrix outside cells alongside epithelial-to-mesenchymal transition. Substantial research nowadays focuses on identifying novel agents capable of inhibiting complex metastatic processes effectively with varying degrees of success. Bioactive plant compounds exert multifaceted effects on various cancer signalling pathways and emerge as promising antimetastatic therapeutic agents very suddenly.

Sulforaphane effectively targets multiple pathways with antimetastatic properties in cruciferous veggies like broccoli fairly quickly. Nuclear factor-kappa B, a transcription factor regulating genes linked with inflammation, cell survival and metastasis, gets inhibited mainly via one obscure mechanism. Sulforaphane downregulates matrix metalloproteinases very effectively, particularly MMP-2 and MMP-9, which are critical for the degradation of ECM and cancer cell invasion. Sulforaphane significantly impairs the migratory capacity of cancer cells and invasion into surrounding tissues by simultaneously suppressing NF-κB activity and MMP. Sulforaphane significantly reduces metastatic spread in lung cancer models and diminishes it remarkably in prostate cancer and breast cancer setups. Berberine, a compound found in various Berberis plants, shows significant anti-metastatic activity modulating epithelial-mesenchymal transition fairly effectively in several studies (Kaiser et al, 2021).

Berberine quashes EMT by stifling transforming growth factor-beta and Wnt/β-catenin signalling pathways crucial for the induction of EMT. Berberine restores epithelial markers like E-cadherin very effectively and downregulates vimentin and N-cadherin in cancer cells, reversing EMT very aggressively. Effects have manifested remarkably in experimental liver cancer models, surprisingly in gastrointestinal cancer models and also very frequently in nasopharyngeal ones. Sulforaphane and berberine exemplify bioactive compounds disrupting crucial cancer metastasis mechanisms quite effectively through various obscure, somewhat entangled molecular pathways. Phytochemicals in the diet show promise as antimetastatic agents targeting various pathways like NF-κB and EMT-associated signalling very naturally. Novel dietary regimens or pharmacological treatments incorporating these compounds may drastically curb cancer spread and boost patient survival rates in the very longterm (Kaiser et al, 2021).

4.6. Epigenetic Modulation: Reversing Aberrant Gene Expression

Epigenetic regulation involves heritable yet reversible changes in gene expression happening rather mysteriously without profoundly altering underlying DNA sequence. Non-coding RNA regulation and histone modifications alongside DNA methylation play crucial roles remarkably within normal cellular functions. Malignant transformation gets facilitated rather slowly by epigenetic dysregulation in cancer which fosters silencing of tumour suppressor genes and activates oncogenes. Epigenetic alterations are potentially reversible unlike genetic mutations making them rather attractive targets for novel highly promising therapeutic strategies.

Phytochemicals have emerged as very potent modulators of epigenetic machinery, offering cancer prevention avenues and innovative treatment strategies quietly (Al Aboud et al, 2025).

Sulforaphane exhibits potent epigenetic activity as a naturally occurring isothiocyanate found abundantly in cruciferous veggies like broccoli and cauliflower ordinarily. It inhibits histone deacetylases HDACs rather quietly, enzymes that remove acetyl groups from histone tails leading to gene silencing. Sulforaphane fosters histone acetylation by suppressing HDAC activity thereby reactivating silenced tumour suppressor genes in a more open chromatin state. Sulforaphane markedly downregulates DNA methyltransferases very frequently in tumour suppressor gene promoter regions undergoing aberrant hypermethylation rather stealthily (Al Aboud et al, 2025). Dual action restores normal epigenetic patterns and induces cell cycle arrest apoptosis and differentiation in various cancer cell lines including prostate cancer models. Resveratrol a polyphenol often found very abundantly in grapes and some berries exerts surprisingly robust epigenetic effects quite frequently.

Reactivation of silenced genes involving apoptosis and cell cycle regulation occurs rather quietly downstream of modulation of DNA methylation and histone acetylation. Resveratrol inhibits DNMTs and alters activity of histone acetyltransferases very significantly alongside HDACs contributing significantly to a more balanced epigenetic landscape. Tumour suppressive functions get restored subsequently and modifications lead suppression of oncogenic signaling quite effectively afterwards normally. Resveratrol quite effectively demonstrates such properties in various malignancies including leukemia and colon cancer and some breast tumours. Bioactive plant compounds rather effectively reprogram cancer epigenome highlighting profound capacity for epigenetic modulation within malignant cells collectively. Sulforaphane and resveratrol weirdly impede cancer progression deeply by reversing epigenetic silencing of tumour suppressor genes and inhibiting oncogene expression massively. Compounds like these may provide an accessible non-toxic long-term strategy for controlling cancer when incorporated into various therapeutic regimens or diets. Investigation of phytochemical epigenetics might unlock new avenues complementing conventional oncology treatments very effectively with surprising ease nowadays.

5. Antioxidant and Anti-inflammatory Effects of Phytochemicals in Chemoprevention

Tumourigenesis progresses haphazardly via intricate mechanisms fueled largely by heritable predispositions and exogenous stressors including lousy dietary patterns and torpid physical activity. Oxidative stress and chronic inflammation play central roles vigorously in initiating carcinogenic processes under diverse pathological conditions often remarkably. Reactive oxygen species generated during normal cellular metabolism or by environmental insults can badly damage lipids proteins and DNA in cells. Unrepaired damage can very rapidly lead genomic instability and activation of various oncogenic pathways rather quickly over a long period. Relentless cytokine secretion and growth factors create a pro-tumourigenic environment fostering cell proliferation and metastasis from chronic inflammation (Wang et al, 2025).

Phytochemicals exhibit profoundly potent antioxidant properties naturally in various fruits and veggies making them ostensibly promising cancer chemoprevention agents. Compounds effectively neutralise ROS and remarkably boost the activity of endogenous antioxidant enzymes like superoxide dismutase and glutathione peroxidase. Quercetin and curcumin vigorously scavenge free radicals and upregulate antioxidant response elements through activation of Nrf2 pathway remarkably. Phytochemicals effectively modulate various signaling pathways involved very deeply in inflammation including nuclear factor-kappa B and inducible nitric oxide synthase (Wang et al, 2025).

Gingerol from ginger and curcumin from turmeric suppress NF-κB activation markedly decreasing expression of pro-inflammatory cytokines like TNF-α and IL-6. Phytochemicals profoundly disrupt inflammatory cascades, reducing chronic inflammation that supports tumour growth very effectively and boosting survival marginally in patients. Phytochemicals simultaneously cultivate a hostile biochemical milieu for carcinogenesis via profoundly anti-inflammatory actions and markedly antioxidant effects. Compounds significantly contribute to prevention of malignant transformation by restoring cellular redox balance and inhibiting various inflammatory mediators thereby suppressing tumour progression. Consuming phytochemical-rich foods fairly regularly can offer a very natural way of mitigating cancer risk and enhancing overall well-being substantially. Ongoing research slowly unravels molecular mechanisms whereby phytochemicals profoundly exert protective effects offering valuable insight for development of novel chemopreventive agents from plants.

5.1. Oxidative Stress and Cancer

Reactive oxygen species surge wildly beyond bodily capacity and get neutralized somewhat naturally by antioxidants everyday. Reactive oxygen species such as superoxide anions and hydroxyl radicals are generated fairly frequently during normal cellular metabolic processes. Excess ROS production wreaks havoc on cellular components such as DNA and proteins ultimately leading to carcinogenesis and very severe genomic instability. Body relies heavily on endogenous antioxidants like superoxide dismutase alongside glutathione and exogenous antioxidants obtained very effectively from diet. Phytochemicals like polyphenols and carotenoids play a crucial role mitigating oxidative stress thereby preventing DNA damage linked with various cancer onsets (Bardaweel et al, 2018).

Potent antioxidants scavenge ROS thereby encourage bodily defenses significantly modulating cellular pathways deeply entangled in oxidative stress responses. Flavonoids like quercetin and kaempferol are powerful antioxidants found abundantly in fruits and vegetables and various teas. Quercetin-like flavonoids abound in numerous fruits while kaempferol powerfully combats oxidation in sundry teas and vegetables remarkably well. Carotenoids including beta-carotene and lycopene are potent antioxidants found in colorful fruits and veggies thereby reducing mutation risk slowly (Bardaweel et al, 2018).

Flavonoids markedly induce expression of antioxidant enzymes like superoxide dismutase thereby encourage endogenous defense mechanisms very effectively in body. Beta-carotene lycopene and lutein are potent antioxidants found abundantly in vibrantly colorful fruits and some vegetables. Resveratrol found in grapes and berries exhibits strong antioxidant properties by effectively scavenging ROS and reducing DNA damage caused by oxidation. Lycopene rich in tomatoes has been shown rather effectively reducing oxidative damage somewhat peculiarly inside prostate cancer cells.

5.2. Chronic Inflammation and Cancer

Chronic inflammation fosters cancer development rather aggressively and progression happens subsequently with notable rapidity in a most unsettling manner subsequently. Chronic inflammation persists very obstinately fostering a tumourigenic milieu quite unlike acute inflammation that rapidly dissipates after removal of harmful stimuli. Cancer development unfolds via multiple stages with inflammatory cells playing crucial roles from initiation onwards towards eventual metastasis. Prolonged inflammation spawns reactive oxygen species and nitrogen radicals that ravage DNA fueling pathways supporting tumour growth quite aggressively.

Pro-inflammatory cytokines like tumour necrosis factor-alpha spur inflammation-associated cancer alongside interleukin-6 enzymes such as cyclooxygenase-2 and nuclear factor-kappa B transcription factors. NF-κB orchestrates expression of multiple genes heavily involved in inflammation proliferation metastasis and somewhat irregular angiogenesis. Activation of these pathways continuously has been tenuously linked with various cancers of colon and pancreas and stomach and liver among sundry maladies. Phytochemicals present in various plant-based foods possess rather promising anti-inflammatory properties that modulate cancer-promoting processes with some efficacy. Turmeric rhizomes harbor curcumin quite deeply as one of nature's most extensively researched anti-inflammatory compounds apparently (Mao et al, 2025).

NF-κB activation gets suppressed thereby very significantly downregulating expression of TNF-α IL-6 and COX-2 under sundry conditions rather mysteriously. Curcumin thwarts specific mediators thereby mitigating inflammation and disrupting pathways that promote tumour cell proliferation and neovascularization simultaneously inside tissues. Inflammation plays a significant pathogenic role in pancreatic cancers and effects have been notably observed particularly there. Gingerol a pungent phenolic compound found abundantly in ginger rather effectively exhibits fairly comparable anti inflammatory effects these days. COX 2 expression gets very significantly throttled and synthesis of pro-inflammatory prostaglandins plummets substantially within affected tissues (Mao et al, 2025). Gingerol disrupts chronic inflammatory signals fueling cancer progression heavily in gastric and colorectal cancers by downregulating NF-κB activity.

Sulforaphane very much targets inflammatory pathways crudely derived from cruciferous veggies like broccoli and kale rather effectively every single time. It crudely suppresses expression of IL-1β and IL-6 and blocks activation of NF-κB quite effectively in various pathways alongside COX-2. Actions taken together remarkably enhance bodily defence against cancerous cell proliferation and mitigate inflammatory conditions that foster tumourigenesis quite effectively. Phytochemicals with anti-inflammatory properties act very effectively nowadays as a natural strategy to disrupt inflammatory signalling underlying various cancers. Incorporating them into plant-based diets may yield profoundly protective outcomes and enhance cancer prevention strategies alongside various therapeutic interventions effectively today.

5.3. Phytochemicals in Chemoprevention

Phytochemicals wield considerable chemopreventive potential by modulating myriad cancer-related pathways effectively in diverse biological settings all at once very rapidly. Anti-inflammatory activities and antioxidant properties synergize rather effectively reducing molecular damage that fuels cancer initiation and rapid progression. Oxidative stress and chronic inflammation are very tightly interconnected with reactive oxygen species vigorously activating inflammatory signaling pathways while inflammation generates copious ROS production. Vicious cycles fuel epigenetic alterations largely through very severe DNA damage and tumour-promoting microenvironments beset by immune dysregulation. Phytochemicals are oddly well-suited for breaking this vicious cycle through multifaceted mechanisms key in cancer prevention efforts evidently (Jang and Lee, 2023).

Resveratrol very frequently exemplifies a dual role being a polyphenolic compound found in red grapes and various berries and peanuts. It very effectively upregulates endogenous antioxidant enzymes like superoxide dismutase and catalase while neutralizing reactive oxygen species as a potent antioxidant. Resveratrol exerts anti-inflammatory effects by simultaneously suppressing expression of TNF-α IL-6 and COX-2 key mediators within tumour microenvironment very effectively. Resveratrol quite effectively inhibits activation of NF-κB a transcription factor governing expression of numerous genes deeply embedded in inflammatory responses and mechanisms that promote cell survival (Jang and Lee, 2023). Tumour progression markedly slows in breast and colon cancer due largely to combined effects that significantly reduce cancer initiation risk. Epigallocatechin-3-gallate EGCG and other green tea polyphenols display unusually broad chemopreventive effects rather effectively in various contexts. EGCG radically scavenges free radicals thereby heavily reducing oxidative stress at cellular level. It very significantly inhibits NF-κB pathway thereby decreasing expression of inflammatory cytokines and enzymes such as COX-2 and iNOS nitric oxide synthase (Zoi et al, 2024). EGCG appears rather promising against liver cancers skin malignancies and pancreatic ones where oxidative mechanisms play very pivotal roles largely. Phytochemicals having antioxidant and anti-inflammatory properties remarkably boost efficacy of conventional chemotherapy and improve therapeutic index quite significantly. Compounds may significantly enhance treatment outcomes by shielding normal tissues from chemotherapy-induced oxidative damage and subsequent nasty inflammation very effectively. Phytochemicals with antioxidant activity and anti-inflammatory properties represent a potent natural arsenal in chemoprevention of various cancers very effectively nowadays. Very much backing their inclusion in dietary strategies and development as adjunct cancer therapies are critical pathways disrupted during tumourigenesis. Future research must explore their synergistic effects quite deeply in various clinical settings very much fully harnessing their therapeutic potential.

5.4. Synergistic Effects with Conventional Cancer Therapies

Phytochemicals offer promising benefits alongside conventional cancer therapies owing largely to heretofore well-documented roles in preventing various cancer forms effectively. Chemotherapy remains a cornerstone of cancer treatment alongside radiotherapy but effectiveness gets severely compromised by nasty side effects and acquired drug resistance. Phytochemicals possessing extraordinary antioxidant properties and anti-inflammatory effects are being harnessed slowly in novel oncology treatment regimens remarkably enhancing therapeutic efficacy. Curcumin a polyphenolic compound derived from Curcuma longa has been studied extensively for enhancing cancer cells' sensitivity to chemotherapeutic agents and radiation therapy rather thoroughly.

Modulating multiple signaling pathways like NF-κB and PI3K/Akt involved in drug resistance lowers cancer cell death threshold very significantly thereby. Curcumin boosts bioavailability of drugs at tumour sites drastically by altering tumour microenvironment quite significantly and increasing vascular permeability rather rapidly. Curcumin's anti-inflammatory and antioxidant properties remarkably shield non-cancerous tissues from collateral damage caused by chemotherapy and radiotherapy very effectively. This dual action makes it rather promising as adjuvant therapy for treating various malignancies including breast cancer and pancreatic tumours very effectively (Zoi et al, 2024). Gingerol exhibits potent chemotherapeutic effects in various studies on ginger's principal bioactive compound yielding surprisingly efficacious results quite frequently. Gingerol somewhat concurrently boosts cytotoxic effects of chemo agents like cisplatin and doxorubicin while mitigating oxidative stress in healthy tissues. Gingerol remarkably modulates COX-2 expression and reduces production of pro-inflammatory cytokines thereby significantly contributing to its protective effects. Sulforaphane present fairly abundantly in cruciferous vegetables exhibits wildly synergistic effects when paired with meds like 5-fluorouracil very effectively (Zoi et al, 2024). It very significantly boosts anticancer efficacy of such agents by messing with cancer cell proliferation pathways and survival mechanisms and shields normal cells simultaneously by triggering Nrf2-dependent antioxidant defenses.

Phytochemicals act significantly as modifiers of biological response, enhancing therapeutic index of conventional treatments in a rather remarkable manner. They provide a fairly holistic approach, enhancing the efficacy of cancer drugs and greatly reducing treatment-related toxicity very effectively overall. Consuming turmeric, ginger green tea and cruciferous veggies rich in phytochemicals provides a fairly natural complementary strategy for enhancing cancer treatment efficacy successfully. A future rife with modified oncology practices and very futuristic medical interventions gets underscored heavily by an integrative approach nowadays.

6. Phytochemicals and DNA Repair

Cellular homeostasis maintenance relies heavily on DNA integrity and staves off malignant cellular transformation quite gradually over time. The genome suffers unrelenting assault from endogenous sources spawned during metabolism and exogenous agents like ultraviolet radiation from outside. Stressors very frequently induce DNA lesions like base modifications and crosslinks or single-strand breaks and occasionally double-strand breaks. Inefficiently repairing such damage fosters genomic instability a putative hallmark of most cancers that develop stealthily over an extended period. New evidence quite dramatically underscores phytochemicals' capacity for encourage DNA repair processes thereby diminishing genetic mutation rates and furnishing crucial cancer prevention.

Polyphenols and flavonoids modulate enzymes involved in DNA repair pathways like base excision repair quite effectively and alter their expression greatly. Compounds heavily influence expression of genes responsible for DNA repair and modulate various transcriptional regulators alongside epigenetic modifiers simultaneously. Resveratrol markedly enhances expression of BRCA1 and RAD51 genes crucial for repairing DNA double-strand breaks through homologous recombination in grapes and berries. Resveratrol ramps up p53 a tumour suppressor protein that regulates expression of various DNA repair genes and brings cell cycle to screeching halt before division. Epigallocatechin gallate shields genomic integrity somewhat effectively by neutralizing ROS and upregulating OGG1 a crucial glycosylase in base excision repair pathways heavily (Borsoi et al, 2024). EGCG modulates signaling pathways such as ATM/ATR very effectively under oxidative stress conditions that detect DNA damage and coordinate repair responses. Curcumin markedly enhances activity of NER enzymes by upregulating genes such as XPA and ERCC1 very effectively. Curcumin modulates epigenetic factors such as DNA methyltransferases and histone deacetylases playing crucial roles in silencing genes repairing DNA during carcinogenesis. Curcumin very effectively restores normal DNA repair function in precancerous and cancerous cells by reversing significant epigenetic alterations (Borsoi et al, 2024). Sulforaphane an isothiocyanate present in cruciferous veggies triggers expression of detoxifying enzymes very effectively through Nrf2-Keap1 pathway thereby markedly reducing DNA adduct formation and enhancing genomic stability.

Phytochemicals strengthen DNA repair mechanisms fidelity thereby serving as potent cancer chemoprevention agents naturally with huge biological impact. Restoration of damaged repair pathways and suppression of mutagenesis underscores their considerable therapeutic potential in rather precarious genomic settings generally. Foods rich in phytochemicals consumed regularly may remarkably safeguard genome stability and offer protection against initiation of cancer and its progression.

6.1. DNA Repair Mechanisms: A Brief Overview

Crucial utterly remains preservation of genomic integrity for normal cellular function and prevention of diseases like cancer happens thereby usually. Cells have evolved intricate DNA repair pathways remarkably quickly in response to endogenous threats and exogenous agents like highly reactive oxygen species. DNA lesions in diverse forms get detected and fixed by these mechanisms thereby thwarting mutations and major chromosomal reshuffling or cellular transformation altogether. Base Excision Repair pathway fixes small non-helix-distorting base lesions quite effectively and operates as a crucial DNA repair mechanism primarily. Oxidative base damage alongside alkylation events happen frequently during normal cellular metabolism from ROS generated quite erratically.

Damaged base recognition and excision occur via DNA glycosylases in BER pathway followed by end processing and gap filling then ligation restores DNA integrity. Nucleotide Excision Repair pathway excels at removing bulky DNA lesions that frequently distort helical structures very significantly under various circumstances. Thymine dimers and DNA adducts formed from ultraviolet radiation or environmental carcinogens like polycyclic aromatic hydrocarbons occur very frequently nowadays. NER functions through two sub-pathways; global genomic NER scans entire genome for damage while transcription-coupled NER swiftly repairs lesions in actively transcribed genes. Damage recognition triggers a convoluted series of events that culminates in excision of a short damaged oligonucleotide segment and subsequent repair synthesis happens later (Krokan and Bjørås, 2013).

DNA damage forms that are extremely cytotoxic are embodied in nasty double-strand breaks which crucial repair mechanisms fix essentially very effectively. Homologous Recombination fixes double-strand breaks flawlessly with a sister chromatid serving as template whereas Non-Homologous End Joining directly ligates broken DNA ends frequently introducing mutations. Choice among pathways depends on cell cycle phase and nature of DNA damage that occurs abruptly inside cells (Krokan and Bjørås, 2013). Mismatch Repair system rectifies base-base mismatches and small insertion-deletion loops that evade proofreading during DNA replication somewhat finally. Microsatellite instability thrives amidst MMR dysfunction heightening risk very significantly nowadays for Lynch syndrome-associated colorectal cancer and certain other cancers. Failure of DNA repair mechanisms severely compromises genomic fidelity and fosters instability a hallmark characteristic that enables cancer progression very rapidly nowadays. Crucial insights emerge from understanding various quirky repair mechanisms offering heaps of therapeutic opportunities for exploiting glaring defects in tumour cells.

6.2. Phytochemicals in Modulating DNA Repair Pathways

Phytochemicals sourced from plants lately garner recognition for possessing antioxidant properties and directly influencing DNA repair mechanisms. Compounds exert protective effects against cancer partly by influencing signalling pathways and gene expression networks that detect DNA damage somewhat irregularly. Phytochemicals substantially enhance genomic stability by modulating DNA repair pathways thereby mitigating oncogenic mutation risk and gross chromosomal aberrations. Sulforaphane, an isothiocyanate found abundantly in cruciferous veggies like broccoli and cabbage, is one of the most studied phytochemicals in these contexts. Sulforaphane very effectively kickstarts the nuclear factor erythroid 2–related factor 2 signalling pathway, a central cellular antioxidant defence regulator (Lagunas-Rangel and Bermúdez-Cruz, 2020).

Nrf2 activation triggers upregulation of myriad genes encoding DNA repair enzymes like glycosylases involved in base excision repair and various excision endonucleases. Cells respond remarkably well now with enhanced DNA repair capacity, reducing mutation rates very substantially, and cancer risk drops thereby. Resveratrol very effectively modulates DNA repair being a polyphenol found mostly in grapes red wine peanuts and various berries. Resveratrol has been shown to stimulate the homologous recombination pathway a relatively error-free process for repairing DNA double-strand breaks fairly accurately (Lagunas-Rangel and Bermúdez-Cruz, 2020). Activation of ataxia-telangiectasia mutated and ATM and Rad3-related kinases thereby trigger pivotal sensors in DNA damage response pathways rapidly. Upon activation various kinases trigger a plethora of phosphorylation events culminating in recruitment of HR repair proteins BRCA1 and RAD51 at DNA damage sites. Resveratrol fosters efficient HR repair thereby preserving chromosomal stability and thwarting genomic alterations that fuel aggressive cancer progression quite effectively. Phytochemicals somewhat effectively serve as modulators of DNA repair in various cellular contexts very irregularly across diverse biological systems. Phytochemicals enhance intrinsic DNA repair mechanisms, affording protection quite effectively against various malignancies and their nasty progression over time. Molecular targets are being investigated heavily which could spawn novel cancer prevention routes via dietary means and adjunct oncology therapies.

6.3. Phytochemicals and Oxidative DNA Damage Repair

Oxidative stress ravages genomic stability inducing multifarious lesions crucial in cancer development downstream of pivotal molecular pathways. Oxidative stress arises endogenously from normal cellular processes and exogenously via pollutants radiation and carcinogens directly damaging nucleic acids . 8-oxo-dG namely 8-oxo-2'-deoxyguanosine constitutes a prevalent lesion often causing G-to-T transversions if going unrepaired fortunately rarely. Accumulation of such mutations may kickstart carcinogenesis rapidly or drive tumour progression somewhat erratically over time within affected cells. Efficient repair of oxidative DNA damage plays a crucial role remarkably well in cancer prevention under some physiological conditions. Phytochemicals mitigate mutagenic consequences very effectively through antioxidant capacities and modulating specific pathways for DNA repair under oxidative stress (Reuter et al, 2010).

Curcumin a vibrant yellow polyphenolic compound extracted from turmeric exhibits robustly antioxidant properties in numerous lab settings within various living organisms. Curcumin very effectively modulates base excision repair pathway correcting oxidative DNA lesions way beyond mere ROS scavenging activity. Curcumin markedly upregulates expression and activity of DNA glycosylases like OGG1 which recognizes 8-oxo-dG on damaged DNA strands vigorously. Curcumin enhances recruitment of downstream BER proteins thereby facilitating repair of oxidative lesions and restores DNA integrity fairly effectively. Curcumin effectively thwarts carcinogenesis by derailing early molecular events precipitating cancerous transformations and mitigating DNA mutation burden rather significantly (Reuter et al, 2010).

Epigallocatechin-3-gallate or EGCG and other green tea catechins have been flagged as very potent modulators of oxidative DNA damage repair. EGCG a major polyphenolic constituent abundant in green tea Camellia sinensis exhibits radical scavenging activity effectively influencing DNA repair pathways. EGCG markedly enhances expression of poly ADP-ribose polymerase an enzyme intricately involved in recognizing single-strand DNA breaks and initiating repair via BER pathway becomes: Poly ADP-ribose polymerase expression gets markedly enhanced by EGCG which plays a crucial role in repair via BER pathway for single-strand DNA breaks. EGCG modulates SIRT1 activity vigorously a NAD+-dependent deacetylase regulating several DNA repair factors and it contributes significantly to chromatin remodeling greatly at sites of DNA damage (Alam et al, 2024). Collectively these actions remarkably enhance cellular defenses against oxidative damage and foster genomic stability under wildly varied physiological conditions. Phytochemicals such as curcumin or EGCG greatly enhance efficiency of endogenous repair systems and directly neutralize ROS thereby offering dual protection against oxidative DNA damage. Findings ostensibly substantiate their putative role in thwarting oncogenesis by mitigating genotoxic stress and upholding genome fidelity utterly in cells.

6.4. Phytochemicals and DNA Double-Strand Break Repair

Genetic damage manifests notoriously in DNA double-strand breaks ranking among most pernicious forms of mutation within cellular contexts quite frequently. DSBs severely disrupt continuity of both DNA strands thereby threatening cell viability and genomic integrity unlike easily fixed single-strand breaks. Unrepaired DSBs or sloppily mended ones can trigger chromosomal translocations deletions and aneuploidy genetic aberrations strongly associated with oncogenic processes. Cells very heavily rely on homologous recombination and non-homologous end joining pathways somewhat randomly to counteract various nasty effects. HR flawlessly employs a sister chromatid as template for repair whereas NHEJ quite often rapidly introduces small mutations through some template independent process.

Emerging research suggests phytochemicals modulate cellular pathways thereby encourage cellular repair capacity and significantly contributing to prevention of various cancers naturally. Lycopene a carotenoid abundant in tomatoes and red fruits naturally influences HR pathway positively with varying degrees of efficacy. Lycopene significantly boosts expression and functionality of crucial HR mediators such as BRCA1 and BRCA2 which play pivotal roles in recognizing DNA double-strand breaks and recruiting RAD51 recombinase facilitating accurate strand exchange during DNA repair processes. Elevated levels of certain tumour suppressor genes significantly enhance accuracy of double-strand break repair thereby mitigating risk of chromosomally unstable cancer cells. Lycopene enhance HR hence reinforcing a role in chemoprevention by marginally ameliorating cellular responses amidst replication stress and oxidative genomic damage (Rudzińska et al, 2023).

Berberine a wonky isoquinoline alkaloid from Berberis species ramps up key facets of DNA damage response system mostly in contexts involving nasty double-strand breaks. Activation of ATM and Chk2 occurs when berberine is present and these central mediators of DDR sense lesions and kick off repair processes downstream very quickly. Activation of ATM triggers phosphorylation of various repair proteins and orchestrates repair via HR or NHEJ in many different cellular settings. Berberine effectively stimulates certain kinases thereby enhancing cell capacity for detection and resolution of double-strand breaks and significantly reducing mutation rates. Berberine possibly facilitates stabilization of key tumour suppressor p53 deeply involved in DNA repair and apoptosis reinforcing its protective role against carcinogenesis further (Rudzińska et al, 2023). Phytochemicals like lycopene and berberine remarkably exhibit an uncanny ability modulating complex molecular machinery responsible for repairing DNA double-strand breaks. Compounds naturally play crucial roles maintaining genomic stability and mitigating cancer risk by activating key DDR pathways deeply within cells. Incorporating them into therapeutic regimens may yield benefits adjunctively in cancer prevention and treatment downstream over time.

6.5. Epigenetic Regulation and DNA Repair

Genomic stability hinges precariously on epigenetic tweaks that recalibrate gene expression without altering underlying DNA sequence essentially forever . DNA methylation histone acetylation and histone methylation significantly tweak chromatin accessibility and rope in DNA repair machinery at damaged sites very heavily. Dysregulation of epigenetic marks severely impairs function or expression of key DNA repair genes thereby vigorously promoting mutagenesis and cancerous tumour development rapidly. Phytochemicals intriguingly modulate epigenetic regulators very significantly enhancing DNA repair capacity and substantially contribute to prevention of cancer. Sulforaphane a naturally occurring isothiocyanate present in cruciferous veggies like broccoli garnered significant attention recently for various epigenetic effects supposedly (López-Gil et al, 2023).

Histone deacetylases get inhibited through a primary mechanism of action that rather quietly leads to condensed chromatin and transcriptional repression. Sulforaphane fosters histone acetylation very effectively by suppressing activity of HDAC enzymes resulting in quite relaxed chromatin structure. Enhanced chromatin accessibility very efficiently facilitates swift recruitment of DNA repair proteins at sites damaged by oxidation. Sulforaphane modulates activity of DNA methyltransferases namely enzymes that add methyl groups onto cytosine residues buried deep within DNA. Sulforaphane restores silenced tumour suppressor genes and DNA repair enzymes by quashing aberrant DNA methylation thereby markedly enhancing genomic surveillance very efficiently (López-Gil et al, 2023).

Resveratrol a polyphenolic compound present mainly in red grapes and peanuts exerts influence on epigenetic pathways via SIRT1 activation heavily downstream. SIRT1 gets involved in chromatin remodeling very differently from classical HDACs and responds sporadically to various obviously stressful cellular signals. Resveratrol triggers SIRT1 activation quite rapidly promoting deacetylation of histones or DNA repair proteins thereby facilitating localization and functional DNA damage response properly in cells. SIRT1 modulates double-strand breaks and oxidative lesions effectively thereby influencing repair pathways like base excision repair and homologous recombination. Resveratrol markedly enhance cellular capacity to detect genotoxic insults and subsequently resolves them by modulating chromatin dynamics and activating repair proteins very effectively. Various phytochemicals modulate epigenetic mechanisms rather intricately representing a crucial dimension of their overall chemopreventive properties very significantly. Sulforaphane epigenetically regulates expression of DNA repair genes and reduces mutation accumulation thereby contributing significantly to cancer prevention alongside resveratrol.

6.6. Synergistic Effects of Phytochemicals in DNA Repair

Phytochemicals deployed together have somewhat unexpectedly surfaced as a novel promising stratagem encourage bodily defenses against oncogenesis and genomic instability rather effectively. Phytochemicals display marked antioxidant properties and interactions among them amplify such effects greatly in a multitude of convoluted biological processes. Phytochemicals provide curiously robust protection against highly genotoxic stress by intricately modulating molecular pathways crucial for recognizing DNA damage and subsequent reparative mechanisms quite effectively. Curcumin and sulforaphane interact very effectively exemplifying phytochemical synergy in diverse biological systems with considerable flair (Rudzińska et al, 2023).

Turmeric-derived curcumin potently modulates base excision repair pathway thereby substantially enhancing activity of DNA glycosylases recognizing oxidized and alkylated DNA bases. Sulforaphane triggers Nrf2 signaling pathway upregulating myriad detoxifying enzymes deeply involved in base excision repair and nucleotide excision repair processes. Together these compounds stimulate a far more robust DNA repair response rather than being used singly at any given time. Curcumin and sulforaphane given together markedly improve repair of oxidative DNA damage and reduce frequency of mutagenic events in preclinical models. Obviously curcumin and sulforaphane exhibit synergistic effects in many natural cases not merely confined to those two compounds. Various flavonoids like quercetin and carotenoids such as lycopene simultaneously target multiple repair systems alongside polyphenols including epigallocatechin gallate (Rudzińska et al, 2023).

Quercetin possibly boosts mismatch repair pathway whereas lycopene has been strongly tied in enhancing homologous recombination and EGCG curiously supports base excision repair pathway via upregulation of PARP activity. Complementary actions remarkably alleviate DNA damage burden across various lesion types and reinforce genome stability very effectively under stress conditions. Far-reaching consequences emerge surreptitiously beneath findings. Diverse plant-based compounds rich in phytochemicals could robustly support endogenous DNA repair and substantially decrease cancer risk mechanisms. This approach might offer quite an effective low toxicity adjunct therapy alongside conventional cancer treatments particularly for people beset by nasty environmental genotoxins. Phytochemicals' synergistic action very effectively boosts efficacy of DNA repair via multiple complex mechanisms simultaneously in various cellular contexts. Further investigation into such interactions will clarify their therapeutic potential and pave way for cancer prevention dietary strategies very thoroughly.

7. Targeting Cancer Pathways with Plant-Based Compounds

Molecular signaling pathways regulating normal cell functions get disrupted and cancer development unfolds rapidly with proliferation and sly immune evasion. Aberrantly activated pathways very much directly lead unbridled cell division and metastasis into surrounding tissues of bodily organs rather haphazardly. Targeted therapies often harness synthetic drugs showing considerable success against specific cancer types yet efficacy frequently gets thwarted by off-target effects and drug resistance. Phytochemicals offer complementary strategy for modulating cancer pathways with less toxicity deriving from bioactive compounds found in various plant-based contexts occasionally. Phytochemicals display multifaceted mechanisms interfering with dysregulated cellular pathways simultaneously in a complex biological milieu rather effectively nonetheless.

Curcumin a compound found rather abundantly in turmeric modulates NF-κB pathway very critically in cancer cells affecting inflammation and cell survival heavily influencing new blood vessel formation. Curcumin suppresses expression of pro-inflammatory cytokines and anti-apoptotic proteins by inhibiting NF-κB activation thereby promoting cancer cell death sensitizing tumours quite effectively for conventional therapies. Resveratrol a polyphenol found in various berries grapes and other plants inhibits PI3K/Akt/mTOR signaling cascade quite effectively in certain tumour cells. Resveratrol blocks this axis heavily inhibiting angiogenesis and resulting in markedly reduced tumour cell proliferation with increased apoptosis. EGCG from green tea severely disrupts EGFR and MAPK pathways badly impairing growth signals in various cancer cell types rather effectively (Sharifi-Rad et al, 2020).

Sulforaphane and other isothiocyanates very effectively exert anticancer effects through various biochemical pathways by modulating Keap1-Nrf2 axis obviously. This pathway plays crucial roles defense against oxidative stress and in detoxifying carcinogens within cells very effectively under certain conditions. Sulforaphane vigorously activates Nrf2 resulting in rapid induction of phase II detoxifying enzymes and antioxidant proteins thwarting DNA damage swiftly. Pleiotropic effects are exhibited collectively by these plant-based compounds on various cancer-related signaling network nodes with remarkable efficacy apparently. Tumour cells get selectively targeted while sparing normal tissues making them ridiculously attractive nowadays for integration into cancer prevention therapy quite surprisingly. Mechanistic insights gained underscore therapeutic potential of phytochemicals and spur development of novel formulations derived from plants for use alongside existing cancer therapies (Sharifi-Rad et al, 2020).

7.1. Inhibition of Cell Cycle Progression

Cell cycle unfurls through a gnarled sequence of occurrences involving spurts of growth intermittently and DNA replication preceding eventual cell division. Crucial checkpoints for genomic integrity maintenance are very central normally within cellular processes obviously. Malignant cells frequently bypass regulatory checkpoints enabling unchecked proliferation quite rapidly and severe genetic damage accumulates subsequently with hectic velocity. Cancer prevention heavily relies on targeting cell cycle as pivotal strategy and therapy now emerges rather effectively consequently. Bioactive compounds derived from plants have shown considerable potential modulating cell cycle thereby suppressing tumourigenesis and restoring certain regulation quite effectively (Mercadante and Kasi, 2025).

Quercetin and kaempferol have been extensively studied as phytochemicals in various fruits and vegetables richly endowed with such flavonoids. Compounds induce cell cycle arrest fairly readily at multiple phases with prominent effect at G1/S transition where cells commit DNA synthesis. Quercetin exerts effect by downregulating cyclin D1 and cyclin E simultaneously upregulating p21^Cip1 while downregulating cyclin-dependent kinases like CDK2 very effectively. DNA synthesis gets stifled rapidly halting cell proliferation thereby. Kaempferol hinders CDK activity thereby inducing G1 arrest or G2/M arrest in various cellular contexts with disparate cell types. Curcumin a polyphenolic compound derived from Curcuma longa rhizome profoundly disrupts quirky cell cycle regulation mechanisms rather eccentrically (Mercadante and Kasi, 2025). Curcumin rather haphazardly induces G1-phase arrest in various cancer cell lines by suppressing cyclin D1 expression and CDK4 quite effectively. Curcumin boosts expression of tumour suppressor proteins p21^Cip1/WAF1 and p53 crucial in enforcing cell cycle checkpoints under intense genotoxic stress conditions. Effects accumulate rapidly in tumour cells fostering senescence and they become heavily sensitized to apoptosis with markedly reduced cellular proliferation. Novel plant-based compounds severely disrupt machinery governing cell cycle progression offering a promising approach for restraining malignant cell growth very effectively. Phytochemicals induce cell cycle arrest selectively in tumour cells but spare normal ones thereby underscoring their potential as viable cancer management alternatives.

7.2. Induction of Apoptosis: Targeting Survival Pathways

Programmed cell death plays a vital role in eliminating superfluous cells thereby preserving homeostasis deeply within most bodily tissues usually. Malignant cells survive genetic abnormalities and cytotoxic stimuli rather robustly by evading apoptosis quite effectively under various adverse conditions. Oncological research nowadays zeroes in on rekindling apoptosis pathways inside diverse cancer cells via modified therapeutic regimes very intently. Phytochemicals from various plants have lately garnered attention owing largely to their selective modulation of apoptotic pathways in tumour cells. Apoptosis occurs via intrinsic pathway rooted deeply in mitochondria and extrinsic pathway mediated by death receptors basically. Bcl-2 family proteins very tightly regulate mitochondrial membrane integrity and variably release cytochrome c under some rather unusual conditions (Elmore S, 2007).

Extrinsic pathway entails death receptors such as Fas and TRAIL receptors that trigger caspase cascades downstream very rapidly upon activation. Executioner caspases caspase-3 -6 and -7 serve as final effectors utterly dismantling cell in both pathways rather thoroughly. Sulforaphane potently induces apoptosis rapidly in various cancerous cell lines found abundantly in cruciferous veggies like broccoli. Activation of p53 a crucial tumour suppressor protein sensing cellular stress effectively exerts pro-apoptotic effect mainly via very robust mechanisms and DNA damage occurs. Upregulation of pro-apoptotic targets like Bax and PUMA by p53 promotes mitochondrial dysfunction extensively within stressed cellular environments. Sulforaphane amplifies activation of initiator caspases like caspase-9 and executioner caspases yielding apoptotic cell death very much ultimately (Elmore S, 2007). Sulforaphane remarkably exhibits huge selectivity toward transformed cells offering significant therapeutic advantages by effectively sparing normal cells. Resveratrol very effectively induces apoptosis as another well-characterized phytochemical abundant in grapes berries and red wine naturally. Resveratrol modulates Bcl-2 family proteins vigorously by upregulating pro-apoptotic Bax versus anti-apoptotic Bcl-2 thereby promoting mitochondrial outer membrane permeabilization quite effectively. Release of cytochrome c into cytosol from mitochondria triggers apoptosome formation followed by caspase-9 activation and subsequent caspase-3 activation very rapidly. Resveratrol very effectively inhibits survival pathways like PI3K/Akt and NF-κB thereby sensitizing cancer cells further towards various apoptotic stimuli. Various plant-based compounds effectively restore apoptotic responses within cancer cells nowadays underscoring their considerable potential collectively. Sulforaphane and resveratrol target molecular defects very precisely in survival signaling networks thus offering a very slick multi-pronged strategy for tumour regression.

7.3. Targeting Inflammation

Chronic inflammation increasingly manifests as a pivotal factor underlying cancer development very much everywhere in various bodily tissues and organs. Tumour-supportive microenvironments emerge quite rapidly from intense inflammatory processes generating reactive oxygen species that wildly promote angiogenesis and slyly facilitate immune evasion. Cyclooxygenase-2 alongside nuclear factor-kappa B fosters tumourigenesis very crucially with cytokines like interleukin-6 or tumour necrosis factor-alpha from persistent inflammation. Dietary phytochemicals modulate signaling pathways offering a promising cancer prevention therapy quite effectively subsequently for overall health benefits. Curcumin abundantly found in turmeric Curcuma longa is one of most extensively studied anti-inflammatory phytochemicals. Much of its anti-cancer activity lies in inhibition of NF-κB signaling pathway rather mysteriously across diverse cellular contexts (Greten and Grivennikov, 2019).

NF-κB regulates expression of numerous genes deeply involved in inflammation and remarkably promotes cell survival or proliferation downstream of signaling pathways. NF-κB gets constitutively activated very sloppily in various cancer types leading rather robustly to production of pro-inflammatory mediators supporting tumour growth. Curcumin heavily suppresses NF-κB activation by strongly inhibiting IκB kinase thus preventing degradation of IκB a potent inhibitor of NF-κB thereby retaining it in cytoplasm. Curcumin downregulates pro-inflammatory genes such as TNF-α and IL-6 thereby significantly contributing to less tumour-permissive microenvironment effectively. 6-Gingerol a highly active ginger component exhibits potent anti-inflammatory properties largely owing to abundant certain phytochemicals present in Zingiber officinale (Greten and Grivennikov, 2019).

Gingerol exerts anti-cancer effects partly by inhibiting COX-2 a wonky enzyme synthesizing pro-inflammatory prostaglandins in various bodily processes fairly regularly. COX-2 overexpression occurs frequently in various malignancies and heightens cell proliferation resisting apoptosis whilst forming metastasis quite rapidly. Gingerol suppresses COX-2 expression thereby reducing prostaglandin E2 levels quite vigorously a mediator enhancing tumour progression and promoting immune suppression. Gingerol has been shown fairly recently to hinder NF-κB signaling and further attenuate inflammatory responses somewhat effectively in various malignant tissues. Phytochemicals show considerable promise nowadays in targeting cancer-associated inflammation quite effectively and obviously really under certain conditions. Compounds such as curcumin and gingerol tweak crucial molecular pathways and suppress pro-tumourigenic inflammation very effectively enhancing efficacy of standard treatments. Novel cancer management approaches will be significantly aided by further probing molecular targets of anti-inflammatory phytochemicals effectively.

7.4. Angiogenesis Inhibition: Preventing Tumour Blood Supply

New blood vessels erupt rapidly from existing vasculature under diverse pathological and normal conditions such as cancer. Tumour survival and metastasis are aggressively fueled by angiogenesis furnishing requisite nutrients and growth factors rather haphazardly in a malignancy context. Tumours turn rock solid then get severely oxygen-starved around 1–2 mm^3 and kickstart rather frantic blood vessel recruiting signals surprisingly quickly. Several phytochemicals exhibit potent anti-angiogenic properties in oncology mainly by inhibiting tumour neovascularization rather effectively these days. Epigallocatechin gallate ranks among heavily studied natural angiogenesis inhibitors found abundantly in Camellia sinensis commonly known as green tea. EGCG exerts anti-angiogenic effect largely by downregulating vascular endothelial growth factor expression a crucial mediator in various angiogenesis processes (Lugano et al, 2020).

VEGF binds receptors on endothelial cells stimulating cell proliferation and new vessel formation quite rapidly therein and migration occurs subsequently. EGCG quite effectively suppresses VEGF gene transcription thereby inhibiting this pathway and disrupts interaction between VEGF and VEGFR rather remarkably. EGCG effectively hinders endothelial cell tube formation and migration impairing structural processes necessary for angiogenesis suddenly in various contexts. Tumour vascularization gets impeded by these collective effects thereby significantly slowing growth and potential metastasis under fairly specific conditions. Lycopene a bright red carotenoid predominantly found in tomatoes Solanum lycopersicum exhibits very potent anti-angiogenic properties fairly effectively (Lugano et al, 2020). Degradation of extracellular matrix components happens through its mechanism very much facilitating endothelial cell invasion during angiogenesis notably via inhibition of matrix metalloproteinases MMP-2 and MMP-9.

Lycopene quite effectively limits extracellular matrix remodeling and significantly attenuates endothelial cell migration alongside capillary tube formation by suppressing MMP activity. Lycopene rather effectively mitigates oxidative stress and inflammation which are upstream activators of angiogenic signaling thereby diminishing subsequent cascade further downstream. EGCG and lycopene inhibit angiogenesis nowadays quite effectively in cancer therapy through a rather multifaceted somewhat obscure approach. Compounds disrupt vascular support quite effectively not only curtailing nutrient delivery rapidly for growing tumours but also wrecking metastatic potential of cancerous cells. Very much nontoxic means for encourage cancer prevention exist readily and adjunctive treatment regimens get somewhat effective supplementary support. Research expands therapeutic potential of compounds in oncology remarkably through novel insights into obscure molecular targets and unexpected synergy with treatments.

7.5. Metastasis Inhibition

Cancer cells veer off course from original tumours and disseminate erratically via bodily networks forming anomalous outgrowths in distant organs subsequently. Mortality related to cancer stems from a cascade of intricate biological events involving rapid local invasion and subsequent intravasation into bloodstream. Breakdown of extracellular matrix enables tumour cells to invade surrounding tissue readily and epithelial-to-mesenchymal transition markedly boosts cancer cell motility. Several phytochemicals exhibit promising anticancer properties by disrupting key metastatic pathways rather vigorously in various bodily systems simultaneously. Sulforaphane a rather potent isothiocyanate present in cruciferous vegetables emerges rapidly as quite an effective inhibitor of metastasis in various studies. Suppression of matrix metalloproteinases especially MMP-2 and MMP-9 enzymes that degrade components of basement membrane and extracellular matrix happens mainly via a singular mechanism (Martin et al, 2013).

Cancer cells invade surrounding tissues with remarkable efficacy due partly to proteolytic activities which crucially foster metastatic spread. Sulforaphane stabilizes ECM rather effectively by downregulating MMP expression and activity thwarting cancer cell migration and invasion very subtly. Sulforaphane possibly disrupts NF-κB signaling a pathway heavily tied up in transcription of various MMP genes and tumour progression weirdly enough. Berberine a bioactive compound extracted from various Berberis species profoundly shows significant anti-metastatic effects in multiple experimental cancer models. Epithelial cancer cells acquire mesenchymal traits fairly quickly when inhibition of epithelial-to-mesenchymal transition occurs notably via this cellular program (Martin et al, 2013). Berberine suppresses EMT markers like N-cadherin and vimentin while restoring epithelial markers including E-cadherin in cells rapidly undergoing epithelial transition. It very strongly inhibits transforming growth factor-beta signaling a central regulator of epithelial-mesenchymal transition in many cellular contexts normally. Berberine greatly reduces metastatic potential of cancer cells mostly in hepatic tumours and gastrointestinal cancers by reversing epithelial mesenchymal transition. Sulforaphane disrupts key molecular mechanisms of metastasis rather effectively through plant-based properties and berberine too does this quite disruptively. Disrupting cellular motility and ECM remodeling along with EMT presents a rather promising albeit unorthodox stratagem for effectively curbing cancer dissemination. Bioactive phytochemicals infused into treatment protocols enhance metastasis control and offer lower toxicity profiles versus most conventional cancer medications.

7.6. Epigenetic Modulation: Reversing Aberrant Gene Expression

Epigenetic regulation exerts intricate control over gene expression remarkably preserving underlying DNA sequence without any alteration as a vital mechanism. Epigenetic abnormalities drastically fuel tumourigenesis in various cancerous contexts by silencing tumour suppressor genes and activating sundry oncogenes simultaneously thereafter often. Epigenetic alterations include DNA methylation and histone modifications and dysregulation of various non-coding RNAs making them rather attractive therapeutic targets ostensibly reversible unlike genetic mutations altogether. Very potent anti-cancer effects are exerted by various phytochemicals derived from plants which tweak epigenetic marks restoring gene expression normally. Sulforaphane occurs abundantly in cruciferous veggies like broccoli and gets extensively studied in labs very frequently nowadays globally (Al Aboud et al, 2023).

Sulforaphane infamously throttles histone deacetylases and DNA methyltransferases deeply entwined in epigenetic gene silencing machinations via obscure molecular pathways. Sulforaphane potently inhibits HDACs thereby encourage histone protein acetylation and giving rise to relaxed chromatin structure that facilitates tumour suppressor gene activation. Downregulating DNMT activity prevents hypermethylation of gene promoters thereby reversing silencing of genes crucial for cell cycle control and DNA repair mechanisms. Epigenetic changes restore expression of genes such as p21 and PTEN thereby rather effectively enhancing cellular defense against malignancy. Resveratrol exerts significant epigenetic effects markedly enhanceed by its presence in grapes and red wine having anti-cancer properties (Al Aboud et al, 2023).

Resveratrol rather bizarrely flips on sirtuins particularly SIRT1 a very esoteric class III histone deacetylase intricately entangled in chromatin remodeling with DNA repair. Resveratrol triggers SIRT1 very quickly resulting in deacetylation of some histones and transcription factors that favor expression of genes involved heavily in apoptosis. Resveratrol modulates various non-coding RNAs including microRNAs known to regulate expression of oncogene and tumour suppressor genes post-transcriptionally quite effectively. Sulforaphane and resveratrol readily reprogram epigenetic landscapes gone haywire in cancer cells with remarkable efficacy and unusual specificity apparently. Their influence on chromatin structure contributes significantly to growth inhibition and sensitizes cells rapidly to various chemotherapeutic agents fairly quickly. Epigenetic dysregulation characterizes many cancers so plant-based epigenetic modulators represent a promising avenue for chemoprevention and adjunctive cancer therapy. Investigation into such compounds might spur creation of non-toxic therapies aimed at epigenetics for sundry cancers fairly effectively down the line (Atwell et al, 2015).

8. From Plant to Prevention

Cancer remains a behemoth of a global health threat with incidence and mortality rates skyrocketing despite myriad advances in medical tech and treatment modalities. Cancer therapies like surgery or radiotherapy often prove very effective when disease is caught fairly early on in certain instances. Treatments frequently entail ghastly side effects and steep price tags yet yield minimal efficacy in cancers having metastasized or reached an advanced stage. Global focus has shifted very rapidly toward cancer prevention strategies that markedly reduce risk long before any clinical manifestation occurs. Cancer chemoprevention has burgeoned rapidly as a strangely proactive paradigm stressing deployment of assorted natural and synthetic compounds thwarting carcinogenesis. Phytochemicals are bioactive non-nutritive compounds found in various fruits vegetables and whole spices garnering quite significant attention as potent chemopreventive agents nowadays slowly (Nwosu N, 2024).

Flavonoids polyphenols alkaloids terpenoids and a slew of glucosinolates fall under diverse chemical classes comprised by these compounds. Modulating cellular signaling pathways rather effectively makes them fairly attractive for cancer prevention interventions involving regulation of gene expression. Phytochemicals exert very potent anti-cancer effects through a myriad of convoluted cellular pathways very effectively indeed underground. Several compounds exhibit markedly potent antioxidant properties thereby effectively neutralizing reactive oxygen species and minimizing oxidative DNA damage a key mutagenesis initiator. They act as anti-inflammatory agents suppressing chronic inflammation known to facilitate tumour promotion and progression very significantly over fairly long periods. Recently curcumin in turmeric and resveratrol in grapes have been shown effectively inhibiting various pro-inflammatory transcription factors like NF-κB or STAT3 (Nwosu N, 2024).

Phytochemicals effectively induce cell cycle arrest and promote apoptosis whilst inhibiting angiogenesis and metastasis essential hallmarks of most cancers. Sulforaphane lurking in cruciferous veggies and epigallocatechin gallate extracted rather haphazardly from green tea target these processes through molecular machinations. Phytochemicals very frequently reactivate silenced tumour suppressor genes and alter histone modification patterns drastically in various epigenetic cellular processes. Phytochemicals present a remarkably compelling avenue for cancer prevention due mainly to broad-spectrum activity and relatively low toxicity inherently. Research progression potentially unlocks possibilities for embedding compounds within diet plans or transmuting them into groundbreaking medicines thereby lessening worldwide cancer incidence rates significantly. Further exploration remarkably elucidates their role in modern oncology practices through synergistic interactions with various conventional therapies nowadays very effectively.

8.1. Phytochemicals: Natural Protectors with Potent Bioactivity

Phytochemicals synthesized by plants are non-nutritive bioactive compounds ostensibly part of elaborate defense systems against stressors like ultraviolet radiation and herbivory apparently. Secondary metabolites heavily influence flavor and aroma of various plant-based foods while playing a critical mitigating role in human health against diseases like cancer. Polyphenols flavonoids terpenoids and carotenoids are studied extensively for chemopreventive properties alongside various alkaloids in very diverse classes basically. Their antioxidant capacity enables scavenging reactive oxygen species rather effectively in various cellular contexts alongside reactive nitrogen species.

Highly reactive ROS accumulation triggers oxidative stress precipitating DNA damage and protein oxidation fuelling carcinogenesis initiation quite rapidly and progression. Phytochemicals mitigate oxidative stress effectively serving as crucial modulators of cellular homeostasis under diverse physiological states quite remarkably. Polyphenols encompass a vast array of compounds including flavonoids like quercetin and catechins and stilbenes such as resveratrol with phenolic acids notably curcumin. Multiple mechanisms underlie protective effects exerted by these compounds including neutralization of free radicals and enhancement of endogenous antioxidant enzymes notably superoxide dismutase (Liu et al, 2020).

Nrf2 and other redox-sensitive signaling pathways get modulated very effectively at exactly same time with considerable efficacy. Quercetin and epigallocatechin gallate EGCG suppress oxidative stress profoundly in various cancer cells and somewhat recklessly influence cell cycle progression or apoptosis.β-carotene lycopene lutein and zeaxanthin are categorized under carotenoids and known generally for potent antioxidant activity as lipid-soluble pigments. Lycopene found abundantly in tomatoes and red fruits inhibits proliferation of prostate and breast cancer cells by reducing oxidative DNA damage (Liu et al, 2020).

β-carotene supports immune function and protects against oxidative injury but its supplementation effects vary wildly across different population groups.β-carotene a precursor of vitamin A enhance immune function quite vigorously and protects against oxidative injury rather effectively in diverse populations. β-carotene a precursor of vitamin A vigorously enhance immune function and protects diverse populations rather effectively against oxidative injury.

8.2. Mechanisms of Action

Cells hurtle through frenzied growth phases and DNA replication then division within a process ordinarily regulated tightly by various subtle mechanisms. Multiple checkpoints vigilantly monitor DNA integrity at G1/S and G2/M transitions under normal physiological conditions halting cell cycle progression if anomalies surface. Cancer often witnesses regulatory mechanisms badly subverted resulting in cells proliferating quickly rather uncontrollably and at an alarming rate nonetheless. Phytochemicals exert anticancer effects largely by restoring control over cell cycle progression and quite effectively inhibit expansion of malignant cell populations. Phytochemicals induce cell cycle arrest effectively at multiple phases halting cancer cell growth suddenly and exhibit antiproliferative effects very effectively.

8.2.1. Modulation of the Cell Cycle

Cell cycle regulation hinges precariously on modulation of cyclins and cyclin-dependent kinases alongside endogenous inhibitors like p21 or p27 basically. Quercetin a flavonoid found extensively in foods like apples and red onions has been studied rather thoroughly for various antiproliferative effects. Quercetin induces cell cycle arrest very effectively at G1/S transition mainly in various cancer models of colon breast and lung in vitro. Downregulation of cyclin D1 occurs alongside inhibition of CDK2 and CDK4 enzymes crucial for DNA synthesis initiation effectively. Disruption thwarts retinoblastoma protein phosphorylation halting S phase progression effectively suppressing cell division with unbridled efficacy quite remarkably (Casagrande and Darbon, 2011).

Curcuma longa's principal curcuminoid curcumin has shown strikingly potent influence over cell cycle progression dynamics very effectively in spice turmeric. Curcumin inhibits cyclin D1 expression and CDK4 but upregulates p21^Cip1/Waf1 a universal inhibitor binding various cyclin-CDK complexes very effectively . Arrest at G1 phase happens owing largely to such dual modulation thereby severely impairing proliferation in various types of cancer cells from breast prostate pancreas colon. Phytochemicals such as quercetin enhance integrity of cell cycle checkpoints and suppress propagation of tumour cells fairly selectively through multiple obscure mechanisms (Casagrande and Darbon, 2011). Compounds exhibit minimal cytotoxicity in normal cells effectively highlighting potential utility in cancer chemoprevention and adjunctive therapeutic regimes quite broadly.

8.2.2. Induction of Apoptosis

Programmed cell death or apoptosis eliminates damaged cells effectively under diverse physiological conditions with surprising efficacy in cellular homeostasis maintenance. It plays a vital role in tissue remodeling and prevents malignant transformation quietly enough amidst somewhat erratic immune system function. Malignant cells thrive under genomic turmoil and external stressors by deftly evading apoptosis thus fuelling tumour growth and stubbornly resisting therapy. Revitalizing apoptotic mechanisms within malignant cells nowadays stays a paramount therapeutic objective for thwarting and treating cancer with fervor. Phytochemicals have emerged as rather promising agents capable of reactivating dormant pathways through diverse molecular signalling very effectively (Elmore S, 2007).

Sulforaphane a compound found in cruciferous veggies like broccoli quite obviously exhibits very well documented pro-apoptotic activity in various cells. Sulforaphane swiftly activates tumour suppressor protein p53 which becomes central regulator of various cellular responses under stress or DNA damage. p53 induces expression of pro-apoptotic genes like Bax and PUMA heavily contributing to mitochondrial outer membrane permeabilization upon activation. Disruption of mitochondria precipitates release of cytochrome c into cytoplasm sparking activation of caspases like caspase-9 and caspase-3 executing cell death rapidly. Sulforaphane rather effectively quashes anti-apoptotic signals contributing significantly to selectivity for cancerous cells and saves normal ones (Elmore S, 2007).

Resveratrol a polyphenolic compound abundant in grapes red wine and peanuts has demonstrated considerable ability to promote apoptosis in various cancer cell types including colon cancer. Modulation primarily of Bcl-2 family proteins governing mitochondrial integrity under various conditions occurs quite effectively through its mechanism of action. Resveratrol quite effectively downregulates anti-apoptotic protein Bcl-2 stabilizing mitochondrial membrane and upregulates pro-apoptotic Bax protein promoting membrane permeabilization. Shift in Bax/Bcl-2 ratio facilitates release of cytochrome c initiating intrinsic apoptotic cascade rather quickly deep within cells (Elmore S, 2007).

Resveratrol effectively modulates various cellular pathways enhancing apoptotic potential quite downstream through suppression of NF-κB and activation of p53. Sulforaphane and resveratrol very effectively rekindle apoptosis in cancerous cells under some very specific conditions with considerable potency. Modulation of intrinsic death pathways enables selective targeting of malignant cells and underscores huge potential as remarkably effective natural chemopreventive compounds. Probing these obscure mechanisms further might very quickly yield novel cancer prevention strategies based on phytochemicals and fairly innovative adjunctive therapies.

8.2.3. Anti-inflammatory Effects

Cancers arise from chronic inflammation increasingly recognized as a major catalyst for furious progression of various nasty malignancies recently. Inflammatory responses vigorously foster genetic mutations creating a microenvironment supportive of tumours and promoting proliferation of cells rapidly. Cytokines such as tumour necrosis factor-alpha and interleukin-6 alongside enzymes like cyclooxygenase-2 and 5-lipoxygenase play quite a crucial role evidently. Nuclear factor-kappa B and other transcription factors regulating expression of genes deeply involved in oncogenesis are suddenly activated by molecules. Phytochemicals exhibit diverse bioactivity and show promise in disrupting inflammatory pathways thereby significantly aiding cancer chemoprevention efforts under various conditions. Recently worldwide anti-inflammatory properties of curcumin a principal curcuminoid from spice turmeric Curcuma longa have been extensively studied.

Curcumin chiefly targets NF-κB signaling pathway frequently hyperactive in sundry tumour types and plays a pivotal role in sustaining inflammatory milieu surrounding tumours. Curcumin very effectively hampers phosphorylation and subsequent degradation of IκBα a protein preventing nuclear translocation of transcription factor NF-κB. Curcumin very effectively blocks NF-κB activation leading downregulation of target genes like TNF-α and sundry adhesion molecules including IL-6 COX-2. Tumour cell proliferation invasion and survival are quite significantly reduced under various pathological conditions by suppressing inflammatory signaling very effectively (Olivera et al, 2012).

Gingerol wields potent anti-cancer effects rather abundantly in Zingiber officinale being a pungent phenolic compound with markedly anti-inflammatory properties. Gingerol fiercely impacts cyclooxygenase and lipoxygenase pathways involving synthesis of pro-inflammatory lipid mediators through two major enzymatic reaction cascades. Gingerol specifically inhibits COX-2 an inducible enzyme overexpressed in various cancer types closely linked with tumourigenic processes in some cellular contexts. Gingerol suppresses COX-2 expression quite effectively and reduces production of prostaglandins key mediators of inflammation pain tumour progression slowly (Olivera et al, 2012). Gingerol inhibits 5-LOX an enzyme catalyzing formation of leukotrienes another inflammatory mediator class heavily tied in cancer pathogenesis . Curcumin and gingerol illustrate vividly how phytochemicals found in diet modulate signaling of inflammation very effectively at multiple levels and suppress tumour-promoting inflammation. They interfere with upstream regulators and downstream effectors of inflammation positioning them as promising agents for cancer prevention potentially alongside conventional therapies.

8.2.4. Inhibition of Angiogenesis

New blood vessels form sporadically from preexisting vasculature mainly during embryonic development and wound healing and frequently in cancer. Tumour angiogenesis enables rapid supply of oxygen and nutrients necessary for metastasis via newly formed vessels facilitating swift proliferation. Neovascularization gets tightly regulated by a delicate balance between pro-angiogenic factors and anti-angiogenic ones with vascular endothelial growth factor acting as a potent mediator very effectively. Tumours frequently hijack normal processes by ramping up VEGF and other angiogenic signals resulting in snarled vascular networks that facilitate metastasis and proliferation vigorously. Several phytochemicals from plants exhibit anti-angiogenic activity and targeting angiogenesis emerges as critical strategy in cancer therapy nowadays (Saman et al ,2020).

Epigallocatechin gallate or EGCG has been studied fairly extensively in recent years for anti-cancer properties found in green tea. EGCG markedly downregulates VEGF expression in cancer cells thereby interfering vigorously with VEGF signaling that spurs endothelial cell proliferation and new vessel formation. EGCG quite effectively impairs downstream signaling crucial for angiogenesis by binding VEGF receptors and inhibiting their phosphorylation. EGCG potently quashes hypoxia-inducible factor-1α expression a transcriptional regulator that ramps up VEGF production under abysmally low oxygen tension severely impairing tumour angiogenic initiation. Lycopene a non-provitamin A carotenoid exists mostly in tomatoes and other red or orange fruits having very potent anti-angiogenic properties. Lycopene hinders angiogenesis via modulating matrix metalloproteinases' activity; these enzymes degrade extracellular matrix facilitating new blood vessel formation (Saman et al , 2020).

Lycopene downregulates MMP-2 and MMP-9 upregulated in many tumours fostering breakdown of basement membranes surrounding stroma very aggressively. Lycopene disrupts structural remodeling needed for angiogenesis vigorously inside cells by inhibiting expression and activity of MMP quite effectively. Phytochemicals such as EGCG and lycopene markedly suppress tumour angiogenesis through various highly complex molecular signaling pathways normally. Impairment of tumour vascular supply by them significantly enhance efficacy of chemoprevention very substantially in many cancerous tissues. Incorporating such compounds into dietary regimens promises non-toxic cancer prevention strategies very effectively alongside potentially cost-effective supplementary treatments.

8.3. Clinical and Epidemiological Evidence

Epidemiological and clinical research mostly substantiates a significant role for phytochemicals in cancer prevention and also adjunctive therapeutic measures effectively. Sundry populations worldwide exhibit markedly reduced cancer incidence when consuming diets rich in whole grains and fruits alongside various spices. Regular consumption of phytochemical-rich foods can evidently influence cancer risk complementing mechanistic insights gained from various lab research at population level. Individuals with extremely high dietary flavonoid intake had markedly lower risk of certain cancers especially lung cancer according to a study published in Journal of National Cancer Institute. Inverse association remained significant after adjustment for confounding variables like smoking habits and overall dietary quality essentially (Rudzińska et al, 2023).

Flavonoids like quercetin abound in various citrus fruits and catechins are found copiously in plant-based foods such as green tea berries and onions. Antioxidant properties and somewhat enigmatic anti-proliferative effects likely exert considerable influence on protective outcomes within diverse cellular environments quietly. Phytochemicals show therapeutic promise abundantly in numerous trials demonstrating curative properties under various rather unusual medical conditions quite effectively. Lately curcumin a bioactive compound present in turmeric has garnered considerable attention among cancer patients with various malignancies being researched quite extensively. Curcumin supplementation deemed safe in numerous Phase I trials involving patients with precancerous lesions largely suppressing tumour markers significantly and reducing inflammation (Rudzińska et al, 2023).

Curcumin markedly tampers with crucial molecular targets such as NF-κB and p53 in colorectal cancer yielding reduced tumour cell proliferation. Patients harbouring colorectal adenomas exhibited significant reductions in aberrant crypt foci after receiving curcumin treatment for thirty days quite remarkably. Extensive preclinical research and various human trials have recently studied green tea catechins particularly epigallocatechin gallate EGCG quite thoroughly nowadays. Daily supplementation with green tea extract significantly lowers progression to cancer in men with high-grade prostatic intraepithelial neoplasia versus placebo group. Phytochemicals exert multifaceted protective effects during various carcinogenesis stages and may very significantly enhance conventional treatment outcomes remarkably. Very urgently larger more long-term studies are necessary for establishing optimal dosages and treatment durations with various other kinds of therapies.

8.4. Phytochemicals and Synergistic Effects with Conventional Therapies

Phytochemicals have been harnessed with conventional cancer treatments recently emerging as promising adjuncts and encourage efficacy remarkably in clinical settings nowadays. Phytochemicals rather effectively exhibit chemopreventive potential on their own and synergistic action with various treatments adds valuable dimension somewhat surprisingly. Phytochemicals modulate multiple signaling pathways involved in drug resistance apoptosis and oxidative stress effectively under various abnormal physiological conditions. Curcumin principal bioactive component of turmeric has been rather extensively studied for sensitizing tumour cells effectively to chemotherapeutic agents like doxorubicin. Curcumin markedly enhances cancer cells' susceptibility to apoptosis triggered by conventional pharmaceuticals downregulating nuclear factor kappa B and various anti-apoptotic factors (Choudhari et al, 2020).

Curcumin very quietly exerts antioxidant effects in normal cells thereby significantly mitigating chemotherapy toxicity and encourage treatment tolerability overall. Green tea catechins epigallocatechin gallate very effectively display synergistic effects quite frequently with chemotherapy and very much enhance radiotherapy treatments. EGCG reportedly boosts efficacy of cisplatin and doxorubicin among other standard chemo agents in malignancies like breast prostate and lung cancer very effectively. Simultaneously DNA repair enzymes get inhibited and oxidative stress reduction occurs alongside enhancement of cell cycle arrest and apoptosis. EGCG has been shown remarkably effective in protecting healthy tissues from radiation damage thereby rendering it very valuable in radiotherapy. Resveratrol and genistein phytochemicals have surprisingly reversed stubborn chemoresistance by energetically modulating key molecular pathways like PI3K/Akt signalling and STAT3 (Choudhari et al, 2020).

Epigenetic regulators get influenced by such compounds thereby reactivating tumour suppressor genes silenced earlier and responsiveness generally improves with treatment. Phytochemicals assail cancer cells on multiple fronts exhibiting pleiotropy and thwarting tumours' heterogeneity with remarkable effectiveness quite adaptably. They seem very effective long term alongside standard treatments owing largely to their relatively low toxicity. Phytochemicals comprise a potent class of adjunctive agents that significantly contribute to cancer prevention and markedly augment conventional cancer therapies. Integrating phytochemicals into clinical cancer protocols may yield remarkably effective outcomes and substantially improve quality of life for patients quite considerably.

9. Conclusion

Phytochemicals have emerged rather promisingly as potent chemopreventive agents through diverse multifaceted mechanisms operating at various obscure molecular strata. Compounds occurring naturally in fruits and plant-based foods have shown ability to interfere with various stages of carcinogenesis progression quite effectively. Modulating various signaling pathways and inhibiting oxidative stress heavily influences gene expression positioning them as crucial cancer prevention players . Phytochemicals such as flavonoids exert anti-cancer effects via multiple pathways rooted deeply in intricate biological mechanisms and cellular responses simultaneously. Cell proliferation gets stifled very thoroughly and apoptosis induction happens rapidly alongside thorough suppression of angiogenesis and metastasis being entirely blocked.

Phytochemicals abundantly exhibit antioxidant properties by neutralizing reactive oxygen species and encourage cellular detoxification through activation of transcription factors like Nrf2. Curcumin and resveratrol sway key regulatory molecules such as NF-κB p53 and MAPKs thereby effectively facilitating homeostasis and DNA repair. Phytochemicals significantly influence epigenetic activity by altering DNA methylation and histone modifications that effectively suppress oncogene expression or reactivate tumour suppressor genes. Dietary phytochemicals wield fairly long-lasting protective effects nowadays and enhance conventional cancer therapies quite effectively through epigenetic modulations underground. Challenges persist quietly in harnessing benefits of phytochemicals for clinical use amidst unfulfilled promise festering menacingly in background shadows. Further research seems necessary owing largely to issues like nonuniform dosing and wildly variable individual responses stemming from very low bioavailability.

Nanoformulations and synergistic combinations of phytochemicals are being explored presently for overcoming limitations and enhancing therapeutic efficacy. Phytochemicals offer a vital very natural cancer prevention strategy with fairly low toxicity reducing risk rather effectively somewhat. Their capacity for targeting multifaceted pathways simultaneously aligns rather well with cancer biology's labyrinthine nature under most ordinary circumstances very ordinarily. Phytochemicals will probably assume a rather pivotal role gradually in integrative oncology as our understanding of preventive health deepens profoundly over time. Unlocking full potential requires further interdisciplinary research and developing evidence-based dietary recommendations that therapeutically harness chemopreventive properties of plants very effectively.

References

Al Aboud NM, Tupper C, Jialal I. Genetics, Epigenetic Mechanism. [Updated 2023 Aug 14]. In: StatPearls [Internet]. Treasure Island (FL): StatPearls Publishing; 2025 Jan-. Available from: https://www.ncbi.nlm.nih.gov/books/NBK532999/

Alam M, Gulzar M, Akhtar MS, Rashid S, Zulfareen, Tanuja, Shamsi A, Hassan MI. Epigallocatechin-3-gallate therapeutic potential in human diseases: molecular mechanisms and clinical studies. Mol Biomed. 2024 Dec 27;5(1):73. doi: 10.1186/s43556-024-00240-9. PMID: 39725830; PMCID: PMC11671467.

Atwell LL, Beaver LM, Shannon J, Williams DE, Dashwood RH, Ho E. Epigenetic Regulation by Sulforaphane: Opportunities for Breast and Prostate Cancer Chemoprevention. Curr Pharmacol Rep. 2015 Apr 1;1(2):102-111. doi: 10.1007/s40495-014-0002-x. PMID: 26042194; PMCID: PMC4450146.

Bardaweel SK, Gul M, Alzweiri M, Ishaqat A, ALSalamat HA, Bashatwah RM. Reactive Oxygen Species: the Dual Role in Physiological and Pathological Conditions of the Human Body. Eurasian J Med. 2018 Oct;50(3):193-201. doi: 10.5152/eurasianjmed.2018.17397. PMID: 30515042; PMCID: PMC6263229.

Barnum KJ, O'Connell MJ. Cell cycle regulation by checkpoints. Methods Mol Biol. 2014;1170:29-40. doi: 10.1007/978-1-4939-0888-2_2. PMID: 24906307; PMCID: PMC4990352.

Borsoi FT, Neri-Numa IA, de Oliveira WQ, de Araújo FF, Pastore GM. Dietary polyphenols and their relationship to the modulation of non-communicable chronic diseases and epigenetic mechanisms: A mini-review. Food Chem (Oxf). 2022 Dec 13;6:100155. doi: 10.1016/j.fochms.2022.100155. PMID: 36582744; PMCID: PMC9793217.

Casagrande F, Darbon JM. Effects of structurally related flavonoids on cell cycle progression of human melanoma cells: regulation of cyclin-dependent kinases CDK2 and CDK1. Biochem Pharmacol. 2001 May 15;61(10):1205-15. doi: 10.1016/s0006-2952(01)00583-4. PMID: 11322924.

Chavda VP, Patel AB, Mistry KJ, Suthar SF, Wu ZX, Chen ZS, Hou K. Nano-Drug Delivery Systems Entrapping Natural Bioactive Compounds for Cancer: Recent Progress and Future Challenges. Front Oncol. 2022 Mar 29;12:867655. doi: 10.3389/fonc.2022.867655. PMID: 35425710; PMCID: PMC9004605.

Chen J. The Cell-Cycle Arrest and Apoptotic Functions of p53 in Tumour Initiation and Progression. Cold Spring Harb Perspect Med. 2016 Mar 1;6(3):a026104. doi: 10.1101/cshperspect.a026104. PMID: 26931810; PMCID: PMC4772082.

Chen M, Li M, Budai MM, Rice AP, Kimata JT, Mohan M, Wang J. Clearance of HIV-1 or SIV reservoirs by promotion of apoptosis and inhibition of autophagy: Targeting intracellular molecules in cure-directed strategies. J Leukoc Biol. 2022 Nov;112(5):1245-1259. doi: 10.1002/JLB.4MR0222-606. Epub 2022 Mar 31. PMID: 35362118; PMCID: PMC9522917.

Choudhari AS, Mandave PC, Deshpande M, Ranjekar P, Prakash O. Phytochemicals in Cancer Treatment: From Preclinical Studies to Clinical Practice. Front Pharmacol. 2020 Jan 28;10:1614. doi: 10.3389/fphar.2019.01614. Erratum in: Front Pharmacol. 2020 Feb 28;11:175. doi: 10.3389/fphar.2020.00175. PMID: 32116665; PMCID: PMC7025531.

Didier AJ, Stiene J, Fang L, Watkins D, Dworkin LD, Creeden JF. Antioxidant and Anti-Tumour Effects of Dietary Vitamins A, C, and E. Antioxidants (Basel). 2023 Mar 3;12(3):632. doi: 10.3390/antiox12030632. PMID: 36978880; PMCID: PMC10045152.

Elmore S. Apoptosis: a review of programmed cell death. Toxicol Pathol. 2007 Jun;35(4):495-516. doi: 10.1080/01926230701320337. PMID: 17562483; PMCID: PMC2117903.

El-Saadony MT, Yang T, Korma SA, Sitohy M, Abd El-Mageed TA, Selim S, Al Jaouni SK, Salem HM, Mahmmod Y, Soliman SM, Mo'men SAA, Mosa WFA, El-Wafai NA, Abou-Aly HE, Sitohy B, Abd El-Hack ME, El-Tarabily KA, Saad AM. Impacts of turmeric and its principal bioactive curcumin on human health: Pharmaceutical, medicinal, and food applications: A comprehensive review. Front Nutr. 2023 Jan 10;9:1040259. doi: 10.3389/fnut.2022.1040259. PMID: 36712505; PMCID: PMC9881416.

Fishbein A, Hammock BD, Serhan CN, Panigrahy D. Carcinogenesis: Failure of resolution of inflammation? Pharmacol Ther. 2021 Feb;218:107670. doi: 10.1016/j.pharmthera.2020.107670. Epub 2020 Sep 3. PMID: 32891711; PMCID: PMC7470770.

Greten FR, Grivennikov SI. Inflammation and Cancer: Triggers, Mechanisms, and Consequences. Immunity. 2019 Jul 16;51(1):27-41. doi: 10.1016/j.immuni.2019.06.025. PMID: 31315034; PMCID: PMC6831096.

Gu M, Ren B, Fang Y, Ren J, Liu X, Wang X, Zhou F, Xiao R, Luo X, You L, Zhao Y. Epigenetic regulation in cancer. MedComm (2020). 2024 Feb 19;5(2):e495. doi: 10.1002/mco2.495. PMID: 38374872; PMCID: PMC10876210.

Hossain MS, Wazed MA, Asha S, Amin MR, Shimul IM. Dietary Phytochemicals in Health and Disease: Mechanisms, Clinical Evidence, and Applications-A Comprehensive Review. Food Sci Nutr. 2025 Mar 19;13(3):e70101. doi: 10.1002/fsn3.70101. PMID: 40115248; PMCID: PMC11922683.

Jang JH, Lee TJ. Mechanisms of Phytochemicals in Anti-Inflammatory and Anti-Cancer. Int J Mol Sci. 2023 Apr 26;24(9):7863. doi: 10.3390/ijms24097863. PMID: 37175569; PMCID: PMC10177803.

Jiang H, Shang X, Wu H, Huang G, Wang Y, Al-Holou S, Gautam SC, Chopp M. Combination treatment with resveratrol and sulforaphane induces apoptosis in human U251 glioma cells. Neurochem Res. 2010 Jan;35(1):152-61. doi: 10.1007/s11064-009-0040-7. Epub 2009 Aug 15. PMID: 19685289; PMCID: PMC2821708.

Kaiser AE, Baniasadi M, Giansiracusa D, Giansiracusa M, Garcia M, Fryda Z, Wong TL, Bishayee A. Sulforaphane: A Broccoli Bioactive Phytocompound with Cancer Preventive Potential. Cancers (Basel). 2021 Sep 25;13(19):4796. doi: 10.3390/cancers13194796. PMID: 34638282; PMCID: PMC8508555.

Kamaraju S, Drope J, Sankaranarayanan R, Shastri S. Cancer Prevention in Low-Resource Countries: An Overview of the Opportunity. Am Soc Clin Oncol Educ Book. 2020 Mar;40:1-12. doi: 10.1200/EDBK_280625. PMID: 32239989; PMCID: PMC7935443.

Krokan HE, Bjørås M. Base excision repair. Cold Spring Harb Perspect Biol. 2013 Apr 1;5(4):a012583. doi: 10.1101/cshperspect.a012583. PMID: 23545420; PMCID: PMC3683898.

Lagunas-Rangel FA, Bermúdez-Cruz RM. Natural Compounds That Target DNA Repair Pathways and Their Therapeutic Potential to Counteract Cancer Cells. Front Oncol. 2020 Nov 19;10:598174. doi: 10.3389/fonc.2020.598174. PMID: 33330091; PMCID: PMC7710985.

Lan T, Chen L, Wei X. Inflammatory Cytokines in Cancer: Comprehensive Understanding and Clinical Progress in Gene Therapy. Cells. 2021 Jan 8;10(1):100. doi: 10.3390/cells10010100. PMID: 33429846; PMCID: PMC7827947.

Li K, Deng Z, Lei C, Ding X, Li J, Wang C. The Role of Oxidative Stress in Tumourigenesis and Progression. Cells. 2024 Mar 2;13(5):441. doi: 10.3390/cells13050441. PMID: 38474405; PMCID: PMC10931308.

Liu S, Liu J, Wang Y, Deng F, Deng Z. Oxidative Stress: Signaling Pathways, Biological Functions, and Disease. MedComm (2020). 2025 Jul 1;6(7):e70268. doi: 10.1002/mco2.70268. PMID: 40599237; PMCID: PMC12209598.

López-Gil L, Pascual-Ahuir A, Proft M. Genomic Instability and Epigenetic Changes during Aging. Int J Mol Sci. 2023 Sep 19;24(18):14279. doi: 10.3390/ijms241814279. PMID: 37762580; PMCID: PMC10531692.

Lugano R, Ramachandran M, Dimberg A. Tumour angiogenesis: causes, consequences, challenges and opportunities. Cell Mol Life Sci. 2020 May;77(9):1745-1770. doi: 10.1007/s00018-019-03351-7. Epub 2019 Nov 6. PMID: 31690961; PMCID: PMC7190605.

Ma C, Gurkan-Cavusoglu E. A comprehensive review of computational cell cycle models in guiding cancer treatment strategies. NPJ Syst Biol Appl. 2024 Jul 5;10(1):71. doi: 10.1038/s41540-024-00397-7. PMID: 38969664; PMCID: PMC11226463.

Mao H, Zhao X, Sun SC. NF-κB in inflammation and cancer. Cell Mol Immunol. 2025 Aug;22(8):811-839. doi: 10.1038/s41423-025-01310-w. Epub 2025 Jun 25. PMID: 40562870; PMCID: PMC12310982.

Martin TA, Ye L, Sanders AJ, et al. Cancer Invasion and Metastasis: Molecular and Cellular Perspective. In: Madame Curie Bioscience Database [Internet]. Austin (TX): Landes Bioscience; 2000-2013. Available from: https://www.ncbi.nlm.nih.gov/books/NBK164700/

Mercadante AA, Kasi A. Genetics, Cancer Cell Cycle Phases. [Updated 2023 Aug 14]. In: StatPearls [Internet]. Treasure Island (FL): StatPearls Publishing; 2025 Jan-. Available from: https://www.ncbi.nlm.nih.gov/books/NBK563158/

Nishida A, Andoh A. The Role of Inflammation in Cancer: Mechanisms of Tumour Initiation, Progression, and Metastasis. Cells. 2025 Mar 25;14(7):488. doi: 10.3390/cells14070488. PMID: 40214442; PMCID: PMC11987742.

Nwosu N. Cancer: A Disease of Modern Times? Cureus. 2024 Nov 28;16(11):e74666. doi: 10.7759/cureus.74666. PMID: 39735050; PMCID: PMC11681836.

Olivera A, Moore TW, Hu F, Brown AP, Sun A, Liotta DC, Snyder JP, Yoon Y, Shim H, Marcus AI, Miller AH, Pace TW. Inhibition of the NF-κB signaling pathway by the curcumin analog, 3,5-Bis(2-pyridinylmethylidene)-4-piperidone (EF31): anti-inflammatory and anti-cancer properties. Int Immunopharmacol. 2012 Feb;12(2):368-77. doi: 10.1016/j.intimp.2011.12.009. Epub 2011 Dec 22. PMID: 22197802; PMCID: PMC3372981.

Parrish AB, Freel CD, Kornbluth S. Cellular mechanisms controlling caspase activation and function. Cold Spring Harb Perspect Biol. 2013 Jun 1;5(6):a008672. doi: 10.1101/cshperspect.a008672. PMID: 23732469; PMCID: PMC3660825.

Rahman MA, Hannan MA, Dash R, Rahman MH, Islam R, Uddin MJ, Sohag AAM, Rahman MH, Rhim H. Phytochemicals as a Complement to Cancer Chemotherapy: Pharmacological Modulation of the Autophagy-Apoptosis Pathway. Front Pharmacol. 2021 May 7;12:639628. doi: 10.3389/fphar.2021.639628. PMID: 34025409;

PMCID: PMC8138161.

Randisi F, Perletti G, Marras E, Gariboldi MB. Green Tea Components: In Vitro and In Vivo Evidence for Their Anticancer Potential in Colon Cancer. Cancers (Basel). 2025 Feb 13;17(4):623. doi: 10.3390/cancers17040623. PMID: 40002218; PMCID: PMC11853328.

Reuter S, Gupta SC, Chaturvedi MM, Aggarwal BB. Oxidative stress, inflammation, and cancer: how are they linked? Free Radic Biol Med. 2010 Dec 1;49(11):1603-16. doi: 10.1016/j.freeradbiomed.2010.09.006. Epub 2010 Sep 16. PMID: 20840865; PMCID: PMC2990475.

Rudzińska A, Juchaniuk P, Oberda J, Wiśniewska J, Wojdan W, Szklener K, Mańdziuk S. Phytochemicals in Cancer Treatment and Cancer Prevention-Review on Epidemiological Data and Clinical Trials. Nutrients. 2023 Apr 14;15(8):1896. doi: 10.3390/nu15081896. PMID: 37111115; PMCID: PMC10144429.

Saman H, Raza SS, Uddin S, Rasul K. Inducing Angiogenesis, a Key Step in Cancer Vascularization, and Treatment Approaches. Cancers (Basel). 2020 May 6;12(5):1172. doi: 10.3390/cancers12051172. PMID: 32384792; PMCID: PMC7281705.

Selvaraj S, Sun Y, Sukumaran P, Singh BB. Resveratrol activates autophagic cell death in prostate cancer cells via downregulation of STIM1 and the mTOR pathway. Mol Carcinog. 2016 May;55(5):818-31. doi: 10.1002/mc.22324. Epub 2015 Apr 27. PMID: 25917875; PMCID: PMC4624064.

Shankar S, Kumar D, Srivastava RK. Epigenetic modifications by dietary phytochemicals: implications for personalised nutrition. Pharmacol Ther. 2013 Apr;138(1):1-17. doi: 10.1016/j.pharmthera.2012.11.002. Epub 2012 Nov 16. PMID: 23159372; PMCID: PMC4153856.

Sharifi-Rad J, Rayess YE, Rizk AA, Sadaka C, Zgheib R, Zam W, Sestito S, Rapposelli S, Neffe-Skocińska K, Zielińska D, Salehi B, Setzer WN, Dosoky NS, Taheri Y, El Beyrouthy M, Martorell M, Ostrander EA, Suleria HAR, Cho WC, Maroyi A, Martins N. Turmeric and Its Major Compound Curcumin on Health: Bioactive Effects and Safety Profiles for Food, Pharmaceutical, Biotechnological and Medicinal Applications. Front Pharmacol. 2020 Sep 15;11:01021. doi: 10.3389/fphar.2020.01021. PMID: 33041781; PMCID: PMC7522354.

Singh BN, Shankar S, Srivastava RK. Green tea catechin, epigallocatechin-3-gallate (EGCG): mechanisms, perspectives and clinical applications. Biochem Pharmacol. 2011 Dec 15;82(12):1807-21. doi: 10.1016/j.bcp.2011.07.093. Epub 2011 Jul 30. PMID: 21827739; PMCID: PMC4082721.

Singh N, Baby D, Rajguru JP, Patil PB, Thakkannavar SS, Pujari VB. Inflammation and cancer. Ann Afr Med. 2019 Jul-Sep;18(3):121-126. doi: 10.4103/aam.aam_56_18. PMID: 31417011; PMCID: PMC6704802.

Tungmunnithum D, Thongboonyou A, Pholboon A, Yangsabai A. Flavonoids and Other Phenolic Compounds from Medicinal Plants for Pharmaceutical and Medical Aspects: An Overview. Medicines (Basel). 2018 Aug 25;5(3):93. doi: 10.3390/medicines5030093. PMID: 30149600; PMCID: PMC6165118.

van Helden YG, Keijer J, Heil SG, Picó C, Palou A, Oliver P, Munnia A, Briedé JJ, Peluso M, Franssen-van Hal NL, van Schooten FJ, Godschalk RW. Beta-carotene affects oxidative stress-related DNA damage in lung epithelial cells and in ferret lung. Carcinogenesis. 2009 Dec;30(12):2070-6. doi: 10.1093/carcin/bgp186. PMID: 19638427.

Wang H, Khor TO, Shu L, Su ZY, Fuentes F, Lee JH, Kong AN. Plants vs. cancer: a review on natural phytochemicals in preventing and treating cancers and their druggability. Anticancer Agents Med Chem. 2012 Dec;12(10):1281-305. doi: 10.2174/187152012803833026. PMID: 22583408; PMCID: PMC4017674.

Wang M, Xiao Y, Miao J, Zhang X, Liu M, Zhu L, Liu H, Shen X, Wang J, Xie B, Wang D. Oxidative Stress and Inflammation: Drivers of Tumourigenesis and Therapeutic Opportunities. Antioxidants (Basel). 2025 Jun 15;14(6):735. doi: 10.3390/antiox14060735. PMID: 40563367; PMCID: PMC12189506.

Yao Y, Dai W. Genomic Instability and Cancer. J Carcinog Mutagen. 2014;5:1000165. doi: 10.4172/2157-2518.1000165. PMID: 25541596; PMCID: PMC4274643.

Zafar A, Khatoon S, Khan MJ, Abu J, Naeem A. Advancements and limitations in traditional anti-cancer therapies: a comprehensive review of surgery, chemotherapy, radiation therapy, and hormonal therapy. Discov Oncol. 2025 Apr 24;16(1):607. doi: 10.1007/s12672-025-02198-8. PMID: 40272602; PMCID: PMC12021777.

Zoi V, Kyritsis AP, Galani V, Lazari D, Sioka C, Voulgaris S, Alexiou GA. The Role of Curcumin in Cancer: A Focus on the PI3K/Akt Pathway. Cancers (Basel). 2024 Apr 18;16(8):1554. doi: 10.3390/cancers16081554. PMID: 38672636; PMCID: PMC11048628.

Chapter 11

Clinical Nutritional Support in Oncological Treatment

Praneeth Juvvi[1], Sheetanshu Gupta[2*], Sarfraj Ahmad Siddiqui[3] and Lokesh Kumar Mishra[4]

[1]Department of Food Processing Technology, College of Food Technology-Central Agricultural University, Imphal, Manipur, India
[2]Department of Food Safety and Quality Assurance, College of Food Technology, Central Agricultural University (CAU), Imphal, Manipur, India
[3]Department of Biochemistry, King George's Medical University, U.P., India
[4]Department of BPME, College of Agriculture, Central Agricultural University (CAU), Imphal, Manipur, India

Abstract

Nutritional support significantly enhances the effectiveness of cancer treatment, and patient outcomes often improve substantially during and after therapy in many cases. Modified nutritional regimens crucially play a pivotal role throughout cancer treatment cycles, deeply addressing myriad oncology ward challenges with considerable precision. Chemotherapy precipitates severely debilitating side effects like anorexia alongside radiation, which negatively impacts the efficacy of cancer treatment. The importance of nutritional assessment surfaces early on for optimising treatment plans, and the implications of such effects are discussed thoroughly in this chapter. Nutritional support encompasses various modalities like enteral nutrition and parenteral nutrition, playing crucial roles in sustaining bodily functions vigorously and thwarting cachexia effectively, alongside alleviating nasty side effects attributed mostly to harsh treatment. Omega-3 fatty acids and protein significantly support immune function by reducing severe inflammation with considerable efficacy. Nowadays personalized nutrition in oncology is rigorously tailored for individual metabolic profiles and various cancer types rather meticulously. Optimal nutritional care hinges crucially on oncologists collaborating very closely with dietitians, as highlighted in various recent research and sundry case studies.

Keywords: Nutritional Therapy, Cachexia, Tumour Metabolism, Parenteral Nutrition, Oncology Dietetics, Symptom Management

DOI: 10.1201/9781042010387-11

1. Introduction

Innovations in chemotherapy and radiotherapy are offering new hope for patients undergoing targeted therapies, with significant advancements emerging quite recently. Treatments frequently yield nasty side effects that culminate in malnutrition and badly ravaged overall health, impacting patients' lives very severely afterwards. Clinical nutrition assumes vital significance in oncological care, being now an integral part of cancer treatment plans for frail patients. Nutrition plays a pivotal role in encouraging therapeutic efficacy during cancer treatment while reducing heinous side effects fairly significantly amidst bodily turmoil. Cancer-related malnutrition manifests insidiously with subtle weight loss and ghastly muscle wasting alongside deficiencies in crucial proteins or various vitamins. Tumour burden and metabolic changes spawn nutritional challenges, partly due to treatment side effects and drastically lowered food consumption overall.

Cancer treatments brutally ravage usual metabolic routes, resulting in greatly heightened expenditure of energy and unbridled catabolism that fuels precipitous loss of weight and skeletal muscle wasting very rapidly. Tumour-driven systemic inflammation muddies nutritional support somewhat rapidly as it fuels muscle catabolism and suppresses protein synthesis in hosts. Nutritional deficits are mitigated daily with striking efficacy, thereby remarkably lessening cancer's ravaging impact on patient health during treatment. Multifaceted interventions target malnutrition in cancer patients quite effectively and treat it with varying degrees of efficacy afterwards sometimes. Interventions are tailored for each patient individually with specific needs involving oral nutrition support or enteral nutrition via tube feeding, and parenteral nutrition is administered intravenously (Law ML, 2022).

Maintaining overall nutritional status quite effectively most of the time relies heavily on adequate caloric intake and supplementation with various micronutrients and protein. Meticulous routine screening and thorough assessment for nutritional support are necessitated by early detection and management of malnutrition generally. Clinicians very effectively wield tools like Patient-Generated Subjective Global Assessment and Malnutrition Universal Screening Tool nowadays for devising treatment plans and assessing malnutrition severity. Nutritional support nowadays frequently entails meticulous management of cancer treatment side effects, rather critically. Chemotherapy induces severe nausea, vomiting, and mouth sores very frequently, while radiotherapy drastically alters taste perception, reducing nutrient uptake significantly. Immunotherapy and targeted therapies frequently precipitate nasty gastrointestinal symptoms like diarrhoea and constipation with considerable ferocity in many patients (Kesari and Noel, 2023).

Nutritional support strategies must judiciously assess treatment regimen severity and the patient's compromised ability to ingest nutrients without exacerbating dire side effects. The crucial issue of managing cancer cachexia persists quietly in oncological nutritional care, beset by mystifying weight loss and debilitating muscle fatigue. Cachexia nowadays frequently correlates with bleak prognosis and diminished tolerance for cancer treatments, making management an utmost priority. Heightened metabolic demands and plummeting nutrient intake fuel systemic inflammation that drives this nasty condition very aggressively underground daily. Pro-inflammatory cytokines such as TNF-α and IL-6 drive muscle degradation fairly quickly during the development of cachexia with alarming rapidity.

Cachexia treatment involves a multifaceted strategy entailing high-calorie diets and oral nutritional supplements, alongside pharmacological interventions such as appetite stimulants sometimes. Nutritional counselling incorporated into cancer treatment remarkably improves patient outcomes substantially over time in a rather natural manner. Educating patients about food choices remarkably well during meal planning phases helps manage symptoms and optimise nutritional intake effectively. Patients undergoing treatment may benefit from small, frequent meals, high-calorie snacks and liquid nutritional supplements, which help ensure adequate intake. Emotional distress, depression, and anxiety often further severely reduce appetite and badly complicate eating behaviours during nutritional counselling sessions lacking sufficient psychosocial support mechanisms (Arends et al, 2021).

Enteral nutrition or tube feeding and parenteral nutrition, namely IV nutrition, frequently become necessary for patients struggling mightily with oral nutritional deficiencies. People afflicted with cancers of head or neck and gastrointestinal malignancies often struggle mightily swallowing nutrients due to ravages of intense treatment. Enteral nutrition through feeding tubes delivers essential nutrients directly into stomach or intestines in exceedingly complicated and particularly dicey health situations apparently. Parenteral nutrition supplies essential nutrients directly into veins generally reserved for patients with severe gut problems like bowel blockages or massive surgical removals.

Crucial interventions maintain nutritional status and support recovery but effectiveness hinges somewhat unpredictably on underlying disease state with various comorbidities. Patients with virulent cancers or receiving arduous treatments may necessitate very specialized dietary interventions quite frequently these days. Tailoring nutritional support mostly according to disease stage and cancer type while factoring in patient preferences necessitates quite specific regimen. Recent research underscores significance of tailored nutrition in oncology where patients nutritional requirements fluctuate remarkably across diverse demographic groups. Clinicians now grasp how quirky genetic factors and individual responses to nutrition badly affect cancer progression and treatment efficacy very irregularly. Cancer treatment recovery gets optimized very effectively when healthcare providers develop super precise nutrition plans using genetic profiles and metabolic data (Mercier et al, 2022).

Nutritional support for oncology patients undergoing holistic management serves some very vital purpose beyond merely serving meals for cancer sufferers. Nutrition profoundly affects physical facets of cancer treatment and psychosocial well-being of patients undergoing arduous therapy regimes simultaneously. Nutritional status significantly boosts treatment tolerance and enhances life quality while substantially mitigating risk of various nasty complications down the line. Cancer treatments evolve rapidly now with nutrition playing a vital role in sustaining patients throughout their incredibly arduous ordeal. Oncology clinical nutritional support encompasses multifaceted components crucial for managing malnutrition and mitigating effects of cancer cachexia effectively enhancing cancer treatment outcomes. Cancer treatment research emerging rapidly will be scrutinized heavily alongside myriad challenges clinicians face whilst providing effective care nutritionally for patients necessitating collaboration across multiple disciplines. Furnishing fairly comprehensive insight into clinical nutritional support as a vital facet of modern oncology care enhance patient outcomes remarkably well nowadays.

2. The Role of Nutrition in Enhancing Cancer Treatment Outcomes

Cancer treatment entails a plethora of therapeutic strategies including chemotherapy and radiotherapy or surgery with immunotherapy in diverse combos very frequently. Malignant cells are targeted by such interventions which wreak havoc on tissues thereby precipitating plethora of debilitating side effects unfortunately. Malnutrition occurs frequently under certain circumstances as a serious aftermath of disease and treatments that severely undermine nutritional status unfortunately. Patients suffer terribly from anorexia and nausea alongside mucositis resulting in significant weight loss fostering severe malnutrition and cachexia very quickly. Malnutrition drastically impairs immune function and wound healing gets delayed somewhat reducing tolerance for therapy which diminishes quality of life negatively influencing treatment outcomes (Anand et al, 2022).

Nutrition plays a pivotal role in mitigating complications rather effectively under specific conditions and encourage somewhat sluggish clinical responses very fairly. Adequate nutrition very effectively enhance cancer treatment outcomes by enhancing patients' resilience and maintaining lean body mass very substantially. Toxicity related to treatment further exacerbates oxidative stress somewhat irregularly and inflammatory responses already elevated within tumour microenvironment. Protein-energy malnutrition occurs frequently among cancer patients and associates with heightened morbidity and starkly elevated mortality rates suddenly. Muscle wasting and subsequent immune suppression nowadays must be offset rather vigorously by ensuring adequate caloric intake and sufficient protein consumption effectively (Anand et al, 2022).

Diets comprising high-quality proteins and essential amino acids such as leucine rather effectively support muscle synthesis during chemotherapy and reduce inflammation very significantly. Micronutrients such as vitamin A enhance antioxidant defense mechanisms very effectively alongside DNA repair and immune function quite naturally underground. Phytochemical-rich dietary patterns like Mediterranean and plant-based diets may remarkably improve treatment outcomes and tolerance very well these days. Diets rich in bioactive compounds modulate cellular pathways and synergize very powerfully with anticancer agents reducing damage caused by oxidation significantly. Tumours are being sensitized effectively nowadays through nutritional strategies such as ketogenic diets and intermittent fasting sparing normal cells effectively.

Registered dietitians should be deeply involved in oncology care teams for thorough nutritional assessment and swift intervention during complex treatment planning processes. Tailored nutritional care remarkably supports physiological needs very well and significantly contributes to emotional well-being effectively during treatment. Nutritional therapy integration into oncology practice embodies a vital aspect of fairly comprehensive cancer care with multifaceted approach inherently. Enhancing treatment efficacy substantially occurs in cancer patients with optimized nutritional status ultimately yielding better quality of life and improved survival.

2.1. Nutritional Support During Cancer Treatment

Nutritional support plays a crucial role in management of cancer patients undergoing aggressive daily treatment regimens with extreme intensity. Therapies like chemotherapy wreak havoc on metabolic balance quite significantly while targeting malignant cells and impairing nutritional intake drastically meanwhile. Nausea vomiting mucositis anorexia altered taste and smell dysphagia and gastrointestinal disturbances emerge greatly reducing subsequent nutrient absorption and food intake. Malnutrition and cancer cachexia characterized by drastic weight loss and muscle wasting occur frequently in patients with advanced stage cancer exhibiting systemic inflammation.

Malnutrition severely undermines physical strength life quality and strongly correlates with dire clinical outcomes like treatment intolerance rampant infections and very prolonged hospital stays. A meticulously crafted nutritional regimen sustains patients' functional capacity effectively and enhance bodily resilience against strain induced by rigorous treatment protocols. Aggressive cancer treatment induces remarkably catabolic state which often necessitates extremely high calorie and very high protein dietary regimen. Protein preserves lean body mass remarkably well and supports immune function thoroughly amidst various physiological processes like tissue repair mechanisms ordinarily. Lean meats eggs and legumes rich in high-quality protein should be eaten daily in most meals fairly easily almost everywhere. Protein and calorie supplements may be given rather liberally when patients aren't getting enough nutrients orally meeting their specific bodily needs (Saunders and Smith, 2010). Healthy fats significantly boost energy intake particularly in patients struggling with eating sizable meals or having severely diminished appetites. Foods such as avocados and nut butters provide energy dense nutrition remarkably well and olive oil fosters satiety very effectively. Omega-3 fatty acids found mainly in salmon and mackerel also occur in flaxseeds chia seeds and various fish oil supplements with profoundly anti-inflammatory properties. Fatty acids possibly mitigate inflammatory responses associated with cancer cachexia and have been researched fairly extensively for potentially boosting appetite stability (Saunders and Smith, 2010). Personalized proactive nutritional support stands as a cornerstone of comprehensive cancer care nowadays entirely within quite varied treatment protocols effectively. Strategic dietary changes tailored quite specifically to patient needs can significantly mitigate adverse effects of cancer therapy during treatment.

2.2. Nutrition and Immune Function in Cancer Patients

Crucial defense mechanism against rapidly proliferating cancerous cells is served by immune system and it plays pivotal role in various cancer therapies effectiveness. Chemotherapy and radiotherapy treatments significantly damage immune function over time in most patients undergoing these harsh therapies quite badly. Therapies often target rapidly proliferating cells like bone marrow cells resulting in leukopenia and severely compromised host defenses subsequently. Cancer patients face heightened vulnerability to opportunistic infections alongside markedly delayed wound healing and reduced tolerance for treatment very frequently nowadays. Malnutrition common among cancer patients further severely exacerbates immune suppression. Essential nutrient deficiency can severely hobble innate immunity and adaptive immune system functionality very drastically under certain circumstances naturally.

Energy deficits and protein-calorie malnutrition severely impair macrophage function natural killer cell activity and various lymphocyte responses diminishing bodily defenses against tumour cells fiercely. Optimal nutritional support effectively mitigates dire consequences via enhanceed immune function offering considerable safeguard against myriad infections and nasty diseases. Vitamin C and vitamin E exhibit potent antioxidant properties and play crucial roles upholding immune function during cancer treatment remarkably well. Vitamin C and E effectively scavenge reactive oxygen species generated during various cancer therapies in rather excessive amounts quite frequently. They very effectively shield immune cells from damage by mitigating oxidative stress and encourage overall functionality in a somewhat irregular manner. Vitamin C boosts production of white blood cells vigorously including neutrophils and lymphocytes while vitamin E supports cell-mediated immunity rather effectively (Ibrahim et al, 2017).

Vitamin D plays a crucial role in regulating innate immunity and adaptive immunity through extensively profound immunomodulatory effects. It enhance pathogen-fighting effects of monocytes hugely and macrophages help regulate production of inflammatory cytokine very effectively meanwhile. Elevated serum vitamin D correlates with better cancer prognosis including lower infection incidence and robust immunotherapy response in certain patient populations. Selenium serves remarkably well as a crucial cofactor in many enzymatic reactions pivotal for modulating immune function alongside zinc typically. Zinc remarkably facilitates DNA synthesis underneath cellular surfaces and enhances immune cells structural integrity during wound healing processes very effectively (Ibrahim et al, 2017). Selenium a vital component of selenoproteins effectively enhance antioxidant defense systems protecting immune cells very thoroughly from oxidative damage. Deficiency in either mineral strongly correlates with lymphocytes functioning poorly and subsequently greatly heightened susceptibility to infection occurs. Crucial micronutrient intake profoundly impacts immune resilience during cancer treatment extremely effectively fundamentally. Specific nutritional interventions markedly enhance immune response and enhance oncological treatment efficacy substantially while improving patient tolerability quite remarkably.

2.3. Antioxidants and Cancer Treatment: A Double-Edged Sword?

Antioxidants occur naturally in fruits vegetables nuts and whole grains and neutralize reactive oxygen species quite effectively. Antioxidants play protective roles under normal physiological conditions by thwarting cellular damage linked intricately to oxidative stress often implicated in various cancers. Antioxidants play a somewhat contentious role during various cancer treatments often fraught notoriously with complex controversy under certain circumstances. Chemotherapy and similar conventional cancer treatments exert cytotoxic effects by generating reactive oxygen species that damage rapidly dividing cells very severely. Malignant cells are targeted effectively by this mechanism but normal tissues get harmed brutally leading to severe side effects like organ toxicity.

Antioxidants effectively shield healthy tissues from damage by neutralizing excess free radicals generated during treatment reducing toxicity greatly. Concerns have been raised that antioxidants possibly shield cancer cells from ROS-mediated damage and somewhat diminish treatment efficacy rather oddly. High-dose antioxidant supplementation with vitamin C and β-carotene may blunt certain chemotherapeutic agents' effectiveness by meddling with mechanisms of oxidative stress rather quietly. Antioxidants derived from whole foods are deemed very safe and super beneficial yet isolated antioxidant supplements warrant extreme caution during various cancer treatments. Leafy greens and whole grains harbour diverse bioactive compounds naturally in rather balanced physiologically favourable doses alongside some citrus fruits and berries (Zahra et al, 2021).

Antioxidant rich foods enhance endogenous defense systems very effectively without swamping them or undermining therapeutically induced oxidative stress. Maintaining a diet rich in antioxidant-containing foods during treatment remains very much always safe and advisable for most people undergoing therapy. Supplementation with hefty doses of isolated antioxidants warrants careful scrutiny individually rather haphazardly under vastly different and often unpredictable circumstances. Patients undergoing treatment ought consult specialists in oncology and experts in nutrition before starting supplements thereby sidestepping pernicious interactions with chemotherapy (Zahra et al, 2021). Antioxidants yield crucial health benefits yet their application during cancer treatment necessitates tailoring judiciously based on sound empirical evidence.

2.4. The Role of Dietary Fibre in Cancer Prevention and Recovery

Dietary fibre a non-digestible constituent of plant-based edibles plays a rather crucial role in gut health maintenance and impacts various physiological processes altering cancer risk profoundly. Mounting epidemiological evidence and some clinical data strongly support a markedly reduced risk of various malignancies with high dietary fibre intake especially for colorectal cancer. Fibre remarkably improves intestinal function and modulates gut microbiota whilst facilitating excretion of some carcinogens and reducing systemic inflammation very effectively. Fibre exists mainly in soluble forms and insoluble ones primarily nowadays. Soluble fibre present in oats and apples dissolves quite rapidly in water forming a gel-like substance slowing digestion down very significantly (Fu et al, 2022).

Soluble fibre fosters metabolic conditions somewhat inhospitable tumour growth by heavily mitigating blood glucose and significantly diminishing insulin resistance associated with cancer. Soluble fibre serves as fermentable substrate for colonic microbiota thereby promoting production of short-chain fatty acids like butyrate very effectively underground. Butyrate possesses anti-inflammatory properties and exhibits profoundly anti-neoplastic effects by inducing apoptosis very effectively in colon cancer cells. Insoluble fibre present in whole grains nuts veggies adds bulk to stool and accelerates intestinal transit thereby diluting potential carcinogens lurking deep within colon (Fu et al, 2022). Mechanical cleansing action remarkably reduces colorectal carcinogenesis risk alongside effectively improving bowel regularity with considerable efficacy. Prebiotic fibres such as inulin and fructooligosaccharides found abundantly in garlic onions leeks and asparagus stimulate beneficial gut bacteria growth selectively around Bifidobacterium and Lactobacillus species. Diverse microbes thriving in a balanced gut microbiome effectively enhance mucosal immunity and significantly reduce pro-inflammatory cytokines. Patients with cancer having robust gut microbiota often exhibit better responses to immune checkpoint inhibitors and experience relatively fewer gastrointestinal side effects during such treatment.

Diets high in fibre substantially support healing during cancer recovery by restoring gut microbiota equilibrium and mitigating chronic nasty inflammation very effectively. Dietary fibre may facilitate weight management quite effectively and regulate metabolic hormones which contributes significantly to long-term cancer survivorship overall. Dietary fibre represents a vital nutritional component crucial obviously for cancer prevention effectively in various obscure ways. Fibre-rich plant foods remarkably benefit individuals recovering from cancer or at risk by encourage treatment responses and promoting gut health.

2.5. Personalized Nutrition in Cancer Care

Personalized nutrition represents a rapidly evolving frontier in oncology emphasizing modified diets shaped by genomic profiles cancer specifics and lifestyle factors usually. Personalized nutrition in cancer care seeks modified nutritional solutions addressing peculiar physiological anomalies and heightened metabolic requirements of individual patients thereby significantly boosting treatment efficacy. Fairly effectively nowadays personalized nutrition involves targeted nutrient supplementation remarkably mitigating various medical treatment side effects quite often. Glutamine a conditionally essential amino acid somewhat effectively reduces severity of chemotherapy-induced mucositis and debilitating inflammation occurs in gastrointestinal tract lining. Glutamine fuels enterocytes and supports robust immune function thereby potentially mitigating treatment complications and facilitating uninterrupted therapy under highly stressful conditions normally.

Nutrigenomics sheds novel light on how distinct genetic variations inside individuals very radically sway reactions to particular diets comprising sundry nutrients. Genetic variations in MTHFR seriously impact folate metabolism, thereby altering cancer risk and treatment efficacy, mandating genotype-guided folate intake guidelines very urgently. Genetic variations like those found in SOD2 and GPX1 hugely impact response to antioxidant-rich diets during cancer treatment quite significantly. Precision nutrition plans emerge from integrating nutrigenomic data into clinical practice and are simultaneously super preventive and remarkably therapeutic. Molecular tumour profiling alongside biomarkers indicating inflammation or oxidative stress influences adjustments made roughly according to metabolic needs and native microbiome composition. Such an approach aligns nutrition closely with precision medicine principles, allowing healthcare providers to recommend diets that support general health and contribute substantially towards therapeutic processes (Sharma and Dwivedi, 2017). Personalised nutrition interventions must very carefully consider behavioural and cultural psychosocial determinants during design phases, aside from biological factors. Nutritional support requires cooperation among healthcare professionals like oncologists and dietitians, providing feasible evidence-based dietary advice for patients quite effectively. Personalised nutrition might overhaul cancer care measures radically by tailoring dietary regimes closely around specific quirks in patient biology. Personalised nutrition significantly enhances immune function, thereby serving as a vital adjunct for conventional oncology and supporting recovery with better clinical outcomes (Sharma and Dwivedi, 2017).

3. Nutritional Strategies to Support Cancer Patients During Therapy

Cancer therapy frequently exacts a hefty physiological toll on patients, not just via cytotoxic effects but also through woefully debilitating metabolic aftereffects. Surgical interventions and chemotherapy often beget a slew of debilitating side effects like nausea, mucositis and unrelenting fatigue very suddenly. Malnutrition and weight loss stem from severely impaired food intake, hampering nutrient absorption and ravaging immune function, which then badly affects cancer therapy outcomes. Nutritional strategies ought to be deliberately woven into cancer care as a vital component right alongside various oncology treatment protocols. Strategies must be tailored for each patient based on disease type, stage, treatment protocol, nutritional deficiencies and quite severe symptoms obviously (Anand et al, 2022).

Prevention and management of cancer cachexia becomes primary during nutritional therapy for cancer treatment, marked by progressive weight loss and muscle wasting. Energy-dense diets rich in protein are often recommended afterwards for naturally supporting tissue repair and effectively maintaining lean body mass. Protein sources such as fortified oral nutritional supplements and legumes can be emphasised right alongside lean meats and a variety of dairy products. Meals eaten frequently in small portions and enriched with healthy fats from sources such as nuts or olive oil really help patients with poor appetite meet their energy needs. Apparently, drastic changes in diet aimed squarely at alleviating nasty symptoms are utterly essential for people plagued by such issues daily. Patients queasy with nausea tend to tolerate bland foods or cold food rather well, while soft textured super moist foods ease discomfort in folks suffering mucositis (Anand et al, 2022).

Taste enhancement techniques, such as using herbs or acidic flavouring agents like lemon juice, may surprisingly counteract dysgeusia and greatly boost food palatability. Patients exhibiting profuse vomiting or diarrhoea and prone to sudden renal complications must be monitored extremely carefully for hydration status. Incorporating functional foods teeming with omega-3 fatty acids and certain probiotics and prebiotics may hugely modulate inflammation and somewhat enhance immune competence effectively. Oncologists work closely with registered dietitians throughout treatment, ensuring heavily evidence-based nutritional care remains very much continuous. Proper nutritional support amplifies patients' tolerance for gruelling therapy and markedly fosters faster recuperation with significantly improved overall treatment compliance.

3.1. Optimizing Caloric and Protein Intake

Maintaining sufficiently high caloric intake daily and consuming enough protein remains foundational in nutritional management of patients with cancer. Cancer treatments heap massive metabolic stress on bodily functions precipitating negative energy balance and rapid protein degradation very quickly. Treatment-related symptoms such as anorexia and mucositis exacerbate these effects rapidly by diminishing dietary intake and further fuelling severe malnutrition. Unintentional weight loss greatly diminishes quality of life severely impairing immune function or substantially increasing mortality risk with muscle wasting. Very much throughout therapy high-calorie dietary strategies rich in protein are generally recommended during various cancer treatments. Energy-dense foods containing healthy fats from sources like avocados and nuts or olive oil greatly benefit patients having reduced appetite (Gangadharan et al, 2017).

Omega-3 fatty acids found in fatty fish like salmon and flaxseeds have been shown exerting profoundly anti-inflammatory effects during severely catabolic states. Protein intake stays crucial for upkeep of skeletal muscle and supports mending of tissue while remarkably preserving functionality of immune systems very well. Daily protein needs frequently skyrocket far beyond typical dietary recommendations during treatment with active systemic inflammation or pronounced muscle wasting underway. Lean meats poultry fish eggs and dairy products like Greek yogurt are rich sources of high-quality protein from legumes and soy products such as tofu. Oral nutritional supplements or protein-enriched beverages may be necessary for patients struggling mightily to meet protein targets through usual dietary intake (Gangadharan et al, 2017).

Supplements often furnish extra calories or branched-chain amino acids and sometimes provide specialized nutrients like leucine supporting muscle protein synthesis quite vigorously in athletes. Proper timing boosts meal planning effectiveness remarkably well overall during any given period. Patients can meet protein and energy needs effectively by consuming frequent small nutrient-rich meals roughly every few hours, almost always. Regular assessment by a clinical dietitian alongside nutritional counselling ensures dietary plans adapt rapidly with each patient's changing needs during intensive treatment. Proactive nutritional strategies optimize intake of calories and protein, preserving physiological resilience in cancer patients and markedly supporting treatment response.

3.2. Managing Side Effects through Nutritional Adjustments

Chemotherapy elicits many nasty side effects severely impairing nutritional status with gastrointestinal symptoms flaring up quite frequently and uncomfortably. Nutritional strategies tailored to individuals play a pivotal role in markedly enhancing quality of life and improving tolerance of treatment. Vomiting and nausea often manifest unfortunately in many patients following radiation therapy and chemotherapy treatments as commonly reported adverse effects. Grossly inadequate caloric intake occurs very regularly alongside anorexia and food aversions with symptoms manifesting frequently in such cases. Patients are advised eating bland meals frequently in small portions low in fat that are ridiculously easy afterwards to digest properly. Bananas rice applesauce and toast comprising BRAT diet gets frequently touted for being ridiculously gentle on most gastrointestinal tracts.

Greasy food and pungent eats may worsen symptoms so steering clear of such victuals utterly matters in most cases ordinarily. Ginger, a natural antiemetic, has been shown in various clinical studies very effectively reducing chemotherapy-induced nausea and can be had as tea. Dysgeusia often manifests alongside certain brutal chemotherapeutic agents and radiation treatments targeting head region with some alarming frequency. Patients frequently bemoan rather bizarre metallic tastes or bland flavors which render sustenance unpalatable and markedly exacerbate anorexia nervosa. Dietary strategies overcoming dysgeusia involve enhancing flavor very heavily with natural herbs and very acidic stuff like lemon juice or ridiculously salty seasonings.

Tart foods and citrus fruits very effectively stimulate salivation and quite remarkably heighten perception of taste. Using utensils made from stainless steel or plastic might minimize unpleasant sensations triggered by highly reactive metal surfaces rather effectively. Xerostomia plagues patients receiving head radiation therapy quite severely and swallowing gets really impaired affecting the enjoyment of food badly. Strategies alleviating xerostomia involve encouraging frequent water sips using saliva substitutes and consuming soft foods like creamy smoothies or yogurt daily. Sugar-free lozenges very effectively stimulate residual salivary gland function inside mouth enhancing oral moisture quite obviously nowadays. Adequate hydration with oral rehydration solutions, sporadically used, largely keeps mucosal integrity intact and facilitates absorption of nutrients effectively. Nutritional adjustments crucially maintain intake during therapy based largely on each patient's side-effect profile under a specific therapeutic regimen. Registered dietitians guide a proactive somewhat flexible approach that alleviates treatment related symptoms and supports optimal nutrition during entire cancer care process.

3.3. Supporting Immune Function through Micronutrient Intake

Risky chemotherapy regimens frequently yield profound immunosuppression making patients extremely vulnerable to opportunistic bacterial infections quite rapidly afterwards normally. Cancer therapies become remarkably effective when optimal immune function is maintained during treatment thereby reducing risk of infection substantially. Key micronutrients boasting antioxidant properties play a crucial role daily in encourage immune resilience remarkably well under normal circumstances. Vitamin C remarkably acts as a potent antioxidant deeply entangled in various roles within human immunity ostensibly in many bodily processes. It very effectively enhance proliferation and function of various immune cells including neutrophils lymphocytes and natural killer cells under certain obscure conditions (Safdar et al, 2011).

Vitamin C substantially enhance epithelial barrier function and facilitates neutralization of reactive oxygen species spawned during inflammation induced by certain treatments. Citrus fruits and strawberries, along with kiwis, bell peppers and broccoli, boasting exceptionally high vitamin C content, sit alongside various leafy greens. Vitamin E rather effectively shields immune cells from oxidative damage and somewhat irregularly modulates production of sundry inflammatory cytokines, meanwhile. T-cell function gets enhanced quite vigorously, and antibody responses ramp up significantly. Nuts like almonds seeds spinach and various vegetable oils serve naturally as abundant food sources (Safdar et al, 2011).

Vitamins C and E have shown an ability somewhat unusually quite effectively mitigating oxidative stress related at surprisingly rather high dietary levels. Vitamin D plays a crucial albeit somewhat obscure role in modulating immune responses by influencing the activity of various innate cells very effectively. It promotes differentiation of monocytes into macrophages and enhance microbicidal activity very vigorously while modulating inflammatory responses quite irregularly. Survival outcomes are markedly improved with sufficient vitamin D levels whilst infection rates dwindle significantly amongst cancer patients fiercely battling various malignancies. Fatty fish such as salmon or sardines, and fortified dairy products and egg yolks serve as decent dietary sources virtually everywhere nowadays. Supplementation may be necessary for cancer patients severely deficient in vitamin D particularly those with appallingly poor dietary habits or limited exposure to sunlight.

Zinc plays a crucial role greatly in development of immune cells particularly in proliferation and function ofT lymphocytes and B lymphocytes. It plays somewhat significantly role in DNA synthesis quietly and rather profoundly in wound healing bodily processes. Meat and shellfish provide rich sources of zinc whereas legumes whole grains and seeds supply it abundantly in various obscure ways. Selenium another vital trace element significantly contributes to antioxidant defense via selenoproteins and effectively enhance humoral immunity in various ways. Selenium abounds in brazil nuts and seafood whereas whole grains furnish a rich stash of this vital nutrient remarkably well (Wessels et al, 2017). Cancer treatment outcomes improve remarkably well with incorporation of balanced micronutrient-rich diets reinforcing overall immune competence very effectively. Collaboration with a clinical dietitian guarantees fulfillment of vital nutritional needs thereby deftly circumventing glaring shortfalls and overzealous supplementation in patients.

3.4. Preventing Dehydration and Supporting Electrolyte Balance

Cancer treatments such as chemotherapy wreak havoc on bodily fluids and electrolytes resulting in very nasty side effects extremely often. Treatment-related complications such as severe vomiting and nasty mucositis often result in significant fluid loss reducing oral intake substantially risking dehydration. Severe imbalances can grossly disrupt organ function rather quickly and exacerbate fatigue substantially increasing rates of hospitalization and limiting tolerance for treatment. Proactive strategies maintaining hydration and electrolyte balance are crucial components of cancer nutrition care under such uniquely challenging circumstances essentially. Dehydration drastically impairs circulatory volume and reduces clearance of chemotherapy drugs thereby greatly increasing risks of severe toxicity very quickly (Naidu et al, 2004).

Clinicians and dietitians should encourage patients drink fluids regularly throughout day based heavily on individual body weight and severity of symptoms. Patients experiencing nausea tolerate clear liquids remarkably well such as filtered water or diluted fruit juices very frequently obviously. Very beneficial oral rehydration solutions and low-sugar sports drinks replace fluids and electrolytes in severe gastrointestinal distress cases effectively. Coconut water serves as a naturally occurring rich in potassium and magnesium substitute suitable for patients preferring rather unprocessed beverages. Gelatin-based snacks or ice chips provide extra hydration options for patients battling nasty mucositis or struggling with swallowing very badly. Electrolytes like sodium potassium magnesium and chloride are vital essentially for neuromuscular function maintaining acid-base balance and facilitating intracellular signaling (Naidu et al, 2004).

Cancer patients on platinum-based chemotherapies or diuretics are especially susceptible to hypokalemia hyponatremia and hypomagnesemia particularly with parenteral nutrition or when corticosteroids are administered. Regularly incorporating foods rich in electrolytes into one's diet seems crucial for maintaining optimal bodily functions effectively over time. Bananas oranges and sweet potatoes contain copious amounts of potassium while leafy greens rank surprisingly high as stellar sources naturally. Magnesium can be obtained readily from various sources including nuts seeds whole grains legumes and avocados are notably rich in it. Cancer patients experiencing excessive losses from vomiting or diarrhea may need temporary sodium boosts and salted snacks can be very helpful. Very individualized fluid management gets guided effectively through various assessments like lab values and blood pressure monitoring of hydration status. Caregivers and patients must be schooled rather extensively on recognizing signs of dehydration such as dizziness or dark colored urine very quickly. Crucial for physical well-being in cancer patients undergoing treatment slowly is maintaining hydration and electrolyte balance for optimizing therapeutic efficacy.

3.5. Fibre-Rich Diet for Digestive Health

Cancer treatments such as chemotherapy yield unpleasant gastrointestinal side effects including diarrhea within the gastrointestinal tract and nasty inflammation too. Symptoms can severely impact patient's life quality and badly compromise nutritional status treatment adherence and overall recovery quite slowly afterwards. Dietary fibre plays crucial roles in maintaining gastrointestinal function and it prominently figures in supportive nutrition therapy for patients undergoing oncology treatment. Dietary fibre gets categorized broadly into soluble and insoluble types both playing distinctly crucial roles in overall health of digestive mechanisms. Soluble fibre dissolves in water fairly quickly forming a rather gel-like substance and softens stools very effectively during constipation.

Beneficial gut bacteria feast on it, producing short-chain fatty acids such as butyrate with profoundly anti-inflammatory properties thereby promoting overall gut health. Oats barley apples and carrots are decent sources of soluble fibre alongside legumes and psyllium husk virtually everywhere. Insoluble fibre adds bulk very quickly and speeds up intestinal transit thereby benefiting patients stuck with opioid pain meds-induced constipation. Whole grains nuts and seeds bran comprise foods rich in insoluble fibre and rather fibrous veggies like kale or spinach are quite notable. Eating these foods regularly, when tolerated, very effectively supports normal bowel function and minimizes gastrointestinal discomfort somewhat over time. Tailoring fibre recommendations according to specifics of each patient and myriad symptoms matters very darn much however (Ioniță-Mîndrican et al, 2022).

Patients with radiation-induced enteritis or severe diarrhea and mucositis may need temporary reduction in fibre intake mostly insoluble fibre avoiding further bowel distress. Low-residue diets are often recommended under close clinical supervision in rather unusual cases obviously with some very strict monitoring. Fibre-rich foods introduced gradually alongside plenty of fluids help restore bowel regularity very effectively in patients afflicted with stubborn constipation. Fibre kicks in rapidly as a prebiotic fueling beneficial gut microbiota growth which plays some part in modulating immunity and vigorously absorbing nutrients. Emerging evidence suggests quite significantly a diverse gut microbiome very often enhances efficacy of some immunotherapies in various cases (Ioniță-Mîndrican et al, 2022). Cancer care incorporates a well-balanced fibre-rich diet that helps mitigate treatment-related digestive issues thereby contributing significantly overall recovery.

3.6. Tailored Nutritional Approaches: A Personalized Strategy

Cancer isn't a one-size-fits-all disease and treatment for it doesn't necessarily work wholly effectively on every patient every time. Nutritional needs during cancer therapy vary drastically and must be tailored rather carefully for each patient in a distinct clinical context. Genetic predispositions alongside comorbidities influence patient responses to foods differently based on baseline nutritional status and varying metabolic demands under specific treatment modalities. Personalized nutrition plans become utterly essential for garnering optimal support throughout cancer care of each individual with modified tailored specifics. Oncology personalized nutrition starts thoroughly assessing nutritional status with various anthropometric measurements and analyzing dietary intake very meticulously. Oncology dietitians can recommend modified strategies that help stave off malnutrition or manage anorexia very effectively under various circumstances (Barrera S, Demark-Wahnefried, 2009).

Patients undergoing head and neck radiation therapy may develop severe mucositis and dysphagia necessitating soft diets or pureed food and occasionally enteral nutrition via feeding tubes becomes necessary. Patients with gastrointestinal cancers may benefit from low-residue diets during treatment and then reintroduce fibre-rich foods slowly as tolerated afterwards. Others might require extremely calorie dense formulas particularly when snacking covers barely half their daily energy needs so oral supplements can be super helpful. Nutritional genomics advances have opened fresh avenues very recently for super personalized nutrition surprisingly and with considerable fanfare nowadays. Fairly well understood gene-nutrient interactions can somewhat predict individual responses to foods and inform selection of various therapeutic interventions effectively.

Metabolic alterations like cancer cachexia or insulin resistance render highly individualized approaches crucial in such complex clinical contexts obviously. Tailored interventions involve adjusting macronutrient composition or supplementing quite effectively with specific nutrients like glutamine and branched-chain amino acids. Tailored nutritional support greatly enhances medical treatment efficacy and remarkably improves functional status in patients suffering from various chronic ailments. Cancer patients heal effectively under intensive therapy while receiving requisite nutrition and participating actively in their own recovery process. Personalized nutrition represents a crucial frontier evolving rather slowly within cancer treatment as a vital component of multidisciplinary oncology care remarkably.

4. Managing Treatment Side Effects

Potent tools against cancer such as chemotherapy and surgery, frequently exact harsh tolls on patients both physically and emotionally. Nausea and vomiting erupt simultaneously with drastically altered taste or smell, while mucositis manifests severely in patients plagued by extreme fatigue. Unaddressed complications devolve precipitously into malnutrition or cachexia and severely suppress immune function rather quickly in most clinical cases. Nutritional support serves vitally as a cornerstone in cancer care frameworks remarkably enhanceed by various measures highly supportive of patient needs. Nutrition preserves lean body mass remarkably and enhance immune function effectively while maintaining fluid balance subsequently facilitating repair of tissue thereafter. Well-nourished patients fare markedly better with therapy yielding fewer complications and they recover swiftly with decidedly better psychosocial outcomes reported long afterwards (Lalla et al, 2008).

Nutrition rather effectively serves as therapeutic adjunct enhancing cancer treatment tolerability very significantly in various very challenging clinical oncology contexts. Brutal treatments often yield painstakingly nuanced side effects that can be somewhat alleviated for patients undergoing therapy with dietary strategies carefully tailored. Patients plagued by queasiness or premature satiety derive benefit from tiny bland meals featuring stuff like rice bananas or dry toasted whole wheat bread. Foods become remarkably delectable when infused with lemon essence or some exotic herbs especially for people undergoing drastic taste changes usually. Mucositis alleviates rather quickly with soft bland food and avoidance of acidic or devilishly spicy foods very much every time. Targeted micronutrient support becomes necessary fairly often when managing debilitating symptoms effectively over quite a prolonged period of time (Lalla et al, 2008).

Deficiencies in vitamins like D or B-complex alongside minerals such as zinc can severely worsen treatment-related fatigue and greatly impair immune function. Supplementation coupled with timely assessment plays a profoundly protective role in patients beset by risk of severe dietary deficiencies or malabsorption issues. Proactive nutritional intervention under guidance of an oncology trained dietitian transforms patient's treatment experience rather dramatically very effectively sometimes. Furnishing various tools markedly enhances outcomes and empowers patients remarkably well while undergoing many therapies with swift recovery afterwards. Cutting-edge cancer therapies yield remarkably holistic treatment outcomes these days with personalized nutrition deeply embedded in standard oncology care.

4.1. Managing Nausea and Vomiting

Cancer patients undergoing brutal chemotherapy sessions often suffer terribly from nausea and very debilitating vomiting side effects ensue subsequently. Symptoms spawn physical angst influencing food consumption heavily leading often to malnourishment and drastic weight loss with dehydration occurring simultaneously. Unrelenting nausea that goes unmanaged can detrimentally impact overall prognosis by significantly contributing to malnutrition and delaying subsequent treatment cycles. Targeted nutritional strategies obviously enhance patient resilience throughout grueling therapy sessions and mitigate such debilitating symptoms effectively. Radically altering meal patterns helps manage nausea stemming from diverse causes via a fundamentally dietary approach apparently with varied success.

Patients are urged nowadays rather vigorously to eat small meals frequently like five or six daily in place of three square meals. Mitigating overdistension exacerbates nausea feelings really badly in stomach. Frequent small meals stabilize blood sugar levels and mitigate gastric irritation thereby diminishing nausea somewhat severely at times rather unpredictably. Ginger has garnered considerable acclaim for its anti-emetic properties and is used extensively alongside chemotherapy as a nutritional remedy nowadays. Gingerol and shogaol in ginger exert quite potent effects by modulating serotonin receptors deep within gastrointestinal tract very effectively. Ginger consumption manifests diversely in various forms like fresh tea or chews and capsules and gets blended rather subtly into smoothies (Kahleova et al, 2014).

Ginger use doesn't hinder anticancer medication efficacy according fairly well to some rather conclusive recent clinical studies on various subjects. Meal size and specific botanicals known remarkably well for quelling nausea play a vital role alongside food selection in many instances. Plain rice and bananas and toast are usually well tolerated but applesauce and boiled potatoes less frequently induce nasty nasty nausea. Patients are warned not to eat pungent foods or rich food that rather badly exacerbates gastrointestinal misery in some instances. Serving food at room temperature may quite effectively reduce odor intensity and make it more tolerable rather effectively. Sipping clear liquids slowly after meals in fairly well ventilated areas enhances comfort quite significantly and very effectively alleviates discomfort. Cancer treatment tolerance improves markedly when healthcare providers combine nutritional strategies and lifestyle tweaks allowing patients sustain energy remarkably (Kahleova et al, 2014).

4.2. Combating Loss of Appetite

Cancer patients undergoing treatment often face an insidious challenge known as anorexia which manifests as sudden substantial appetite loss. Chemotherapy radiation therapy some medications psychological distress and cancer itself occasionally drastically alter taste perception triggering it in various unexpected ways suddenly. Anorexia drastically curtails overall caloric intake and spurs muscle wasting and sarcopenia fatigue and generally delays recovery afterwards. Nutritional strategies implemented proactively ensure patients get essential nutrients needed for healing effectively and tolerate treatment fairly well afterwards. Eating energy-dense foods rich in protein nowadays can be a sound strategy for effectively mitigating loss of appetite in many individuals. Nutrient-dense foods cram vital nutrients into tiny servings rather crucial for patients really struggling with surprisingly meager appetites daily.

Smoothies provide nutrition very effectively in a highly customizable form and are quite palatable most of the time anyway. A smoothie blends remarkably well with seeds nut butters milk or various plant-based alternatives packing macronutrients and micronutrients into a compact nutritious format. Blends can be fortified with calorie boosters like avocado or flaxseed oil and honey if tolerated very well generally. Very effectively stimulating food intake involves offering people variety and autonomy in their eating experiences almost every single time. Fostering autonomy in patients through diverse culinary options can greatly enhance mealtime experience significantly under various circumstances normally. Consuming food steeped in nostalgic cultural heritage can very significantly boost palatability and fairly effectively knock down psychological barriers.

Meals served in pleasant surroundings should look very good and foster positive associations with eating most of time. Munching frequently on calorie-rich superfoods substantially ramps up total energy consumption without huge repasts or elaborate meal prep being necessary. Nuts and nut butters pack concentrated nutrition into tiny servings while hard-boiled eggs and rich dairy products are generally well tolerated. Snacks get stockpiled for weird moments when hunger hits hard suddenly at very inopportune times mostly with extreme ferocity. Medical nutrition therapy often entails oral nutritional supplements or potent appetite stimulants when drastic weight loss occurs very rapidly. Food-first approaches remain foundational care aiming zealously rather to restore enjoyment of eating and preserve substantial muscle mass throughout ordeal treatment.

4.3. Preventing and Managing Weight Loss (Cachexia)

Patients with advanced malignancies frequently suffer quite remarkably from progressive weight loss and muscle atrophy accompanied by debilitating fatigue every single day. Cachexia triggers various profound metabolic changes leading rapidly in muscle wasting and grave inflammation that often defy conventional nutritional interventions entirely. Targeted nutritional interventions remain crucial in alleviating severe impacts remarkably well whilst preserving patients' strength and life quality rather effectively overall. Preserving lean body mass remarkably enhance resilience against harsh medical regimens and maintains mobility very effectively particularly in skeletal muscle. Protein plays a crucial yet oft overlooked role in upkeep of muscle and bodily functions rather effectively under various physiological conditions evidently. Patients oughta wolf down super high-quality protein sources like lean meats fish eggs or soy-based food at virtually every meal (Law et al, 2022).

Oral nutritional supplements and protein powders bridge dietary gaps for patients struggling mightily with oral intake delivering leucine and other amino acids essential. High caloric intake becomes crucial obviously under certain dire circumstances aside sufficient protein for averting further debilitating energy deficits. Foods rich in nutrients such as avocados or fortified beverages can substantially boost caloric intake without adding bulk normally in meals. Frequent consumption of small meals and snacks throughout day manages food intake effectively while significantly reducing burden of eating. Enteral nutrition may be warranted in very advanced cachexia cases where heinous treatment sequelae drastically impede oral intake or tumour burden lingers heavily (Law et al, 2022). Patients get enough calories and vital nutrients through this method thereby preventing malnutrition and supporting treatment success overall very effectively . Formulation of enteral feeds very much needs matching quite closely with specific clinical needs of an individual under registered dietitian guidance. Nutritional intervention initiated at diagnosis slows cachexia progression remarkably and substantially improves outcomes for patients significantly over time. Nutrition forms the cornerstone of multimodal cachexia management effectively when paired alongside physical activity with various anti-inflammatory therapeutic tactics.

4.4. Managing Dry Mouth (Xerostomia)

Xerostomia or dry mouth often arises after radiation therapy ravages head and neck area making swallowing very darn difficult. Dry mouth amplifies risk of nasty oral infections very significantly over time and hampers patient's capacity for proper nutrition . Hydration remains key for managing dry mouth effectively. Proper hydration plays a crucial role in managing dry mouth effectively under most circumstances rather quietly. Drink plenty of water and consume moist foods such as creamy soups yogurt and smoothies very frequently every single day saliva substitutes or sugar-free gum can stimulate production of saliva effectively. Coconut water alongside oral rehydration solutions maintains tricky electrolyte balance thoroughly hydrating body extremely well afterwards in somewhat mysterious ways. Patients should avoid spicy salty or acidic foods which can irritate mouth and worsen sensation of dryness very badly.

4.5. Managing Diarrhea and Constipation

Cancer treatment ravages digestive systems badly often precipitating diarrhea or obstinate constipation and subsequently dehydration becomes severe very quickly. Nutritional strategies must be devised properly and implemented effectively for managing debilitating health issues with considerable success ordinarily diarrhea sufferers may benefit from a low-fibre diet that reduces irritation in the digestive tract. Patients experiencing diarrhea may be prescribed a very low-fibre diet thereby reducing irritation in their digestive tract somewhat slowly. Foods such as bananas or applesauce are fairly easily digestible and very effectively mitigate diarrhea with boiled potatoes being somewhat helpful too. Constipation sufferers need a considerable boost in fibre intake (McQuade et al, 2016). Electrolyte-rich fluids such as clear broths or sports drinks rapidly replenish lost fluids in dehydrated people with considerable efficacy ordinarily. Patients suffering, from constipation on other hand essentially require a very badly needed boost in fibre intake very desperately.

4.6. Addressing Fatigue and Low Energy

Debilitating fatigue frequently manifests in patients undergoing cancer therapy exhibiting unusually low energy levels subsequently. Patients struggle very frequently nowadays undertaking daily tasks, with significant difficulty and eating becomes a major ordeal quite often. Nutritional strategies properly implemented alongside rest can help manage debilitating fatigue over time. Iron-rich foods like lean meats and leafy greens prevent anemia a common cause of fatigue in cancer patients. Lean meats and fortified cereals rich in iron can help combat anemia a significant energy-sapping issue in cancer patients quite effectively meanwhile whole grains sweet potatoes and legumes loaded with complex carbs provide energy sustainably. Diagnosing anemia often prompts doctors to recommend oral iron supplements for varying durations and at somewhat irregular intervals.

4.7. Psychological and Emotional Support through Nutrition

Independent clauses joined by conjunctions like and but or yet should not typically be separated by commas unnecessarily. Cancer treatment precipitates emotional turmoil somewhat negatively impacting patients' relationships with food in ways that manifest very insidiously over time. Caregivers can ameliorate patients eating experience and diminish mealtime stress by serving up frequent small meals in a fairly relaxed atmosphere. Nutritional support mitigates cancer treatment side effects substantially constituting a crucial element in current patient care regimes very effectively nowadays. Nutrition plays a vital role quite significantly in bodily strength and supporting immunity somewhat by mitigating nasty symptoms like dry mouth or digestive issues. Cancer patients receive modified dietary plans from an oncology nutrition specialist registered dietitian helping them retain optimal nutrition and mitigate harsh side effects substantially.

5. Personalized Nutrition in Oncology

Oncology has lately adopted precision medicine a paradigm shift that individualises treatment very the effectively nowadays based on a patient's peculiar genetic profile. Holistic cancer treatment now incorporates personalized nutrition quite effectively alongside various groundbreaking medical discoveries rather surprisingly every now and then. Nutritional needs fluctuate vastly among patients owing largely to cancer type and stage of disease alongside various metabolic factors. Personalized nutrition optimizes therapeutic outcomes remarkably well by aligning dietary interventions with individual characteristics and boosts patient quality of life drastically. Traditional nutritional strategies frequently falter when pitted against modified dietary requirements of diverse patient populations presenting suddenly with peculiar health issues (Krzyszczyk et al, 2018).

Patients undergoing head and neck radiation struggle mightily with dysphagia necessitating soft bland foods while others on immunotherapy face debilitating fatigue fueled by inflammation. Modified dietary plans are concocted reckoning with sundry factors for patients undergoing swift medical flux or wildly divergent treatment responses. Genomic and metabolic profiling scrutinizes this approach intensely nowadays with further refinement under extremely close scrutiny mostly. Novel studies indicate specific gene-nutrient interplay drastically affects patient metabolism of various bioactive compounds and antioxidants found in certain foods. Folate-rich supplements could confer substantial benefits on patients exhibiting rare genetic variations that affect metabolism of folate very significantly. Gut microbiome composition plays a crucial role in absorption of nutrients and modulation of immune responses helping clinicians recommend probiotic-rich foods quite specifically (Krzyszczyk et al, 2018).

Personalized nutrition reckons with a slew of factors beyond just bodily wellness incorporating deeply psychosocial elements weirdly rooted in certain cultural milieus. Nutrition care plans are woven with considerable comfort usually incorporating patient preferences and quirky emotional eating behaviors very carefully. Dietitians possessing oncology nutrition savvy play a crucial role alongside oncologists and nurses in cancer care with patients very intensely. Modified approaches remarkably tailored quite specifically utterly eclipse generic dietary guidelines altogether in oncology favouring personalized nutrition very effectively. Nutritionally supporting patients fairly effectively throughout their cancer journey involves a very dynamic strategy that incorporates individual needs and various biomedical data . Integrating nutrition into precision oncology nowadays will be essential for achieving highly effective cancer care centered around patients as field rapidly evolves.

5.1. The Need for Personalized Nutrition in Cancer Care

Cancer treatment involves modified decisions made according specific patient's diagnosis including tumour type and stage alongside overall health and genetic predispositions quite frequently nowadays. Nutritional care must be tailored effectively supporting complex treatment regimens with utmost care in wildly varying individual circumstances every time. Cancer patients' nutritional needs fluctuate quite wildly under influence of specific cancer treatments such as chemotherapy or surgery and ensuing nasty side effects. Grueling therapy sessions brutally confront cancer patients with harsh realities that generalized dietary recommendations often falter woefully in tackling head-on. A patient undergoing grueling chemotherapy might battle debilitating nausea and anorexia necessitating energy dense meals fairly easy on stomach (Caccialanza et al, 2016).

Patients receiving radiation therapy near head and neck may develop xerostomia and dysphagia requiring intake of soft or very moist foods. Personalized nutrition offers rather nuanced approach integrating patient's genetic background and clinical status into development of highly tailored dietary plan. Tailoring interventions quite meticulously supports nutritional sufficiency and substantially enhance patients' capacity for coping with rather grueling therapeutic protocols. Personalized nutrition evolves dynamically with a patient's condition adjusting rapidly shifts in appetite and gastrointestinal function throughout entire cancer care trajectory (Caccialanza et al, 2016). Customization at such level frequently makes quite a difference between declining nutritionally fast and maintaining functional health remarkably well in many cases.

Hiring a registered dietitian with oncology nutrition expertise rather effectively implements highly individualized evidence-based strategies in various clinical settings nowadays. Personalized nutrition in cancer care isn't some fancy luxury ultimately but rather a stark raving necessity for survival basically. Tailoring dietary intake quite precisely around personal variables can enhance tolerance and enhance immune response mitigating numerous treatment-related complications overall.

5.2. Key Elements of Personalized Nutrition in Oncology

Personalized nutrition in oncology hinges on grasping multifaceted factors that heavily influence nutritional requirements of individual patients somewhat differently. Stuff like that gets listed here. These include:

a. Cancer Type and Stage

Cancer type profoundly influences nutritional requirements dictating specific dietary interventions that effectively support various clinical outcomes during treatment periods. Cancer progresses swiftly and treatments intensify drastically altering bodily metabolic demands significantly over time in rather complex and various ways. Crucial aspects of comprehensive oncology care evidently involve tailoring nutritional strategies based on disease stage and organ system fairly precisely. Various cancers wreak havoc on bodily functions in profoundly different manners often entailing drastically dissimilar physiological consequences and terrible reactions occur. Colorectal cancer manifests with symptoms like diarrhea and constipation alongside quite severe bloating due largely to ravaging effects on gastrointestinal tract (Mercier et al, 2022).

Tumour presence or harsh chemotherapy aftermath and surgical removal of bowel portions may yield such problems due to radiation side effects. Nutritional strategies in such patients typically involve drastically altering fibre intake by boosting soluble fibre for relatively regulated bowel movements or slashing insoluble fibre content in acute diarrhea cases and post-surgical strictures simultaneously narrowing. Fluid and electrolyte balance must be monitored very closely in patients suffering from severe diarrhea that persists for quite some time. Breast cancer typically doesn't directly ravage digestive systems but often manifests with systemic treatment side effects like chemo-induced fatigue and profound muscle wasting. Preserving lean body mass thoroughly and supporting tissue repair becomes utterly essential with increased protein intake in such peculiar cases (Mercier et al, 2022).

Omega-3 fatty acids vitamin D and antioxidants might be super beneficial rather slowly in mitigating inflammation and oxidative stress linked with grueling disease treatment. Aggressive stages of cancer develop swiftly and patients suffer severe weight loss and drastically altered metabolic states quite suddenly. Malnutrition gets combated rather effectively through energy-dense foods and supplements sustaining functional capacity very nicely in high-calorie diets. Dietitians and oncologists craft quirky highly personalized nutrition plans addressing severe disease-related nutritional deficiencies and treatment side effects rather effectively nowadays. Customized plans remarkably enhance immune function and foster accelerated wound recovery after surgical procedures with life quality improving quite noticeably afterwards. Cancer therapy gets very darn personalized and nutritional interventions must evolve rapidly matching complex patient needs dynamically with each quirky case.

b. Treatment Protocol

Cancer care utilizes multifaceted treatment regimens including chemotherapy or radiation therapy exerting disparate physiological impacts on nutritional requirements and food tolerance very significantly. Creating modified nutrition plans in sync with specific treatment regimens demands subtly nuanced grasp of myriad understated consequences extremely carefully. Cancer treatments nowadays frequently entail chemotherapy brutally disrupting normal gastrointestinal function quite widely across various medical settings. It can lead very frequently quite unpleasantly to nasty side effects like vomiting or severe constipation and diarrhea too. Such symptoms drastically curtail food intake very badly and undermine overall nutritional balance with somewhat deleterious effects on health. Frail stomachs of chemotherapy patients benefit from calorie-dense food rich in protein and surprisingly easy on digestive systems most of time.

Nutritional supplements orally or enterally administered may be required fairly often in patients experiencing protracted treatment regimens or battling lackluster appetite quite severely. Radiation therapy blasted mercilessly at head neck or torso poses thorny dietary conundrums very suddenly and wreaks havoc on bodily functions badly. Patients may experience nasty oral mucositis and xerostomia terribly or dry mouth extremely badly with esophagitis from severe radiation exposure altering bowel habits significantly. Mouth sores or ridiculously dry mucosa cause head and neck cancer patients considerable distress with chewing and swallowing very laboriously. A rather bland diet very soft and quite moist becomes recommended in fairly unusual cases nowadays with some frequency apparently. Nutrient-dense liquids such as smoothies help people maintain sufficient intake easing digestive discomfort fairly remarkably under certain conditions. Texture-modified diets or temperature-modified ones may be required fairly often under very certain specific circumstances ensuring tolerability and food safety (Ferreira et al, 2020).

Nutritional needs after surgery fluctuate quite radically depending on extent and site of intervention undertaken. Surgeries such as esophagectomy or gastrectomy on gastrointestinal tract severely impair digestion requiring highly specialized regimens or sometimes parenteral nutrition for recovery afterwards. Immunotherapy and targeted therapies though less cytotoxic still frequently cause very debilitating side effects like pronounced fatigue and nasty gastrointestinal issues. Wildly fluctuating metabolic demands and utterly bewildering tolerance levels in some individuals may necessitate highly adaptable nutritional strategies on occasion (Ferreira et al, 2020). Nutritional care coupled with appropriate cancer treatment type and intensity remarkably enhances physiological resilience and boosts life quality very significantly.

c. Nutritional Status and Pre-Treatment Assessment

Thorough nutritional assessment prior cancer treatment initiation is ostensibly foundational component of comprehensive oncology care in many cancer centers nowadays. Nutritional status at diagnosis profoundly affects patient response to therapy and overall prognosis markedly with heightened risk of nasty complications arising. Designing tailored nutritional interventions relies heavily on evaluating indicators like muscle mass and body mass index based on recent dietary habits. Undernourished patients face heightened vulnerability rapidly during aggressive cancer treatments and those at risk of malnutrition suffer brutally. Insufficient caloric consumption precipitates muscle degeneration thereby heightening odds of protracted hospital stays due partly to treatment interruptions and dose tapering.

Early initiation of nutritional support via oral supplements or enteral feeding markedly boosts energy intake and slashes risk of infection fairly significantly. Prehabilitation entailing nutritional and physical prep before medical interventions nowadays often gets recommended for encourage readiness and sundry outcomes quite effectively. Overweight or obese patients need modified nutrition plans weirdly tailored specifically under unique circumstances for their own sake basically. Excess adiposity fuels chronic low-grade inflammation and insulin resistance whilst perturbing hormone metabolism thus heightening risk of recurrence and poorer treatment outcomes. Weight management during cancer treatment should be undertaken rather warily lest muscle loss and nasty nutrient deficiencies ensue subsequently (Adeyinka et al, 2022).

Eating patterns rich in nutrients remain a focus for thoroughly supporting overall metabolic health and mostly preserving lean body mass. Physical activity should rather vigorously complement nutritional strategies whenever possible significantly enhancing functional capacity. Malnutrition Screening Tool and Patient-Generated Subjective Global Assessment effectively facilitate early detection of patients at risk in clinical settings. Nutritional status changes can be detected through periodic assessments throughout treatment course enabling timely adjustments for optimal care planning purposes (Adeyinka et al, 2022).

Pre-treatment nutritional assessments done thoroughly empower clinicians delivering highly personalized care aligned with each patient's unique physiological status and long-term health. Addressing modifiable risk factors proactively with evidence-based dietary interventions remarkably lays groundwork for cancer treatment that is both effective and compassionate.

d. Genetic Profile and Nutrigenomics

Nutrigenomics evolves rapidly entwining genetic data deeply into dietary planning with profoundly impactful ramifications for specialists in cancer nutrition. Nutrigenomics delves deeply into intricate relationships between nutrients and genes examining influence of genetic makeup on dietary response variably. Very closely cancer care's personalized approach enables fairly targeted dietary strategies aligning with patient's metabolic profile and treatment regimen. Nutrigenomics has myriad applications in oncology especially when identifying gene-nutrient interactions that drastically alter therapeutic outcomes or influence nutrient metabolism heavily. Polymorphisms in MTHFR gene play a crucial role in folate metabolism and may heavily influence patient processing of folate from dietary sources or supplements quite variably.

Folate plays a dual role somewhat mysteriously in DNA synthesis and methylation for breast cancer patients necessitating extremely cautious evaluation of MTHFR status. Genetic variants within cytochrome P450 enzyme family specifically CYP2D6 and CYP3A4 affect metabolism of various chemotherapeutic agents altering efficacy markedly and toxicity profiles. Nutrients or certain food components drastically inhibit or conversely very frequently enhance drug metabolism in patients with reduced-function polymorphisms. Tweaking diet very effectively minimizes wonky interactions between certain drugs and nutrients like cruciferous veggies or St John's Wort supplements. Nutrigenomics sheds light very deeply into inflammatory responses and oxidative stress pathways alongside efficiency of nutrient transporters critical in cancer progression (de la Torre Guzmán et al, 2025).

People with certain SOD2 gene variants may benefit greatly from eating nutrient-dense foods like dark berries and various nuts extremely regularly. Precision nutrition plans deeply rooted in genetics and pharmacogenomics involve healthcare professionals crafting extremely personalized diets for each patient with unique genetic profiles. Nutrigenomic data synergizes with lifestyle biochemical markers and clinical factors empowering oncology nutrition practitioners with strikingly personalized strategies very effectively nowadays. Genetic profiling integration into cancer nutrition care sparks a seismic shift toward precision oncology where dietary tweaks are proactively modified very remarkably for a patients distinct biological makeup greatly enhancing resilience and mitigating toxicity (de la Torre Guzmán et al, 2025).

5.3. Personalized Nutrition for Common Cancer Treatment Side Effects

Nausea and vomiting remain distressing side effects mostly of chemotherapy and somewhat of radiation therapy when brain or gut is targeted fiercely. Malnutrition dehydration and drastically reduced quality of life overall result from severe compromise of dietary intake heavily. Tailored dietary interventions play a crucial role in mitigating nasty side effects throughout very rigorous medical treatment regimens and sustaining quite adequate nutrition. Tailored dietary strategies kick in very quickly overnight by drastically altering meal patterns very effectively. Patients reap huge rewards by noshing on tiny food quite often across entire day rather than downing three whopping meals sluggishly. This approach prevents gastric distention which can trigger nausea or exacerbate it suddenly under fairly specific and somewhat unusual circumstances. Bland foods very low in fat are ridiculously easy on stomach and often tolerated well like rice or boiled potatoes plain toast (PDQ_Cancer, 2025).

Milder options serve as nutritional foundation rather effectively during acute nausea episodes and lessen gastric irritation very substantially. Ginger and other functional foods show rather promising results in extremely obscure studies lately with some supplements yielding surprisingly good outcomes. Ginger harbors bioactive constituents such as gingerol and shogaol exhibiting markedly antiemetic effects under diverse circumstances with considerable efficacy. Ginger supplementation in capsule form rather effectively mitigates chemotherapy-induced nausea without obviously compromising efficacy of treatment very significantly. Ginger consumed thirty minutes prior to meals can remarkably enhance effectiveness of personalized dosing strategies very well in certain instances (PDQ_Cancer…., 2025).

Hydration matters rather critically in a fairly significant way very often. Vomiting and decreased oral intake can quickly deplete bodily fluids exacerbating fatigue severely and impairing organ function in many dire cases. Personalized hydration strategies must incorporate various clear fluids like water broth and slightly diluted fruit juices and electrolyte-rich oral rehydration solutions. Healthcare providers may suggest intravenous fluid therapy or close monitoring of electrolytes in patients experiencing severe vomiting to maintain physiological equilibrium. Patients should ultimately steer clear of pungent aromas and spicy food or edibles having jarring textures with overpowering flavors sometimes.

Nutritional counseling helps devise a highly tailored meal plan reflecting patient preferences and tolerances fairly effectively with pinpointed triggers. Modified nutritional approaches remarkably enhance treatment adherence and patient comfort significantly by mitigating nausea and enhancing overall nutritional status effectively. Pharmacologic approaches paired with early dietary changes and some very innovative behavioral methods offer patients robust support throughout grueling cancer treatment.

a. Taste Changes and Dry Mouth

Radiation therapy causes devastation on patient taste buds and mouths become parched making mealtime a cumbersome ordeal very frequently. Customized meal plans potentially alleviate such problems by recommending succulent soft eats like luscious soups blended beverages and pulpy potatoes that are swallowable easily and utilizing saliva replacements and mouth rinses reduces dryness sensation and boosts oral comfort. Flavor-enhancing spices like lemon, garlic, and herbs to counteract altered taste perceptions.

b. Weight Loss and Muscle Wasting

Cancer treatment often triggers cachexia and muscle wasting marked by drastic weight loss and debilitating fatigue rather quickly afterwards. Consuming high-calorie protein-rich food such as lean meats fish and dairy products alongside protein supplements helps preserve muscle mass remarkably well actually. Energy-dense foods like avocados nuts and full-fat dairy meet caloric needs very effectively without filling up on huge portions. Resistance training or physical activity as part of the nutrition plan to support muscle preservation.

5.4. The Role of Dietitians and Healthcare Teams

Personalized nutrition in oncology succeeds largely due to involvement of a diverse healthcare team with registered dietitians playing a very pivotal role. Specialized oncology dietitians possess extensive clinical knowledge practically assessing complex nutritional challenges faced by cancer patients under wildly diverse medical conditions and various treatment protocols. Assessing body composition and food intake alongside gastrointestinal function laboratory markers and various psychosocial factors thoroughly by a dietitian involves evaluating patient's nutritional status deeply. Thorough assessments devise personalized nutrition plans geared towards markedly enhancing patient health outcomes substantially during lengthy periods. Dietitian works alongside oncologists and nurses very closely during treatment and integrates nutritional care into overall treatment plan very effectively (Food and Nutrition Board, 2016). Dietary recommendations synchronize with a patient's regimen during heightened nutritional risk periods such as intensive chemotherapy and major surgical recovery. Dietitian swiftly modifies nutritional regimen incorporating texture altered diets oral supplements or enteral nutrition for patients experiencing nasty side effects like severe anorexia. Dietitians play a vital role educating patients and empowering them with knowledge about navigating dietary challenges through wise food choices during cancer treatment. Personalized counseling fosters dietary adherence remarkably well and builds trust between patient and healthcare team over time in a fairly effective manner (Food and Nutrition Board…, 2016).

Dietitians heavily promote unorthodox eating habits during patient recovery ostensibly reducing risk of recurrence and fostering long-term health benefits somewhat effectively. Recommendations may involve diets rich in fibre alongside unorthodox strategies for coping with subsequent metabolic disturbances and considerable weight fluctuation afterwards. Personalized nutrition integrated into cancer care represents significant advancement remarkably supporting patients undergoing therapy with fairly hopeful outcomes. Dietitians and healthcare teams fashion nutrition into a fluid adaptive tool encourage treatment tolerance deeply within cancer sufferers very effectively.

6. Integrating Nutritional Support with Conventional Cancer Treatments

Cancer treatment brutally taxes bodily functions downstream resulting in a gamut of severely debilitating physiological aftereffects and occasionally manifests quite unpredictably. Chemotherapy and targeted agents eradicate malignant cells yet wreak havoc on healthy tissues provoking nasty side effects like anorexia and debilitating fatigue. Malnutrition frequently sets in rapidly when severe complications gravely impair patient nutrition thereby diminishing treatment efficacy and significantly ratcheting up morbidity. Nutritional support meshes rather seamlessly with conventional cancer treatments serving essentially as cornerstone of comprehensive oncologic care nowadays effectively.

Nutritional support crucially maintains energy balance and enhance immune function remarkably after cancer therapy preserving lean body mass quite effectively. Patients receiving early customized nutritional support tend to suffer less frequently from severe infections and endure fewer interruptions in treatment. Extensive gastrointestinal surgeries or severe mucositis from head and neck radiotherapy necessitate enteral or parenteral nutrition when oral feeding falters badly. Nutritional interventions somewhat effectively modulate inflammation and oxidative stress, two key processes intricately involved in cancer progression or treatment toxicity.

Diets rich in antioxidants and omega-3 fatty acids can possibly aid counteracting cellular damage caused by therapy whilst encourage recovery quite systemically. Protein-rich diets help stave off cachexia and sarcopenia linked with dismal outcomes in clinical settings rather frequently nowadays apparently. Nutritional care integration unfolds uniquely per individual necessitating collaboration between oncologists and dietitians alongside nurses under vastly different circumstances effectively. Nutritional screening happens routinely before treatment starts and then dietary strategies get adjusted as patients progress rather slowly (de Castro et al, 2022). Tailoring nutritional interventions somewhat vaguely with cancer type treatment regimen side effects and patient preferences in mind ensures best possible support throughout arduous journey. Personalized nutritional support remarkably enhances patients' physical and emotional well-being within conventional cancer treatment yielding enhanced survival outcomes quite significantly. Oncology evolves rapidly toward precision medicine, and nutrition stands out as a vital component of comprehensive cancer care these days.

6.1. The Role of Nutrition in Cancer Treatment

Stuff gets numbered very arbitrarily sometimes underground. Cancer treatments such as chemotherapy brutally ravage bodily systems inducing myriad nasty side effects like vomiting fatigue and drastic weight loss suddenly. Malnutrition and muscle wasting seep in surreptitiously when heinous side effects make ingesting adequate nutrients extremely arduous for debilitated patients. Nutritional needs remaining unmet render body highly susceptible to treatment-related complications and whittle down therapy effectiveness significantly over time. Nutritional support plays a crucial role in remarkably mitigating deleterious effects encourage immune response fairly well during various tissue repair processes. Protein-rich food preserves muscle mass very effectively in such dicey situations, while calorie-dense foods prevent undesirable weight loss meanwhile. Vitamins, minerals, and antioxidants somewhat vigorously enhance immune response and very effectively shield cells from damage caused by chemotherapy and radiation. Patients become remarkably resilient in therapy when cancer treatment's harsh nutritional demands are mitigated effectively, and overall well-being improves fairly markedly.

6.2. Managing Treatment Side Effects with Nutrition

Nutrition remarkably alleviates chaotic bodily repercussions during cancer therapy treatment very well amidst grave bodily turmoil obviously rather effectively. Personalized nutrition regimens alleviate symptoms and enhance patient capacity for nourishment during arduous medical treatments fairly effectively these days. Some treatment side effects are listed below and nutritional support weirdly alleviates them very effectively nowadays with some decent results apparently.

a. Nausea and Vomiting

Chemotherapy spawns nausea and vomiting notoriously under radiation therapy ravaging a patient's eating capacity significantly. Rather severe nutritional deficiencies alongside nasty electrolyte imbalances and dehydration tend to develop very rapidly from these symptoms. Small frequent meals comprising bland, easy-to-digest fare such as toast rice bananas or applesauce can help calm the stomach and alleviate nausea. Ginger and peppermint are known for their anti-nausea properties and can be included in the diet in the form of ginger tea or ginger chews. Hydration is critical to prevent dehydration. Ginger and peppermint possess anti-nausea properties and can be consumed as ginger tea or in the form of ginger chews quite effectively.

b. Loss of Appetite and Weight Loss

Cancer patients frequently endure inexplicable weight loss and appetite suppression mainly due to brutal side effects of rigorous treatment regimens. Prolonged weight loss particularly muscle wasting dubbed cachexia severely hampers treatment efficacy and negatively impacts recovery overall. High-calorie foods rich in protein are crucial for maintaining muscle mass and staving off further debilitating weight loss (Ni and Zhang, 2020). High-protein foods dense with calories play a crucial role in maintaining muscle mass and thwarting drastic weight loss in individuals struggling terribly. Oral nutritional supplements furnish extra calories and protein in cases where people can't manage eating enough food normally.

c. Dry Mouth (Xerostomia)

Patients undergoing radiation therapy near head or neck area often suffer terribly from dry mouth making swallowing extremely difficult sometimes. Malnutrition gets exacerbated by woefully inadequate oral intake further worsening overall nutritional status significantly. Patients should eat soft moist foods like yogurt smoothies or soups that are easier swallowed. Hydration is key to alleviating dryness, so encouraging patients to sip water regularly or drink electrolyte-replenishing drinks can help keep the mouth moist. Saliva substitutes and sugar-free gum can stimulate saliva production, offering relief from the discomfort caused by dry mouth.

d. Digestive Issues

Chemotherapy precipitates nasty bouts of diarrhea or constipation occasionally and nasty gastritis can occur alongside radiation therapy treatments. Digestive issues often spawn considerable unease and amplify dehydration risk while badly impairing absorption of various vital nutrients. Increasing fibre intake through food like whole grains fruits and veggies can foster bowel regularity for constipation woes. Increasing fibre intake through foods like whole grains fruits and veggies can very effectively promote bowel regularity in constipation sufferers. A low-fibre diet comprising bananas white rice and boiled potatoes may be recommended for diarrhea patients to reduce gut irritation. Proper hydration remains essential virtually always under most circumstances.

6.3. Boosting Immune Function through Nutrition

Cancer treatment severely debilitates immune systems leaving patients woefully vulnerable to nasty opportunistic infections thereby grossly compromising overall health. Proper nutrition enhance immune response remarkably and facilitates bodily reaction vigorously against disease under medical care quite effectively. Vitamins like vitamin C and minerals such as zinc play crucial roles in supporting immune function with selenium and vitamin D. Vitamins and minerals like vitamin C and zinc play crucial roles in encourage immune function effectively alongside selenium and vitamin D. Omega-3 fatty acids found in fatty fish flaxseeds and chia seeds have anti-inflammatory properties and can help modulate immune response very well. A balanced diet rich in whole foods, including fruits, vegetables, whole grains, and lean proteins, helps reduce inflammation and support overall immune health (Janakiram et al, 2016).

6.4. Personalized Nutritional Plans for Cancer Patients

Cancer patients have highly varied dietary needs shaped by factors such as tumour type treatment protocols and pre-existing medical conditions quite ordinarily. Personalized nutrition figures prominently in cancer care optimization by tailoring dietary advice according to specific patient needs very effectively. A registered dietitian boasting oncology nutrition expertise assesses patient nutritional status and identifies potential deficiencies then creates a customized diet plan supporting treatment and improving quality of life greatly. Nutritional assessments before, during, and after treatment can help monitor progress, adjust nutrient intake, and prevent complications such as malnutrition and muscle wasting.

6.5. Integrating Nutritional Support into Cancer Treatment Plans

Dietary interventions effectively integrated into cancer treatment plans nowadays maximally benefit patients receiving nutritional support very successfully overall. Oncologists and dietitians work very closely alongside various healthcare pros ensuring nutritional aid gets incorporated effectively into patient care quite frequently nowadays. Nutrition counseling happens alongside chemo or radiation therapy helping patients cope with nasty side effects and maintain some semblance of proper nutrition (Mercier et al, 2022). Nutritional supplements, including protein shakes and oral rehydration solutions, can be used to support patients who have difficulty meeting their nutritional needs through food alone. Nutritional supplements like protein shakes and oral rehydration solutions support patients struggling to meet nutritional needs through diet alone ordinarily. Patients receiving chemotherapy or radiation therapy benefit greatly from nutrition counseling which helps them manage dietary needs and mitigate awful side effects. Nutritional supplements like protein shakes and oral rehydration solutions support patients struggling mightily to meet dietary needs through food alone (Mercier et al, 2022). Cancer care nowadays remarkably involves nutritional support seamlessly amalgamated with conventional treatments, playing a vital role overall quite effectively.

7. Optimizing Immune Function and Recovery Through Clinical Nutrition

Cancer therapies such as chemotherapy profoundly weaken immune systems, rendering patients highly susceptible to nasty infections and nasty treatment complications. Aggressive treatment regimens often induce serious immunosuppression nowadays, posing quite a formidable challenge in oncology care alongside malignancy itself. Clinical nutrition has emerged rather significantly as a crucial strategy encourage immune function and thereby enhancing recovery with reduced rates of complication very markedly. Therapeutic deployment of nutrients and modified diets grounded in evidential guidelines maintains physiological homeostasis rather effectively during protracted sickness episodes. In oncology going beyond basic energy and protein requirements involves strategically incorporating nutrients modulating immune responses quite intricately and inflammatory processes.

Vitamins A C D, and E alongside zinc selenium and iron, play crucial roles supporting development of various immune cells remarkably well. Nutrient deficiencies abound among cancer patients, mostly owing to drastically reduced dietary intake or surging metabolic needs severely weakening immune function. Macronutrients play quite a crucial role rather effectively in optimizing immune function under various physiological conditions. Adequate protein intake vitally supports the synthesis of various immunoglobulins and cytokines deeply involved in immune regulation and tissue repair processes. Omega-3 fatty acids present in fish oil and some unusual plant-based sources exhibit potent anti-inflammatory properties that drastically curb hyperactive immune responses and severely diminish chronic inflammation frequently worsened by harsh cancer regimens (Talib et al, 2024).

Gut microbiota plays a pivotal role orchestrating immune function, which influences local immunity erratically and enhances systemic responses somewhat mysteriously. Probiotics teamed with prebiotics and dietary fibre very effectively maintain intestinal barrier integrity by promoting the growth of beneficial microbes. Modulating immune response occurs rather effectively thereby reducing infection risk, especially in patients with tenuous or severely compromised immunity. Personalized clinical nutrition ought to be integrated very early on into oncology care fairly seamlessly and effectively with considerable success down line (Talib et al, 2024). Optimal immune support relies heavily on oncologists collaborating with nursing staff through timely interventions and very thorough regular nutritional assessments. Targeted nutritional regimens effectively enhance cancer therapies and significantly enhance clinical outcomes for patients enduring arduous treatment protocols.

7.1. Nutritional Deficiencies and Immune Suppression in Cancer

Malnutrition hits cancer patients very hard, variably depending on cancer type and specific regimen of treatment, quite seriously in many cases. Cancer precipitates severely catabolic state beset by heightened systemic inflammation and profound metabolic dysregulation, alongside skeletal muscle atrophy eventually. Gastrointestinal disturbances and altered taste perception accompany severely compromised oral intake and nutrient absorption due to nasty treatment-related side effects. Macro and micronutrient deficiencies occur very frequently due largely to certain risk-heightening factors having deleterious effects on immune function directly. Malnutrition linked with cancer often precipitates a significantly impaired immune response manifesting rather severely in most such cases.

Essential nutrients play crucial roles in maintaining the integrity of physical barriers like skin and mucosa, and encourage the activity of various immunological pathways vigorously. Subclinical nutrient deficiencies disrupt various physiological processes rather significantly beneath overt symptoms often with quite detrimental effects overall. Inadequate protein intake severely impairs production of immunoglobulins and cytokines whilst energy deficits often badly compromise leukocyte function delaying tissue repair slowly. Deficiencies in vitamins A and E alongside minerals like zinc are especially pernicious for bodily functions overall very significantly (Munteanu and Schwartz, 2022). Vitamin A plays a crucial role in maintaining epithelial barrier function remarkably well and enhance mucosal immunity with great effectiveness. Vitamin C substantially enhance phagocyte activity and oxidative burst capacity whereas vitamin D plays an ostensibly immunomodulatory role influencing innate and adaptive responses variably. Vitamin E acts very intensely as antioxidant shielding immune cells heavily from oxidative stress during inflammatory episodes. Selenium plays a crucial role in antioxidant defense systems and regulation of inflammatory pathways while zinc fuels thymic hormone function T-cell maturation and wound healing rapidly (Talib et al, 2024). Iron necessary for immune cell proliferation must be balanced carefully as both deficiency and overload can severely impair immunity quite drastically. Nutritional deficiencies caught early play a remarkably crucial role in oncology care since such nutrients remarkably maintain immune integrity very well. Comprehensive nutritional assessments should be woven thoroughly into patient care plans prior to treatment and sporadically throughout entire therapy sessions. Identified deficiencies should be tackled pronto via dietary counseling or oral supplementation and enteral nutrition sometimes becomes necessary later on. Correcting nutritional deficits restores immune competence rather significantly and improves tolerance of treatment while reducing complications related to infection overall. Nutritional intervention ought to be regarded as a foundational component of immune support in cancer management right from square one, basically.

7.2. Macronutrient Support: Energy and Protein Requirements

Crucially supporting immune function and metabolic balance a cornerstone of clinical oncology nutrition involves ensuring intake of adequate macronutrients. Energy and protein are crucial especially for cancer patients as metabolic demands of disease and aggressive treatment get markedly heightened rapidly. Cancer imposes catabolic stress leading rapidly to muscle protein degradation and it contributes rather insidiously to cachexia with increased resting energy expenditure. Energy intake fuels metabolic demands heavily in immune cells reliant on glucose or fatty acids for producing energy during diverse immune responses. Severe caloric deficiency markedly impairs leukocyte function and hampers recovery from nasty infections substantially over a prolonged period. Precise calculation of individualized caloric needs depends on various factors including patient age physical activity level disease progression and specifics of treatment regimen. Energy needs typically span 25-35 kcal/kg/day but may surge erratically upwards in hypermetabolic states under intense treatment. Protein plays a vital role rather crucially in immunonutrition apparently with fairly significant consequences under certain physiological conditions (Fukuda et al, 2020). Immunoglobulins cytokines and complement proteins rely heavily on it as a fundamental block mediating quite effective immune defense responses underground. Adequate protein consumption supports immune cell growth remarkably well and helps preserve lean muscle mass closely linked with overall resilience naturally.

Cancer patients need 1.2 grams protein per kilogram body weight daily or up to 2 grams based on disease severity and presence of cachexia. Very robust immune competence obviously hinges on high-biological-value proteins such as egg-derived ones and fish for synthesis. Oral nutritional supplements or enteral nutrition may become necessary fairly often when treatment side effects or anorexia significantly hinder oral intake (Fukuda et al, 2020). Clinicians effectively enhance patients' immune responses remarkably by integrating energy-focused interventions into oncology care and preserving physical function substantially. Crucial support fuels long-term survivorship remarkably well afterwards and substantially enhances quality of life during short-term recovery phases too.

7.3. Micronutrients

Micronutrients play a vital role in regulating immune system function and essential vitamins along with trace minerals are crucial. Aggressive treatment regimens in oncology often severely compromise immune competency making adequate intake of specific micronutrients crucially important. Micronutrient deficiencies can very severely exacerbate immunosuppression and increase susceptibility to nasty infections thereby tanking overall treatment outcomes rather badly. Vitamin D gets studied extensively nowadays in cancer-related immunonutrition and remains one of the most crucial micronutrients. It plays a dual role by encourage innate immunity vigorously and adaptive immune responses are regulated very effectively, preventing excessive inflammation (Gombart et al, 2020). Low serum 25(OH)D levels correlate with heightened risk of various cancers, including breast and prostate cancer and poorer overall outcomes.

Vitamin D supplementation possibly reduces infection risk markedly and enhances responsiveness variably under certain conditions to some immunotherapies, apparently. Vitamin C acts extremely powerfully as an antioxidant, effectively mitigating oxidative stress and encouraging immune cell function very robustly indeed. It enhances neutrophil activity and natural killer cells, thereby markedly improving innate immune responses and adaptive ones quite rapidly. Cancer patients undergoing chemotherapy or radiotherapy often suffer precipitous depletion of vitamin C levels, resulting in significant oxidative stress simultaneously. Replenishing vitamin C somewhat effectively maintains mucosal barrier integrity overall and supports faster recovery by reducing inflammation (Gombart et al, 2020). Zinc plays a crucial role in thymic development and maturation of T-lymphocytes, effectively maintaining mucosal barriers very subtly underneath epithelial layers.

Zinc deficiency severely impairs cytokine production and phagocytic activity alongside lymphocyte proliferation, which become hallmarks of profoundly weakened immunity. Ostensibly, low zinc levels correlate with delayed wound healing and unduly prolonged hospital stays among patients undergoing oncology treatment. Supplementation guided by serum zinc concentrations restores immune competence fairly effectively and reduces myriad nasty complications arising subsequently. Selenium remarkably well shields immune cells from oxidative damage and quietly modulates inflammation within bodily systems under normal circumstances. It enhances T-cell function significantly and enhances natural killer cell activity markedly contributing effectively to immunosurveillance against tumours. Selenium possibly mitigates chemotherapy agent toxicity quite effectively and enhance overall antioxidant capacity remarkably well in diverse clinical settings. Supplementation must be very carefully tailored based on individual deficiencies and clinically observed symptoms alongside various obviously crucial laboratory assessments. Cancer therapy demands supervision from healthcare professionals for micronutrient repletion ensuring immune support optimally rather than haphazardly during treatment periods.

7.4. Anti-Inflammatory and Immunomodulatory Nutrients

Cancer progression typically entails chronic inflammation as a crucial characteristic and major obstacle for immune recovery after treatment, almost invariably. Tumour microenvironment abounds with inflammation, fostering immunosuppression and cancer cell survival whilst hindering normal tissue repair somewhat imperfectly. Modulating inflammation via dietary interventions presents a promising complementary approach in cancer care very effectively these days. Certain bioactive compounds and nutrients exhibit potent anti-inflammatory actions effectively restoring immune balance with considerable supporting evidence available nowadays. Omega-3 fatty acids, namely eicosapentaenoic acid and docosahexaenoic acid, are polyunsaturated fats found abundantly in fatty fish like salmon and mackerel and also occur in flaxseeds, walnuts and marine algae.

Fatty acids morph into peculiar lipid mediators brutally suppressing inflammation and downregulating nasty cytokines like interleukin-6 vigorously beneath tumour necrosis factor-alpha. Omega-3 supplementation has shown considerable benefits in cancer patients encourage tolerance of treatment and mitigating cachexia-related muscle loss. Ongoing clinical trials suggest omega-3s may strangely meld with immunotherapy by cultivating a somewhat less suppressive tumour microenvironment, rather haphazardly. Probiotics and prebiotics orchestrate gut integrity effectively while substantially shaping systemic immune response quietly from behind the scenes (Sundrarjun et al, 2004). Beneficial microbes largely from the genera Lactobacillus and Bifidobacterium enormously colonize gut enormously, enhancing mucosal immunity very effectively nowadays.

Prebiotics such as inulin and fructooligosaccharides act as fermentable substrates for microbes, thereby vigorously promoting microbial growth and substantial metabolic activity. Modulation of immune cells, such as Tregs, deep within bodily tissues by gut microbiota happens rather effectively, inhibiting systemic inflammation. Oncology research nowadays very deeply explores the modulation of gut microbiota for potentially boosting the efficacy of chemotherapy and lessening gastrointestinal toxicity. Polyphenols exhibit remarkably strong antioxidant properties in various plant-based foods such as berries and green tea alongside turmeric extracts. Recently curcumin from turmeric and epigallocatechin gallate found in green tea have been shown to inhibit nuclear factor-kappa B and several signaling pathways (Sundrarjun et al, 2004). Compounds interact vigorously with various immune cells promoting considerable anti-tumour activity and encourage recovery remarkably in badly affected tissues. Bioactive nutrients can be harnessed very effectively through diet or evidence-based supplementation under supervision of qualified clinicians ensuring safety in oncology settings.

7.5. Nutrition and Post-Treatment Recovery

Recovery signifies a pivotal moment in care continuum after cancer treatment ceases and patients embark on gradual physiological recuperation and tumultuous emotional readjustment slowly afterwards. Lingering fatigue and sarcopenia frequently emerge afterwards chemotherapy or surgery halts bringing novel quandaries alongside neurocognitive changes and gastrointestinal distress. Nutritional interventions facilitate cellular repair and enhance psychological resilience very effectively during this period with considerable success. Replenishing micronutrients and antioxidant reserves depleted during grueling treatment becomes primary nutritional goal rather quickly in recovery phase afterward. Vitamins A C D E and B-complex alongside minerals like iron magnesium selenium often remain woefully suboptimal post-treatment largely due to impaired gut absorption.

Lean proteins and healthy fats abundantly available in whole foods generally foster systemic healing and restore equilibrium very effectively. Restoring lean body mass remains crucial especially for patients experiencing severe weight loss due to treatment induced cachexia quite frequently nowadays. Daily protein intakes of 1.2 grams per kilogram body weight or slightly higher remain crucial post recovery depending somewhat on existing muscle reserves. Eggs and fish are high-quality protein sources that alongside resistance-based exercise remarkably improve strength and ramp up muscle synthesis significantly. Cognitive changes dubbed chemo brain manifest with ferocity suddenly in post-treatment settings alongside anxiety and depression fairly frequently. Omega-3 fatty acids EPA and DHA alongside B-vitamins like B6 B9 and B12 plus magnesium rather effectively support neurocognitive function and mood (Cava et al, 2017). Professionally guided supplementation or a diet carefully selected with some forethought may effectively provide these essential nutrients effectively under certain conditions.

Personalized nutrition guidance very effectively reinforces healthy eating habits during survivorship and tackles nagging gut issues or appetite fluctuations rather successfully. Structured nutrition education coupled with behavior change strategies empowers patients greatly to stick rather tenaciously to cancer-protective diets and reduces recurrence risk significantly enhancing overall quality of life. Nutrition acts as restorative mechanism deeply fostering resilience beyond treatment for long-term wellness and forging a bridge quite holistically.

7.6. Personalized and Interdisciplinary Approaches

Cancer treatment demands a super tailored strategy rooted deeply in evidence utterly diverging from run-of-mill dietary recommendations for overall wellbeing. Cancer patients have diverse dietary needs shaped significantly by tumour type treatment regimen and other lifestyle factors simultaneously. Nutrition care gets tailored super carefully for each persons distinct clinical status and gets adapted rapidly throughout treatment phases and recovery afterwards quickly. Personalized nutrition planning remove comprehensively with assessments including validated nutritional screening tools anthropometric measurements dietary evaluations and laboratory biomarkers alongside other evaluative processes. Data addressing energy protein needs and specific nutrient tweaks informs individualized care plans based on patient symptomatology and micronutrient repletion status slowly.

Registered dietitians specializing in oncology nutrition play a crucial role in multidisciplinary cancer care teams with various other disciplines involved simultaneously. They work intimately alongside oncologists, nurses, pharmacists, psychologists and rehab specialists ensuring nutritional regimens align very seamlessly with overall care plans. Dietitians vigilantly monitor patient progress amidst fluctuations in appetite or gut function and tweak nutritional regimens according lab values like serum albumin levels. Emerging technologies vastly improve clinical applications of precision nutritional care furthered rapidly nowadays by advancements in nutrigenomics and metabolomics. Nutrigenomics probes intricately genetic makeup's influence on nutrient metabolism and dietary responsiveness, thereby facilitating prediction of most salubrious or deleterious dietary components for modulating immune responses in patients.

Genetic polymorphisms in enzymes like MTHFR badly impact folate utilization necessitating rather personalized dietary changes with quite significant long-term health consequences. Metabolomic profiling examines a vast array of tiny molecular metabolites present in blood or urine and tissue somewhat insightfully. Such data informs decisions on nutrient timing and supplementation involving immunonutrients like glutamine or omega-3s fairly effectively under certain clinical circumstances (Hiraoka and Kagawa, 2017). Radically improving immune outcomes quite significantly and encouraging patient empowerment deeply is achieved by deeply integrating clinical nutrition into oncology care overall. Patients morph into proactive partners very quickly in most cases when armed with modified dietary plans during their recuperation process. Patient-centered care models prove crucial very effectively during survivorship enhancing quality of life while minimising odious complications, rather surprisingly.

8. Nutritional Interventions in Cancer Care

Cancer persists as a major global health issue with far-reaching consequences for patients' overall well-being and survival rates worldwide. Tumour burden directly impacts patients severely, while treatment modalities like chemotherapy and radiation disrupt nutritional status through anorexia and malabsorption mechanisms quite harshly. Such disruptions frequently precipitate unintentional weight loss and sarcopenia alongside compromised immune function negatively impacting treatment tolerance very badly overall. Nutritional interventions tailored specifically are emerging as crucial strategies nowadays in addressing challenges with wildly varying degrees of success. Tailored nutrition plans optimizing macronutrients and micronutrients with oral supplements or enteral nutrition sometimes vigorously mitigate nasty toxicities effectively. Evidence suggests that adequate nutrition during cancer therapy significantly enhance treatment adherence and slashes hospitalization rates over considerable periods of time.

Nutritional care profoundly impacts quality of life and measurably affects overall wellbeing remarkably in many rather significant respects every day. Patients receiving modified nutritional counsel frequently report somewhat substantial increments in vitality and gut comfort emotionally and surprisingly quite rapidly afterwards. Alleviating nutrition-related side effects mercifully promotes a greater sense of control and diminishes psychological stress throughout grueling treatment process very effectively. Anti-inflammatory foods and omega-3 fatty acid supplements alongside symptom-targeted meal planning have shown promise in reducing fatigue pain and depression heavily influencing quality of life in cancer populations. Malnutrition persistently correlates with grim outcomes in various malignancies exhibiting heightened morbidity treatment disruptions and woeful survival statistics.

Nutritional support remarkably improves clinical outcomes quite significantly over time in patients at high risk of muscle wasting or sarcopenia. Nutritional interventions play a vital role very comprehensively in cancer care nowadays with varied complex regimens being implemented. They play a pivotal role enhancing quality of life very effectively by supporting metabolic demands for cancer patients with long-term prognosis. Clinical nutrition integration into standard oncology practice remains very essential for advancing patient-centered care effectively around their specific needs.

8.1. Malnutrition and Its Prognostic Significance

Malnutrition frequently slips under the radar as complication in oncology afflicting substantial numbers of cancer patients at disparate stages very frequently. Epidemiological data suggest cancer patients undergoing treatment often suffer greatly from nutritional decline severely down to outright cachexia or mild undernutrition. Cancer-related malnutrition arises from ghastly amalgamation of factors like anorexia ravaging oral intake and systemic inflammation ratcheting up metabolic demands quite furiously. Malnutrition manifests starkly in cancer patients not just as somewhat minor collateral damage but as independently prognostic indicator of outcome. A sizable body of convincing clinical evidence indicates malnutrition strongly correlates with very adverse outcomes in various oncology patients (Muscaritoli et al, 2017). Tissue repair gets severely hampered and drug metabolism slows significantly alongside badly weakened immune defenses mainly with chemotherapy or radiotherapy treatments.

Prolonged hospitalization happens with higher healthcare utilization driven by nasty complications like stubborn infections and delayed wound healing very frequently. Dose reductions or treatment interruptions become increasingly likely thereby potentially jeopardizing efficacy and resulting in markedly suboptimal disease control. Survival rates plummeted markedly across various cancer types including gastrointestinal malignancies and lung cancers and head and neck tumours became dismal. Sarcopenia entails gradual deterioration of skeletal muscle mass and strength typically manifesting in patients sporting remarkably stable or elevated body weight. Sarcopenia correlates strongly with markedly diminished functional capacity and heightened toxicity from treatment while yielding generally poor response to therapy (Muscaritoli et al, 2017). Early identification and targeted intervention warrant attention now that this entity has gained widespread recognition clinically as distinct very much everywhere.

Nutritional risk screening early on ought be routine in oncology care given its profoundly impactful prognosis, mostly for patients. Patient-Generated Subjective Global Assessment utilized alongside Malnutrition Universal Screening Tool criteria and Global Leadership Initiative on Malnutrition, can identify patients at risk substantially. Early nutritional interventions greatly enhance quality of life through dietary counseling supplementation or enteral nutrition sometimes administered very quickly. Nutritional management plays a crucial role in cancer care, essentially always optimizing prognosis and encourage patient care very comprehensively.

8.2. Nutritional Interventions and Their Role in Enhancing Quality of Life

Life quality remarkably encompasses myriad aspects of well-being, including physical vitality and social connections, with functional capability intricately underlying them. Profound disruptions ravage cancer patients across multiple domains, owing largely to woefully subpar nutrition severely hampering their already arduous recovery. Nutrient-rich diets containing B vitamins, magnesium and omega-3 fatty acids yield measurable gains in reviving quality of life remarkably across diverse realms. Personalized nutritional interventions fused into oncology care fuels muscle upkeep and enhance immunity, thus diminishing fatigue and enabling patients to sustain autonomy (Nayak et al, 2017). Adequate nutrition revives energy metabolism and alleviates symptoms of anxiety and depression and improves mood, sleep and cognitive clarity very significantly. Tryptophan rich foods have been linked to improvements in psychological well-being and alleviating debilitating symptoms of various psychological disorders effectively. Tailored diets can minimise nausea, constipation, mucositis, and taste alterations, all of which commonly affect food intake and enjoyment during treatment. Food is a social anchor in many cultures. Tailored diets can minimize nausea and other issues like mucositis that commonly plague patients during treatment affecting food intake very significantly (Nayak et al, 2017). Food serves as a social anchor deeply embedded in various cultures worldwide often acting as a catalyst for community bonding.

8.3. Impact on Treatment Tolerance and Completion

Cancer patients undergoing lengthy therapeutic protocols often exhibit greatly varied tolerance of intensive treatment regimens based on their nutritional status. Targeted therapies, chemotherapy and radiotherapy impose considerable physiological stress, often exacerbating malnutrition very badly in patients undergoing such harsh treatments. Malnourished patients are markedly more susceptible to treatment-related issues like hematologic toxicity or infections and gastrointestinal dysfunction necessitating dose reductions prematurely. Well-nourished patients display greatly enhanced physiological resilience, enabling completion of prescribed therapy sans debilitating toxicities and better maintaining functional status.

Tumour shrinkage occurs frequently in these patients alongside markedly improved disease control rates often resulting in significantly favorable outcomes. Nasty side effects largely get sidestepped resulting in fewer unplanned hospital admissions for them usually. Nutrition has a profoundly positive effect on treatment outcomes and quality of life seems significantly better in various clinical studies. Nutritional interventions seem very crucial overall for treatment success apparently. High-protein oral nutritional supplements preserve lean body mass effectively during therapy vital for maintaining metabolic homeostasis and fostering proper immune response. Formulas enriched with omega-3 fatty acids like EPA and DHA very effectively curb systemic inflammation and boost muscle protein synthesis factors (Fukuda et al, 2025).

Nutritional effects reverberate profoundly inside specific malignancies namely gastrointestinal cancers such as colorectal and esophageal tumours where surgical interventions severely disrupt normal digestion often afterwards. Profound cachexia and anorexia occur frequently in lung cancers and pancreatic cancer often exhibits satiety rather unpredictably too. Mucositis dysphagia and xerostomia often severely complicate oral intake hugely in head and neck cancers making nutrition quite a behemoth challenge. Tailored nutritional intervention maintained throughout cancer treatment substantially improves physical outcomes and mitigates anxiety fatigue with perceived burden somewhat alleviated (Fukuda et al, 2025). Nutritional adequacy markedly enhance pharmacokinetics and pharmacodynamics of various chemotherapeutic agents reinforcing its crucial role in therapeutic success. Optimal nutritional status enhances treatment efficacy significantly in patients undergoing rigorous therapy protocols and curtails various nasty complications suddenly.

8.4. Targeted Nutritional Strategies

Nutritional interventions are broadly categorized into preventive, supportive and therapeutic strategies. Preventive nutrition entails screening patients at diagnosis and providing early dietary counseling for those deemed at risk. Supportive nutrition targets patients experiencing nutritional decline with interventions like oral nutritional supplements enteral nutrition or parenteral nutrition when needed very urgently. Therapeutic nutrition focuses on modulating tumour biology and host metabolism. Therapeutic nutrition aims at modulating tumour biology alongside host metabolic processes deeply within bodily systems. Supportive nutrition targets patients beset by serious nutritional decline with interventions like oral nutritional supplements or parenteral nutrition when deemed absolutely necessary.

8.5. Survivorship and Long-Term Outcomes

Nutritional interventions play a crucial albeit somewhat surprising role in survivorship beyond active treatment phases with decidedly varying degrees of success. A healthy post-treatment diet can greatly mitigate risk of cancer recurrence and support normalization of weight managing lingering debilitating effects. Plant-forward diets rich in fruits whole grains correlate with markedly reduced cancer mortality in sizable prospective analyses stemming from EPIC cohort and Nurses' Health Study. Nutrition plays a crucial role increasingly in management of comorbidities as cancer patients live longer facing myriad conditions like cardiovascular disease and osteoporosis.

8.6. Interdisciplinary Care and Future Directions

Oncologists and registered dietitians work alongside psychologists in wildly diverse teams necessitating integration of nutrition into standard care very effectively. Patient evaluations should partly comprise routine nutritional assessment tools like Patient-Generated Subjective Global Assessment or Malnutrition Screening Tool over time initially. Fresh frontiers in personalized nutrition are being opened rather quietly nowadays by advances in nutrigenomics and metabolomics down various uncharted paths. These tools enable clinicians tailor interventions based on individual genetic profiles and metabolic states alongside microbiome composition thereby improving precision markedly.

Nutritional interventions have become utterly foundational in modern cancer care rather than playing a somewhat ancillary supporting role. Clinical nutrition significantly enhances patient outcomes by preventing treatment interruptions and encourage quality of life improving prognosis remarkably thereby. Modified nutritional support integrated across cancer care continuum empowers patients effectively from diagnosis through various survivorship phases obviously. Advances in research steadily unfold new opportunities for oncology care heavily reliant on nuanced understanding of nutrition with evidence-based interventions.

9. Conclusion

Nutritional support plays a pivotal role in cancer patient care by enhancing quality of life and reducing treatment complications significantly nowadays. Cancer therapies are getting sophisticated fast so supportive strategies must evolve quickly with clinical nutrition standing out as a vital intervention often underutilized strangely enough. Assessing and managing nutritional status throughout cancer care continuum remains vitally important underscoring a crucial consideration now. Metabolic disturbances and sarcopenia often arise from disease progression or its treatment significantly impacting outcomes for patients badly. Nutritional risk correlates strongly with protracted recovery periods and heightened susceptibility to opportunistic infections and dose-limiting toxicities decreasing overall survival rates significantly. Early identification of patients at risk and timely individualized nutrition interventions are essential in evidence-based care for oncological patients apparently.

Various nutritional support strategies are available including dietary counseling and oral supplements alongside enteral nutrition and parenteral nutrition options . Interventions must be tailored carefully according to cancer type treatment modality and personal preferences of each patient under varying clinical conditions. Oncologists dietitians nurses and pharmacists in multidisciplinary care teams play a crucial role implementing effective nutrition plans with considerable continuity effectively. Emerging disciplines such as immunonutrition and precision nutrition heavily influenced by microbiome studies, offer vast potential for significantly enhancing clinical outcomes (Akbulut G, 2011). Sophisticated nutrient blends potentially enhance therapeutic effectiveness very significantly through mitigating inflammatory responses and propping up immune function remarkably well. Very robust clinical validation and some sort of standardization beforehand is crucial for widespread adoption of these approaches really now.

Nutritional support caters largely for cancer patient physiological needs and enhance psychosocial well-being thereby empowering them very significantly in their care. Holistic benefits robustly reinforce nutrition's value as a clinical tool and means of promoting dignity and resilience during exceptionally grueling cancer treatments. Clinical nutritional support stands firmly as a core component in modern oncology practice rather than an adjunct quite effectively nowadays. Research advances steadily shedding light on convoluted nexus among diet and metabolism ultimately informing modified nutritional regimens within standard oncology treatment protocols largely nowadays. Investing heavily in clinical nutrition infrastructure education and cross-disciplinary collaboration yields superior long term oncological outcomes advancing patient centered care remarkably.

References

Adeyinka A, Rouster AS, Valentine M. Enteral Feeding. [Updated 2022 Dec 26]. In: StatPearls [Internet]. Treasure Island (FL): StatPearls Publishing; 2025 Jan-. Available from: https://www.ncbi.nlm.nih.gov/books/NBK532876/

Akbulut G. New perspective for nutritional support of cancer patients: Enteral/parenteral nutrition. Exp Ther Med. 2011 Jul;2(4):675-684. doi: 10.3892/etm.2011.247. Epub 2011 Apr 1. PMID: 22977559; PMCID: PMC3440777.

Anand U, Dey A, Chandel AKS, Sanyal R, Mishra A, Pandey DK, De Falco V, Upadhyay A, Kandimalla R, Chaudhary A, Dhanjal JK, Dewanjee S, Vallamkondu J, Pérez de la Lastra JM. Cancer chemotherapy and beyond: Current status, drug candidates, associated risks and progress in targeted therapeutics. Genes Dis. 2022 Mar 18;10(4):1367-1401. doi: 10.1016/j.gendis.2022.02.007. Erratum in: Genes Dis. 2024 Jan 20;11(4):101211. doi: 10.1016/j.gendis.2024.101211. PMID: 37397557; PMCID: PMC10310991.

Arends J, Strasser F, Gonella S, Solheim TS, Madeddu C, Ravasco P, Buonaccorso L, de van der Schueren MAE, Baldwin C, Chasen M, Ripamonti CI; ESMO Guidelines Committee. Electronic address: clinicalguidelines@esmo.org. Cancer cachexia in adult patients: ESMO Clinical Practice Guidelines☆. ESMO Open. 2021 Jun;6(3):100092. doi: 10.1016/j.esmoop.2021.100092. PMID: 34144781; PMCID: PMC8233663.

Barrera S, Demark-Wahnefried W. Nutrition during and after cancer therapy. Oncology (Williston Park). 2009 Feb;23(2 Suppl Nurse Ed):15-21. PMID: 19856583; PMCID: PMC2770876.

Caccialanza R, Pedrazzoli P, Cereda E, Gavazzi C, Pinto C, Paccagnella A, Beretta GD, Nardi M, Laviano A, Zagonel V. Nutritional Support in Cancer Patients: A Position Paper from the Italian Society of Medical Oncology (AIOM) and the Italian Society of Artificial Nutrition and Metabolism (SINPE). J Cancer. 2016 Jan 1;7(2):131-5. doi: 10.7150/jca.13818. PMID: 26819635; PMCID: PMC4716844.

Cava E, Yeat NC, Mittendorfer B. Preserving Healthy Muscle during Weight Loss. Adv Nutr. 2017 May 15;8(3):511-519. doi: 10.3945/an.116.014506. PMID: 28507015; PMCID: PMC5421125.

de Castro GS, Andrade MF, Pinto FCS, Faiad JZ, Seelaender M. Omega-3 Fatty Acid Supplementation and Its Impact on Systemic Inflammation and Body Weight in Patients With Cancer Cachexia-A Systematic Review and Meta-Analysis. Front Nutr. 2022 Jan 31;8:797513. doi: 10.3389/fnut.2021.797513. PMID: 35174197; PMCID: PMC8841833.

de la Torre Guzmán SR, Pelayo-Chávez B, García-Muro AM, Soto-Reyes E, Sánchez-López JY. The Role of Folic Acid in DNA Methylation and Breast Cancer. Int J Vitam Nutr Res. 2025 Mar 28;95(2):26221. doi: 10.31083/IJVNR26221. PMID: 40298153.

Ferreira IB, Lima EDNS, Canto PPL, Gontijo CA, Maia YCP, Pena GDG. Oral Nutritional Supplementation Affects the Dietary Intake and Body Weight of Head and Neck Cancer Patients during (Chemo) Radiotherapy. Nutrients. 2020 Aug 20;12(9):2516. doi: 10.3390/nu12092516. PMID: 32825254; PMCID: PMC7551746.

Food and Nutrition Board; Health and Medicine Division; National Academies of Sciences, Engineering, and Medicine. Examining Access to Nutrition Care in Outpatient Cancer Centers: Proceedings of a Workshop. Washington (DC): National Academies Press (US); 2016 Aug 26. 2, Current Knowledge and Status of Nutrition Practices in Oncology Outpatient Care. Available from: https://www.ncbi.nlm.nih.gov/books/NBK384589/

Fu J, Zheng Y, Gao Y, Xu W. Dietary Fibre Intake and Gut Microbiota in Human Health. Microorganisms. 2022 Dec 18;10(12):2507. doi: 10.3390/microorganisms10122507. PMID: 36557760; PMCID: PMC9787832.

Fukuda K, Osumi H, Shimozaki K, Chin K, Ogura M, Fukuoka S, Udagawa S, Yoshino K, Tamba M, Wakatsuki T, Shinozaki E, Yamaguchi K, Ooki A. Impact of early tumour shrinkage on survival outcomes in patients with HER2-positive advanced gastric cancer treated with trastuzumab deruxtecan in third- or later-line settings. Therap Adv Gastroenterol. 2025 Apr 24;18:17562848251333538. doi: 10.1177/17562848251333538. PMID: 40297207; PMCID: PMC12035244.

Fukuda T, Tanaka M, Yamazaki M, Marunaka Y, Fukui M. Standard medical nutrition therapy of 25 kcal/kg ideal bodyweight/day often does not reach even resting energy expenditure for patients with type 2 diabetes. J Diabetes Investig. 2020 May;11(3):626-632. doi: 10.1111/jdi.13167. Epub 2019 Nov 28. PMID: 31659860; PMCID: PMC7232290.

Gangadharan A, Choi SE, Hassan A, Ayoub NM, Durante G, Balwani S, Kim YH, Pecora A, Goy A, Suh KS. Protein calorie malnutrition, nutritional intervention and personalized cancer care. Oncotarget. 2017 Apr 4;8(14):24009-24030. doi: 10.18632/oncotarget.15103. PMID: 28177923; PMCID: PMC5410360.

Gombart AF, Pierre A, Maggini S. A Review of Micronutrients and the Immune System-Working in Harmony to Reduce the Risk of Infection. Nutrients. 2020 Jan 16;12(1):236. doi: 10.3390/nu12010236. PMID: 31963293; PMCID: PMC7019735.

Hiraoka M, Kagawa Y. Genetic polymorphisms and folate status. Congenit Anom (Kyoto). 2017 Sep;57(5):142-149. doi: 10.1111/cga.12232. Epub 2017 Jul 20. PMID: 28598562; PMCID: PMC5601299.

Ibrahim MK, Zambruni M, Melby CL, Melby PC. Impact of Childhood Malnutrition on Host Defense and Infection. Clin Microbiol Rev. 2017 Oct;30(4):919-971. doi: 10.1128/CMR.00119-16. PMID: 28768707; PMCID: PMC5608884.

Ioniță-Mîndrican CB, Ziani K, Mititelu M, Oprea E, Neacșu SM, Moroșan E, Dumitrescu DE, Roșca AC, Drăgănescu D, Negrei C. Therapeutic Benefits and Dietary Restrictions of Fibre Intake: A State of the Art Review. Nutrients. 2022 Jun 26;14(13):2641. doi: 10.3390/nu14132641. PMID: 35807822; PMCID: PMC9268622.

Janakiram NB, Mohammed A, Madka V, Kumar G, Rao CV. Prevention and treatment of cancers by immune modulating nutrients. Mol Nutr Food Res. 2016 Jun;60(6):1275-94. doi: 10.1002/mnfr.201500884. Epub 2016 Mar 9. PMID: 26833775; PMCID: PMC6038926.

Kahleova H, Belinova L, Malinska H, Oliyarnyk O, Trnovska J, Skop V, Kazdova L, Dezortova M, Hajek M, Tura A, Hill M, Pelikanova T. Eating two larger meals a day (breakfast and lunch) is more effective than six smaller meals in a reduced-energy regimen for patients with type 2 diabetes: a randomised crossover study. Diabetologia. 2014 Aug;57(8):1552-60. doi: 10.1007/s00125-014-3253-5. Epub 2014 May 18. Erratum in: Diabetologia. 2015 Jan;58(1):205. doi: 10.1007/s00125-014-3411-9. PMID: 24838678; PMCID: PMC4079942.

Kesari A, Noel JY. Nutritional Assessment. [Updated 2023 Apr 10]. In: StatPearls [Internet]. Treasure Island (FL): StatPearls Publishing; 2025 Jan-. Available from: https://www.ncbi.nlm.nih.gov/books/NBK580496/

Krzyszczyk P, Acevedo A, Davidoff EJ, Timmins LM, Marrero-Berrios I, Patel M, White C, Lowe C, Sherba JJ, Hartmanshenn C, O'Neill KM, Balter ML, Fritz ZR, Androulakis IP, Schloss RS, Yarmush ML. The growing role of precision and personalized medicine for cancer treatment. Technology (Singap World Sci). 2018 Sep-Dec;6(3-4):79-100. doi: 10.1142/S2339547818300020. Epub 2019 Jan 11. PMID: 30713991; PMCID: PMC6352312.

Lalla RV, Sonis ST, Peterson DE. Management of oral mucositis in patients who have cancer. Dent Clin North Am. 2008 Jan;52(1):61-77, viii. doi: 10.1016/j.cden.2007.10.002. PMID: 18154865; PMCID: PMC2266835.

Law ML. Cancer cachexia: Pathophysiology and association with cancer-related pain. Front Pain Res (Lausanne). 2022 Aug 22;3:971295. doi: 10.3389/fpain.2022.971295. PMID: 36072367; PMCID: PMC9441771.

McQuade RM, Stojanovska V, Abalo R, Bornstein JC, Nurgali K. Chemotherapy-Induced Constipation and Diarrhea: Pathophysiology, Current and Emerging Treatments. Front Pharmacol. 2016 Nov 3;7:414. doi: 10.3389/

fphar.2016.00414. PMID: 27857691; PMCID: PMC5093116.

Mercier BD, Tizpa E, Philip EJ, Feng Q, Huang Z, Thomas RM, Pal SK, Dorff TB, Li YR. Dietary Interventions in Cancer Treatment and Response: A Comprehensive Review. Cancers (Basel). 2022 Oct 20;14(20):5149. doi: 10.3390/cancers14205149. PMID: 36291933; PMCID: PMC9600754.

Munteanu C, Schwartz B. The relationship between nutrition and the immune system. Front Nutr. 2022 Dec 8;9:1082500. doi: 10.3389/fnut.2022.1082500. PMID: 36570149; PMCID: PMC9772031.

Muscaritoli M, Lucia S, Farcomeni A, Lorusso V, Saracino V, Barone C, Plastino F, Gori S, Magarotto R, Carteni G, Chiurazzi B, Pavese I, Marchetti L, Zagonel V, Bergo E, Tonini G, Imperatori M, Iacono C, Maiorana L, Pinto C, Rubino D, Cavanna L, Di Cicilia R, Gamucci T, Quadrini S, Palazzo S, Minardi S, Merlano M, Colucci G, Marchetti P; PreMiO Study Group. Prevalence of malnutrition in patients at first medical oncology visit: the PreMiO study. Oncotarget. 2017 Aug 10;8(45):79884-79896. doi: 10.18632/oncotarget.20168. PMID: 29108370; PMCID: PMC5668103.

Naidu MU, Ramana GV, Rani PU, Mohan IK, Suman A, Roy P. Chemotherapy-induced and/or radiation therapy-induced oral mucositis--complicating the treatment of cancer. Neoplasia. 2004 Sep-Oct;6(5):423-31. doi: 10.1593/neo.04169. PMID: 15548350; PMCID: PMC1531648.

Nayak MG, George A, Vidyasagar MS, Mathew S, Nayak S, Nayak BS, Shashidhara YN, Kamath A. Quality of Life among Cancer Patients. Indian J Palliat Care. 2017 Oct-Dec;23(4):445-450. doi: 10.4103/IJPC.IJPC_82_17. PMID: 29123353; PMCID: PMC5661349.

Ni J, Zhang L. Cancer Cachexia: Definition, Staging, and Emerging Treatments. Cancer Manag Res. 2020 Jul 9;12:5597-5605. doi: 10.2147/CMAR.S261585. PMID: 32753972; PMCID: PMC7358070.

PDQ Cancer Information Summaries [Internet]. Bethesda (MD): National Cancer Institute (US); 2002-. Nausea and Vomiting Related to Cancer Treatment: Patient Version. 2025 May 9. Available from: https://www.ncbi.nlm.nih.gov/books/NBK65850/

Safdar A, Bodey G, Armstrong D. Infections in Patients with Cancer: Overview. Principles and Practice of Cancer Infectious Diseases. 2011 Jan 4:3–15. doi: 10.1007/978-1-60761-644-3_1. PMCID: PMC7122113.

Saunders J, Smith T. Malnutrition: causes and consequences. Clin Med (Lond). 2010 Dec;10(6):624-7. doi: 10.7861/clinmedicine.10-6-624. PMID: 21413492; PMCID: PMC4951875.

Sharma P, Dwivedi S. Nutrigenomics and Nutrigenetics: New Insight in Disease Prevention and Cure. Indian J Clin Biochem. 2017 Oct;32(4):371-373. doi: 10.1007/s12291-017-0699-5. Epub 2017 Sep 22. PMID: 29062169; PMCID: PMC5634986.

Sundrarjun T, Komindr S, Archararit N, Dahlan W, Puchaiwatananon O, Angthararak S, Udomsuppayakul U, Chuncharunee S. Effects of n-3 fatty acids on serum interleukin-6, tumour necrosis factor-alpha and soluble tumour necrosis factor receptor p55 in active rheumatoid arthritis. J Int Med Res. 2004 Sep-Oct;32(5):443-54. doi: 10.1177/147323000403200501. PMID: 15458276.

Talib WH, Ahmed Jum'AH DA, Attallah ZS, Jallad MS, Al Kury LT, Hadi RW, Mahmod AI. Role of vitamins A, C, D, E in cancer prevention and therapy: therapeutic potentials and mechanisms of action. Front Nutr. 2024 Jan 11;10:1281879. doi: 10.3389/fnut.2023.1281879. PMID: 38274206; PMCID: PMC10808607.

Wessels I, Maywald M, Rink L. Zinc as a Gatekeeper of Immune Function. Nutrients. 2017 Nov 25;9(12):1286. doi: 10.3390/nu9121286. PMID: 29186856; PMCID: PMC5748737.

Zahra KF, Lefter R, Ali A, Abdellah EC, Trus C, Ciobica A, Timofte D. The Involvement of the Oxidative Stress Status in Cancer Pathology: A Double View on the Role of the Antioxidants. Oxid Med Cell Longev. 2021 Aug 5;2021:9965916. doi: 10.1155/2021/9965916. PMID: 34394838; PMCID: PMC8360750.

Chapter 12

Post-Treatment Nutritional Strategies: Recurrence Prevention and Survivorship

Sarfraj Ahmad Siddiqui[1], Sheetanshu Gupta[2*], Ng. Joykumar Singh[3], and Praneeth Juvvi[4]

[1]Department of Biochemistry, King George's Medical University, U.P., India
[2]Department of Food Safety and Quality Assurance, College of Food Technology, Central Agricultural University (CAU), Imphal, Manipur, India
[3]Department of Food Process Engineering, College of Food Technology, Central Agricultural University (CAU), Imphal, Manipur, India
[4]Department of Food Processing Technology, College of Food Technology-Central Agricultural University, Imphal, Manipur, India

Abstract

Cancer survivors benefit enormously from dietary tactics post treatment, which significantly mitigate recurrence risk and enhance overall long-term health outcomes greatly. Diet plays a crucial role in facilitating recovery in numerous cases and thwarting subsequent oncological relapse, apparently. Certain nutrients markedly curtail inflammatory responses, and emerging evidence indicates that dietary patterns significantly impact cancer recurrence more than rigorous exercise routines. Plant-based diets and Mediterranean eating habits remarkably promote healthy weight and balance the gut microbiome very effectively in many individuals. Polyphenols play crucial roles in supporting cellular repair remarkably while vitamin D enhances immune function significantly in myriad obscure ways effectively. Cancer survivors need modified nutrition plans factoring in diverse health profiles, treatment history and survivorship issues like cardiovascular disease or diabetes, amidst complex needs. Targeted nutritional approaches markedly enhance quality of life post-treatment for cancer survivors and significantly mitigate recurrence risk afterwards.

Keywords: Recurrence Prevention, Survivorship, Post-Treatment Nutrition, Immune Modulation, Metabolic Health, Dietary Biomarkers

1. Introduction

Oncological care now fixates squarely on long-term survivorship issues owing largely to early detection breakthroughs and innovative treatment modalities boosting cancer patient survival rates. Cancer survivors

DOI: 10.1201/9781042010387-12

contend with a multitude of vexing physical and emotional sequelae long after treatment terminates in a haphazard somewhat disquieting fashion. Cancer recurrence risk and long-term health outcome management are paramount concerns in such situations almost invariably very carefully. Nutritional strategies after treatment play a rather crucial role in preventing recurrence and remarkably encourage long-term survivorship very naturally afterwards. Nutrition has garnered considerable attention recently owing largely to its potential role in mitigating cancer recurrence risk and encourage post-treatment health outcomes quite remarkably.

Cancer therapy patients often exhibit drastic changes in eating habits and metabolic functions largely owing to harsh treatment side effects. Taste alterations and muscle wasting or cachexia occur alongside fatigue loss of appetite and gastrointestinal distress severely impairing nutritional adequacy. Survivors must focus intently on nutritional recovery after treatment regaining optimal health rather quickly and reducing likelihood of cancer recurrence somewhat. New studies underscore significance of dietary regimens in sustaining overall wellness and diminishing likelihood of subsequent malignancies or relapse over time. Numerous studies investigate links between eating habits and recurrence of cancer because specific dietary patterns significantly influence outcomes very heavily nowadays. Survivors of cancer frequently show markedly reduced rates of recurrence and vastly improved survival on diets replete with fruits and leaner proteins usually (Peixoto da Silva et al, 2020).

Diets laden with ultra-processed foodstuffs and saturated fats correlate strongly with dire outcomes and elevated risk of chronic maladies like cardiovascular disease. Post-treatment dietary interventions have rather profound bearings on long-term cancer control and aren't simply about rectifying weight deficits afterwards. Nutrition heavily influences cancer recurrence by regulating key metabolic pathways deeply involved in cell proliferation and significantly modifying immune function (Juul et al, 2021). Cancer development and recurrence are linked very frequently with chronic inflammation alongside dysregulated cellular metabolism and insulin resistance. Upping fibre intake and noshing on anti-inflammatory food can significantly slash the risk of tumour regrowth by modulating certain cellular pathways quietly. Fibre-rich foods drastically improve gut health and modulate levels of insulin-like growth factor 1 driving proliferation of cancer cells quite rapidly.

Polyphenols found in foods such as exotic fruits and green tea exhibit potent anti-inflammatory properties mitigating oxidative stress that fuels cancer recurrence rampantly. Nutritional strategies employed post-treatment can remarkably thwart muscle wasting in cancer survivors effectively with somewhat quirky approaches afterwards often. Muscle loss persists way after treatment ends especially in people diagnosed with advanced stage cancers or subjected very intensively to chemotherapy lately. Muscle mass upkeep matters hugely for overall bodily function and survival rather crucially and also boosts physical prowess quite remarkably. Diets fostering protein synthesis fairly quickly with ample essential amino acids can help curb muscular breakdown and boost recovery afterwards vigorously (Mileo and Miccadei, 2016). Decent nutrition paired with regular physical activity has been shown to markedly enhance overall quality of life in some cancer survivors rather convincingly.

Nutrition plays a vital supporting role quite effectively in immune system function across areas of intense human physiological turmoil. Dodgy chemotherapy and intense radiation often ravage immune systems mercilessly leaving patients extremely vulnerable to heinous opportunistic infections and sepsis quite rapidly afterwards. Survivors may experience prolonged immune dysregulation very slowly after treatment and cancer recurrence risk increases significantly due to this. Micronutrients like vitamin D or zinc play a crucial role in modulating immune response and restore immune function very effectively. Adequate intake of these nutrients substantially improves overall health post-treatment by fostering a better immune response and reducing infection risk. Nutritional interventions are crucial yet addressing psychosocial aspects of survivorship remains very vital with fervor simultaneously in many cases (Munteanu and Schwartz, 2022).

Cancer survivors often harbour deep unease afterwards as post-treatment care kicks in awkwardly with gnawing fear of recurrence hanging precariously overhead. Psychological challenges severely hamper motivation for nutritious food undermining appetite and overall wellbeing very badly in some cases every day. Nutrition therapy with psychosocial support education and counseling helps patients cope with survivorship's heavy emotional toll fostering remarkably healthy eating habits. Survivors thoroughly adopting sustainable lifestyle changes can positively impact long-term health and reduce recurrence likelihood significantly over a considerable period. Personalized nutrition nowadays represents quite a promising research area in nutrition after treatment fairly extensively. Personalized nutrition endeavors deliberately tailor dietary recommendations according to individual genetic factors influencing cancer prognosis in each cancer survivor very specifically. Modified dietary plans are formed by melding genetic profiles alongside lifestyle factors and metabolic assessments quite intricately encourage health outcomes (Al Harrasi et al, 2025).

Cancer survivors receive highly targeted nutritional interventions nowadays from healthcare providers leveraging advances in nutrigenomics alongside effective clinical nutrition practices. Nutritional strategies after treatment play a vital role in cancer care with focus on diet's significant influence on preventing recurrence and survivorship outcomes utterly. Nutrition modulates myriad key processes including inflammation very significantly and metabolic regulation happens alongside immune function with muscle preservation occurring simultaneously. Evidence-based dietary interventions like whole foods and anti-inflammatory diets will be highlighted for cancer survivors having vastly different needs. Challenges and opportunities implementing effective nutritional strategies post-treatment will be discussed highlighting quite crucial multidisciplinary collaboration for supporting cancer survivors toward long-term health.

2. The Role of Nutrition in Cancer Survivorship

Cancer survival rates have improved markedly across many types owing largely to advancements in detection early on and therapies highly targeted. Global cancer survivors have grown substantially worldwide exceeding 43 million individuals according to data released recently by World Health Organization. Shifts in demographics have triggered drastic rethink of survivorship care that extends clinical gaze far beyond treatment into fairly comprehensive post-treatment support afterwards slowly. Nutrition remarkably fosters recovery and restoration of physical well-being after severe illness and aids secondary disease prevention effectively. Cancer survivors often struggle mightily with lingering disease aftermath and harsh treatment side effects like utterly debilitating fatigue and sporadic metabolic woes. Survivors frequently encounter elevated risk of comorbidities such as cardiovascular disease or diabetes and osteoporosis in many subsequent instances (Thun et al, 2010).

Carefully crafted nutritional strategies tailored somewhat specifically for an individual's particular health status and intricate cancer history foster long-term health benefits greatly. Evidence accumulating rapidly suggests dietary patterns heavily influence cancer recurrence and overall mortality significantly across various contexts clinically (Thun et al, 2010). Diets rich in whole grains fruits and veggies with lean proteins and healthy fats found in Mediterranean patterns have been associated with markedly improved survival. Survivors of breast cancer frequently display notably lower mortality rates on diets comprising mostly whole foods and plenty of nutrients. Colorectal and prostate cancer survivors eating mostly plant-based diets rich in healthy fats also exhibit lowered survival rates and cancer-related mortality. Consuming copious amounts of heavily processed foodstuffs and foods laced with saturated fats appears linked with very dismal health outcomes and heightened risk of secondary malignancies across multiple research endeavors.

Crucial nutritional guidance persists for weight management largely because obesity and post-treatment weight gain remain modifiable risk factors in several cancer types. Sarcopenia manifests as loss of muscle mass and strength but can be somewhat mitigated through generous protein consumption alongside excessive physical activity. Nutrition plays therapeutically relevant roles in cancer survivorship and warrants ongoing dietary counseling as part of highly structured care plans typically. Oncology specialists in dietetics play a crucial role providing sage evidence-based counsel among survivors with evolving complex needs remarkably sustainably. Survivorship emerges as distinct phase in cancer care continuum and nutrition must be reckoned cornerstone of holistic recovery now very much. Integration into long-term care models remarkably improves survival outcomes and quality of life well beyond cancer treatment afterwards surprisingly.

2.1. Nutritional Needs During Survivorship

Survivorship phase ensues subsequently after active cancer treatment concludes marking a crucial juncture of physiological recuperation alongside protracted health maintenance gradually. Cancer survivors often wrestle with nasty aftereffects such as debilitating fatigue and gut issues long after treatment has wrapped up completely. Cancer type and treatment modality heavily influence nutritional requirements during survivorship alongside residual organ function and various pre-existing comorbid conditions. Personalized nutrition supports recovery effectively and significantly enhances quality of life while preventing recurrence with a carefully tailored regimen. Optimizing macronutrient intake becomes crucial for meeting surging tissue repair demands and supporting immune restoration vigorously alongside rehabilitation efforts physically (Thong et al, 2022). Protein is vital for maintaining lean body mass slowly over time and supports immune reconstitution nicely and promotes wound healing rapidly.

Daily intake recommendations fluctuate wildly between 1.0 g/kg and 1.5 g/kg according to activity levels or some clinical status in individuals. Adequate carbohydrate intake fuels energy metabolism vigorously, while healthy fats like omega-3 fatty acids somewhat mitigate inflammation supporting cardiovascular well-being. Micronutrients play a vital role very crucially in bodily recovery after intense exertion or super stressful life events. Vitamin D remains glaringly crucial for bone health yet deficiency persists alarmingly among survivors with scant sun exposure or prior chemotherapy treatments. B-complex vitamins especially B6 and B12 coupled with folate play crucial roles in neurological health and manufacture of red blood cells. Iron enhances hematologic recovery rapidly while magnesium plays a crucial role in neuromuscular function and orchestrates stress response very effectively (Thong et al, 2022).

Mitigating lingering symptoms such as fatigue involves correcting nutrient deficiencies through supplementation or drastic dietary changes very effectively sometimes. Hydration and electrolyte balance crucially matter in survivorship care often woefully neglected especially for folks sporting colostomies or suffering radiation-induced bowel chaos with resultant chronic fluid depletion. Boosting hydration and nutrient absorption occurs with encouragement of small meals and use of isotonic oral rehydration solutions while emphasizing soluble fibre greatly improves gut function. Survivorship nutrition must be proactive addressing biological sequelae alongside lifestyle challenges and deep emotional tribulations during long grueling recovery periods. Robust dietary interventions integrated into post-treatment care significantly boost overall health results giving patients agency in fairly lengthy recovery journeys afterwards.

2.2. Weight Management and Body Composition

Cancer survivors often put on weight inexplicably during treatment or afterwards, particularly with hormone-related cancers such as breast cancer and prostate cancer. People struggling with severe gastrointestinal cancers or cachexia face a mighty uphill battle regaining muscle mass amidst severe malnutrition naturally.

Visceral weight gain correlates strongly with heightened systemic inflammation and insulin resistance thereby significantly heightening risk of disease recurrence. Loss of muscle mass, known as sarcopenia, contributes heavily to frailty and diminished mobility, precipitating lower survival rates markedly in affected individuals. Customized dietary regimes ought to fairly effectively promote maintenance of a healthy weight and preservation of lean body mass simultaneously. Balanced macronutrient distribution and moderate caloric control frequently facilitate desired outcomes via resistance training and fairly intense physical activity. Crucially minimizing excess fat accumulation supports overall metabolic health, rather effectively under certain conditions. Resistance training significantly impacts overall health, while numerous factors converge with physical activity playing a substantial role.

2.3. Reducing Risk of Recurrence Through Diet

Mounting evidence quite rapidly underscores the significant impact that long-term eating habits have on mitigating risk of relapse or onset of new cancers. Evidence suggests nutrition influences long-term outcomes significantly in oncology as a modifiable behavioral factor playing a pivotal role now. Cancer survivors in several observational studies exhibit markedly reduced recurrence and fairly strong correlations with specific dietary choices enhancing survival rates. World Cancer Research Fund and American Institute for Cancer Research issued guidelines promoting dietary patterns marked by copious veggie consumption recently.

Foods rich in antioxidants phytochemicals and anti-inflammatory compounds may inhibit carcinogenesis very effectively and remarkably promote hormonal balance quite naturally. Survivors are advised against consuming red and processed meats sugar refined carbs high-fat dairy products alcohol and ultra-processed foods very much altogether these days. Tumour progression gets spurred by elevated circulating growth factors like IGF-1 alongside gut dysbiosis and insulin resistance often develops simultaneously. A plethora of sizable cohort studies steadily increasing in number nowadays backs these recommendations with empirical evidence gathered quite rapidly (Flore et al, 2022). Women participating in Womens Healthy Eating and Living Study saw massive drops in mortality rates from consuming copious amounts of veggies and whole grains. Survivors of colorectal and prostate cancer showed markedly improved disease-free survival overall when adhering closely to Mediterranean dietary patterns generally. Dietary approaches quite effectively manage comorbidities related to treatment like obesity and cardiovascular disease or insulin resistance sometimes rather well. Survivors skillfully maintain protective dietary habits long term with regular counseling on nutrition and modification of behaviour strategies. A nutrient-dense diet rich in plants forms cornerstone of care after treatment with growing recognition of its potential for significantly reducing recurrence.

2.4. Managing Long-Term Side Effects with Nutrition

Cancer survivorship often lingers way beyond remission, encompassing myriad physical and metabolic aftereffects stemming heavily from preceding grueling treatment protocols. Survivors frequently endure nagging bone demineralization problems and gastrointestinal disturbances alongside chronic fatigue and chemo induced peripheral neuropathy rather severely. Nutrition plays a crucial role modulating inflammation and supporting physiological recovery afterwards effectively by addressing various nutritional deficiencies very quickly. Survivors frequently report chronic fatigue which can be effectively alleviated somewhat by targeted employment of specific nutritional strategies. Deficiencies in iron and vitamin B12 or folate are often implicated and should be rectified quickly with dietary changes or supplements. Eating iron-rich foods like lean red meat and dark leafy greens with B-complex vitamins supports erythropoiesis and boosts mitochondrial energy quite effectively (Ebede et al, 2017).

Cognitive dysfunction persists for years post-treatment fairly often nowadays and chemo brain is what many people still call it loosely. Evidence emerging rapidly nowadays suggests omega-3 fatty acids and B vitamins possibly support cognitive performance heavily by reducing neuroinflammation greatly. Eating foods like fatty fish and nuts with whole grains possibly yields greatly beneficial synergistic effects on cognitive function very regularly nowadays. Neurotoxic chemotherapies causing peripheral neuropathy might be somewhat alleviated by consuming omega-3 fatty acids and various anti-inflammatory nutrients very effectively. Flaxseeds walnuts and marine oils or clinically supervised supplementation may prove very beneficial for some people under fairly specific circumstances (Ebede et al, 2017). Treatment-induced gut dysbiosis rather mysteriously worsens gastrointestinal symptoms like bloating and discomfort alongside altered bowel habits fairly frequently.

Eating prebiotic fibres present in onions and bananas and probiotic-rich foods like yogurt and fermented veggies may help restore microbial balance and enhance immunity. Bone demineralization occurs frequently in patients undergoing androgen deprivation therapy or very aggressively treated with aromatase inhibitors necessitating reinforcement of dietary calcium and vitamin D. Leafy greens and fortified plant-based milks effectively maintain bone mineral density alongside dairy products and sun exposure or supplementation preventing fractures. Registered dietitians play a pivotal role in crafting modified dietary regimens based on individual symptoms and laboratory findings with great meticulousness. Survivors can very effectively adopt dietary patterns alleviating long-term side effects and supporting recovery alongside overall health maintenance very thoroughly.

2.5. Psychological and Social Aspects of Eating

Psychosocial dimensions of eating gain profound significance slowly in post-treatment phase of cancer survivorship over a considerable period of time. Food carries deep emotional and symbolic significance quietly resonating with cultural identity beyond nutritional value very profoundly. Eating frequently stirs up recollections in cancer survivors who endured nausea during treatment and harbored apprehensions about their gastrointestinal health afterwards . Survivors entering recovery often retain lingering associations that markedly sway appetite and food preferences altering overall dietary habits significantly. Fear of recurrence influences eating habits very strangely at times drastically altering food choices in many individuals (Philip and Merluzzi, 2016). Survivors frequently harbour profound unease around eating foods labelled potentially carcinogenic such as red meat or sugar without substantial proof existing. Restrictive diets often severely compromise nutritional adequacy resulting obsessively in food intake monitoring with no balance whatsoever.

Binge eating and emotional eating manifest haphazardly as maladaptive coping strategies amidst trauma of cancer diagnosis and subsequent treatments. Nutritional care involves emotional well-being consideration rather effectively alongside physiological needs via quite an integrative approach addressing sundry psychological facets. Mindful eating with sensory engagement and awareness cultivates a far healthier relationship with food and remarkably reduces overall anxiety levels. Survivors keenly heed hunger pangs and savor eating experiences deeply while shedding guilt tied up with problematic food choices (Philip and Merluzzi, 2016). Cultural factors play a rather crucial role somewhat surprisingly in shaping behaviors and attitudes deeply rooted in social norms. Culturally relevant food options strengthen emotional connections while identity and communal ties teeter precariously on very fine edge.

Survivors tend maintain healthy diets when personal faith-based eating habits are honored and care plans embody long-held quirky cultural legacies. Survivors acquire hands-on skills and shake off feelings of loneliness quite rapidly in intensely structured group sessions run by experienced dietitians. Empathy rooted approach surprisingly fosters empowerment and dispels myths around anti-cancer diets with cultural competence playing quite a crucial supporting role. Nutrition care thoroughly enhance emotional fortitude and overall well-being in cancer survivors by tackling psychological issues with considerable depth very effectively.

2.6. The Role of Healthcare Providers and Survivorship Clinics

Cancer care's paradigm shift towards embracing long-term survivorship tasks, healthcare providers nowadays with addressing multifaceted needs of survivors increasingly. Nutrition stands out as vital pillar of survivorship care and remains woefully underutilized amidst plethora of other very pressing disparate needs. Evidence heavily influences recovery and overall life quality while impacting functional status variably and modulating recurrence risk somewhat unpredictably. Survivorship care models must formally integrate nutrition incredibly urgently now under various circumstances across different healthcare settings. Oncologists and rehab specialists must prioritize nutritional evaluation very much everywhere as a standard component in post-treatment patient assessments. Routine screening should be implemented very quickly identifying individuals at risk of malnutrition and other dietary deficiencies facilitating early intervention.

Patient-Generated Subjective Global Assessment or Malnutrition Screening Tool can effectively support such processes in diverse clinical settings very obviously. Registered dietitians with oncology expertise should be deeply embedded in patient rehabilitation programs after treatment as part of survivorship care teams. Registered dietitians furnish modified nutrition guidance crucial for cancer survivors struggling intensely with therapy-related issues like swallowing difficulties or food aversions (Abbott et al, 2016). Dietitians empower patients with practical meal planning skills and label reading expertise thus greatly reducing confusion around many obscure food choices. Survivorship clinics foster veritable hotbeds for multidisciplinary care delivery encompassing nutrition and physical rehab alongside rigorous medical surveillance afterwards often with psychological support. Clinics serve as hubs where patients receive services that restore function and prevent comorbidities thereby greatly enhancing overall well-being very much nowadays.

Healthy behaviors may be reinforced sparingly through group-based education programs and cooking demonstrations alongside support groups of peers. Survivorship care becomes increasingly formalized nationwide and nutrition must be acknowledged as core element of care rather than some ancillary afterthought. Nutritional support ongoing markedly improves various outcomes including fatigue and surprisingly bone health or cardiovascular risk quite significantly alongside psychosocial adjustment. Survivors in modified nutrition programs often report heightened satisfaction with care and feel rather empowered managing their health matters very effectively nowadays. Clinical nutrition gets woven into survivorship pathways very remarkably optimizing most long-term health outcomes afterwards very well essentially. Focusing squarely on nutritional care enormously helps survivors thrive way beyond cancer years and greatly enhances their overall well-being subsequently (Abbott et al, 2016).

3. Nutritional Guidelines for Preventing Recurrence in Cancer Patients

Recovery signifies a pivotal stage afterwards active cancer treatment ceases and patients undergo gradual physiological healing and rather turbulent emotional readjustment slowly over time. Ending treatments like chemotherapy brings relief yet spawns fresh hurdles including lingering fatigue and neurocognitive changes afterwards often with significant sarcopenia. Nutritional interventions facilitate cellular overhaul and enhance psychological resilience quite effectively during this sensitive period with somewhat surprising outcomes. Replenishing micronutrients and antioxidant reserves severely depleted during grueling medical treatment stays a crucial nutritional goal in recovery. Vitamins A C D E and B-complex alongside minerals like iron magnesium selenium often remain woefully suboptimal post-treatment largely due to heightened metabolic demand. A nutrient-dense diet consisting mainly of veggies and fruits along with whole grains lean proteins and super healthy fats can restore bodily equilibrium naturally (Ganz et al, 2011).

Rebuilding lean body mass stays vital, particularly for patients affected by treatment-induced cachexia or substantial weight loss. Protein needs remain largely elevated during recovery with recommended intakes fluctuating greatly from 1.2 g/kg/day up to roughly 1.5 g/kg/day for individuals sporting disparate baseline muscle mass and vastly different activity levels. Eggs and fish are high-quality protein sources that alongside resistance-based physical activity markedly enhance muscle synthesis and counteract treatment-related fatigue. Cognitive changes nicknamed chemo brain alongside anxiety and depression often surface irregularly in post-treatment settings these days with some frequency. Magnesium and B-vitamins like B6 B9 and B12 along with omega-3 fatty acids EPA and DHA support mood regulation rather effectively (Ganz et al, 2011).

Personalized supplementation or meticulous dietary planning under expert guidance overseen by a qualified healthcare professional can yield desired results effectively. Tailored nutrition guidance reinforces healthy eating habits persistently in survivorship phase and addresses nagging symptoms such as gastrointestinal distress or aversive taste perceptions rather effectively. Tactics involving structured nutrition education and behavior modification empower patients maintaining cancer-protective diets thereby markedly enhancing overall life quality and reducing recurrence risk. Nutrition serves as restorative remedy and bridges deeply into survivorship fostering long-term wellness far beyond typical treatment timelines very effectively.

3.1. Foundations of an Anti-Recurrence Diet

Crucial foundational dietary principles effectively support prevention of cancer recurrence and manage comorbidities like cardiovascular disease diabetes and obesity related to treatment. Mediterranean diet has lately gained considerable prominence owing largely to effects on various pathways related rather intimately with cancer development processes. Dietary pattern remarkably rich in monounsaturated fats from olive oil and omega-3 fatty acids from various sources like fish and flaxseeds modulates chronic systemic inflammation effectively. Pro-inflammatory markers such as C-reactive protein and interleukin-6 are downregulated heavily via dietary patterns rich in phytonutrients. Oxidative stress gets mitigated rather effectively via enhanced intake of vitamin C and E alongside selenium and polyphenols found abundantly in diverse plant foods (Muscogiuri et al, 2022).

Tumour growth gets influenced heavily by insulin signaling relevant in insulin resistance particularly in cancers like breast and colorectal cancer recurrence. Plant-based diversity fairly rich in such nutrients ensures prebiotic fibres and bioactive compounds that gut microbiota thrive on quite vigorously. A healthy microbiome plays a crucial role in maintaining immune homeostasis profoundly influencing response to therapy and cancer outcomes remarkably longterm. Restricting certain food intake possibly fostering tumour growth is very crucial as well apparently. Processed meats contain nitrites and nitrates that form rather nasty carcinogenic compounds under some very unusual circumstances fairly readily (Muscogiuri et al, 2022). Heavy drinking markedly heightens risk of recurrence in cancers of head neck and breast as well as colorectal ones with moderate boozing posing seriously grave risks in hormone sensitive cancers.

Ultra-processed foods bursting with sodium and dodgy additives have been linked rather alarmingly with inflammation and increased cancer mortality rates. Practical application entails a rainbow on plate strategy very effectively maximizing phytonutrient diversity with whole foods in an impressively straightforward manner. Swapping refined grains like white rice for quinoa or brown rice utterly transforms nutritional intake rather subtly making a huge difference. Swapping animal fats for extra virgin olive oil or avocado oil usually proves a sound move nowadays in most culinary contexts. Meals centered on legumes ought to feature prominently in diets maybe three or four times a week with intermittent fasting occasionally thrown in. Nutritional foundations underpin integrative survivorship care quite naturally when paired with regular exercise stress management and diligent medical follow-up afterwards.

3.2. Body Weight and Recurrence Risk

Rigorous weight management plays a crucial role in mitigating risk of cancer recurrence fairly effectively amidst survivorship with significant impacts. Visceral adiposity correlates with poorer survival rates in malignancies such as breast cancer and heightened recurrence risk in colorectal tumours. Excess adipose tissue acts as a rambunctious endocrine organ pumping out sundry bioactive molecules including adipokines and cytokines that nurture a pro-tumourigenic milieu. Obesity fuels cancer progression largely via insulin resistance and ramped up insulin levels spuriously triggering rampant cell proliferation (Pati et al, 2023).

Chronic low-grade systemic inflammation fuels tumour growth wildly marked by surges in interleukin-6 and tumour necrosis factor-alpha production. Estrogen synthesized copiously in adipose tissue fuels aggressive recurrence of hormone receptor-positive breast cancers driven by sex hormone dysregulation. Obesity-associated immune dysfunction compromises bodily functions severely and malignant cells evade eradication quite effectively under such circumstances (Pati et al, 2023). Survivors oughta target optimal body mass index range while dodging drastic weight reduction and severely limiting calorie intake that utterly decimates overall wellbeing. Optimizing body composition sometimes necessitates resistance-based physical activity and very high dietary protein intake roughly around 1.0–1.2 g/kg/day or even higher occasionally.

Nowadays a very balanced approach towards somewhat sustainable caloric control is highly recommended. Survivors must keenly focus on nutrient-dense whole foods like veggies fruits and whole grains while drastically cutting back on junk foods. Mindful eating habits and at least 150 minutes of moderate exercise weekly support long-term weight maintenance very effectively over time. Incorporating regular dietary assessments and anthropometric evaluations into follow-up care enables early identification of weight-related risks and facilitates timely modified interventions. A healthy body weight greatly reduces risk of recurrence and markedly enhance life quality enhancing overall physical function in cancer survivors.

3.3. Role of Specific Food Groups and Nutrients

a. Fruits and Vegetables

Fruits and veggies crucially factor into most diets geared to thwart recurrence of various cancer types rather effectively nowadays. Phytochemical-rich plant-based foods modulate oxidative stress and inflammation vigorously with multifaceted protective effects on immune function substantially every day. Fruits and vegetables consumed in high amounts correlate with reduced cancer recurrence risk and markedly improved overall survival in various tumour types notably breast cancer. Antioxidant properties inherent in various fruits neutralize reactive oxygen species quite effectively damaging DNA and impeding mechanisms underlying carcinogenesis rapidly (Hossain et al, 2025).

Polyphenols and flavonoids alongside vitamin C have shown considerable promise in curtailing oxidative stress rather irregularly tweaking cellular signaling that influences apoptosis. Broccoli and kale contain heaps of glucosinolates that morph into very bioactive compounds inside human bodies fairly readily. Preclinical studies suggest these compounds very effectively induce phase II detoxifying enzymes and inhibit carcinogen-activating enzymes or so researchers reckon. Malignant cells undergo apoptosis swiftly under treatment (Hossain et al, 2025). Estrogen metabolism modulation subsequently quashes hormone-driven tumour growth remarkably down line. Fruits contain both soluble fibre and insoluble fibre which supports gut health and promotes beneficial microbiota diversity abundantly inside human gut vigorously.

Production of short-chain fatty acids like butyrate occurs fairly quickly and SCFAs possess anti-inflammatory properties and become anti-tumourigenic virtually overnight. High-fibre diets correlate strongly with markedly enhanced insulin sensitivity and drastically reduced systemic inflammation thereby further lowering recurrence risk significantly. Survivors ought to gobble a diverse array of vibrantly colored edibles daily aiming for five servings with penchant for organic seasonal produce.

b. Whole Grains and Dietary Fibre

Whole grains and dietary fibre play a pivotal role in cancer survivorship nutrition largely by mitigating recurrence risk and fostering long term health outcomes subsequently becomes: Dietary fibre and whole grains mitigate recurrence risk and foster long term health outcomes subsequently in cancer survivorship nutrition. Oats and brown rice teem with complex carbs and phytochemicals fueling overall metabolic regulation and fostering robust unusually healthy outcomes remarkably. Eating whole grains yields numerous benefits with fibre content substantially encourage gastrointestinal health and playing a significant role in estrogen regulation (Klobodu et al, 2024). Crucial albeit oft overlooked metabolic pathways fuel progression of hormone-sensitive malignancies like breast cancer and endometrial tumours very significantly. Soluble dietary fibre and insoluble fibre promote bowel regularity deeply within colon regions and enhance microbial fermentation quite profoundly.

Fermentation yields short-chain fatty acids like butyrate exhibiting profoundly anti-inflammatory properties in various obscure contexts and ostensibly anti-carcinogenic effects rather remarkably. Butyrate remarkably supports intestinal barrier integrity and suppresses tumour cell proliferation effectively while modulating immune responses of gut-associated lymphoid tissue. Survivors of colorectal cancer often exhibit markedly lower recurrence risk with high dietary fibre intake according to some recent epidemiology research. Higher total fibre intake from cereals has been linked quite frequently with reduced mortality from various causes and some forms of cancer (Klobodu et al, 2024). Colorectal cancer survivors boosting fibre intake after getting diagnosed in Nurses Health Study had remarkably lower mortality rates overall in follow-up studies. Fibre plays a crucial role systemically in reducing inflammation and improves insulin sensitivity thereby contributing significantly to weight management with markedly better cancer outcomes.

Fibre binds excess estrogens very effectively via gastrointestinal tract in cancers driven by hormone fluctuations and thwarts wildly circulating levels thereby lowering tumour growth quite significantly. Nowadays survivors of cancer are strongly advised daily consumption of around 25 to 30 grams of dietary fibre very much everywhere. Daily intake ought to be fairly replete with abundance of fruits nuts seeds legumes and veggies alongside whole grains. Consuming whole foods with minimally processed rough grain products preserves fibre effectively and boosts nutrient density in various very healthy diets.

c. Healthy Fats

Dietary fats plays a very important role in cancer survivorship with quality of consumed fat being way more crucial than sheer quantity overall. Consuming massive quantities of unsaturated fats present in nuts seeds and fatty fish might effectively reduce inflammatory responses and alter cancer pathways somewhat. Fatty fish like sardines and salmon as well as flaxseeds contain omega-3 fatty acids possessing profoundly anti-inflammatory properties that have garnered attention lately. Fatty acids like eicosapentaenoic acid or docosahexaenoic acid suppress pro-inflammatory cytokines significantly influencing gene expression involved in cell proliferation in various models. Omega-3 intake has been rather strongly tied to enhanced tolerance of chemo and reduced cachexia in survivors of sundry cancers. Omega-3s might mitigate recurrence risk quite substantially in breast and colorectal cancers albeit large-scale human trials remain sorely needed still (Bojková et al, 2020).

Consumption of saturated fats present in red meat and full-fat dairy products readily fosters carcinogenesis by promoting inflammation and insulin resistance. Diets extremely high in such fats strongly correlate with higher recurrence rates and poorer survival outcomes mostly in hormone-sensitive prostate and breast cancers. Cancer survivors receive dietary advice emphasizing replacement of saturated and trans-fats with monounsaturated fats present abundantly in olive oil and assorted nuts. Snacking liberally on nuts or seeds and devouring fatty fish at least twice weekly yield super fabulous results very quickly (Bojková et al, 2020). Fat intake balancing significantly enhance cancer survivorship whilst greatly contributing to overall cardiovascular health and cognitive function in quite surprising ways.

d. Red and Processed Meats

Processed meat consumption and red meat intake have been fairly strongly linked mainly to higher risks of colorectal and prostate cancer recurrence. Red meats encompass beef and lamb quite obviously while processed meats include products preserved by smoking with various chemical preservatives like bacon. Carcinogenic potential of such meats gets attributed haphazardly to murky mechanisms and sundry compounds found therein rather nebulously. Cooking red meat at scorching temperatures either by grilling or pan-frying forms nasty compounds like polycyclic aromatic hydrocarbons and heterocyclic amines. Processed meats harbor nitrates and nitrites that act as preservatives and potentially morph into N-nitroso compounds highly carcinogenic in human bodies (Aykan NF, 2015). Epidemiological research and meta-analyses rather quietly unearthed a link between consumption of red processed meat and various cancer outcomes dose-dependently.

Processed meats get classified by World Health Organization's cancer research agency as carcinogenic substances and red meat falls under probably carcinogenic category. Classifications stem from robust evidence linking consumption strongly with heightened risk of colorectal cancer in numerous epidemiological studies worldwide recently. Processed meat consumption possibly fuels chronic inflammation in cancer survivors thereby dampening immune surveillance and gut health suffers greatly. Cancer survivors face heightened recurrence risk when consuming diets heavy with saturated fats found lurking in processed food and red meats. Cancer survivors are advised limiting red meat intake roughly 18 ounces per week and avoiding processed meats whenever possible (Aykan NF, 2015). Legumes and nuts offer protein-rich alternatives devoid of noxious substances inherent in processed meat products sourced from animals. Adopting certain dietary practices robustly supports cancer risk reduction and aligns remarkably well with broader health guidelines for overall cardiovascular wellness offering numerous long-term quality benefits.

e. Added Sugars and Refined Carbohydrates

High consumption of refined carbs and added sugars has been increasingly linked with poor cancer outcomes and heightened risk of recurrence lately. Sweetened drinks and baked goods harbour hidden carbs that fuel metabolic chaos and smoldering inflammation fostering cancer growth rather quickly. Foods boasting a high glycemic index get digested rapidly and absorbed recklessly leading spikes in glucose levels and insulin surges in bloodstream. Hyperinsulinemia persists stubbornly and may bump up IGF-1 levels a hormone spurring cell proliferation and inhibiting cell death processes underlying various cancers oddly. Insulin resistance gets very gnarly with a ton of refined carbs in your diet and pro-inflammatory cytokines surge alongside oxidative stress (Iqbal et al, 2025). High sugar consumption and refined carb intake detrimentally affect cancer survivorship significantly enough to cause worry in numerous cohort studies observed lately.

Higher dietary glycemic load strongly correlates with mortality rates among survivors of breast and colorectal cancer especially for cancer-specific deaths. Beverages sweetened with copious fructose and possessing scant nutrients have been linked rather strongly to obesity and hepatic steatosis and systemic inflammation presaging cancer recurrence often. Cancer survivors are very strongly urged nowadays to drastically cut down consumption of added sugars lurking in energy drinks and ultra-processed snacks. Women ought to extremely strictly limit daily added sugar intake 25 grams or six teaspoons and men should similarly curb theirs at 36 grams or nine teaspoons (Iqbal et al, 2025). Survivors oughta prioritize complex carbs like whole grains oats quinoa brown rice and whole wheat alongside legumes including lentils beans chickpeas really well.

Apples berries and fibre-rich pears provide sustained energy and valuable micronutrients along with remarkably stable blood glucose levels. Sweet potatoes and beets rich in phytochemicals and dietary fibre play protective roles remarkably in immune regulation and overall digestive health. Such foods help mitigate systemic inflammation rather effectively too apparently. Cancer survivors remarkably enhance metabolic health by wisely opting for carbs thus significantly enhancing long-term remission prospects and overall wellness.

3.4. Alcohol Consumption and Cancer Recurrence

International Agency for Research on Cancer slaps Group 1 carcinogen label on alcohol suggesting very strong evidence of human carcinogenicity exists. Consumption of it has been weirdly linked and strongly correlated with development of various nasty malignancies especially breast and esophagus cancers. New findings savagely sink the idea that drinking small amounts of alcohol yields heart benefits for cancer survivors with no clear-cut safe limit whatsoever. Modest alcohol consumption has been linked with heightened risk of recurrence and disease progression in survivors of hormone-sensitive malignancies such as breast cancer. Alcohol consumption particularly surges circulating estrogen levels thereby fueling growth in estrogen receptor-positive cancers quite vigorously nowadays. More than 100000 breast cancer survivors participated in a meta-analysis that showed significantly higher risk of breast cancer recurrence and mortality with excessive weekly alcohol consumption typically over three or four drinks (Testino G, 2011).

Alcohol fuels oxidative stress heavily and badly impairs immune function disrupting intestinal barrier function potentially enhancing inflammation systemically. Acetaldehyde forms DNA adducts readily and interferes significantly with mechanisms of DNA repair thus promoting mutagenesis quite essentially in cells. Alcohol significantly hinders drug metabolism from a clinical standpoint particularly in survivors undergoing hormonal therapies or medications metabolized largely by liver enzymes (Testino G, 2011). Interference can diminish efficacy of treatment or amplify toxic effects of drugs thereby further complicating long-term management quite significantly. American Society of Clinical Oncology and American Institute for Cancer Research vehemently promote total abstinence from booze among cancer survivors nowadays.

Women ought limit daily consumption one standard drink and men possibly two standard drinks though such limits rarely appear safe for cancer patients undergoing intensive treatments. Survivors are prodded rather quietly to explore herbal remedies and infused elixirs which foster social bonding without entirely sacrificing wellbeing nowadays. Dietitians and oncologists offer crucial education helping survivors grasp risks and make informed decisions about consuming alcohol very effectively afterwards.

3.5. Gut Microbiome and Immune Modulation

Gut microbiome has emerged fairly suddenly as a central player at interface between nutrition immunity and cancer biology nowadays. Trillions of microorganisms including archaea and fungi inhabit gut microbiota influencing numerous physiological processes quite deeply inside human body. Cancer survivors may benefit greatly from diverse microbial ecosystems that play a pivotal role in reducing recurrence risk remarkably and encourage overall health. Regulatory T-cell activity gets promoted with gut microbiota in balance maintaining immune tolerance and preventing inflammation chronically quite effectively. A robust microbiome substantially enhances immune system's ability to detect residual tumour cells and destroy them supporting long-term cancer remission very effectively (Shreiner et al, 2015). Microbial metabolites such as short-chain fatty acids exhibit profoundly anti-inflammatory properties and butyrate displays markedly anti-carcinogenic effects notably within various tissues.

SCFAs maintain intestinal barrier integrity fairly well and inhibit growth of potentially pathogenic microbes thereby reducing systemic inflammation quite effectively. Gut microbiome modulates efficacy and toxicity of various cancer therapies significantly under certain conditions with varying degrees of impact apparently. Microbial diversity correlates positively with responses to chemotherapy and immune checkpoint inhibitors in several rather robust studies conducted quite recently. Microbial composition imbalance characterizing dysbiosis can severely undermine immune function and cultivates inflammation thereby markedly reducing treatment responsiveness. Remarkably healthy microbiome resilience is fostered very effectively inside human gut by diverse dietary strategies playing a crucial supportive role (Shreiner et al, 2015). Garlic and onions being prebiotic-rich foods contain non-digestible fibres that very effectively stimulate growth of beneficial gut bacteria selectively. Fermented foods such as yogurt kefir kimchi sauerkraut tempeh and miso harbor live microorganisms dubbed probiotics that boost microbial diversity remarkably.

Mitigating factors that disrupt microbiota matters equally under normal circumstances ordinarily meanwhile some measures are taken quite effectively already. Eating ultra-processed foods alongside high-fat low-fibre diets and consuming artificial sweeteners can very drastically alter microbial composition sometimes negatively. Survivors ought to target a diet fairly rich in fibre-dense foods and stuff that fosters very favorable gut environments naturally. Gut-friendly dietary practices remarkably enhance gastrointestinal health and enhance systemic immunity overall alongside metabolic balance in survivorship care contexts effectively (Rondinella et al, 2025). Nutritional interventions aimed squarely at gut health optimization will become vital very soon in survivorship care personalized deeply.

3.6. Supplements: Use with Caution

Cancer survivors driven by desire rather haphazardly utilize various dietary supplements to rectify perceived nutritional deficiencies and enhance bodily defenses somewhat. Evidence-based guidance advocates cautious approach meanwhile marketers in supplement industry hawk products touted as ridiculously natural and extremely super beneficial. Certain supplements may strikingly heighten recurrence risk in specific cancer cohorts and not be entirely innocuous rather unexpectedly at all. Supplementation with high doses of antioxidant compounds such as vitamin E and selenium often fails to deliver expected benefits in large-scale studies. Antioxidants occasionally quash reactive oxygen species tangled up in cancer cell apoptosis thus undermining efficacy of chemotherapy heavily reliant on oxidative stress.

High-dose beta-carotene supplementation was associated very convincingly with increased risk of lung cancer in trials involving smokers apparently. Supplements can drastically alter metabolism of certain therapeutic agents significantly in some cases or interact very badly with prescription medications. St John's Wort badly interferes with metabolism of various chemotherapeutic medications being a fairly common herbal remedy for mood disorder treatment typically. Unsupervised supplement use during survivorship may carry some gnarly unforeseen consequences fairly frequently under various obscure circumstances very often . Leading cancer organizations such as World Cancer Research Fund strongly advise getting essential nutrients from whole foods in a balanced diet (Middha e6t al, 2019).

Whole foods furnish vitamins minerals and an array of bioactive phytochemicals fibre and surprisingly healthy fats that support immune function synergistically. Supplementation becomes utterly necessary sometimes and proves positively crucial mercifully in other rather obscure cases down the line apparently. Survivors with documented deficiencies such as vitamin D or iron owing largely to malabsorption from treatment may benefit greatly from targeted supplementation. Routine blood work and nutritional assessments prove vital in identifying such needs fairly accurately most times with a reasonable degree of precision. Supplements play a somewhat ancillary role in survivorship when judiciously utilized but should never wholly supplant a nutrient-dense dietary regimen (Middha e6t al, 2019). Survivors should consult a registered dietitian or healthcare provider before starting some supplement regimen for utmost safety aligned with personal health goals.

3.7. Individualized and Culturally Sensitive Approaches

Cancer survivorship encompasses myriad needs and profoundly varied experiences yielding drastically disparate outcomes for individuals so affected thereby quite frequently. A one-size-fits-all dietary regimen fails miserably nowadays in addressing complex nutritional needs of cancer survivors rather ineffectively. Tailoring essential nutrition care around cultural contexts and various psychological factors supports recovery and minimizes longterm risk of recurrence very effectively. Personalized nutrition must reckon with cancer type stage and uniquely gnarled metabolic malaises spawned by each malignancy and befuddling side effects from therapy. Survivors of head and neck cancers frequently grapple with dysphagia or warped taste sensations impacting food intake rather drastically.

Colorectal cancer survivors may require twists in dietary fibre and fluid consumption largely due to bowel resection or ostomy management issues. Previous treatments like chemotherapy and radiation or hormonal therapy greatly alter bone density and gastrointestinal function holistically during dietary planning. Chronic disease states such as cardiovascular disease necessitate meticulous coordination between cancer survivorship care and diabetes management very carefully. Nutritional plans must balance cancer-related needs with broader health priorities ensuring every aspect of a survivor's overall health remains adequately addressed. Socioeconomic status and murky cultural nuances radically shape eating habits while very obscure psychosocial dynamics affect access fairly significantly. Survivors from diverse ethnic backgrounds may cling stubbornly to time-honoured dietary practices that should be respected greatly in subsequent treatment plans.

Cultural competence in nutritional counseling fosters trust deeply and enhance adherence remarkably supporting a survivor's personal identity with cherished core values unwaveringly. Forging sustainable diet interventions hinges crucially on recognizing hurdles such as food scarcity and woefully meager access to nutritious edibles. Registered dietitians specializing in oncology play crucial roles very much always on survivorship care teams with other supremely skilled medical professionals. Survivors get highly personalized meal plans crafted by specialists with unusual training who carefully factor in evolving personal needs and quirky preferences. Survivorship clinics staffed with such professionals guarantee remarkably dynamic nutritional guidance thoroughly personalized for each patient stays readily available. Nutrition serves remarkably as cornerstone of holistic cancer survivorship in the end with quite astonishing efficacy naturally. Culturally sensitive interventions remarkably empower survivors reclaiming agency over health in various settings and optimize clinical outcomes very effectively. Personalized nutrition becomes crucial in survivorship care quietly underscoring intricacies of clinical science amidst cancer survivors lived tumultuous experiences (Hundal et al, 2025).

4. Key Nutrients in Post-Treatment Recovery and Long-Term Health

Cancer care's post-treatment recovery phase signifies a pivotal juncture of physiological recuperation and radical reconstitution of the immune system, slowly thereafter. Survivors frequently struggle with debilitating exhaustion and severe muscle deterioration, often alongside bone degeneration after gruelling treatments like brutal chemotherapy. Nutrition plays a foundational role in encouraging recovery processes remarkably every single day and fosters substantially long-term health benefits afterwards thoroughly. Specific nutrients robustly fortify tissue repair and enhance immune response, safeguarding against disease relapse and the onset of ancillary health issues. Crucial nutrients for cancer survivors' recovery are thoroughly highlighted in this vital section, with a focus on sustained wellness.

4.1. Protein

Protein rapidly serves as fundamental block for tissue regeneration in cancer survivors post-treatment. Surgery or radiation triggers heightened metabolic demand and often precipitates inflammatory stress alongside severe malnutrition marked by protein energy depletion rapidly. Protein plays a crucial role naturally during recovery afterwards largely due to its pivotal role as a macronutrient facilitating slow bodily repairs. Adequate protein intake is necessary for swiftly mending ravaged tissues badly damaged by intense radiation or mangled surgical wounds. Treatment heavily suppressing immune competence often necessitates rapid synthesis of requisite immune cells and immunoglobulins under certain peculiar circumstances (Jin et al, 2023). Rebuilding lean muscle mass crucially facilitates functional recovery and boosts metabolic efficiency very effectively during prolonged rehab processes somewhat significantly.

Cancer-related sarcopenia manifests as profound skeletal muscle mass loss impairing physical function significantly boosting mortality risk very substantially afterwards. Survivors generally require 1.2 grams protein per kilogram body weight daily or substantially more depending on activity level and individual bodily needs. Physiological demands surge remarkably during cancer treatment necessitating intake substantially higher than 0.8 g/kg/day recommended for generally healthy adults afterwards. Protein sources remarkably abundant in essential amino acids normally take precedence quite heavily over others for various bodily functions. Lean animal proteins like poultry and fish alongside eggs are included basically with low-fat dairy products such as milk or cheddar cheese. Quinoa nuts and seeds effectively supplement plant-based proteins like lentils and soy-based products namely tofu and rather unusually tempeh (Jin et al, 2023).

Protein distribution throughout each day matters greatly for optimizing muscle protein synthesis effectively over fairly long periods of time apparently. Spreading protein consumption around 20-30 grams per meal possibly enhances anabolic response and reduces muscle wasting quite notably in elderly patients. Protein integration with physical rehab alongside strength training remarkably stimulates subsequent muscle rebuilding and significantly enhance overall outcomes afterwards very well. Survivors with nasty metabolic issues or severe renal impairment ought very safely consult a clinician very safely for tailored protein recommendations. Protein acts therapeutically in survivorship crucially restoring physiological function and fostering long-term wellness quite effectively promoting recovery slowly afterward in many cases.

4.2. Omega-3 Fatty Acids: Anti-inflammatory and Muscle-preserving Effects

Omega-3 fatty acids especially EPA and docosahexaenoic acid crucially support recovery overall and general health subsequently in many survivors of cancer. Long-chain polyunsaturated fatty acids exhibit surprisingly potent anti-inflammatory effects remaining particularly valuable during some rather crucial post-treatment phases. Cancer therapies often unleash brutal systemic inflammation that subsequently festers heavily inside patients contributing enormously to debilitating fatigue and tissue damage and gut-wrenching cachexia. Omega-3s thwart nasty effects fairly effectively by inhibiting cytokines like TNF-α and IL-6 amidst emerging somewhat dubious health trends. They promote anti-inflammatory eicosanoids and resolvins quite significantly under certain conditions with varying degrees of efficacy naturally (Freitas and Campos, 2019).

Omega-3s substantially enhance T-cells under specific circumstances, thereby very effectively enhancing immune surveillance and regulatory activity significantly downstream. Muscle protein synthesis gets facilitated very effectively by them while degradation gets thwarted in super catabolic states such as cancer cachexia. Evidence piles up quickly, indicating omega-3s substantially enhance tolerance of exhausting chemotherapy regimens and significantly mitigate cancer-related fatigue, enhancing tumour response markedly. Higher omega-3 intake has been linked tenuously, somewhat enigmatically with improved survival rates across diverse cancer types with markedly reduced recurrence risk overall. EPA and DHA exhibit neuroprotective effects stabilizing mood significantly benefiting survivors struggling mightily with cognitive decline or severe depressive episodes (Freitas and Campos, 2019).

Salmon and mackerel teem with EPA and DHA omega-3 fatty acids very abundantly in fatty fish categories. Flaxseeds furnish copious alpha-linolenic acid in diets very abundantly while chia seeds provide it lavishly. Algal oil supplements often pack a hefty dose of DHA. Human body converts ALA into EPA and DHA at pitifully low rates so therapeutically most times people prefer direct sources heavily. Daily intake of combined EPA and DHA by cancer survivors varies greatly across various studies ranging wildly from 1 gram up to 3 grams. Omega-3 supplementation should be guided extremely cautiously by healthcare providers in individuals with bleeding disorders or those concurrently taking anticoagulant medications. Omega-3 fatty acids work mystifyingly well as nutritional agents in survivorship care mitigating inflammation very effectively with very decent therapeutic outcomes.

4.3. Vitamin D: Immune Support, Bone Health, and Beyond

Vitamin D wields multifaceted influence over cancer survivors' overall well-being functioning far beyond its oft-quoted impact on skeletal metabolism remarkably. Potential far-reaching implications for cancer progression have been lately recognized with its influence on immune regulation and controlling inflammation. Cancer survivors often suffer vitamin D deficiency partly because harsh chemotherapy treatments cause mucosal injury and reduce sun exposure drastically. Deficiency may severely undermine immunity and fuel inflammation thereby contributing alarmingly rather to osteopenia or osteoporosis in cancer survivors mostly. Vitamin D plays crucial physiological roles in survivorship remarkably well by enhancing innate immunity and encourages adaptive immune responses very significantly (Kennel and Drake, 2013).

Vitamin D supports macrophage activation and modulation of T-cell responses thereby encourage resistance slowly to various nasty infections over time. Vitamin D may substantially aid immunosurveillance of residual tumour cells effectively. It plays a vital role maintaining skeletal health crucial for survivors on aromatase inhibitors or undergoing androgen deprivation therapy with glucocorticoids. Vitamin D very effectively downregulates pro-inflammatory cytokines and upregulates anti-inflammatory mediators helping manage chronic inflammation frequently observed in cancer recovery contexts. Serum levels of 25-hydroxyvitamin D are ostensibly linked with lower cancer recurrence and mortality rates mostly in breast cancers and prostate cancer (Kennel and Drake, 2013). Cancer survivors frequently require vitamin D supplementation despite eating fatty fish such as sardines and salmon very regularly nowadays.

Egg yolks surprisingly harbor considerable amounts of vitamin D mostly within their yellow centers. Plant-based milks and cereals fortified with essential nutrients serve as vital sources seemingly overnight. Sunlight very effectively triggers synthesis under certain skin conditions. Regular serum checks are typically mandated. Clinicians often target serum 25(OH)D levels roughly between 40-60 ng/mL for optimal benefit above that minimum threshold of 30 ng/mL. Typical daily supplementation ranges from 1000 IU and goes up to fairly high doses of 2000 IU although higher amounts are sometimes administered. Vitamin D stands out very much solely as crucial micronutrient in survivorship care vital for skeletal health and supporting immunity rather robustly (Browning and Cowieson, 2014). Targeted supplementation alongside highly personalized monitoring makes a significant difference remarkably enough in outcomes of survivors with some frequency obviously.

4.4. B Vitamins: Energy Metabolism and Cognitive Health

B-complex vitamins form a cluster of water-soluble micronutrients crucial for energy metabolism and DNA synthesis especially in red blood cell formation. Cancer survivors badly need optimal B vitamin status largely owing to treatment-related fatigue and chemo brain with compromised nutrient absorption subsequently. Key B vitamins massively comprise thiamine aka B1 which supports metabolism of carbohydrates and proper nerve function remarkably down the line. Debility often arises from deficiencies that starkly impair neurocognitive faculties resulting in quite a marked precipitous decline. Riboflavin or B2 and Niacin aka B3 play crucial roles very much everywhere in mitochondrial energy production via oxidative phosphorylation. Pyridoxine or vitamin B6 synthesizes neurotransmitters like serotonin and dopamine and GABA fairly effectively within human brain chemistry (Hanna et al, 2022).

Folate B9 and Cobalamin B12 play a crucial role in DNA repair and formation of red blood cells remarkably. Vitamin deficiencies severely impair cellular regeneration and homocysteine levels surge becoming a serious risk factor for cardiovascular health. Cancer treatments such as chemotherapy and targeted therapies severely damage mucosa in the gastrointestinal tract impairing absorption of B vitamins like folate. Individuals who have undergone gastric resections or bowel surgery and survivors of gastrointestinal or hematologic cancers are especially susceptible nowadays. Overt or subclinical deficiencies in B vitamins may fairly significantly exacerbate persistent fatigue neuropathy and cognitive dysfunction over rather long periods obviously. Survivorship meal planning should heavily emphasize diverse sources of B vitamins found naturally in various kinds of wholesome foodstuffs (Hanna et al, 2022). Leafy greens such as spinach are super beneficial and whole grains like brown rice quinoa and oats pack plenty of essential nutrients.

Legumes encompass lentils and various sorts of black beans rather exotically. Dairy products serve as a fairly reliable source of essential nutrients underground. Nuts and seeds provide nourishment quite abundantly for human health. Supplementation may be necessary quite often in individuals having gastrointestinal issues or absorption problems such as pernicious anemia occurring sporadically. Debilitating fatigue frequently manifests in individuals with specific underlying conditions but nutritional interventions often prove ineffective surprisingly enough. Supplementation ought to be guided by thorough clinical evaluation and lab tests like serum B12 levels or folate readings avoiding potential toxicity. B vitamins play a pivotal role in resilience after grueling cancer treatment and facilitate recovery with relative rapidity subsequently (Polak et al, 2015). Nutrients encourage mitochondrial function and DNA integrity help survivors regain vitality rather quickly afterwards with noticeably improved mental clarity.

4.5. Antioxidants: Cellular Protection and Immune Regulation

Antioxidants comprise diverse micronutrients and phytochemicals neutralizing reactive oxygen species byproducts of normal metabolism often markedly elevated during cancer treatments like chemotherapy or radiation therapy suddenly. Oxidative stress rampantly precipitates DNA damage and protein dysfunction fuelling chronic inflammation that spurs carcinogenesis wildly and fosters cancer progression. Vitamin C or ascorbic acid a very potent water-soluble antioxidant plays crucial role in collagen synthesis and supports immune cell function greatly. It facilitates iron absorption readily in many individuals alongside anemia and may help alleviate fatigue somewhat effectively thereby. Tocotrienols and tocopherols comprising vitamin E remarkably shield cellular membranes from oxidative stress and modulate T-cell-mediated immunity awkwardly alongside inflammation (Singh et al, 2018).

Selenium acts remarkably as a cofactor for glutathione peroxidase quite naturally a major antioxidant enzyme produced endogenously within human bodily systems. Selenium plays crucial roles rather quietly in thyroid hormone regulation and enhance immune surveillance with significant efficacy. Cancer survivors often suffer unusually high oxidative stress long afterwards largely due to lingering inflammation and badly impaired mitochondrial function. Adequate antioxidant intake from whole foods might very significantly enhance tissue repair mechanisms rapidly and help restore redox balance. Fruits such as berries and citrus pack plenty of vitamin C and polyphenols while leafy greens and sweet potatoes abound with various carotenoids. Almonds and sunflower seeds rich in vitamin E and selenium contain antioxidants mostly found in various other nuts (Lee et al, 2025).

Some whole grains provide polyphenols and assorted trace minerals very effectively underneath various circumstances ordinarily. Turmeric and green tea are very potent sources of antioxidants derived from plants obviously in various very significant ways. Excessive supplementation of isolated antioxidants in high doses may be contraindicated problematically in some cancer survivors with various complicating health issues. Mega-dose antioxidants possibly undermine therapeutic effects of certain chemotherapies and radiation therapy by reducing cell death mediated by reactive oxygen species quite significantly. Survivors ought prioritize antioxidant-rich whole foods rather than popping supplements unless medical experts have indicated otherwise very strongly today. Antioxidants ostensibly serve as crucial bulwark against oxidative stress plaguing survivors of various cancers with fairly impressive effectiveness. Naturally people can safely boost cellular integrity and tissue recovery by consuming richly diverse plant-based foods.

4.6. Iron and Magnesium: Rebuilding Vital Reserves

Cancer survivors often grapple with severely depleted nutrient stores mostly due to systemic inflammation and gastrointestinal dysfunction alongside significant blood loss. Essential nutrients such as iron or magnesium are crucial for cellular function and energy metabolism in humans generally notably. Iron plays a crucial role in hemoglobin synthesis facilitating mitochondrial respiration effectively and encourage DNA synthesis via oxygen delivery mechanisms. Cancer survivors often develop anemia especially iron-deficiency anemia after undergoing chemotherapy or radiation or surgeries with massive blood loss involved. Utter fatigue and profoundly disorienting dizziness or severely impaired cognitive function manifests reducing life quality significantly in rather inexplicable ways (Inglis et al, 2024). Eating foods rich in iron such as lean red meat and seafood replenishes iron stores quickly from highly bioavailable heme sources. Lentils beans tofu and spinach are non-heme iron sources along with quinoa and some fortified breakfast cereals very much everywhere nowadays.

Eating foods extremely rich in vitamin C like bell peppers strawberries and various citrus fruits in a meal boosts non-heme iron absorption markedly. Tea and coffee along with calcium supplements can conversely inhibit iron uptake so they ought to be consumed separately from iron rich meals. Iron supplementation may be necessary in diagnosed deficiency cases but healthcare providers should guide it very carefully avoiding nasty gastrointestinal side effects and potential overload. Magnesium plays crucial role in myriad enzymatic reactions exceeding 300. Magnesium plays a crucial role in energy production inside cells facilitating ATP synthesis remarkably. Function of muscle and nerve heavily relies utterly on it. Magnesium is utilized significantly by DNA repair mechanisms and replication processes occur with considerable reliance on it quietly. Magnesium play a crucial role in maintaining blood glucose levels and regulating blood pressure under various physiological conditions (Inglis et al, 2024). Prolonged diarrhea from radiation therapy or surgery and platinum-based chemotherapies such as cisplatin can very frequently result in hypomagnesemia.

Fatigue and arrhythmias unfold alongside muscle cramps or irritability and disturbed sleep patterns often manifest with considerable frequency. Magnesium intake comes mainly from dietary sources like nuts and certain seeds including almonds and rather nutritious pumpkin seeds. Brown rice and oats along with other whole grains contain loads of magnesium naturally. Legumes like black beans are loaded heavily with magnesium. Spinach and other dark leafy greens boast unusually high magnesium content rather remarkably in their deeply hued leaves. Supplementation under strict clinical supervision may be warranted in cases of severe persistent deficiency though dietary sources should remain primary.

4.7. Phytochemicals and Fibre: Long-Term Protection

Phytochemicals and dietary fibre offer protection against cancer recurrence and comorbidities rather significantly in cancer survivorship contexts over fairly long periods. Bioactive compounds and non-digestible carbs significantly contribute to physiological homeostasis and regulation of molecular pathways deeply involved in carcinogenesis. Very much myriad biological activities relevant alongside some immune system support are exhibited evidently by naturally occurring compounds found in various plant-based foods. Flavonoids and carotenoids prominently manifest alongside glucosinolates polyphenols stilbenes naturally in diverse categorizations of notable compounds. Broccoli and kale veggies contain glucosinolates that very effectively break down into isothiocyanates inhibiting carcinogen activation fairly significantly (Kotecha et al, 2016).

Isothiocyanates fairly quickly suppress various pro-inflammatory signaling pathways and remarkably enhance several antioxidant defense systems in biological organisms. They swiftly promote apoptosis of aberrant cells and fairly strongly inhibit formation of new blood vessels. Multiple mechanisms modulate immune cell signaling deeply over time and affect gene expression irregularly at various cellular levels. Tumour-promoting pathways like NF-κB are vigorously suppressed beneath metastatic lesions and progression gets thoroughly inhibited. Detoxification enzymes get promoted significantly through diverse mechanisms by these compounds acting fairly rapidly with varying degrees of efficacy (Kotecha et al, 2016). Berries and grapes harbour anthocyanins and resveratrol while green tea furnishes catechins like EGCG exhibiting chemopreventive properties in numerous preclinical studies.

Turmeric abundant in curcumin has garnered considerable attention lately owing largely to markedly anti-inflammatory effects and hindering cell proliferation remarkably well. Dietary fibre plays a crucial role somewhat surprisingly in promoting long-term health very effectively after cancer treatment of various forms. Whole grains legumes fruits and veggies contain soluble and insoluble fibres that beneficially impact gut health and systemic physiology in myriad obscure ways. Key functions involve enhancing fecal bulk irregularly and bowel regularity often improves markedly with considerable variation in outcomes sometimes observed afterwards. Gut microbial diversity gets boosted remarkably alongside production of short-chain fatty acids such as butyrate in varying concentrations suddenly (El-Saadony et al, 2023). Glucose and insulin responses after eating stay remarkably in check very effectively beneath a typically tolerable threshold.

Carcinogenic compounds get bound very quickly and then get excreted with remarkable facility in bodily waste rather effortlessly. Estrogen metabolism undergoes modulation particularly in hormone-sensitive cancers where it ostensibly matters greatly under certain circumstances. Daily consumption of over 25 grams fibre correlates with lower recurrence rates and mortality especially among breast cancer survivors quite remarkably. Diets rich in vibrantly colored vegetables foster hefty phytochemical and fibre intake which synergistically promotes anti-inflammatory and anti-carcinogenic environments internally in bodily tissues. Cancer survivors can markedly enhance long-term outcomes by integrating specific dietary components into a tailored nutrition regimen very consistently over several years.

5. Dietary Modifications for Strengthening the Immune System After Cancer Treatment

Cancer care after treatment gradually unfolds into a critical window of recovery marked rather quietly by reconstitution of immune systems afterwards slowly. Cancer therapies such as chemotherapy exert deeply suppressive effects on immunity by disrupting hematopoietic function and depleting key immune cell populations grossly. Survivors face heightened risk of systemic inflammation and persistent fatigue alongside opportunistic infections and poor wound healing afterwards rather mysteriously. Targeted nutritional interventions enhance remarkably immune resilience and mitigate effectively risks of various infectious agents and neoplastic diseases. Immune cells rely heavily on energy availability and specific nutrients for proper proliferation differentiation and function optimally under various physiological conditions. Protein-energy malnutrition tends to linger throughout cancer treatment and afterwards significantly suppresses innate and adaptive immunity rather badly (Sharma et al, 2024).

A high-protein nutrient-dense diet very effectively supports leukocyte synthesis and boosts antibody production during various tissue regeneration processes. Poultry fish and legumes serve as lean protein sources sufficiently recommended daily around 1.2–2.0 g/kg body weight in elevated metabolic demands typically. Vitamins A, C, D E and B6 along with zinc and iron are vital utterly for proper regulation of immune system. Nutrients foster integrity of epithelial barriers and modulate cytokine signaling significantly influencing activity of various lymphocytes and natural killer cells very profoundly. Eating whole grains nuts and seeds alongside vibrant fruits and veggies practically guarantees very broad coverage of various essential micronutrients (Sharma et al, 2024). Vitamin D plays a very crucial immunomodulatory role when levels are nosediving rapidly and supplementation becomes downright necessary very swiftly. Berries and citrus fruits and leafy greens along with turmeric green tea or fatty fish packed with antioxidants mitigate oxidative stress from cancer treatments.

Certain compounds quite effectively mitigate chronic inflammation a known major contributor of dysfunctional immune response and subsequent cancer recurrence. Gut microbiota health plays a crucial albeit largely inscrutable role in immune education and surveillance through complex bodily mechanisms. Fermented food such as yogurt and kimchi and prebiotic-rich foods like garlic and asparagus boosts short-chain fatty acid production fostering microbial diversity remarkably and gut barrier function gets enhanced and immune homeostasis is maintained decently. Super personalized dietary interventions ridiculously grounded in evidence are often developed in close consultation with oncology-trained dietitians very frequently . Nutritional strategies vigorously strengthen immune mechanisms holistically promoting long-term survivorship remarkably well afterwards and foster recovery with great efficacy.

5.1. Rebuilding Immune Function

Nutrient intake diversity underpins immune functionality precariously sustaining cellular integrity while orchestrating signal transduction pathways rather effectively amidst various bodily processes. Malnutrition and metabolic imbalances severely compromise immune function in cancer survivors heightening susceptibility to nasty infections and delayed healing of wounds. Post-treatment dietary strategies are crucial afterwards for restoration of innate immunity and adaptive immunity becoming fundamentally extremely important. Replenishing depleted micronutrient reserves crucial for immune cell function and cytokine production remains key goal of nutritional intervention here. Sufficient intake of macronutrients rich in high-quality protein supports tissue regeneration and proliferation of immune cells very effectively. Pro-inflammatory and immunosuppressive pathways frequently go awry during cancer progression so modulating them becomes utterly vital.

Nutritional intervention done properly fosters immune homeostasis by restoring gastrointestinal integrity and pivotal microbial diversity simultaneously. Nutrient-dense dietary patterns replete with anti-inflammatory edibles ostensibly undergird robust immune reconstitution fairly effectively over a considerable period. A diet rich in vitamins A and C and minerals zinc and selenium prioritizes whole foods and lean protein with omega-3 fatty acids abundantly. Components act synergistically reducing oxidative stress greatly and facilitate recovery from treatment induced damage via modulation of immune system effectively. Eating a diverse assortment of vibrantly colorful fruits and vegetables provides flavonoids and carotenoids with profoundly potent immunomodulatory effects (Reis et al, 2025). Whole grains legumes and nuts remarkably enhance macro and micronutrient adequacy while fostering gut health via prebiotic properties somewhat effectively.

Fermented foods harbour probiotics that quite effectively enhance mucosal immunity and regulate immune response in a manner highly beneficial overall. Reconstruction of dietary immune function must be tailored quite carefully around individual needs with regard to treatment history and current status. Registered dietitians boasting oncology expertise guarantee dietary recommendations remain firmly rooted in science and very feasible in real life situations. Survivors enhance immune restoration remarkably by tapping into nutrition's healing properties and subsequently mitigate risk of various nasty complications or disease resurgence quite effectively.

5.2. Emphasizing Immune-Enhancing Nutrients

Several nutrients have been identified as critical to immune system function:

a. Protein

Protein intake sufficiently fuels cytokine production and formation of various immune cells at a fairly rapid pace. Survivors after treatment often need roughly 1.2 grams of protein per kilogram daily for tissue repair and they require quite a lot more sometimes up to 1.5 grams. High-quality protein sources include lean meats and poultry and fish and eggs or dairy products or legumes such as lentils and beans.

b. Vitamin A

Vitamin A enhances mucosal barrier function and ramps up activity of T-cells and natural killer cells quite significantly. Foods rich in beta-carotene include carrots sweet potatoes and pumpkins while eggs and liver contain preformed vitamin A naturally.

c. Vitamin C

Vitamin C plays a crucial role in immune homeostasis after cancer treatment recovery processes unfold gradually quite slowly over time naturally. Vitamin C serves crucially as a potent antioxidant in various bodily responses and effectively functions as a water-soluble nutrient. It shields cells quite effectively against oxidative stress fuelled simultaneously by cancer treatments and lingering inflammatory responses in the body. Vitamin C remarkably enhances functional capacity of various key immune cells at cellular level effectively with great efficacy suddenly. It enhances neutrophil chemotaxis vigorously and very rapidly facilitates migration of these cells towards sites of nasty infection or severe injury. Phagocytosis happens very vigorously and neutrophils engulf pathogens with abandon destroying them rapidly in a most enthusiastic manner (Pawlowska et al, 2019).

Vitamin C plays a crucial role in apoptosis and clearance of spent neutrophils thereby supporting resolution of inflammation very quietly preventing tissue damage. Vitamin C fosters lymphocyte proliferation mainly of T-cells extremely central rather crucially to adaptive immunity responses quite effectively. Cancer survivors frequently endure intensified susceptibility quietly over time where immunosuppression lingers substantially long after treatment gradually stops (Pawlowska et al, 2019). Vitamin C plays crucial role in collagen synthesis thereby facilitating wound healing and repair of epithelial barriers against pathogens very effectively. It regenerates other antioxidants like vitamin E and boosts overall antioxidant network rather effectively deep within various bodily systems. Oranges and lemons being citrus fruits rich in vitamin C alongside kiwi strawberries and various berries are fantastic dietary sources essentially.

Red bell peppers are exceptionally packed with it mostly. Broccoli and similar veggies serve as stellar sources of essential nutrients remarkably well inside human diets generally. Cancer survivors are recommended 75–120 mg daily but may benefit from significantly higher intakes owing largely to extremely heighly oxidative stress levels. Whole-food sources usually outdo supplements largely because of broader phytochemical profiles and far superior bioavailability in various nutritional contexts. Supervised supplementation may be warranted in cases of very severe dietary insufficiency or documented deficiency obviously very frequently nowadays. Sufficient vitamin C intake remarkably enhances antioxidant defenses and facilitates healing post treatment thereby supporting immune recovery rather thoroughly.

d. Vitamin D

Vitamin D plays multifaceted crucial role in immune regulation vital for cancer survivors beset by arduous recovery processes lingering afterwards quite problematically. Vitamin D exerts profoundly innate effects and broadly adaptive immunomodulatory actions making it crucial in restoration of immune function after medical treatment. Vitamin D plays a crucial role enhancing innate immunity rather significantly underneath various environmental conditions normally. Production of antimicrobial peptides like cathelicidins and defensins gets stimulated very vigorously in epithelial cells and macrophages encourage defenses against pathogens. Certain peptides ravage bacterial cell membranes brutally and help eradicate viral infections effectively in severely immunocompromised cancer patients.

Vitamin D modulates adaptive immunity effectively by tempering very excessive inflammatory responses simultaneously rather than exacerbating them further downstream. Fostering development of regulatory T cells it suppresses proliferation of pro-inflammatory Th1 and Th17 cells helping prevent chronic inflammation very deeply. Dual action proves highly beneficial post-treatment because systemic inflammation or immune dysregulation often ensue after chemotherapy and radiation therapy or immunotherapy. Cancer survivors often suffer vitamin D deficiency mostly because treatment curtails sun exposure and dietary intake falls woefully short. Suboptimal levels correlate with markedly heightened infection susceptibility and slower tissue repair alongside fatigue and musculoskeletal pain possibly escalating cancer recurrence rates in breast prostate and colorectal cancers (Aranow C, 2011).

Survivors ought to get checked very regularly nowadays for very severe vitamin D deficiency since lots of people apparently lack it badly. Vitamin D production happens rapidly in skin upon being exposed mostly through UVB radiation in sunlight fairly quickly. Fatty fish such as salmon and sardines are typically loaded with it while mackerel sometimes have it in abundance too apparently. Egg yolks and some mushrooms exposed extensively to ultraviolet light are very good sources too beneath surprisingly rich liver extracts. Many people can opt for breakfast cereals and plant-based milk heavily fortified with vitamin D or various dairy products instead. Targets vary greatly among individuals and optimal levels are deemed be within range of 30 to 50 ng/mL occasionally (Aranow C, 2011).

Doses ranging wildly from 1000 IU daily right up to 4000 IU may be necessary to correct deficiencies particularly in people with glaring malabsorption issues or scarce sun exposure. Rebuilding immune resilience necessitates adequate vitamin D intake safely via dietary tweaks or supplementation as deemed necessary over long term.

e. Zinc

Zinc plays a fundamental role in maintaining innate and adaptive immune function making it crucial during recovery from cancer treatment essentially. Its functions in immunity are multifaceted involving cell-mediated responses quite broadly and deeply antioxidant defense mechanisms regulating inflammatory processes. Zinc plays a crucial role in development of various immune cells and activation occurs rapidly in T lymphocytes undergoing differentiation. It serves as a crucial structural component in numerous enzymes and transcription factors guiding T-cell maturation profoundly within thymus and heavily skews balance between Th1 and Th2 helper subsets. Zinc deficiency severely hampers T-cell proliferation and reduces antibody responses thereby heightening vulnerability to nasty infections and damaging epithelial barriers badly (Skrajnowska and Bobrowska-Korczak, 2019).

Zinc plays a crucial role in neutrophils and macrophages function within innate immune system and enhance natural killer cells remarkably. It modulates activity of nuclear factor-kappa B a transcription factor that regulates expression of very nasty pro-inflammatory cytokines thereby exhibiting some surprisingly potent anti-inflammatory properties. Zinc plays a crucial role in mitigating oxidative damage and fostering repair of tissue among cancer survivors with heightened stress levels. Zinc deficiency occurs fairly often among cancer patients and survivors largely due to malabsorption or very woeful nutrition occasionally. Grossly impaired wound healing and drastically altered taste make recovery very complicated sometimes in really messy and highly problematic ways (Skrajnowska and Bobrowska-Korczak, 2019).

A zinc-rich diet ought to be encouraged for recovery of immune function naturally over quite a long period slowly. Foods derived from animals such as beef poultry and shellfish notably oysters naturally offer zinc in highly bioavailable forms. Cashews alongside pumpkin seeds and sesame seeds offer rich sources of minerals found very frequently in lentils and various whole grains. Bioavailability from plant sources tends to be very low mainly due to phytates inhibiting absorption significantly in most cases. Supplementation might be justified in people highly susceptible to zinc deficiency or those having lab-verified subnormal levels generally necessitating dosage between 8 mg daily for upkeep and 40 mg daily under strict medical oversight. High doses of zinc can very quickly impair immune function and badly interfere with copper absorption rather severely. Zinc stays very crucial post-treatment for cancer survivors owing largely to roles in immune modulation and seriously encourage antioxidant defenses (Tokarczyk & Koch, 2025).

f. Selenium

Selenium plays a crucial role in maintaining immune function optimally and defends cells very effectively against oxidative stress. Biological activity manifests mainly via incorporation into quirky proteins called selenoproteins that perform diverse antioxidant roles and weird immunomodulatory functions. Selenium plays a crucial role in activity of glutathione peroxidases and thioredoxin reductases neutralizing reactive oxygen species during inflammatory responses or various cancer treatments effectively. Selenium mitigates oxidative damage effectively during recovery from chemotherapy or radiation supporting immune cell viability very well thereby preserving cellular integrity (Huang et al, 2012).

Selenium quite profoundly influences innate and adaptive immune responses sometimes within various facets of the immune system. It enhances T lymphocyte proliferation vigorously while supporting natural killer cell cytotoxicity and interleukin-2 production gets promoted fervently. Selenium levels high enough have been associated with markedly better vaccine responses suggesting relevance in reconstituting immunity effectively across broader populations. Cancer survivors often have severely compromised selenium status due to gastrointestinal disturbances related to treatment and poor dietary habits heightening oxidative stress. Low selenium levels correlate with substantially diminished immune function and potentially exacerbate adverse clinical outcomes including protracted recuperation and greatly heightened susceptibility to nasty infection (Huang et al, 2012). Selenium deficiency may be linked rather strongly to poor prognosis in various cancers such as lung cancer prostate cancer and others.

Dietary selenium sourced from whole foods like ridiculously rich Brazil nuts supports recovery of immune function naturally over time. Just one Brazil nut provides over 100% of the daily recommended selenium intake surprisingly effortlessly almost every time. Tuna and sardines and shrimp boast rather high bioavailability of nutrients naturally in dwellings beneath ocean surfaces very frequently. Choose surprisingly lean meats like beef or chicken and also turkey for a healthier diet. Brown rice lentils and oats contribute fairly moderate amounts alongside whole grains and various legumes typically found in very standard everyday diets. Selenium intake should be quite judicious or daily consumption above 400 micrograms can trigger nasty gastrointestinal issues associated with selenosis quite rapidly (Huang et al, 2012).

Supplementation should be considered only in individuals with confirmed deficiency under stringent clinical oversight at wildly varying dosages typically around 50 micrograms daily. Selenium evidently plays a rather enigmatic dual role in immune restoration and oxidative protection during recovery post cancer treatment. Balanced nutrition significantly boosts survivors' immune resilience and potentially results in substantially better long-term health outcomes over time remarkably.

5.3. Supporting Gut Health for Immune Balance

Gastrointestinal tract serves centrally as primary site of nutrient absorption and functions crucially for immune activity meanwhile internally. Gut-associated lymphoid tissue harbors approximately 70 to 80 percent of body's immune cells underscoring a rather intricate link between gut health and systemic immunity overall. Harsh chemotherapy brutally disrupts delicate gut balance in patients undergoing cancer treatment with radiation and broad-spectrum antibiotics rampantly. Dysbiosis triggers chronic low-grade inflammation wreaking havoc on barrier function with translocation of microbial products like lipopolysaccharides fairly often (Bemark et al, 2024).

Cancer survivors frequently display severe nutritional deficiencies which this condition worsens by impeding uptake of crucial nutrients necessary for revitalizing immune systems. Restoring a healthy gut microbiome fundamentally is required after treatment for rehabilitating immunity thoroughly in most medical cases obviously. Prebiotic Fibre fuels beneficial microbes rather deeply within gut flora environments every day. Prebiotics being non-digestible fibres selectively foster growth of Bifidobacterium species and Lactobacillus very quietly beneath radar. Foods like onions garlic asparagus bananas rich in prebiotic compounds promote microbial fermentation producing short-chain fatty acids such as butyrate vigorously. SCFAs rather effectively possess anti-inflammatory properties and modulate function of various immune cells within gut-associated lymphoid tissue (Bemark et al, 2024).

Probiotic-rich foods introduce live beneficial microorganisms into GI tract including yogurt kefir kimchi sauerkraut miso and tempeh. Fermentation processes fairly regularly introduce live beneficial microbes into the GI tract through consumption of probiotic-rich foods like kimchi and yogurt. Microbes restore balance fairly vigorously by suppressing pathogenic bacteria growth and substantially encourage mucosal immune responses deep within tissues.

Diets rich in diverse plant-based foods greatly enhance microbiota resilience which is a hallmark of a robust healthy microbiome. Probiotic supplementation possibly enhances quality of life in cancer patients by supporting immune recovery and lessening treatment-related diarrhea fairly significantly. Microbial diversity a hallmark of salubrious gut microbiota is enhanceed remarkably by diets rich in various plant-based foods and nutrients abundantly. Interventional studies alongside epidemiological research indicate that eating diverse plant-based foods thirty or more times weekly often correlates with heightened microbial richness and production of metabolites regulating immune function. Essential plant foods typically comprise fruits legumes whole grains various nuts seeds and herbs very much everywhere around the world. Collectively these dietary tactics facilitate restoration of mucosal immunity and modulate inflammatory responses vital for post-cancer recovery success (Conlon and Bird, 2014).

5.4. Anti-Inflammatory Dietary Patterns

Malignancy itself and grueling treatments such as chemotherapy and radiation therapy often bequeath cancer survivors with nagging low-grade inflammation quite persistently. Sustained inflammation severely hampers immune reconstitution and fuels profound fatigue alongside cognitive dysfunction while driving cancer recurrence and sundry comorbidities including cardiovascular disease. Dietary changes offer a promising non-pharmacological strategy mitigating systemic inflammation and reinstating immune homeostasis slowly in cancer survivors after treatment. Bioactive compounds and certain dietary patterns suppress pro-inflammatory signaling pathways like NF-κB and COX-2 effectively downregulating inflammatory cytokines such as TNF-α (Walker et al, 2022).

Key anti-inflammatory dietary tactics involve emphasis on long-chain omega-3 polyunsaturated fatty acids with inflammation-resolving properties notably EPA and DHA becomes: Dietary tactics for reducing inflammation heavily rely on long-chain omega-3 polyunsaturated fatty acids like EPA and DHA remarkably. They vigorously suppress synthesis of pro-inflammatory eicosanoids and cytokines whilst promoting formation of peculiar pro-resolving mediators quite effectively. Fatty fish such as salmon or mackerel are primary dietary sources rich in certain nutrients alongside flaxseeds chia seeds and walnuts (Walker et al, 2022).

A diet packed with vibrantly colored fruits and veggies provides plenty of vitamin C carotenoids flavonoids and polyphenols that act as potent antioxidants. Vibrant produce loaded with polyphenols and carotenoids serves as potent antioxidants in human diet very effectively every single day. Compounds neutralize reactive oxygen species quite effectively and reduce oxidative stress while modulating gene expression in various inflammatory responses.

Monounsaturated fats from sources like extra virgin olive oil and nuts such as almonds and walnuts support cardiovascular health and lower systemic inflammation. Turmeric rich in curcumin inhibits inflammatory markers experimentally alongside spinach kale broccoli and tomatoes; refined sugars red meats and ultra-processed foods boost production of advanced glycation end products. Consuming pro-inflammatory edibles triggers oxidative stress and activation of inflammatory pathways. Berries and citrus fruits remain crucial anti-inflammatory edibles. Replacing saturated fats with monounsaturated ones from sources like extra virgin olive oil and walnuts greatly supports overall cardiovascular health (Schwingshackl and Hoffmann, 2014). Oleocanthal a phenolic compound found in olive oil exhibits COX-inhibiting effects much like ibuprofen in certain non-steroidal anti-inflammatory pharmaceuticals. Rampant consumption of refined sugars and processed meats triggers production of advanced glycation end products and oxidative stress deep inside human body.

Foods like these tie very strongly with obesity and insulin resistance and microbial dysbiosis which ramps up inflammation significantly. Mediterranean diet exhibits profoundly anti-inflammatory effects and protective outcomes across diverse research studies observationally and sometimes interventionally. Mediterranean diet typically involves very high intake of fruits legumes whole grains and nuts with fish eaten fairly regularly using olive oil. Minimal intake of processed foods and red meat typifies this peculiar eating regimen unusually (Schwingshackl and Hoffmann, 2014). Cancer survivors prone to recurrence should perhaps avoid moderate wine intake altogether or at least not make it a regular habit. It remarkably improves inflammatory biomarkers like CRP and IL-6 and gets linked with reduced cancer mortality and enhanced life quality in survivors.

5.5. Hydration and Detoxification

Cancer survivors require multifaceted restorative interventions subsequently reviving cellular repair and metabolic homeostasis at a fairly slow pace afterwards naturally. Nutritional support and hydration facilitate crucial albeit underappreciated detoxification pathways in various bodily processes remarkably well. Both play crucial roles in encourage immune function and mitigating treatment-related toxicity thereby remarkably promoting overall homeostasis very effectively. Water plays a crucial role in virtually every bodily function ranging from cellular metabolism deeply embedded in cells to broad immunological responses often. Hydration sufficiently facilitates lymphatic circulation in cancer survivors thereby aiding transport of immune cells and waste gets cleared subsequently.

Chemotherapeutic metabolites get flushed out very effectively through renal excretion with sufficient fluid intake basically every single time. Mucosal hydration crucially maintains integrity of respiratory barriers and gastrointestinal tracts supporting first-line immune defense mechanisms effectively always. Fatigue reduction and cognitive clarity are benefits often reported by individuals (Dahlgren et al, 2021). Most adults need roughly 1.5 liters of fluid daily with adjustments made according to body size and surrounding climate conditions normally. Diluted fruit-infused water alongside herbal teas and broths can contribute significantly to total hydration needs despite water being utterly paramount. Survivors having histories of nephrotoxic treatments or ileostomies with various gastrointestinal issues may need frequent precise hydration monitoring and replenishment of electrolytes.

Detoxification happens naturally inside human bodies mainly via liver functioning and kidney processes and somewhat through gut activity and skin too. Liver very rapidly metabolizes xenobiotics through phase I and phase II detoxification mechanisms utilizing various enzymatic pathways effectively eliminating chemo drugs and dietary carcinogens. Broccoli and kale contain sulforaphane that induces glutathione S-transferase and other phase II detox enzymes very effectively in human bodies. Foods rich in such compounds ramp up diverse detoxification processes very quickly by stimulating production of various enzymes necessary for clearance. Consumption of certain veggies like cabbage and Brussels sprouts triggers upregulation of various cytochrome P450 enzymes alongside glutathione synthesis rampantly. Compounds in such foods facilitate other conjugation reactions crucial for effective elimination of toxins and promoting overall bodily well-being subsequently (Hodges and Minich, 2015).

Citrus fruits like lemons and grapefruits contain limonoids and flavonoids that significantly enhance liver enzyme activity and remarkably enhance antioxidant defenses. Green tea fairly significantly modulates immune responses and contains various catechins such as EGCG exhibiting rather potent hepatoprotective properties and anti-inflammatory effects. Garlic and onions are rich in organosulfur compounds that effectively support glutathione production and activate various enzymes very rapidly. Regular consumption of such nutrient-dense foods may very effectively enhance natural detox mechanisms and facilitate swift recovery from oxidative stress. Begin mornings with lukewarm lemony liquid stimulating gut activity and rehydrating bodily tissues very thoroughly down deep every single day. Consume sautéed or steamed cruciferous vegetables daily preferably with generous servings really quite liberally for maximal glucosinolate retention. Swap sugary fizzy beverages for green tea or herbal infusions bursting with polyphenols and remain remarkably hale effortlessly with great ease (Saini et al, 2022).

Urine color and output serve very effectively as non-invasive hydration gauges with light yellow hue signifying adequate hydration fairly obviously. Targeted nutrition fuels immune restoration effectively in cancer survivors by supporting optimal hydration whilst robustly aiding bodily detoxification processes. Simple tactics remarkably boost vitality every day and slash toxic load contributing mightily to long-term survivorship in a most significant manner.

5.6. Lifestyle Integration and Dietary Caution

Cancer survivors often turn desperately to dubious supplements or extremely restrictive diets in a frantic bid for regaining control suddenly over health. High-dose antioxidant supplementation during immune rebuilding may possibly blunt somewhat beneficial oxidative signaling required for activation of certain immune cells. Survivors must prioritize food-first tactics and rely heavily on supplements merely for medically verified deficiencies under oncology-savvy dietitians guidance. Rebuilding resilience after cancer requires deliberately altering diet drastically focusing on nutrient-dense food with anti-inflammatory properties and gut-friendly foods naturally.

A diet comprising whole foods rich in diverse plants vitamins and omega-3s offers most effective path for reconstituting immunity with ample protein. Personalized nutrition regimes coupled with medical consultations and lifestyle guidance facilitate survivors reclaiming vigor rather quickly and lowering recurrence risk substantially. Targeted nutrition incorporated into post-treatment recovery plans becomes vital very much for long-term resilience and overall health outcomes basically.

6. Balancing Macronutrients

Post-cancer recovery entails a multifaceted physiological and immunological recalibration necessitating modified support and intense psychological rehab rather simultaneously alongside targeted interventions underpinning holistic recuperation. Survivor transitioning beyond active treatment often finds nutrition crucial for long-term health and becomes effectively pivotal in prevention of recurrence. Macronutrient balance plays crucial yet haphazard roles somewhat distinctively in physiology after treatment with carbohydrates proteins and fats being vital. Something fluctuated wildly beneath surface. Proteins play a crucial role post-cancer serving as fundamental blocks regenerating tissues rapidly healing nasty wounds and encourage shaky immunity somewhat. Wound healing happens very swiftly with adequate protein consumption and tissue regeneration occurs fairly rapidly under such conditions.

Restoration of immune system entails generating crucial cytokines and immunoglobulins very rapidly for warding off nasty infection effectively. Sarcopenia frequently ensues after chemotherapy and lengthy inactivity periods yet sufficient protein intake may possibly mitigate this debilitating muscle wasting somewhat. Daily protein intake recommendations typically hover around 1.2 grams per kilogram of body weight for relatively sedentary individuals or ramp up drastically to 2.0 grams per kilogram for athletes. Lean meats eggs fish and dairy products alongside legumes quinoa nuts and other plant-based options ought to be incorporated fairly liberally. Spreading protein consumption relatively evenly across meals maximizes muscle protein synthesis and fosters functional recovery afterwards extremely effectively (Mora-Flores et al, 2023).

Complex carbs fuel bodily functions energetically and strangely gut microbes thrive on carbs chosen with foresight almost magically. Complex carbs furnish sustained energy necessary for grueling physical exertion while dietary fibre vigorously promotes gut health with remarkable efficacy. B vitamins and phytonutrients from whole foods are abundant micronutrient carriers found prevalently. Survivors should prioritize low-glycemic carbs rich in fibre such as whole grains starchy veggies legumes and certain fruits richly embedded with nutrients. High-fibre carbs deeply support microbial diversity and regulate glucose metabolism with considerable efficacy in various physiological contexts. Survivors must eat whole foods loaded with phytonutrients and B vitamins very carefully avoiding insulin resistance from processed food (Mora-Flores et al, 2023).

Dietary fat quality impacts hormonal balance deeply within bodily tissues every day and influences inflammation profoundly across various systems. Key strategies involve boosting consumption of unsaturated fats like omega-3 fatty acids from fatty fish and flaxseeds which help suppress pro-inflammatory cytokines profoundly. Fatty acids present in chia seeds and walnuts significantly enhance cardiovascular well-being and neurological health very effectively overall. Curbing consumption of saturated fats found in red meats proves crucial while doing away with trans fats lurking in ultra-processed foods altogether becomes necessary (Muskiet FAJ, 2010). Both are linked with increased systemic inflammation and metabolic issues occur subsequently.

Daily energy intake must derive around 25 to 35 percent from fat with emphasis on monounsaturated fats such as olive oil and avocado. Minimizing sources of noxious lipids is vital for overall health while polyunsaturated fats are beneficial normally in most dietary contexts. Cancer survivors' optimal macronutrient ratios vary greatly depending on numerous factors surrounding their specific condition and overall health status. Macronutrient distribution gets heavily influenced by cancer type and its peculiar stage rather quietly. Metabolic health status factors including diabetes and metabolic syndrome play a rather huge role in determining overall wellbeing somewhat irregularly nowadays (Liuet et al, 2017).

Body composition goals matter rather significantly and muscle gain alongside weight normalization is very crucial for athletic physiques apparently. Rehabilitation status must be factored in alongside activity level which remains very significant. Evidence-backed research suggests daily energy intake should comprise roughly 20 percent or maybe even 30 percent protein. Carbohydrates should comprise roughly 45-55 percent of dietary intake primarily from complex sources like whole grains and vegetables (Liuet et al, 2017). Fats ideally get consumed at around 25 percent or maybe up to 35 percent with emphasis on fairly healthy unsaturated fats. Ongoing assessment by an oncology-trained registered dietitian ensures macronutrient balance stays aligned with rapidly changing recovery goals alongside fluctuating biomarkers.

Therapeutically balancing macronutrients markedly enhances immune competence and promotes healing stabilizing metabolism in cancer survivors with greatly improved long term outcomes. Survivors proactively enhance their recovery trajectory and fortify resilience against disease by individualizing macronutrient intake with emphasis on precise timing of quality nutrients. Optimizing macronutrients ought to be incorporated into standard nutritional advisories within sweeping survivorship care blueprints and various lifestyle adjustments accordingly.

6.1. The Role of Macronutrients in Recovery and Long-Term Health

Simply incrementing a single digit utterly fails. Macronutrients serve distinct physiological functions crucial for survivors of various cancers quite vitally and remarkably effectively post treatment. Proteins are necessary partly through synthesis of immune cells for repairing tissue and regenerating muscle effectively afterwards. Grueling treatments such as chemo leave patients depleted and body mass rebuilding becomes crucial very quickly afterwards obviously.

Body's primary energy source comes from carbohydrates. Carbohydrates serve as primary energy source for various body functions fairly efficiently and fats play crucial roles in cellular signaling pathways. Excessive intake of refined carbs with high glycemic index may fuel chronic inflammation and hyperinsulinemia often linked with cancer recurrence viciously. Polyunsaturated and monounsaturated fats play crucial roles via various anti-inflammatory pathways in cellular signaling and nutrient absorption remarkably well normally.

6.2. Preserving Lean Mass and Supporting Immunity

Cancer treatment protocols often precipitate muscle wasting unnecessarily as a very dismal side effect and debilitation sets in fairly quickly. Sarcopenia has been tenuously linked to heightened fatigue and markedly impaired physical function with survival rates plummeting drastically under grave pathological influence. Protein intake remains utterly fundamental for restoring physical capacity quickly post-treatment and encourage immune function somewhat effectively afterwards generally (Lavalle et al, 2024).

Survivors typically require 1.2–1.5 grams protein per kilogram body weight daily based on their treatment regimen history and overall physical activity. Lean poultry fish and eggs dairy products like Greek yogurt legumes lentils tofu tempeh nuts and seeds are high-quality protein sources ordinarily consumed. Distributing protein fairly evenly across main meals and coupling it with resistance exercise effectively enhance muscle protein synthesis. Functional recovery is aided very effectively thereby (Lavalle et al, 2024).

6.3. Choosing for Glycemic Control and Microbiome Health

Carbohydrates serve as vital fuel but quality of carbs heavily influences numerous health outcomes negatively over an extended period rather mysteriously. Refined carbs and added sugars possibly exacerbate metabolic disturbances such as insulin resistance or systemic inflammation fairly quickly post treatment. Tumour growth and recurrence emerge rapidly inside tissues due to somewhat conducive microenvironments potentially created by these effects very quickly. Cancer survivors ought to focus on low-glycemic fibre-rich carbs from whole grains quinoa and oats legumes rich in nutrients and veggies (Clemente-Suárez et al, 2022).

Complex carbs largely furnish prolonged energy and dietary fibre thereby substantially supporting gut microbiome diversity a factor now frequently linked to immune regulation. They can chow down on root veggies such as sweet potatoes or brown rice and various fruits simultaneously every now and then. These foods very significantly enhance treatment outcomes essentially and numerous bodily functions operate fairly normally with their help. Carbohydrates should ideally make up around 45–55% of daily energy intake adjusted according to individual dietary needs and glycemic response levels (Clemente-Suárez et al, 2022).

6.4. Supporting Cellular Health and Hormonal Balance

Fat remains crucial for recovery and disease prevention in oncology nutrition despite frequently getting a terrible rep rather unfairly. Eating varied fats profoundly impacts metabolic resilience and cardiovascular risk substantially altering inflammation in many different obscure ways suddenly. After cancer treatment dietary fat intake should liberally focus on monounsaturated fats found in olive oil avocados and various types of nuts including almonds. Fatty fish such as salmon or sardines and foods like flaxseeds and walnuts contain crucial omega-3 fatty acids very much everywhere. Oils from plants like canola and flaxseed should be utilized sparingly in cooking and food preparation methods daily. Eating trans fats and loads of saturated fats found in processed meats and red meat probably harms you by fueling inflammation and spiking cholesterol levels way up. Daily calorie intake should comprise around twenty five percent fats with a marked emphasis on quality over quantity rather than sheer volume (Wang and Hu, 2017).

6.5. Individualizing Macronutrient Ratios

Cancer survivors exhibit diverse nutritional requirements and a universally applicable macronutrient ratio doesn't exist for every individual apparently. Oncology-trained registered dietitians devise scrupulously tailored nutrition plans factoring heavily in cancer stage treatment protocols and quirky metabolic variables. Breast cancer survivors on hormone therapy often benefit from eating diets with lower glycemic load and head and neck cancer survivors struggling with swallowing issues require energy-dense soft foods rich in protein.

6.6. Integrating Physical Activity and Nutrient Timing

Macronutrient balance syncs fairly synergistically with daily physical activity quite effectively every day under normal circumstances. Aerobic exercise remarkably improves body composition in frail individuals while resistance training stimulates voracious appetite with heightened insulin sensitivity. Strategic nutrient timing including post-exercise protein intake can effectively enhance muscle repair and modulate immune responses rather quietly afterwards. Small protein-rich meals eaten frequently help survivors maintain energy levels and reduce nasty gastrointestinal issues after treatment rather effectively (Ata et al, 2010).

Balancing macronutrients for cancer survivors involves a very fluid modified approach rather than some formulaic one size fits all solution. People can boost overall longevity quite remarkably by fine-tuning intake ratios of proteins carbs and fats thereby enhancing recuperation and lowering relapse risk substantially. Evidence guided strategic macronutrient intake tailored very specifically serves as a potent tool for survivors thriving vigorously after cancer treatment (Ata et al, 2010).

7. The Impact of Antioxidants and Anti-Inflammatory Foods on Recurrence Risks

Cancer recurrence risk drops drastically nowadays with growing comprehension of dietary influence across cancer care spectrum becoming utterly crucial. Antioxidants and anti-inflammatory foods markedly influence critical cellular pathways deeply implicated in tumour progression within bodily tissues chronically. Dietary factors possibly exert protective effects against recurrence and underlying biological mechanisms are explored thoroughly in this section rather meticulously.

7.1. Oxidative Stress and Inflammation in Cancer Recurrence

Cancer recurrence poses significant thorny clinical challenges; growing evidence underscores crucial roles of oxidative stress in tandem with chronic inflammatory processes. Oxidative stress arises from a drastic disparity between generation of highly reactive oxygen species and endogenous antioxidant defenses that mitigate their effects. ROS function largely as signaling molecules in various cellular processes under normal physiological conditions very much everywhere. Excessive ROS accumulation precipitated by environmental stressors or various metabolic perturbations leads to oxidative damage of nucleic acids and proteins suddenly. Genetic instability fueled by damage spawns oncogenic mutations very rapidly alongside some epigenetic alterations that rather quietly spur tumourigenesis (Reuter et al, 2010).

Chronic inflammation drastically worsens a pro-tumourigenic environment within certain tissues further. Chronic inflammation persists very slowly driven by factors like obesity and tissue injury or sometimes lingering effects of chemotherapy. Prolonged inflammatory state manifests through persistent release of pro-inflammatory cytokines like interleukin-6 and tumour necrosis factor-alpha alongside NF-κB signaling pathway getting activated suddenly. Mediators vigorously promote angiogenesis and inhibit apoptosis thereby enhancing survival of tumour cells quite invasively with increased potential for metastasis. Oxidative stress and inflammation aren't isolated phenomena but rather act synergistically within a vicious damaging cycle almost invariably. Reactive oxygen species spur transcription factors like NF-κB which crank up inflammatory cytokines ferociously and further enhance production quite vigorously (Reuter et al, 2010).

Tumour-promoting microenvironment lingers obstinately via feedback loop after initial treatment thereby heightening recurrence likelihood very significantly over prolonged periods. Researchers and practitioners alike have garnered huge interest in devising strategies rapidly that disrupt this vicious cycle lately with great fervor. Lifestyle interventions especially tweaks in diet are emerging rather rapidly as fairly promising adjuncts of conventional medical therapy nowadays. Diets rich in natural antioxidants like vitamin

C polyphenols and carotenoids may help restore redox balance effectively attenuating inflammatory cellular signaling pathways very thoroughly (Cheng et al, 2020). Nutritional approaches enhance endogenous defense systems quite effectively and reduce oxidative stress in survivors potentially lowering cancer recurrence risk. Unraveling intricate molecular machinations amidst oxidative stress and chronic inflammation remains vital very much for concocting innovative strategies preventing cancer recurrence and enhancing patient prognosis greatly under diverse circumstances.

7.2. Dietary Antioxidants: Mechanisms and Key Sources

Antioxidants crucially counter highly reactive oxygen species that ravage DNA and lipids thereby protecting bodily functions from oxidative damage very effectively. Exogenous antioxidants from dietary sources serve as critical adjuncts while endogenous systems like glutathione peroxidase maintain cellular redox. Oxidative stress frequently spikes rather dramatically in cancer survivors owing largely to cellular damage from intense therapy and stays heightened during recuperation. Various classes of dietary antioxidants remarkably fortify bodily defense systems with vitamin C acting swiftly as a water-soluble ROS scavenger (Manful et al, 2025). It robustly supports immune function and synthesizes collagen very effectively beneath layers of skin and deep within various bodily tissues.

Foods like kiwi bell peppers broccoli strawberries and citrus fruits are remarkably rich sources of essential dietary nutrients. Tocopherols and tocotrienols known collectively as vitamin E serve rather effectively as lipid-soluble antioxidants protecting cell membranes from oxidative damage. Abundant especially in seeds and whole grains it occurs copiously in various nuts and vegetable oils quite naturally. Beta-carotene and lycopene alongside lutein exhibit potent antioxidant properties predominantly in plants exhibiting remarkably vivid pigmentation. They quench singlet oxygen remarkably and modulate myriad immune responses effectively with considerable efficacy in various cellular environments (Manful et al, 2025). Vibrant fruits and veggies such as carrots and leafy greens contain abundance of compounds really beneficial for overall health apparently. Selenium functions as a cofactor for antioxidant enzymes notably glutathione peroxidase which very effectively detoxifies hydrogen peroxide and lipid hydroperoxides in human body.

Selenium occurs naturally in whole grains eggs seafood brazil-nuts and various other foods somewhat mysteriously often appearing in surprising amounts. Polyphenols comprise a diverse array of phytochemicals displaying rather potent antioxidant properties and substantial anti-inflammatory effects under most circumstances ordinarily. Flavonoids occur abundantly in green tea and onions whereas stilbenes such as resveratrol are plentiful mostly in grapes and some berries. Current research underscores benefits of whole-food sources over high-dose antioxidant supplements potentially disrupting delicate redox balance or conflicting with various cancer therapies. Whole foods richly supply antioxidants naturally bundled with fibre and sundry bioactive compounds enhancing bioavailability in a fairly synergistic manner. Cancer survivors benefit greatly from a varied diet comprising mostly plants rich in antioxidants which effectively reduces oxidative stress and supports recovery.

7.3. Anti-Inflammatory Foods and Their Role in Tumour Suppression

Chronic low-grade inflammation remains a very well-recognized factor heavily contributing to progression of various cancers gradually over long periods. Sustained inflammation within tumour microenvironment heavily promotes genetic instability and supports angiogenesis while facilitating immune evasion very effectively inhibiting apoptosis. Tumour necrosis factor-alpha fosters inflammatory conditions vigorously through activation of nuclear factor kappa B transcription factors partly alongside interleukin-1 beta cytokines. Dietary interventions modulate systemic inflammation offering a non-pharmacological tactic vigorously enhancing cancer survivorship outcomes and supporting tumour suppression (Greten and Grivennikov, 2019). Fatty fish like salmon are rich in eicosapentaenoic acid and docosahexaenoic acid which are long-chain omega-3 fatty acids very frequently down there.

Bioactive lipids effectively downregulates cyclooxygenase-2 expression inhibiting arachidonic acid metabolism strongly, and reducing production of various pro-inflammatory eicosanoids. Berries teem with polyphenolic compounds like anthocyanins and ellagic acid which inhibit TNF-α and IL-1β and various other cytokines thereby exhibiting profoundly anti-inflammatory effects. Compounds vigorously act as antioxidants inside bodily tissues reducing oxidative stress that fuels inflammation intensely damaging cells rapidly over time. Turmeric contains curcumin a polyphenol whose anti-inflammatory properties are very extensively documented in folk medicine from ancient times. Curcumin modulates key signaling pathways such as NF-κB and STAT3 thereby exerting heavy inhibitory effects on tumour growth promoting inflammation (Das UN, 2020). Folate fibre and phytochemicals abound in leafy greens like spinach and kale occurring very abundantly in such veggies quite often.

Detoxification pathways get a boost from various components that significantly amp up activity of anti-inflammatory cytokines fostering swift resolution of inflammation. Oats brown rice and quinoa are rich in dietary fibre and magnesium linked with drastically reduced levels of C-reactive protein biomarkers. Nuts like almonds and seeds such as walnuts supply healthy unsaturated fats and plant-based protein while very substantially reducing inflammation. Survivors of breast colorectal and prostate cancers often exhibit significantly enhanced quality of life after wholeheartedly embracing an extremely anti-inflammatory diet. Diets rich in plant-based foods and healthy fats curtail intake of processed items thereby offering quite a viable anti-inflammatory strategy.

7.4. Evidence Linking Antioxidants and Anti-Inflammatory Foods to Recurrence Risk

Chronic low-grade inflammation stays a fairly well-recognized factor contributing heavily to progression of various cancers gradually over lengthy time spans. Sustained inflammation within tumour microenvironment heavily promotes genetic instability and supports angiogenesis whilst facilitating extremely effective immune evasion thereby inhibiting apoptosis very effectively. Tumour necrosis factor-alpha fosters inflammatory conditions vigorously through activation of nuclear factor kappa B transcription factors partly alongside interleukin-1 beta. Dietary interventions significantly modulate systemic inflammation offering non-pharmacological tactics that enhance cancer survivorship outcomes and somewhat effectively support tumour suppression. Fatty fish such as salmon contain eicosapentaenoic acid and docosahexaenoic acid which are long-chain omega-3 fatty acids found fairly often in those waters (Zhao et al, 2021).

Bioactive lipids very effectively downregulate cyclooxygenase-2 expression inhibiting arachidonic acid metabolism strongly and reduce production of pro-inflammatory eicosanoids substantially. Berries are replete with polyphenolic compounds such as anthocyanins and ellagic acid which inhibit TNF-α IL-1β and sundry cytokines thereby exhibiting profoundly anti-inflammatory effects. Compounds act vigorously as antioxidants within bodily tissues effectively mitigating oxidative stress that intensely fuels inflammation and damages cells rapidly. Turmeric contains curcumin a polyphenol whose very extensively documented anti-inflammatory properties have roots in ancient folk medicine practices. Curcumin modulates pivotal signaling pathways like NF-κB and STAT3 thereby exerting profound inhibitory effects on tumour growth heavily promoting inflammation. Phytochemicals and folate abound remarkably in spinach and kale which occur abundantly in leafy green veggies (Das UN, 2020).

Detoxification pathways receive a considerable boost from sundry components that markedly amplify activity of anti-inflammatory cytokines thereby fostering relatively swift resolution of inflammation. Oats brown rice quinoa abound in dietary fibre magnesium ostensibly linked with drastically reduced C-reactive protein biomarker levels under certain conditions. Nuts such as almonds supply healthy unsaturated fats and plant-based protein while very substantially reducing inflammation around bodily tissues naturally everyday. Survivors of breast cancer often exhibit remarkably enhanced quality of life after adopting a decidedly anti-inflammatory diet with fervent dedication. Diets heavy in veggies and healthy fats slash consumption of processed junk thereby offering very viable anti-inflammatory effects overall.

7.5. Practical Considerations and Cautions

Dietary antioxidants and anti-inflammatory foods offer promising benefits in reducing cancer recurrence risk while several important caveats hover menacingly in the background. Antioxidant supplements overused pose primary concern nowadays globally among many experts in health sector very frequently apparently. Supplementation with high doses of isolated compounds such as vitamin E or beta-carotene has been linked to heightened mortality rates among smokers. High doses of antioxidants consumed during aggressive cancer therapy might disrupt oxidative processes underlying chemotherapy's tumour-killing effects potentially undermining radiation treatment efficacy (Wieland et al, 2021). Whole foods remain a safer somewhat more effective alternative for obtaining antioxidants and anti-inflammatory compounds very widely regarded still today. Whole foods harbour an assortment of bioactive compounds including vitamins and phytochemicals that boost nutrient uptake and fortify immunity remarkably.

Supplemental formulations laboriously mimic such an intricate natural balance and numerous studies among diverse populations show broadly protective overall effects. Oncology specialists and nutritionists should extremely effectively stress evidence-based personalized nutrition guidance for cancer survivors very strongly nowadays. Rigid dietary protocols or elimination diets may unnecessarily sometimes drastically reduce quality of life or lead to serious nutrient imbalances. Survivors ought to emphasize wildly diverse food choices very heavily and eat moderately rather than obsess over severely restrictive short-term diets (Wieland et al, 2021). A plant-forward diet rich in veggies fruits whole grains legumes nuts seeds and healthy fats from fatty fish or extra virgin olive oil provides comprehensive cellular repair support. Obviously nutrition plays a crucial role in comprehensive survivorship care alongside other vital stuff very significantly over time.

Maximal benefit stems from integrating dietary strategies with lifestyle interventions like regular physical activity and stress management alongside plenty of sleep. Eating foods rich in antioxidants and anti-inflammatory compounds daily represents a strategy with low risk for aiding recovery from various cancers. Minimally processed natural foods will stay pivotal in survivorship guidelines as grasp of diet's connection with cancer advances rapidly still. Empowering survivors with practical knowledge enhances autonomy greatly and promotes long-term well-being effectively through informed dietary choices made rather obviously.

8. Personalized Nutrition Plans for Cancer Survivors

Novel treatment methods and survivorship care gains traction slowly while breakthroughs in detection help cancer survival rates improve rapidly nowadays. Cancer survivors frequently struggle rather unpredictably with lingering maladies such as fatigue or muscle wasting and various micronutrient deficiencies too. Nutrition plays a pivotal role supporting physiological recovery remarkably well afterwards and enhances overall quality of life in a somewhat profound manner. General dietary guidelines provide a foundation for healthy eating but often fall woefully short for cancer survivors harbouring complex nutritional needs. Personalized nutrition planning offers a rather effective strategy slowly over time by integrating tumour type and various genetic predispositions with treatment modality and metabolic profile. Survivors having undergone gastrointestinal surgery often initially require a low-residue diet whereas some cancer patients might benefit from energy-dense protein-rich meals occasionally. Survivors with hormone-sensitive cancers who are overweight may require modified dietary plans emphasizing anti-inflammatory nutrients under specific conditions (Hussey et al, 2024).

Personalization enables targeted support aligning with medical goals and individual capabilities virtually always in nearly all such instances obviously. Nutrigenomic testing alongside metabolomics and gut microbiome analysis further enhances ability to tailor interventions effectively these days very remarkably. Such technologies may reveal obscure nutrient-gene interactions or microbiota imbalances that deeply influence a survivor's bodily response with certain unusual dietary patterns. Success of modified nutrition plans hinges not only on sound scientific rationale but also on sheer tenacity of survivors to follow recommendations (Hussey et al, 2024). Plans should be co-developed very practically with patients reflecting lifestyle socioeconomic circumstances and psychological readiness for significant somewhat sustainable change.

Personalized nutrition interventions remarkably enhance survivorship care frameworks substantially beyond conventional treatment protocols playing quite a vital role therein. Such plans facilitate recovery remarkably well within each person's idiosyncratic context by addressing fluctuations in metabolic requirements. Oncology professionals collaborating with behavioral health experts very much everywhere will be essential in delivering remarkably effective individualized dietary care for cancer survivors.

8.1. Rationale for Personalized Nutrition in Cancer Survivorship

Cancer survivorship involves a vast array of physiological upheaval and metabolic obstacles differing markedly across a diverse population over time. Various factors spawn these variations including cancer type stage very nasty long-term side effects and presence of comorbid conditions simultaneously. Nutritional needs fluctuate drastically during survivorship largely owing to disparate individual circumstances under wildly different environmental pressures. Tailoring nutrition strategies precisely meets diverse complex needs ensuring remarkably good long-term health outcomes afterwards normally in most cases very effectively. Cancer treatments ravage bodily functions badly and metabolism slows down drastically with severely impaired immune response and gut health suffers terribly.

Tamoxifen and similar endocrine therapies frequently precipitate considerable weight gain in breast cancer survivors fostering elevated risk of cancer recurrence. Gastrointestinal cancer survivors struggle mightily with malabsorption and altered bowel habits after undergoing brutal chemotherapy or extensive surgical resection. Such complications severely impede nutrient absorption and often result in unwarranted weight loss fatigue and diminishing life quality very gradually. Head and neck cancer survivors frequently face numerous grim hurdles such as dysphagia or xerostomia greatly impeding nutritional adequacy substantially every day. Certain individuals may require bizarrely altered sustenance or enteral nutrition support and various interventions for mitigating feeding difficulties and maintaining adequate caloric consumption effectively. Personalized nutrition planning intricately tailors dietary interventions according to each survivor's complex medical history amidst wildly varying personal circumstances.

Tailored methods guarantee nutritional interventions stay physiologically apt and simultaneously practically viable for diverse populations culturally. It enables tweaking macronutrient ratios and encourage micronutrient intake according to a survivor's fluctuating requirements amidst diverse meal schedules and eclectic food choices. Targeting specific dietary deficiencies with personalized plans remarkably enhances physical recovery and boosts immune function effectively while significantly reducing overall inflammation. Such approaches enable proactive risk reduction for secondary diseases and recurrence by addressing modifiable lifestyle factors fairly effectively very often. Surviving cancer daily makes personalized nutrition utterly necessary rather than some fancy luxury for those fighting desperately every day. Nowadays it provides a framework grounded in science that optimizes dietary care effectively in populations centered around patient needs very heterogeneously (Espinosa-Salas et al, 2025).

8.2. Key Components of Personalized Nutrition Planning

Crafting personalized nutrition plans for cancer survivors necessitates thoroughly examining various factors and making frequent adjustments over time. Key components comprise various essential parts include:

a. Medical and Treatment History

Survivor's diagnosis stage and treatment type involving surgery or nasty chemotherapy with extremely debilitating side effects must be thoroughly grasped. Patients undergoing gastrointestinal resections may require changes in fibre intake and chemotherapy induced nausea frequently necessitates bland energy dense food consumption heavily.

b. Nutritional Status Assessment

A comprehensive evaluation encompasses body weight and composition alongside lab markers like vitamin D and B12 and iron levels and appetite. Malnutrition or risk thereof can be identified with tools such as PG-SGA a subjective global assessment somewhat patient-generated.

c. Metabolic and Comorbid Profiles

Individuals beset by multiple health woes make dietary choices heavily influenced by coexisting maladies such as diabetes or kidney dysfunction. Survivors with metabolic syndrome may benefit greatly from anti-inflammatory diets rich in omega-3 fats and numerous phytonutrients very basically.

d. Lifestyle and Behavioral Factors

Daily routines and psychological ties with sustenance sway adherence to diets amidst shifting cultural predilections and spotty food availability always. Behavioral counseling may be crucial under certain circumstances for surmounting aversions to food or eating fueled by deep-seated emotions and terror of relapse.

8.3. Commonly Tailored Dietary Approaches in Survivorship

Specific dietary regimens demonstrably yield various health perks across cancer survivor demographics and get tweaked very frequently for modified clinical applications. Evidence-based frameworks act as springboards enabling clinicians tailor nutritional regimens according peculiar physiological state of survivor and multifaceted treatment goals. Something ostensibly appears awkwardly at the start. Various health practitioners highly tout Mediterranean dietary patterns for cancer survivors and people afflicted with other dreadful debilitating diseases. Mostly featuring high intake of veggies fruits whole grains legumes nuts and olive oil this diet is rich in antioxidants and fibre. Breast cancer survivors and those with colorectal or prostate cancer often subsequently experience drastically reduced rates of recurrence and mortality. Mediterranean diets are tailored meticulously for weight reduction and gut microbiota diversity enhancement alongside support for cardiovascular health generally (Ennouri et al, 2024).

Survivorship care frequently employs predominantly plant-based and vegetarian diets fostering abundant phytonutrient-rich food sources and markedly reduced systemic inflammation. Survivors with hormone-sensitive cancers or insulin resistance find these diets super useful and tweaking them for lean animal proteins is fairly easy. Omega-3 fatty acids and iron matter hugely in effectively designing such plans alongside adequate protein and vitamin B12 intake typically. Survivors with metabolic issues such as insulin resistance may benefit greatly from adopting a low-glycemic diet rich in nutrients and anti-inflammatory properties (Ennouri et al, 2024). Diets like these obsess over slashing processed food and added sugars while fixating rather fervently on whole grains and lean protein sources. Recently they have been shown fairly substantially improving metabolic biomarkers and very remarkably enhancing insulin sensitivity which lowers C-reactive protein levels.

Survivors battling cancer cachexia often linked with gastrointestinal cancers need diets dense with energy and high-quality protein to prevent muscle wasting. Plans often entail ingesting smaller meals frequently and consuming foods altered in texture alongside targeted supplementation fostering tissue reparation and upkeep of lean body mass. Dietary models get applied haphazardly in some real world situations rather infrequently. Frameworks malleable in nature get tweaked according to tolerance levels and severity of symptoms under wildly varying lifestyle constraints and demands. Flexibility very effectively ensures nutritional adequacy while encourage treatment adherence and markedly improving overall survivorship outcomes in many cases.

a. Mediterranean Diet

Survivors of breast prostate and colorectal cancer often exhibit markedly reduced cancer recurrence and mortality on diets very rich in whole grains and legumes with generous amounts of olive oil.

b. High-Protein, Energy-Dense Diets

High-protein diets help severely undernourished survivors preserve lean body mass and enhance immune function in individuals with muscle wasting. Oral nutrition supplements and frequent small meals may be necessary rather slowly under certain complicated circumstances sometimes.

c. Low-Residue or Modified Fibre Diets

Survivors having undergone bowel resections or bearing colostomies may require temporary reduction in fibre intake favoring soluble fibre rather quickly afterwards.

d. Plant-Forward, Low-Glycemic Diets

Survivors with insulin resistance often exhibit markedly improved metabolic markers and reduced inflammation on diets rich in plant-based foods low in refined carbs.

8.4. The Role of Genetics, Microbiome, and Emerging Technologies

Emerging digital health tech rapidly informs modified nutrition plans for cancer survivors backed by genomics and microbiome science nowadays effectively. Innovations enable a fairly precise understanding of individual biology over nutritional requirements and enhance recuperation post-cancer therapy quite effectively nowadays. Nutrigenomics has uncovered specific genetic polymorphisms that influence nutrient metabolism rather significantly potentially altering disease risk very drastically. Variants in MTHFR gene rather significantly impair folate metabolism potentially increasing need for some methylated folate forms very substantially. Variations within VDR gene can very significantly sway vitamin D utilization thus influencing supplementation or sun exposure recommendations rather heavily (Molla and Bitew, 2024). Gene-nutrient interactions influencing glutathione synthesis heavily impact antioxidant intake strategies supporting cellular defense in cancer survivors remarkably well afterwards.

Survivorship nutrition heavily incorporates research on gut microbiome a rapidly evolving area nowadays in various nutritional epidemiological studies. Chemotherapy or antibiotics severely disrupt microbial diversity and composition impacting immune regulation inflammation and absorption of various nutrients rather terribly in many cases. Personalized microbiome analysis can identify deficiencies in beneficial bacteria such as Lactobacillus or overabundance of nasty pathogens guiding modified therapeutic regimens quietly. Probiotics or prebiotics and fibre-rich diets might be included restoring microbial balance and enhancing production of short-chain fatty acids greatly in gut flora. Emerging tech transforms delivery of nutritional care profoundly and revolutionizes monitoring processes significantly with considerable impact on patient outcomes daily. Sleek wearable fitness monitors and quirky mobile apps for super detailed dietary tracking facilitate real-time collection of extremely valuable lifestyle data. These tools pinpoint trends in fatigue and appetite alongside gastrointestinal issues and physical exertion enabling somewhat dynamic pulls in dietary habits rather effectively.

Machine learning algorithms might greatly aid interpretation of complex datasets like genetic markers or microbiome profiles alongside food logs generating highly modified adaptive nutrition recommendations quietly. Cancer survivorship care shifts rapidly from static model to dynamic data-driven approach with these technologies, collectively being utilized. Clinicians offer precision nutrition strategies nuanced by biology and grounded deeply in lived experience of each survivor informed by genomic data.

8.5. Psychosocial and Behavioral Support in Dietary Adherence

Cancer survivorship entails profound dietary modifications grounded rather tenuously in psychological and somewhat obscure social behavioral aspects. Survivors frequently wrestle with angst regarding reoccurrence and sentiments of susceptibility amidst exasperation stemming from befuddling dietary guidance dispensed haphazardly. Motivation and self-efficacy get swayed very heavily by psychosocial factors which ultimately impacts ability to stick with dietary changes over time effectively. Effective nutrition interventions must stem from understanding survivor's lived experience very realistically within various societal contexts . Dietary recommendations must acknowledge diverse cultural norms respectfully and socioeconomic constraints slowly fostering genuinely sustainable changes in eating behavior (Mollica et al, 2025).

Unrealistic plans frequently yield poor adherence and nutritional inadequacy eventually diminishing overall quality of life drastically over time. Registered dietitians specializing quite heavily in oncology nutrition play a crucial role very much everywhere apparently in cancer treatment teams nowadays. Experts provide tailored advice grounded in data that combines personal goals with clinical considerations such as treatment side effects and comorbidities. Dietitians assist survivors in navigating baffling food choices and mitigating symptoms such as dysgeusia or gut issues while slowly gaining confidence in wholesome eating habits. Multidisciplinary collaboration greatly benefits addressing dietary adherence under various normal circumstances effectively across diverse populations somewhat surprisingly. Psychologists and behavioral therapists reinforce positive dietary habits rather quietly in anxious survivors by employing somewhat unorthodox cognitive-behavioral strategies effectively.

Physiotherapists promote physical activity synergistically improving metabolic health and appetite regulation effectively alongside exercise specialists enhancing overall psychological well-being very quietly. Primary care providers and oncology teams play an essential role vigilantly coordinating comprehensive care over time ensuring messaging remains fairly consistent. Regular follow-ups substantially reinforce changes in behavior and facilitate tweaks in nutritional plans promptly as survivors' health status fluctuates very wildly. Cancer survivors face very vexing challenges necessitating fairly thorough support centered on individual needs very regularly in their daily lives. Survivors achieve healthier dietary patterns within integrated care frameworks by getting specialized counseling on nutrition and very intensive behavioral therapy interventions often.

8.6. Monitoring and Adaptation Over Time

Cancer survivorship undergoes drastic transformation over time as shifting health priorities and rapidly changing nutritional needs remarkably collide. Personalized nutrition plans need fairly frequent revisiting and adaptation reflecting physiological status changes treatment outcomes and new comorbidities emerging slowly over time. Iterative cycles involving monitoring and adjustment remain crucial for keeping dietary strategies fairly effective and supportive of overall long term health. Survivors attend numerous follow-up appointments allowing clinicians thoroughly reevaluate drastic fluctuations in body composition caused by treatment aftereffects or rapid aging. Tracking biomarkers such as CRP and various micronutrient levels very effectively yields objective data for refining nutritional interventions in many clinical settings. Regularly tweaking dietary objectives syncs with a survivor's mercurial health status and everyday life amidst ongoing assessments. Survivors slipping into remission might stealthily shift focus from acutely handling brutal treatment aftermath toward thwarting chronic disease with vigilant efforts.

Drastic dietary changes are warranted quite frequently nowadays due to emergence of new symptoms like altered taste preferences or gastrointestinal issues. Ongoing care necessitates identifying budding hurdles fairly often within intricate scenarios and swiftly shifting healthcare environments nowadays with evolving landscapes. Psychosocial stress and financial constraints severely impact adherence requiring nuanced support as evolving food intolerances emerge somewhat problematically. Survivors taking active roles in nutritional health are empowered quite effectively by ongoing educational efforts and sundry motivational boosts nowadays. Sustained behavior change emerges gradually from updated evidence-based resources being provided alongside frequent encouragement of rigorous self-monitoring over long periods.

A lifelong component of comprehensive survivorship care involves personalized nutrition rather than some one-time gimmicky intervention obviously underscoring this dynamic patient-centered approach. Adopting this adaptive model effectively mitigates cancer recurrence risk and markedly enhances overall quality of life afterwards for patients. Personalized nutrition planning emerges nowadays as crucial aspect of holistic cancer survivorship management very much always in many such cases. Nutrition becomes an empowering tool remarkably fostering resilience in cancer survivors with meticulous ongoing monitoring and very close collaboration.

9. Conclusion

Survivorship denotes a precarious juncture in patient's odyssey necessitating meticulous attention towards protracted health quality and prophylaxis against recurrence very vigilantly. Nutrition plays a very crucial albeit somewhat modifiable role in backing these objectives as an oddly empowering factor after all. Dietary interventions grounded in evidence can enhance physiological recuperation and diminish lasting treatment sequelae thereby lowering cancer reoccurrence risk quite markedly. Survivors frequently struggle afterwards with lingering debilitating issues such as deep seated fatigue and disruption of metabolic processes. Targeted nutritional interventions enhance immune response fairly rapidly and strip away systemic inflammation with considerable efficacy ordinarily. Mediterranean dietary patterns rich in whole grains fruits legumes and nuts along with healthy fats yield significantly improved health outcomes surprisingly.

The role of Nutrition unfurls extensively into metabolic fine-tuning and epigenetic influence over pathways intimately linked with cancer development downstream. Phytochemicals alongside omega-3 fatty acids and dietary fibre foster a rather inhospitable biochemical environment for re-emergent tumour cells . Simultaneously cutting back on refined sugars and red meats helps prevent metabolic disturbances notoriously dodgy risk factors for secondary cancers. Incorporating nutrition into comprehensive care plans for survivors matters equally. Tailored nutrition guidance informed by unique risk profiles and existing health issues boosts compliance and somewhat actively emboldens recovery among participants. Registered dietitians involvement in oncology care teams quite often proves crucial and very regular follow-up ensures success of interventions.

Nutrition plays a mighty role quite deeply in cancer care continuum post-treatment where prevention and passable life quality become utterly paramount suddenly. Healthcare providers can substantially support long-term recovery in survivorship planning by adopting evidence-informed dietary patterns reducing cancer recurrence risk. Research evolves steadily and implementation of precision nutrition approaches refines strategies further remarkably ensuring survivors thrive way beyond cancer diagnoses.

References

Abbott J, Teleni L, McKavanagh D, Watson J, McCarthy AL, Isenring E. Patient-Generated Subjective Global Assessment Short Form (PG-SGA SF) is a valid screening tool in chemotherapy outpatients. Support Care Cancer. 2016 Sep;24(9):3883-7. doi: 10.1007/s00520-016-3196-0. Epub 2016 Apr 19. PMID: 27095352.

Al Harrasi SM, Al-Awaisi H, Al Balushi M, Al Balushi L, Al Kharusi S. Fear of Cancer Recurrence and Its Association with Depressive Symptoms Among Adult Omani Female Breast Cancer Survivors. Int J Womens Health. 2025 Aug 21;17:2625–35. doi: 10.2147/IJWH.S541449. PMCID: PMC12377397.

Aranow C. Vitamin D and the immune system. J Investig Med. 2011 Aug;59(6):881-6. doi: 10.2310/JIM.0b013e31821b8755. PMID: 21527855; PMCID: PMC3166406.

Ata SM, Vaishnav U, Puglisi M, Lofgren IE, Wood RJ, Volek JS, Fernandez ML. Macronutrient composition and increased physical activity modulate plasma adipokines and appetite hormones during a weight loss intervention. J Womens Health (Larchmt). 2010 Jan;19(1):139-45. doi: 10.1089/jwh.2009.1472. PMID: 20088670.

Aykan NF. Red Meat and Colorectal Cancer. Oncol Rev. 2015 Dec 28;9(1):288. doi: 10.4081/oncol.2015.288. PMID: 26779313; PMCID: PMC4698595.

Bemark M, Pitcher MJ, Dionisi C, Spencer J. Gut-associated lymphoid tissue: a microbiota-driven hub of B cell immunity. Trends Immunol. 2024 Mar;45(3):211-223. doi: 10.1016/j.it.2024.01.006. Epub 2024 Feb 23. PMID: 38402045; PMCID: PMC11227984.

Bojková, B., Winklewski, P. J., & Wszedybyl-Winklewska, M. (2020). Dietary Fat and Cancer—Which Is Good, Which Is Bad, and the Body of Evidence. International Journal of Molecular Sciences, 21(11), 4114. https://doi.org/10.3390/ijms21114114

Browning LC, Cowieson AJ. Vitamin D fortification of eggs for human health. J Sci Food Agric. 2014 May;94(7):1389-96. doi: 10.1002/jsfa.6425. Epub 2013 Nov 6. PMID: 24114770.

Cheng YQ, Wang SB, Liu JH, Jin L, Liu Y, Li CY, Su YR, Liu YR, Sang X, Wan Q, Liu C, Yang L, Wang ZC. Modifying the tumour microenvironment and reverting tumour cells: New strategies for treating malignant tumours. Cell Prolif. 2020 Aug;53(8):e12865. doi: 10.1111/cpr.12865. Epub 2020 Jun 26. PMID: 32588948; PMCID: PMC7445401.

Clemente-Suárez VJ, Mielgo-Ayuso J, Martín-Rodríguez A, Ramos-Campo DJ, Redondo-Flórez L, Tornero-Aguilera JF. The Burden of Carbohydrates in Health and Disease. Nutrients. 2022 Sep 15;14(18):3809. doi: 10.3390/nu14183809. PMID: 36145184; PMCID: PMC9505863.

Conlon MA, Bird AR. The impact of diet and lifestyle on gut microbiota and human health. Nutrients. 2014 Dec 24;7(1):17-44. doi: 10.3390/nu7010017. PMID: 25545101; PMCID: PMC4303825.

Dahlgren D, Sjöblom M, Hellström PM, Lennernäs H. Chemotherapeutics-Induced Intestinal Mucositis: Pathophysiology and Potential Treatment Strategies. Front Pharmacol. 2021 May 4;12:681417. doi: 10.3389/fphar.2021.681417. PMID: 34017262; PMCID: PMC8129190.

Das UN. Can Bioactive Lipid Arachidonic Acid Prevent and Ameliorate COVID-19? Medicina (Kaunas). 2020 Aug 19;56(9):418. doi: 10.3390/medicina56090418. PMID: 32825011; PMCID: PMC7560027.

Ebede CC, Jang Y, Escalante CP. Cancer-Related Fatigue in Cancer Survivorship. Med Clin North Am. 2017 Nov;101(6):1085-1097. doi: 10.1016/j.mcna.2017.06.007. Epub 2017 Aug 25. PMID: 28992856.

El-Saadony MT, Yang T, Korma SA, Sitohy M, Abd El-Mageed TA, Selim S, Al Jaouni SK, Salem HM, Mahmmod Y, Soliman SM, Mo'men SAA, Mosa WFA, El-Wafai NA, Abou-Aly HE, Sitohy B, Abd El-Hack ME, El-Tarabily KA, Saad AM. Impacts of turmeric and its principal bioactive curcumin on human health: Pharmaceutical, medicinal, and food applications: A comprehensive review. Front Nutr. 2023 Jan 10;9:1040259. doi: 10.3389/fnut.2022.1040259. PMID: 36712505; PMCID: PMC9881416.

Ennouri S, Daoud N, Berrazegua Y, El Benna H, Korbi S, Rachdi H, Mejri N, Labidi S, Boussen H. VARIATIONS IN DIETARY HABITS DURING CANCER TREATMENT: RESULTS OF A CROSS-SECTIONAL SURVEY. Acta Clin Croat. 2024 Apr;63(1):80-88. doi: 10.20471/acc.2024.63.01.10. PMID: 39959318; PMCID: PMC11827403.

Espinosa-Salas S, Gonzalez-Arias M. Nutrition: Micronutrient Intake, Imbalances, and Interventions. [Updated 2023 Sep 21]. In: StatPearls [Internet]. Treasure Island (FL): StatPearls Publishing; 2025 Jan-. Available from: https://www.ncbi.nlm.nih.gov/books/NBK597352/

Flore G, Deledda A, Lombardo M, Armani A, Velluzzi F. Effects of Functional and Nutraceutical Foods in the Context of the Mediterranean Diet in Patients Diagnosed with Breast Cancer. Antioxidants (Basel). 2023 Oct 11;12(10):1845. doi: 10.3390/antiox12101845. PMID: 37891924; PMCID: PMC10603973.

Freitas RDS, Campos MM. Protective Effects of Omega-3 Fatty Acids in Cancer-Related Complications. Nutrients. 2019 Apr 26;11(5):945. doi: 10.3390/nu11050945. PMID: 31035457; PMCID: PMC6566772.

Ganz PA, Kwan L, Stanton AL, Bower JE, Belin TR. Physical and psychosocial recovery in the year after primary treatment of breast cancer. J Clin Oncol. 2011 Mar 20;29(9):1101-9. doi: 10.1200/JCO.2010.28.8043. Epub 2011 Feb 7. PMID: 21300931; PMCID: PMC3083865.

Greten FR, Grivennikov SI. Inflammation and Cancer: Triggers, Mechanisms, and Consequences. Immunity. 2019 Jul 16;51(1):27-41. doi: 10.1016/j.immuni.2019.06.025. PMID: 31315034; PMCID: PMC6831096.

Hanna M, Jaqua E, Nguyen V, Clay J. B Vitamins: Functions and Uses in Medicine. Perm J. 2022 Jun 29;26(2):89-97. doi: 10.7812/TPP/21.204. Epub 2022 Jun 17. PMID: 35933667; PMCID: PMC9662251.

Hodges RE, Minich DM. Modulation of Metabolic Detoxification Pathways Using Foods and Food-Derived Components: A Scientific Review with Clinical Application. J Nutr Metab. 2015;2015:760689. doi: 10.1155/2015/760689. Epub 2015 Jun 16. PMID: 26167297; PMCID: PMC4488002.

Hossain MS, Wazed MA, Asha S, Amin MR, Shimul IM. Dietary Phytochemicals in Health and Disease: Mechanisms, Clinical Evidence, and Applications-A Comprehensive Review. Food Sci Nutr. 2025 Mar 19;13(3):e70101. doi: 10.1002/fsn3.70101. PMID: 40115248; PMCID: PMC11922683.

Huang Z, Rose AH, Hoffmann PR. The role of selenium in inflammation and immunity: from molecular mechanisms to therapeutic opportunities. Antioxid Redox Signal. 2012 Apr 1;16(7):705-43. doi: 10.1089/ars.2011.4145. Epub 2012 Jan 9. PMID: 21955027; PMCID: PMC3277928.

Hundal J, Peshin S, Ghazanfar R, Hayes S, Mansfield S, Sirotin N, Comander A. Implementing Lifestyle Medicine in Cancer Survivorship: A Narrative Review of Global Models. Am J Lifestyle Med. 2025 Jul 12:15598276251359525. doi: 10.1177/15598276251359525. Epub ahead of print. PMID: 40661669; PMCID: PMC12255655.

Hussey C, Hanbridge M, Dowling M, Gupta A. Cancer survivorship: understanding the patients' journey and perspectives on post-treatment needs. BMC Sports Sci Med Rehabil. 2024 Apr 12;16(1):82. doi: 10.1186/s13102-024-00864-y. PMID: 38605386; PMCID: PMC11010277.

Inglis JE, Lin PJ, Kerns SL, Kleckner IR, Kleckner AS, Castillo DA, Mustian KM, Peppone LJ. Nutritional Interventions for Treating Cancer-Related Fatigue: A Qualitative Review. Nutr Cancer. 2019;71(1):21-40. doi: 10.1080/01635581.2018.1513046. Epub 2019 Jan 26. PMID: 30688088; PMCID: PMC6456409.

Iqbal S, Malik ZI, Farooq U, Abid J, Shah HBU, Ahmad AMR. Consumption of Sugar Sweetened Beverages (SSBs) and Breast Cancer: A Narrative Review. Iran J Public Health. 2025 Mar;54(3):489-498. doi: 10.18502/ijph.v54i3.18242. PMID: 40330181; PMCID: PMC12051794.

Jin J, Zhu X, Deng Z, Zhang P, Xiao Y, Han H, Li Y, Li H. Protein-energy malnutrition and worse outcomes after major cancer surgery: A nationwide analysis. Front Oncol. 2023 Jan 17;13:970187. doi: 10.3389/fonc.2023.970187. PMID: 36733308; PMCID: PMC9886875.

Juul F, Vaidean G, Parekh N. Ultra-processed Foods and Cardiovascular Diseases: Potential Mechanisms of Action. Adv Nutr. 2021 Oct 1;12(5):1673-1680. doi: 10.1093/advances/nmab049. PMID: 33942057; PMCID: PMC8483964.

Kennel KA, Drake MT. Vitamin D in the cancer patient. Curr Opin Support Palliat Care. 2013 Sep;7(3):272-7. doi: 10.1097/SPC.0b013e3283640f74. PMID: 23912386; PMCID: PMC3899831.

Klobodu C, Vitolins MZ, Deutsch JM, Fisher K, Nasser JA, Stott D, Murray MJ, Curtis L, Milliron BJ. Examining the Role of Nutrition in Cancer Survivorship and Female Fertility: A Narrative Review. Curr Dev Nutr. 2024 Mar 12;8(4):102134. doi: 10.1016/j.cdnut.2024.102134. PMID: 38584676; PMCID: PMC10997918.

Kotecha R, Takami A, Espinoza JL. Dietary phytochemicals and cancer chemoprevention: a review of the clinical evidence. Oncotarget. 2016 Aug 9;7(32):52517-52529. doi: 10.18632/oncotarget.9593. PMID: 27232756; PMCID: PMC5239570.

Lavalle S, Valerio MR, Masiello E, Gebbia V, Scandurra G. Unveiling the Intricate Dance: How Cancer Orchestrates Muscle Wasting and Sarcopenia. In Vivo. 2024 Jul-Aug;38(4):1520-1529. doi: 10.21873/invivo.13602. PMID: 38936901; PMCID: PMC11215601.

Lee JG, Jang JY, Baik SM. Selenium as an Antioxidant: Roles and Clinical Applications in Critically Ill and Trauma Patients: A Narrative Review. Antioxidants (Basel). 2025 Feb 28;14(3):294. doi: 10.3390/antiox14030294. PMID: 40227249; PMCID: PMC11939285.

Liu AG, Ford NA, Hu FB, Zelman KM, Mozaffarian D, Kris-Etherton PM. A healthy approach to dietary fats: understanding the science and taking action to reduce consumer confusion. Nutr J. 2017 Aug 30;16(1):53. doi: 10.1186/s12937-017-0271-4. PMID: 28854932; PMCID: PMC5577766.

Manful CF, Fordjour E, Subramaniam D, Sey AA, Abbey L, Thomas R. Antioxidants and Reactive Oxygen Species: Shaping Human Health and Disease Outcomes. Int J Mol Sci. 2025 Aug 4;26(15):7520. doi: 10.3390/ijms26157520. PMID: 40806653; PMCID: PMC12347716.

Middha P, Weinstein SJ, Männistö S, Albanes D, Mondul AM. β-Carotene Supplementation and Lung Cancer Incidence in the Alpha-Tocopherol, Beta-Carotene Cancer Prevention Study: The Role of Tar and Nicotine. Nicotine Tob Res. 2019 Jul 17;21(8):1045-1050. doi: 10.1093/ntr/nty115. PMID: 29889248; PMCID: PMC6636175.

Mileo AM, Miccadei S. Polyphenols as Modulator of Oxidative Stress in Cancer Disease: New Therapeutic Strategies. Oxid Med Cell Longev. 2016;2016:6475624. doi: 10.1155/2016/6475624. Epub 2015 Nov 16. PMID: 26649142; PMCID: PMC4663347.

Molla G, Bitew M. Revolutionizing Personalized Medicine: Synergy with Multi-Omics Data Generation, Main Hurdles, and Future Perspectives. Biomedicines. 2024 Nov 30;12(12):2750. doi: 10.3390/biomedicines12122750. PMID: 39767657; PMCID: PMC11673561.

Mollica MA, Doose M, Reed C, Tonorezos E. Defining concepts in cancer survivorship. Cancer. 2025 Aug 15;131(16):e70039. doi: 10.1002/cncr.70039. PMID: 40810248; PMCID: PMC12351516.

Mora-Flores LP, Moreno-Terrazas Casildo R, Fuentes-Cabrera J, Pérez-Vicente HA, de Anda-Jáuregui G, Neri-Torres EE. The Role of Carbohydrate Intake on the Gut Microbiome: A Weight of Evidence Systematic Review. Microorganisms. 2023 Jun 30;11(7):1728. doi: 10.3390/microorganisms11071728. PMID: 37512899; PMCID: PMC10385781.

Munteanu C, Schwartz B. The relationship between nutrition and the immune system. Front Nutr. 2022 Dec 8;9:1082500. doi: 10.3389/fnut.2022.1082500. PMID: 36570149; PMCID: PMC9772031.

Muscogiuri G, Verde L, Sulu C, Katsiki N, Hassapidou M, Frias-Toral E, Cucalón G, Pazderska A, Yumuk VD, Colao A, Barrea L. Mediterranean Diet and Obesity-related Disorders: What is the Evidence? Curr Obes Rep. 2022 Dec;11(4):287-304. doi: 10.1007/s13679-022-00481-1. Epub 2022 Sep 30. PMID: 36178601; PMCID: PMC9729142.

Muskiet FAJ. Pathophysiology and Evolutionary Aspects of Dietary Fats and Long-Chain Polyunsaturated Fatty Acids across the Life Cycle. In: Montmayeur JP, le Coutre J, editors. Fat Detection: Taste, Texture, and Post Ingestive Effects. Boca Raton (FL): CRC Press/Taylor & Francis; 2010. Chapter 2. Available from: https://www.ncbi.nlm.nih.gov/books/NBK53557/

Pati S, Irfan W, Jameel A, Ahmed S, Shahid RK. Obesity and Cancer: A Current Overview of Epidemiology, Pathogenesis, Outcomes, and Management. Cancers (Basel). 2023 Jan 12;15(2):485. doi: 10.3390/cancers15020485. PMID: 36672434; PMCID: PMC9857053.

Pawlowska E, Szczepanska J, Blasiak J. Pro- and Antioxidant Effects of Vitamin C in Cancer in correspondence to Its Dietary and Pharmacological Concentrations. Oxid Med Cell Longev. 2019 Dec 24;2019:7286737. doi: 10.1155/2019/7286737. PMID: 31934267; PMCID: PMC6942884.

Peixoto da Silva S, Santos JMO, Costa E Silva MP, Gil da Costa RM, Medeiros R. Cancer cachexia and its pathophysiology: links with sarcopenia, anorexia and asthenia. J Cachexia Sarcopenia Muscle. 2020 Jun;11(3):619-635. doi: 10.1002/jcsm.12528. Epub 2020 Mar 6. PMID: 32142217; PMCID: PMC7296264.

Philip EJ, Merluzzi TV. Psychosocial issues in post-treatment cancer survivors: Desire for support and challenges in identifying individuals in need. J Psychosoc Oncol. 2016 May-Jun;34(3):223-39. doi: 10.1080/07347332.2016.1157716. Epub 2016 Mar 3. PMID: 26939620; PMCID: PMC4961683.

Polak R, Phillips EM, Campbell A. Legumes: Health Benefits and Culinary Approaches to Increase Intake. Clin Diabetes. 2015 Oct;33(4):198-205. doi: 10.2337/diaclin.33.4.198. PMID: 26487796; PMCID: PMC4608274.

Reis F, Ferreira LMR, Ortega E, Viana S. Nutrition and Gut Microbiota-Immune System Interplay in Chronic Diseases. Nutrients. 2025 Apr 11;17(8):1330. doi: 10.3390/nu17081330. PMID: 40284195; PMCID: PMC12030219.

Reuter S, Gupta SC, Chaturvedi MM, Aggarwal BB. Oxidative stress, inflammation, and cancer: how are they linked? Free Radic Biol Med. 2010 Dec 1;49(11):1603-16. doi: 10.1016/j.freeradbiomed.2010.09.006. Epub 2010 Sep 16. PMID: 20840865; PMCID: PMC2990475.

Rondinella D, Raoul PC, Valeriani E, Venturini I, Cintoni M, Severino A, Galli FS, Mora V, Mele MC, Cammarota G, Gasbarrini A, Rinninella E, Ianiro G. The Detrimental Impact of Ultra-Processed Foods on the Human Gut Microbiome and Gut Barrier. Nutrients. 2025 Feb 28;17(5):859. doi: 10.3390/nu17050859. PMID: 40077728; PMCID: PMC11901572.

Saini RK, Ranjit A, Sharma K, Prasad P, Shang X, Gowda KGM, Keum YS. Bioactive Compounds of Citrus Fruits: A Review of Composition and Health Benefits of Carotenoids, Flavonoids, Limonoids, and Terpenes. Antioxidants (Basel). 2022 Jan 26;11(2):239. doi: 10.3390/antiox11020239. PMID: 35204122; PMCID: PMC8868476.

Schwingshackl L, Hoffmann G. Monounsaturated fatty acids, olive oil and health status: a systematic review and meta-analysis of cohort studies. Lipids Health Dis. 2014 Oct 1;13:154. doi: 10.1186/1476-511X-13-154. PMID: 25274026; PMCID: PMC4198773.

Sharma A, Jasrotia S, Kumar A. Effects of Chemotherapy on the Immune System: Implications for Cancer Treatment and Patient Outcomes. Naunyn Schmiedebergs Arch Pharmacol. 2024 May;397(5):2551-2566. doi: 10.1007/s00210-023-02781-2. Epub 2023 Oct 31. PMID: 37906273.

Shreiner AB, Kao JY, Young VB. The gut microbiome in health and in disease. Curr Opin Gastroenterol. 2015 Jan;31(1):69-75. doi: 10.1097/MOG.0000000000000139. PMID: 25394236; PMCID: PMC4290017.

Singh K, Bhori M, Kasu YA, Bhat G, Marar T. Antioxidants as precision weapons in war against cancer chemotherapy induced toxicity - Exploring the armoury of obscurity. Saudi Pharm J. 2018 Feb;26(2):177-190. doi: 10.1016/j.jsps.2017.12.013. Epub 2017 Dec 19. PMID: 30166914; PMCID: PMC6111235.

Skrajnowska D, Bobrowska-Korczak B. Role of Zinc in Immune System and Anti-Cancer Defense Mechanisms. Nutrients. 2019 Sep 22;11(10):2273. doi: 10.3390/nu11102273. PMID: 31546724; PMCID: PMC6835436.

Testino G. The burden of cancer attributable to alcohol consumption. Maedica (Bucur). 2011 Oct;6(4):313-20. PMID: 22879847; PMCID: PMC3391950.

Thong MSY, van Noorden CJF, Steindorf K, Arndt V. Cancer-Related Fatigue: Causes and Current Treatment Options. Curr Treat Options Oncol. 2020 Feb 5;21(2):17. doi: 10.1007/s11864-020-0707-5. Erratum in: Curr Treat Options Oncol. 2022 Mar;23(3):450-451. doi: 10.1007/s11864-021-00916-2. PMID: 32025928; PMCID: PMC8660748.

Thun MJ, DeLancey JO, Center MM, Jemal A, Ward EM. The global burden of cancer: priorities for prevention. Carcinogenesis. 2010 Jan;31(1):100-10. doi: 10.1093/carcin/bgp263. Epub 2009 Nov 24. PMID: 19934210; PMCID: PMC2802672.

Tokarczyk, J., & Koch, W. (2025). Dietary Zn—Recent Advances in Studies on Its Bioaccessibility and Bioavailability. Molecules, 30(13), 2742. https://doi.org/10.3390/molecules30132742

Walker AK, Chan RJ, Vardy JL. Sustained Mild Inflammation in Cancer Survivors: Where to from Here? JNCI Cancer Spectr. 2022 Jul 1;6(4):pkac054. doi: 10.1093/jncics/pkac054. PMID: 35900189; PMCID: PMC9420042.

Wang DD, Hu FB. Dietary Fat and Risk of Cardiovascular Disease: Recent Controversies and Advances. Annu Rev Nutr. 2017 Aug 21;37:423-446. doi: 10.1146/annurev-nutr-071816-064614. Epub 2017 Jun 23. PMID: 28645222.

Wieland LS, Moffet I, Shade S, Emadi A, Knott C, Gorman EF, D'Adamo C. Risks and benefits of antioxidant dietary supplement use during cancer treatment: protocol for a scoping review. BMJ Open. 2021 Apr 13;11(4):e047200. doi: 10.1136/bmjopen-2020-047200. PMID: 33849858; PMCID: PMC8051392.

Zhao H, Wu L, Yan G, Chen Y, Zhou M, Wu Y, Li Y. Inflammation and tumour progression: signaling pathways and targeted intervention. Signal Transduct Target Ther. 2021 Jul 12;6(1):263. doi: 10.1038/s41392-021-00658-5. PMID: 34248142; PMCID: PMC8273155.

Chapter 13

Precision Nutrition in Oncology: Genetic, Lifestyle, and Individualized Approaches

Sheetanshu Gupta[1], Praneeth Juvvi[2], Lokesh Kumar Mishra[3*], and Ng. Joykumar Singh[4]

[1]Department of Food Safety and Quality Assurance, College of Food Technology, Central Agricultural University (CAU), Imphal, Manipur, India
[2]Department of Food Processing Technology, College of Food Technology-Central Agricultural University, Imphal, Manipur, India
[3]Department of BPME, College of Agriculture, Central Agricultural University (CAU), Imphal, Manipur, India
[4]Department of Food Process Engineering, College of Food Technology, Central Agricultural University (CAU), Imphal, Manipur, India

Abstract

Precision oncology nutrition signifies a profoundly impactful paradigm shift in cancer therapeutics, underscoring modified dietary regimens substantiated by genomic analysis and nuanced tumour morphology. Genomics, alongside epigenetics, is investigated very thoroughly for optimizing cancer treatment via highly tailored nutritional interventions with personalized health info. Genetic factors heavily influence metabolic pathways under specific conditions and play a crucial role in individual responses to various nutrients. This highlights the importance of genomic profiling very closely in identifying dietary needs for cancer patients harbouring super-specific genetic predispositions. Holistically, it addresses facets like stress, sleep and physical activity in modulating treatment response and cancer risk fairly precisely within nutrition. Modified diets vigorously attack cancer cell energetics and inflammation within tumour ecosystems, unfolding novel research into tumour-specific metabolic susceptibilities, augmenting standard treatments. Nutrigenomics probes quite deeply into interactions between nutrients and genes, thereby advancing cancer treatment via highly personalised dietary regimens that enhance immune response, rather effectively nowadays. Precision nutrition's oncology potential flourishes rapidly, leveraging cutting-edge research and some gutsy real-world clinical examples that emphasise highly efficacious modified cancer strategies for prevention and survivorship.

Keywords: Nutrigenomics, Personalized Nutrition, Genetic Profiling, Epigenetics, Cancer Metabolism, Lifestyle Interventions

DOI: 10.1201/9781042010387-13

1. Introduction

Cancer care lately has entered an era of unprecedented advances with therapies evolving rapidly into remarkably targeted highly personalized treatments. Precision nutrition emerges rapidly as a vital oncology strategy alongside precision medicine tailoring treatment specifically according to individual disease characteristics of each patient. Recognition that dietary factors profoundly influence cancer development progression response to treatment and survivorship has lately spurred fairly rapid integration of nutrition into precision medicine. Precision nutrition in oncology gets significantly impacted by genetic predisposition and lifestyle choices substantially reducing cancer recurrence and improving patient outcomes (Rituraj et al, 2025). Precision nutrition involves highly tailored dietary plans influenced largely by an individual's unique genetic profile and various complex environmental factors.

Nutrigenomics evolves quickly with study of gene-diet interactions and clinicians increasingly recognize nutrition doesn't work uniformly for every individual. Nutrition should be meticulously tailored for each cancer patient factoring in their unique genetic makeup and lifestyle habits optimizing health outcomes during treatment. Precision nutrition takes into account genetic quirks and metabolic nuances in individuals much like oncology therapies target specific cancerous cell mutations heavily. Genetic factors profoundly modulate nutrient metabolism remarkably well in individuals and bodily responses vary greatly with specific dietary regimens. Genetic variants profoundly affect absorption of micronutrients such as vitamin D and folate which play crucial roles in preventing various cancers. DNA sequence variations that tweak enzyme function crucial for metabolizing specific dietary components drastically sway cancer risk and therapeutic outcomes very significantly (Farhud et al, 2010).

Personalized dietary regimens devised by clinicians enhance nutrient uptake and metabolic processes furnishing cancer sufferers requisite nutrients and mitigating disease progression quite effectively. People with certain genetic quirks affecting folate metabolism might display a wonky ability to synthesize or use this nutrient so crucial for DNA mending. Such individuals may benefit greatly from increased folate intake or supplementation potentially reducing cancer risk significantly or subsequent recurrence very substantially. Methylenetetrahydrofolate reductase gene polymorphisms may necessitate fastidious monitoring of folate levels lest excessive supplementation somewhat heightens risk of cancer. Genetic profiling enables clinicians intricately tailor dietary interventions optimizing nutrient intake largely according to each patient's peculiar genetic signature (Singar et al, 2024).

Probing gut microbiota within cancer nutrition reveals another deeply complex stratum lurkining eerily beneath surface level in a rather convoluted manner. Trillions of microbes inhabit gut microbiome, playing crucial role in digestion heavily influenced by various dietary habits and affecting overall metabolism quite significantly. Gut microbiome profoundly influences cancer therapy response including chemotherapy and immunotherapy by significantly modulating dietary component metabolism (Ağagündüz et al, 2023). Precision nutrition effectively factors interactions between dietary patterns and gut microbiome rather astutely heightening treatment efficacy whilst somewhat mitigating heinous adverse effects. Probing interactions between probiotics and microbiome sheds considerable light on modified regimens for markedly ameliorating cancer patient outcomes with dietary fibres.

Precision nutrition involves lifestyle behaviors such as physical activity or stress management and various genetic factors alongside very crucial microbial influences. Physical activity markedly improves treatment outcomes in cancer patients and reduces fatigue substantially enhancing immune function remarkably. Modified exercise regimens coupled with tailored nutrition plans mitigate severe weight loss associated with cachexia fairly effectively overall in most cases. Bodily inflammatory responses often dysregulated in cancer patients are mercifully nowadays very significantly influenced by various stress management techniques and good sleep hygiene (Chen et al, 2025). Mind-body therapies like meditation or yoga can naturally enhance metabolism and significantly improve patient quality of life alongside an anti-inflammatory dietary regimen.

Oncology precision nutrition puts great emphasis on thwarting cancer recurrence through highly individualized dietary plans very obviously. Tumour recurrence poses significant challenges post-treatment and nutrition substantially impacts key pathways involved in cancer regrowth these days rather markedly. Phytonutrient-rich diets comprising fruits vegetables and whole grains modulate cellular signaling pathways and epigenetic changes very effectively reducing cancer recurrence. Vitamin D and omega-3 fatty acids in green tea and various berries significantly inhibit tumour angiogenesis and cell proliferation very effectively. Nutrient-rich dietary regimens rather specifically tailored around genetic makeup may thwart cancer reoccurrence and foster survivorship extremely effectively long-term (Reglero et al, 2019). Precision nutrition involves much more than dietary selections or mere food choices with subtleties and complexities inherently embedded. Nutrient intake timing has rather swiftly emerged as consideration quite naturally in some specific contexts lately.

Harmonizing nutrient intake intricately with bodily circadian rhythms involves aligning dietary strategies quite meticulously throughout day and metabolic processes. Studies emerging recently suggest that timing of meals and composition of diet eerily influence metabolism of cancer cells and sensitivity to insulin. Intermittent fasting or time-restricted eating has been shown very effectively encourage metabolic health and may potentially supercharge various cancer therapies rapidly. Precision nutrition might entail incorporating temporal factors thereby furnishing an additional stratum of personalization in modified nutrition regimens supporting cancer care effectively nowadays (Reytor-González et al, 2025). Precision nutrition's intricacies necessitate a very complex strategy in clinical oncology practice fusing expertise of oncologists and metabolic specialists with skilled nutritionists. Skilled practitioners will craft highly tailored nutrition plans informed heavily by genomic analysis and meticulous clinical evaluation under constant patient surveillance.

Genetic sequencing and microbiome profiling offer valuable insights into modified dietary strategies for cancer patients thereby ensuring more holistic cancer care nowadays. Precision oncology nutrition relies heavily on genetic variances somewhat and sundry lifestyle factors informing highly modified dietary strategies that greatly enhance cancer treatment outcomes. Nutrition can be effectively tailored for specific cancer patient needs at various disease stages from prevention through treatment and long-term survivorship. Precision nutrition has a profound impact on cancer care by offering novel pathways that enhance patient health significantly and reduce recurrence overall.

2. Precision Nutrition

Recently cancer care underwent a profound transformation shifting from uniform protocols and embracing personalized approaches tailored around each patient's molecular characteristics. Profound insights into tumour heterogeneity and variability were gained through advances in genomic sequencing and integrative systems biology alongside biomarker profiling. Precision nutrition emerges dynamically alongside developments in personalized medicine integrating genetic and environmental data into dietary recommendations very effectively nowadays. Precision nutrition acknowledges effects of diet on cancer risk progression and survivorship gets modulated intricately by complex gene-nutrient interactions. Genetic polymorphisms deeply affect cellular nutrient metabolism thereby starkly altering individual nutritional needs and susceptibility to carcinogenic diet-related effects rather variably.

Genetic variations like those found in MTHFR hugely impact one-carbon metabolism pathways crucial for DNA synthesis and encourage post-treatment recovery. Gut microbiome significantly modulates inflammation and immune function impacting cancer outcomes variably within diverse ecosystems thereby playing a crucial role. Microbial composition discrepancies significantly impact bioavailability of dietary nutrients and modulate metabolic pathways or immune responses to various chemo agents. Microbiome profiling integration enhances nutritional planning efficacy significantly and mitigates side effects effectively through highly tailored interventions. Epigenetic mechanisms variably shape gene expression alongside psychosocial stressors while lifestyle and toxin exposure heavily influence overall nutritional status (Coppedè et al, 2019).

Precision nutrition integrates multidimensional data creating highly individualized dietary strategies for cancer prevention and enhances therapeutic response rather effectively. Precision nutrition nowadays very effectively offers a biologically informed framework optimizing nutrient intake according to each survivor's genetic makeup uniquely (Coppedè et al, 2019). Modified dietary guidance complements cancer care effectively nowadays and this approach holds promise for vastly improving patient outcomes.

2.1. The Rationale behind Precision Nutrition in Oncology

Cancer manifests fundamentally as a genetic disorder characterized by accumulation of somatic mutations and aberrant signaling pathways governing various crucial cellular processes erratically. Genetic alterations intricately define tumour phenotype and aggressiveness while shaping interindividual differences variably in metabolic pathways under diverse environmental influences. Tumour and host genetic landscapes heavily influence nutritional needs and susceptibility under various diet-related influences on cancer progression quite variably. Genetic polymorphisms intricately exemplify complex nutrient metabolism pathway interplay beneath diverse physiological conditions usually found normally in human bodies. Methylenetetrahydrofolate reductase encoded by MTHFR gene variants powerfully affects folate metabolic pathways deeply intertwined with DNA synthetic processes and methylation (Rivlin et al, 2011).

Genomic instability emerges rather haphazardly from gross deficiencies or aberrant activity rooted in various polymorphisms thereby modifying cancer risk significantly and altering bodily responses to dietary folate supplementation quite dramatically. Variations in vitamin D receptor gene tremendously affect downstream oncogenesis and immune response hugely through altered vitamin D signaling and binding. Variants in genes encoding glutathione S-transferase enzymes such as GSTP1 heavily influence detoxification capacity and awkwardly neutralize reactive oxygen species generated by endogenous metabolism or cancer therapies rather effectively (Rivlin et al, 2011). Traditional dietary guidelines often adopt a one-size-fits-all approach crudely doling out fairly broad nutrient recommendations for sundry populations with underlying genetic differences largely ignored. Guidelines like these possess significant value for public health but may utterly fail accounting for highly personalized nutrient needs influencing cancer risk outcomes drastically. Precision nutrition endeavors bridge this chasm by merging genetic quirks epigenetic markers and metabolic intricacies quite intricately tailoring modified dietary regimens that rather quietly heighten nutrient potency and minimize deleterious outcomes somewhat effectively. Precision nutrition rather effectively enhances therapeutic outcomes by tailoring nutritional strategies around a survivor's biological idiosyncrasies and modulating cancer-related pathways very specifically. Genetically informed approaches herald a new paradigm promising more efficacious supportive oncology care with targeted nutritional precision rather than generic dietary advice.

2.2. Key Genetic Influences on Nutrient Metabolism and Cancer Risk

Genetic variation profoundly influences cancer susceptibility by shaping individual differences in nutrient metabolism and altering bioavailability significantly. Gene-nutrient interactions knowledge furnishes bedrock for modified nutrition strategies squarely targeting cancer prevention or occasionally efficacious management downstream. Methylenetetrahydrofolate reductase gene polymorphisms have been scrutinized thoroughly involving variations harbouring profound physiological ramifications generally in many research studies. MTHFR encodes an enzyme crucially needed for conversion of folate into biologically active 5-methyltetrahydrofolate that participates heavily in DNA methylation processes (Elsamanoudyet al, 2016). Variants like C677T and A1298C drastically impair enzyme activity resulting in markedly elevated homocysteine levels and gross impairment of DNA repair mechanisms occurs.

Alterations can quite dramatically heighten vulnerability to genetic damage and cancer forms rapidly in tissues with swift cell division. MTHFR variants render folate intake critically important so diets rich in folate or supplementation serve as crucial preventive measures for those individuals. Vitamin D receptor gene contains polymorphisms that fairly significantly influence numerous signaling pathways modulating cellular differentiation and apoptosis downstream of immune surveillance. Variants like FokI BsmI and TaqI significantly alter receptor functionality and mess very badly with vitamin D metabolic pathways for cancer. Vitamin D recommendations molded around genetic makeup may significantly amplify protective effects against cancer progression and tumour growth quite effectively. GSTP1 enzyme variability in GST family alters capacity quite significantly to neutralize reactive oxygen species and various carcinogens (Elsamanoudyet al, 2016).

Polymorphic GST activity being knocked out or severely diminished heightens susceptibility to DNA damage triggered by oxidative stress very badly. Antioxidant-rich dietary interventions supplemented with certain phytochemicals may rather effectively support individuals possessing specific GST genotypes these days. Genetic variations profoundly impact metabolism of nutrients such as vitamin B12 or selenium and polyunsaturated fatty acids crucial for DNA integrity. Genetic polymorphisms influencing selenium metabolism can significantly heighten cancer risk by altering selenoprotein activity and impairing antioxidant defenses profoundly (Kadıoğlu et al, 2016). Clinicians tailor dietary recommendations effectively by integrating genomic data into nutritional planning and mitigating various risk factors with optimized nutrient intake. Precision approaches offering targeted interventions that reflect biological individuality of cancer survivors move far beyond generic dietary advice very effectively these days.

a. MTHFR and Folate Pathway

Methylenetetrahydrofolate reductase gene encodes an enzyme that catalyzes conversion of 5,10-methylenetetrahydrofolate into 5-methyltetrahydrofolate crucial for homocysteine remethylation and DNA methylation subsequently. Genomic stability relies heavily on reaction for proper nucleotide synthesis and epigenetic regulation occurs largely through strongly intricate cellular mechanisms. Specific polymorphisms inside MTHFR gene namely C677T and A1298C variants drastically curtail enzyme activity significantly within humans fairly often. C677T variant substantially lowers MTHFR function especially when in homozygous state resulting in seventy percent decrease in availability of methylated folate (Elsamanoudyet al, 2016). Deficiency severely disrupts DNA methylation patterns resulting in hypomethylation and genome instability linked intricately with carcinogenesis development mechanisms.

MTHFR polymorphisms are associated with increased risks of colorectal and breast cancer in individuals with low folate status or deficient in certain B vitamins. Impaired folate metabolism can badly exacerbate DNA damage in populations thereby vigorously promoting tumour initiation and significantly reducing repair capacity. Methylated folate supplementation may vastly boost bioavailability in folks carrying rare MTHFR variants instead of using synthetic folic acid. Optimal folate function gets supported by sufficiently ingesting cofactors like vitamin B6 and B12 involved in one-carbon metabolism thereby significantly lowering cancer risk (Elsamanoudyet al, 2016). Personalized nutrition plans leveraging MTHFR genotyping facilitate modified dietary adjustments tackling genetic anomalies in folate metabolism possibly mitigating oncogenic risks.

b. Vitamin D Receptor (VDR) Polymorphisms

Nuclear hormone receptor gets encoded by vitamin D receptor gene and mediates vitamin D's effects very effectively by regulating gene expression involved in cellular proliferation. Vitamin D exerts anticancer effects by promoting cellular differentiation quite effectively in tumour cells while inducing apoptosis and modulating inflammatory responses. Genetic polymorphisms within VDR gene remarkably alter receptor function under specific physiological conditions and significantly influence downstream signaling pathways. Notable variants such as FokI alter VDR protein structure modulating vitamin D binding affinity very significantly with expression altered drastically downstream. Numerous studies have fairly consistently linked variable vitamin D responsiveness among individuals with polymorphisms in quite diverse populations already. Tenuous epidemiological evidence links certain VDR genotypes very strongly with increased susceptibility to various cancers including prostate cancer breast cancer and colorectal cancer (Haussler et al, 2010).

Certain VDR variants correlate with diminished receptor activity and facilitate carcinogenesis swiftly by impairing cell cycle control regulation thereby fostering tumour progression. Vitamin D supplementation strategies tailored around VDR genotype and serum 25-hydroxyvitamin D levels may optimize status very effectively meanwhile. Tailoring vitamin D intake according some individual genetic profiles might rather effectively improve immune regulation and inhibit tumour cell proliferation markedly (Haussler et al, 2010). Incorporating VDR genotyping into precision nutrition frameworks yields efficacious dietary support for refining vitamin D-related cancer prevention interventions effectively.

c. Glutathione S-Transferases (GSTs)

Glutathione S-transferases effectively safeguard cells from oxidative damage and sundry carcinogenic compounds with considerable efficacy in myriad instances. Enzymes catalyze conjugation of glutathione a tripeptide antioxidant with electrophilic toxins thereby facilitating their rather efficient neutralization and subsequent excretion. GST activity detoxifies reactive oxygen species and environmental carcinogens like polycyclic aromatic hydrocarbons with considerable efficacy under various physiological conditions. GSTP1 GSTM1 and GSTT1 are extensively studied isoforms in relation cancer susceptibility. Single nucleotide variants or gene deletions kinda result in drastically reduced enzyme activity and sometimes complete absence occurs entirely (Mazari et al, 2023).

GSTP1 Ile105Val polymorphism somewhat markedly impairs enzyme catalytic efficiency while homozygous deletions of GSTM1 and GSTT1 genes result in total abrogation of function. Individuals possessing specific genetic mutations exhibit markedly diminished capacity to detoxify carcinogenic substances and frequently fall prey to environmentally induced cancers. Compromised GST function may debilitate cellular defenses against oxidative stress unleashed by chemotherapy and radiation therapy vitiating efficacy of treatment potentially. Certain nutritional adjustments might assuage such hazards very effectively in some cases with varying degrees of success naturally (Mazari et al, 2023). Broccoli and kale contain sulforaphane which induces phase II detoxification enzymes richly in human body under certain conditions.

Phytochemicals present in certain veggies very significantly crank up antioxidant defenses by activating Nrf2 pathway. Sulforaphane and other isothiocyanates rather effectively promote clearance of carcinogens by inducing various GSTs and some other enzymes quite rapidly. People with GST polymorphisms might gain some protective effects heavily from eating sulforaphane-rich foods by boosting residual detox mechanisms and lessening oxidative stress significantly. Personalized nutrition plans incorporating GST genotypes can prioritize higher intake of cruciferous veggies and antioxidant-rich foods thereby strengthening detoxification pathways (Mazari et al, 2023).

2.3. Nutrigenomics and Nutrigenetics in Clinical Cancer Care

Precision oncology nutrition gets undergirded by two closely related albeit distinct disciplines namely somewhat esoteric nutrigenomics and fairly recondite nutrigenetics essentially. Such disciplines cultivate profoundly nuanced understandings of cancer biology interactions with genetic predispositions and dietary patterns allowing much targeted therapeutic interventions effectively nowadays. Nutrigenomics heavily probes influence of nutrients and bioactive dietary compounds on gene expression including genes implicated quite heavily in cancer. Dietary components drastically recalibrate transcription factors and epigenetic marks such as DNA methylation or histone mods altering chromatin structure significantly (Thompson et al, 2023). Curcumin a polyphenol abundant in turmeric and resveratrol found mostly in grapes and red wine modulate expression of several oncogenes effectively.

Compounds like these inhibit signaling pathways such as NF-κB or STAT3 and PI3K/Akt thereby reducing inflammation cell proliferation quite significantly and angiogenesis occurs less. Cancer cells exhibit disrupted gene expression patterns which various quirky epigenetic mechanisms restore very effectively these days with some success normally. Such modulation potentially sensitizes tumours towards conventional therapies and improves treatment response significantly reducing nasty side effects dramatically afterwards. Nutrigenetics examines influence of inherited genetic variations on individual responses to diverse dietary components in markedly different ways sometimes (Thompson et al, 2023). Single nucleotide polymorphisms and other genetic variations often markedly alter efficacy or induce toxicity by influencing absorption rates of various nutrients very frequently.

Genetic variations like MTHFR, VDR, and GSTP1 polymorphisms can slowly influence wildly different nutrient requirements or odd sensitivities, guiding super personalised diet plans over time naturally. Nutrigenetics helps identify patients likely to benefit from customised dietary plans or targeted supplements and potentially harmed by certain nutrient intakes. Nutrigenomic data alongside nutrigenetic info gets integrated into oncology practice, enabling clinicians design highly modified dietary regimens with targeted therapeutics very precisely. Such novel approaches rather effectively alleviate treatment-related side effects nowadays while potentially improving tumour responsiveness under systemic inflammation reduction therapy (Kianiet al, 2022). Precision nutrition enables highly tailored cancer care nowadays by leveraging genetic data and molecular insights very effectively in clinical settings.

2.4. Microbiome-Genetics-Diet Interactions in Cancer

Trillions of microorganisms inhabit gastrointestinal tracts and have surfaced as pivotal modulators of immune function and response mechanisms for cancer therapy. Intricate interactions between microbiome and host genetics, alongside dietary factors, hugely influence cancer progression, treatment efficacy and survivorship outcomes quite significantly. Host genetic variations, particularly in genes governing mucosal immunity, such as NOD2, modulate gut microbiota composition, significantly altering functional capacity. Polymorphisms in NOD2 very badly impair bacterial sensing, and antimicrobial peptide production goes haywire, leading to severe dysbiosis associated with nasty chronic inflammation. Alterations in TLR5 similarly disrupt immune signalling pathways, deeply regulating microbiota-host homeostasis within various bodily environments and other assorted locales (Garget al, 2023).

Diet profoundly shapes microbiome landscape within bodily ecosystems, playing a crucial yet frequently underappreciated role across diverse physiological niches, rather quietly. Beneficial microbes ferment dietary fibres, producing short-chain fatty acids like butyrate having profoundly anti-inflammatory effects and markedly anti-tumourigenic properties in the gut. Prebiotics selectively stimulate beneficial bacteria, while probiotics harbour health-promoting properties, and both revive microbial diversity badly disrupted by harsh cancer treatments. Precision nutrition plans informed by genetic data and microbiome analysis offer promising avenues for enhancing cancer therapy fairly effectively these days (Garget al, 2023). Survivors of gastrointestinal cancers can enhance immune resilience drastically by consuming fibre-rich whole grains and veggies with prebiotic supplementation very effectively. Interventions like these potentially mitigate chemotherapy intolerance and gastrointestinal toxicity stemming from radiotherapy and may significantly lower recurrence risk. Microbiome sequencing and metabolomic profiling advances empower clinicians to monitor microbial shifts in response to diet therapy for making dynamic nutritional adjustments. Precision nutrition leverages microbiome therapeutic potential effectively in comprehensive cancer survivorship care by navigating host genetics and microbial ecology alongside diet.

2.5. Applications in Precision Oncology Nutrition

Precision nutrition embodies a radically novel cancer treatment methodology leveraging modified dietary tweaks calibrated against genomic idiosyncrasies in a person's metabolism. A modified framework integrates effectively at pivotal oncology stages like prevention and active treatment or survivorship to greatly improve life quality. Prevention stays crucial among individuals with heightened genetic susceptibility harbouring BRCA1/2 mutations or rare gene polymorphisms influencing carcinogenesis pathways very significantly in cancer. Diets heavy in micronutrients and antioxidants yet starkly deficient in saturated fat may very effectively counteract nasty genetic predispositions. Diets rich in fruits and whole grains furnish phytochemicals that tweak epigenetic regulation quite effectively, mitigating oxidative stress, thereby stifling tumour initiation potentially (Martínez-Garay and Djouder, 2023).

Precision nutrition leverages genetic and metabolic profiling during active treatment and somewhat effectively improves tolerance, addressing various treatment-related challenges. Cancer therapies often spawn nasty side effects like mucositis or cachexia, and severely compromise immunosuppression, greatly undermining therapy efficacy. Clinicians now prescribe regimens dense with omega-3 fatty acids and polyphenols, effectively mitigating systemic inflammation and causing less oxidative damage. Optimising specific nutrient timing, such as protein distribution, heavily counteracts muscle wasting based on genetic variants that influence various metabolic pathways. Targeted supplementation might enhance immune response somewhat or mitigate underlying deficiencies in various micronutrients without negatively impacting overall efficacy therapeutically (Martínez-Garay and Djouder, 2023). Personalised nutrition strategies with a long-term focus intently on mitigating genetic vulnerabilities during survivorship that significantly contribute to recurrence risk and insulin resistance comorbidities.

Dietary changes rich in methyl donors sustained over time can significantly boost DNA repair and epigenetic stability in folks with faulty folate metabolism. Diets heavy in anti-inflammatory properties enhance immune surveillance very significantly, thereby radically improving life quality and reducing cancer recurrence. Precision nutrition provides a highly personalised regimen intricately linking genetic data and various clinical factors with medical oncology treatment plans effectively. Evidence-based dietary choices tailored within individual biological contexts empower patients while maximising therapeutic efficacy quite effectively simultaneously.

2.6. Limitations and Ethical Considerations

Precision nutrition holds considerable promise for advancing cancer care, but major limitations and very serious ethical concerns remain largely unaddressed. Steep costs associated with comprehensive genetic testing and microbiome analysis pose a formidable barrier, largely nowadays, for many researchers. Such analyses frequently necessitate super-specialised labs and esoteric skillsets not readily available outside rarefied academic or ultra-niche clinical environments. Widespread implementation gets restricted in low-resource settings, raising concerns about stark health disparities in access to modified nutritional advice lately. Scientific understanding of complex gene-diet interactions remains woefully incomplete nowadays despite progress in tangentially related biomedical research fields. Genetics and quirky lifestyle factors simultaneously influence multifactorial dynamic networks embedded deeply in human metabolism and cancer biology.

Nutrigenomic data and microbiome info are increasing rapidly yet remain woefully scant for predicting individual health outcomes or crafting modified dietary regimens. Preliminary findings shrouded in uncertainty necessitate extremely cautious interpretation and studious avoidance of recklessly overpromising hugely beneficial outcomes further down the line. Misuse or misinterpretation of genetic info poses a thorny challenge arguably for stakeholders under certain obscure circumstances, obviously, every now and then. Genetic data might spur unwarranted angst or get exploited by shady outfits peddling dubious nutrigenetic services under the cloak of personalised dietary advice. Precision nutrition's clinical application must be rooted in evidence-based protocols administered by trained professionals skilled at explaining genetic test results with empathy effectively (Kassem et al, 2023). Genetic privacy and data security pose vexing quandaries of utmost gravity nowadays across various spheres with profound ethical implications everywhere. Genetic and microbiome data storage sharing must adhere strictly to confidentiality protocols, preventing unauthorised disclosure and discriminatory practices quite harshly.

Data handling protocols must be delineated explicitly in informed consent processes, respecting patients' autonomy deeply and disclosing parties with potential access. Precision nutrition in oncology often necessitates rather intense collaboration among a diverse range of specialists, including oncologists and data scientists, occasionally with genetic counsellors. Tailored support and realistic goals in culturally relevant counselling effectively foster psychological well-being and promote adherence in patients remarkably well. Precision nutrition represents a seismic paradigm shift from monotonous one-size-fits-all eating advice despite sundry gnarly hurdles and staunch resistance. Integrating genomics and systems biology offers remarkably personalised pathways supporting treatment response and enhancing survivorship outcomes quite effectively nowadays. Embedding nutrition within precision oncology's evolving framework will be crucial for delivering fairly comprehensive cancer care, rather slowly, quite integratively (Kassem et al, 2023).

3. Genetic Profiling in Oncology: Tailoring Diets for Better Outcomes

The emergence profoundly reshaped oncology by prioritising treatment strategies tailored to each patient's genetic makeup and various lifestyle factors. Genetic profiling lies at the heart of evolution, offering piercing insights into tumour-specific mutations fuelling cancer progression, with host genetic variations influencing various metabolic pathways deeply. Harnessing genetic data precipitates a radical paradigm shift towards modified nutrition rather than generic dietary advice, thereby markedly boosting survivorship rates. Nowadays, genetic profiling entails analysis of germline and somatic variants pertinent to various metabolic phenotypes and cancer biology. Polymorphisms in genes like MTHFR drastically alter folate metabolism and DNA methylation, thereby influencing cancer susceptibility and modifying requirements for nutrients substantially (Fujiwara et al., 2023).

Omega-3-rich nutrients and fibre-dense food remarkably support gut flora equilibrium and overall bodily defence mechanisms with tailored suggestions. Precision nutrition rooted deeply in genetic profiling requires concerted effort across various disciplines to ensure safe incorporation of dietary changes within medical treatment regimens. Genetic data incorporation into nutritional care promises remarkably improved cancer outcomes and empowers patients with evidence-based personalised guidance fairly effectively nowadays.

3.1. Understanding Genetic Profiling in Cancer Care

Genetic profiling has surged remarkably in modern oncology, providing critical insights beyond tumour biology and deep into the inherited host genome frequently. Tumour cells harbour specific somatic mutations and germline variants inherited influence physiological responses like nutrient metabolism analyzed via a somewhat novel dual approach. Somatic genetic profiling gets employed routinely, identifying actionable mutations like EGFR in lung cancer or BRCA1/2, typically found in breast cancers. Findings inform modified treatment protocols that boost efficacy remarkably while mitigating adverse side effects fairly effectively in most cases. Germline genetic profiling creeps into cancer care as an increasing frontier with fairly significant implications for survivorship and very nuanced nutritional tweaks. Pharmacogenomics and next-generation sequencing technologies have lately enabled thorough examination of genetic variants influencing biochemical pathways pertinent to cancer treatment response very vigorously nowadays. Genetic polymorphisms rather profoundly affect numerous vital bodily functions, often quite significantly within human physiology every single day. Genetic variants like those found in the MTHFR gene mess with folate usage very badly, thereby hindering DNA synthesis or screwing up methylation patterns. Polymorphisms in enzymes intricately involved in vitamin D metabolic pathways impact calcium homeostasis erratically and enhance immune regulation with unusual efficacy.

Specific genetic profiles modulate DNA repair efficiency significantly, thereby influencing susceptibility markedly to mutagenesis and cancer recurrence in affected cells. Diets rich in antioxidants and methyl donors can possibly support genomic stability remarkably well in individuals harbouring certain genetic predispositions. Genetic variations in hormone receptor signalling pathways potentially heighten cancer risk remarkably under certain dietary conditions or alter tumour progression significantly. Variants impacting cytokine production or immune receptor functionality influence bodily inflammation greatly, and diet plays a supportive role.

Genetic variations within genes that encode antioxidant enzymes such as glutathione S-transferases profoundly impact the body's capacity to neutralise reactive oxygen species. Clinicians and nutrition experts devise modified nutritional regimens by grasping genetic factors underlying each patient's distinct genetic makeup quite thoroughly nowadays. Genetic profiling becomes pivotal in cancer care largely due to novel approaches remarkably enhancing treatment efficacy with astonishingly fewer overall adverse effects.

3.2. Gene–Nutrient Interactions Relevant to Cancer Nutrition

Genetics intricately intertwines with diet, modulating cancer progression risk and response quite significantly under various therapeutic interventions. Gene variants subtly influence nutrient absorption and utilization thereby hindering cellular processes such as DNA repair and immune response very badly. Unravelling intricate gene-nutrient interactions, enables the formulation of tailored dietary plans that remarkably encourage cancer therapy efficacy, these days, very effectively. Stuff gets numbered with surprising ease, usually. Variants C677T and A1298C in the methylenetetrahydrofolate reductase gene significantly diminish enzyme activity responsible for converting folate into biologically active 5-methyltetrahydrofolate. Methylation reactions crucial for DNA synthesis get badly impaired, thereby heightening susceptibility, mostly in breast cancers and colorectal cancer somewhat genomically unstable.

Individuals possessing certain genetic variants may derive considerable benefits from consuming foods rich in 5-MTHF and other vital B vitamins like B6 and B12, which facilitate one-carbon metabolism thoroughly. Variants in the VDR gene markedly impact vitamin D signalling efficacy and subsequently influence calcium absorption and cellular proliferation quite profoundly. Certain genetic variants correlate with heightened prostate, breast and colorectal cancer risks in specific populations rather frequently these days nowadays.

Vitamin D supplementation around VDR genotype and serum 25(OH)D levels very effectively optimises markedly protective effects and enhances immune surveillance very nicely. GST family enzymes like GSTP1, GSTM1, and GSTT1 crucially detoxify various carcinogens and neutralise highly reactive oxygen species very effectively nowadays. Variant alleles can drastically impair enzyme function, thereby heightening susceptibility to oxidative damage and substantially increasing overall cancer risk over time. Sulforaphane and various phytochemicals are found in diets heavy with cruciferous veggies such as broccoli or Brussels sprouts, inducing phase II detox enzymes very effectively.

Cytochrome P450 enzymes like CYP1A1 and CYP2D6 rapidly metabolise various xenobiotics and numerous dietary compounds inside the human body very quickly. Genetic variants in enzymes drastically alter the metabolism of bioactive phytochemicals such as flavonoids and resveratrol, thereby influencing bioavailability and possibly their chemopreventive properties significantly. Genetic polymorphisms that heavily with dietary factors modulate systemic inflammation, crucial in cancer progression involving cytokines like TNF-α and IL-6. Omega-3 fatty acids and curcumin in anti-inflammatory diets might counteract such effects, with efficacy potentially influenced by individual genetic backgrounds. Incorporating knowledge of gene-nutrient interactions into clinical practice facilitates precision nutrition strategies that markedly enhance treatment outcomes for cancer patients.

Folate metabolism is regulated intricately by this crucial enzyme for DNA methylation and subsequent cellular repair processes downstream. MTHFR polymorphisms such as C677T and A1298C significantly impair enzyme efficiency, thereby heightening cancer risk largely due to defective nucleotide synthesis. Affected individuals may benefit greatly from higher intake of methylated folate and vitamin B12, supporting methylation pathways extensively with supplemental choline.

a. CYP1A1 and GSTs (Detoxification Genes)

Genes facilitating phase I detoxification of xenobiotics and carcinogens, alongside certain phase II reactions, help remove toxic substances fairly effectively altogether. Variants in GSTT1, GSTM1, or GSTP1 may markedly impair glutathione activity downstream, thereby significantly increasing oxidative stress. Nutritional strategies boost consumption of cruciferous veggies and selenium-rich foods alongside sulfur-containing amino acids, effectively enhancing detoxification pathways.

b. VDR variant

Variants in the VDR gene strongly affect vitamin D signaling thereby influencing immune regulation pathways and cell proliferation very marginally downstream. People having low VDR activity might require significantly more vitamin D from dietary sources or supplementary means, possibly through various other routes.

Genetic polymorphisms within specific genes potentially predispose individuals to obesity, which subsequently acts as a risk factor for recurring cancer. Tailored nutrition often involves low-glycemic diets and modified exercise regimes, mitigating health risks very effectively under certain conditions.

3.3. Nutrigenomics in Cancer Treatment and Recovery

Nutrition plays a crucial role in supporting immune function effectively and mitigating harsh side effects during active cancer treatment with considerable efficacy. Nutrigenomics offers profoundly insightful revelations for concocting tailor-made nutritional plans eerily attuned to a patient's singular genomic configuration, rather subtly. Clinicians facilitate molecular recovery by integrating genetic information into personalised nutrition plans, thereby somewhat encouraging bodily resilience and mitigating toxic reactions very effectively. Polymorphisms exist in the DPYD gene crucial for metabolising 5-fluorouracil, a widely used chemotherapeutic agent with very nasty side effects sometimes. People with nonfunctional DPYD variants exhibit drastically reduced enzyme activity, resulting in woefully inadequate drug clearance and greatly increased risk of severe toxicity manifesting as mucositis or myelosuppression and diarrhoea.

Nutritional interventions might involve liver-supportive foods like cruciferous veggies and antioxidant-rich stuff while sidestepping compounds that tax hepatic detoxification processes further downstream. SOD2 or superoxide dismutase 2 encodes a crucial mitochondrial enzyme neutralising superoxide radicals spawned by oxidative metabolism and harsh cancer treatments like radiation therapy. Individuals possessing SOD2 variants such as the Val16Ala polymorphism frequently display a greatly reduced ability to detoxify reactive oxygen species, thus elevating tissue damage risk substantially. Consumption of antioxidant-rich edibles like berries alongside green tea and turmeric potentially enhances cellular defence mechanisms rapidly in such persons.

Nutrigenomic insights inform macronutrient distribution, effectively managing issues like cachexia or insulin resistance fairly well under certain circumstances sometimes. People having certain genetic quirks affecting glucose processing might reap benefits from eating foods low in glycemic load or having balanced fatty acid ratios during therapy. Clinicians and registered dietitians can enhance treatment tolerance effectively by tailoring nutritional strategies according to individual genetic profiles, thereby reducing various complication risks. Precision-based approach empowers patients quite actively in their care, yielding stellar oncologic results and markedly improved quality of life possibly.

3.4. Integrating Genetic Profiling into Personalized Diet Planning

Genetic profiling is increasingly being integrated into dietary planning nowadays marking a rather crucial development in oncology precision and personalized nutrition. Clinicians and nutrition professionals devise modified dietary regimens aligned with a patient's molecular blueprint by pinpointing genetic variations influencing metabolic pathways. A rigorous interdisciplinary framework underpins this approach rendering nutritional strategies grounded firmly in evidence and responsive adaptively to patient needs. A single nominal value gets assigned haphazardly in various disparate contexts often quite ostensibly and without much deliberation or forethought. Genetic assessment typically kicks off nowadays by gathering specimens like saliva or blood for analysis of single nucleotide polymorphisms very swiftly. Testing might entail modified nutrigenomic panels homing in on genes related to nutrition such as MTHFR or sweeping whole-exome sequencing for exhaustive genetic profiling.

Crucial data necessary for tailored dietary planning gets yielded effectively by this step. Genetic data sparks collaboration among oncologists and registered dietitians trained in nutrigenomics with genetic counselors interpreting findings extremely meticulously now. Mangled enzyme activity or wonky receptor sensitivity results from SNP variants being linked rather crudely to functional consequences and dietary implications get mapped. A variant in PEMT gene influences choline metabolism heavily and may warrant dietary recommendations surprisingly rich in choline for some people. Genetic data gets crunched really quickly and super personalized dietary plans emerge with heaps of specifics very rapidly nowadays online.

Meal plans get significantly tweaked according to treatment phases like chemotherapy or radiation and recovery phases are heavily modded encourage immune function curbing nasty side effects rapidly. Genetic-based nutrition evolves perpetually underground through intricate vigilant monitoring processes and swift adaptation mechanisms simultaneously. Survivors gingerly navigate various phases of care during treatment progression slowly and regular follow-ups become increasingly essential afterwards really. Lab biomarkers get reevaluated and dietary goals adjusted frequently nowadays alongside thorough symptom tracking reflecting evolving health needs very dynamically. Genetic data integration into diet planning enables a flexible clinically informed personalized nutrition approach across cancer care continuum enhancing therapeutic efficacy greatly.

3.5. Ethical and Practical Considerations

Genetic profiling offers tremendous promise in cancer care personalized nutrition yet poses significant thorny conundrums that demand very careful consideration. Genetic data pose thorny issues surrounding sensitive personal info and are very darn identifying in a very peculiar manner. Robust safeguards must be firmly in place protecting patient privacy and preventing misuse or unauthorized access rather rapidly. Stringent data protection laws like HIPAA or GDPR are very much essential nowadays for maintaining confidentiality everywhere absolutely. Secure data storage practices and informed consent protocols underpin fundamental patient trust partly because transparency regarding genetic information use exists.

Genomic testing remains sporadically available nationwide across diverse populations within various healthcare systems alongside somewhat personalized nutrition services. Availability may be severely curtailed in low-resource settings or underserved locales due largely to geographic constraints and insufficient insurance coverage. Inequity threatens stark widening disparities in cancer outcomes nationwide across diverse populations over lengthy periods of time quite unfortunately. Extensive clinician training in public health programs and reimbursement models, urgently need fostering at policy level through equitable access mechanisms. Genetic results necessitate meticulous interpretation grounded in eclectic knowledge from various obscure fields and highly specialized expertise simultaneously.

Patients might unwittingly misconstrue raw genetic info or fervently adopt unsubstantiated dietary regimens stemming from shaky commercial tests without proper oversight. Patient education and provider training are evidently critical nowadays for optimal healthcare outcomes. Genetic counseling must be deeply embedded alongside evidence-based communication in care models quashing misinformation swiftly and facilitating very informed decisions. Nutrigenomics stays nascent still lacking broad consensus on clinical utility amidst ongoing efforts towards tighter integration with clinical practices. Establishing rigorous guidelines validates nutrigenomic tests and standardizes interpretation of gene-nutrient interactions while designing targeted interventions very carefully nowadays.

Nutrigenomics integration into oncology care requires structured workflows and intense collaboration among highly specialized doctors within electronic health records systems nowadays. Genetic profiling integration into cancer nutrition holds significant potential ethically and practically amidst various sizable and fairly formidable challenges. Clinicians can offer superlative care throughout cancer continuum by tailoring dietary interventions extremely well with individual genetic predispositions from onset of active treatment. Efforts tackling knotty systemic barriers and thorny ethical issues will be crucial in fully leveraging benefits of personalized oncology nutrition as genomics advances at breakneck speed.

4. Lifestyle Factors and Their Role in Personalized Cancer Nutrition Strategies

Modified cancer care models emerge rapidly nowadays and lifestyle factors play a crucial role in shaping nutrition strategies quite dynamically. Molecular profiling and genetic analysis provide crucial insights into a patient's underlying biology but don't occur in some sort of total isolation. Psychosocial factors and environment rather differently modulate patient responses under various circumstances to nutrition and treatment interventions significantly. Addressing such factors enables precision nutrition application across cancer care continuum far more practically in a very sustainable kinda way. Physical activity modulates metabolic health significantly influencing treatment outcomes profoundly in various obscure clinical contexts under certain circumstances apparently.

Exercise remarkably improves insulin sensitivity very significantly in most people and reduces inflammation substantially over time with consistent effort. Nutritional plans must be meticulously tailored alongside patients' diverse activity levels ensuring ample protein for muscle maintenance and bursty energy replenishment. Stress levels severely impact hormonal balance under diverse physiological states and appetite fluctuates wildly while immune function gets heavily compromised. Cortisol levels surge under chronic stress and sleep disturbances spurring inflammation and badly impairing glucose metabolism thereby hindering recovery. Nutritional strategies might incorporate adaptogenic edibles rich in omega-3 fatty acids and magnesium alongside carefully planned meal timing supporting natural circadian rhythm. Psychological well-being plays quite crucial role rather significantly in sticking fairly tenaciously to various dietary regimens every time.

Fear of cancer recurrence and depression may lead to wildly inconsistent daily eating habits or seriously disordered nutritional intake patterns. Mindfulness training and behavioural counselling services alongside nutrition guidance, quite remarkably foster long-term behavioural shifts obviously over an extended period. Socioeconomic factors and deeply ingrained cultural food preferences rather erratically influence the feasibility of dietary interventions across diverse population groups. Personalisation must simultaneously account for food availability and traditional dietary patterns alongside cooking skills and affordability. Nutrition plans reflecting a patient's cultural background tend to be more readily adopted under certain economic situations over long periods.

Lifestyle elements infused into tailored nutrition plans metamorphose rigid regimens into vibrant patient-focused approaches utterly transforming healthcare outcomes with remarkable efficacy nowadays. Nutrition is a deeply personal and profoundly complex phenomenon rooted in biochemical processes and idiosyncratic mores often influenced by mundane habits. Nutritional interventions in cancer care become remarkably efficacious nowadays when lifestyle factors are optimised alongside genetic data and clinical information.

4.1. Why Lifestyle Context Matters in Personalised Nutrition

Cancer nutrition encompasses myriad factors, including biochemical processes and sundry related phenomena functioning irregularly within human bodily systems, rather atypically. Diet unfurls as a befuddling array of processes driven by behavioural tics strongly swayed by whimsical norms and mannerisms moulded gradually. Diets customised haphazardly often result in halfhearted adherence or unexpectedly calamitous health repercussions manifesting slowly over an extended period. Cancer survivors often derive genetic benefits from high-fibre anti-inflammatory foods, but treatment-induced taste changes and nutritionally barren surroundings thwart these benefits somewhat. Personalised nutrition flexibly adapts around lifestyle constraints and peculiar individual capabilities, simultaneously enhancing various physiological outcomes and overall psychological well-being.

4.2. Physical Activity and Energy Balance

Physical activity remains crucial for cancer survivorship efforts generally nowadays. Energy expenditure gets directly hampered, thereby messing with body composition, insulin sensitivity and inflammatory status, influencing nutritional needs rather substantially. Active individuals may need way more protein for muscle recovery and shoring up immune function. Sedentary survivors, especially those with sarcopenic obesity, may benefit from energy-restricted, protein-rich diets to preserve lean mass and reduce adiposity. Sedentary survivors, especially those beset with sarcopenic obesity, may reap huge benefits from protein-rich diets somewhat restricted in energy. Active folks likely necessitate rather elevated protein intake for muscle recovery and maintaining sturdy immune function generally.

4.3. Sleep and Circadian Rhythms

Survivors of cancer often quietly endure rather vexing sleep disturbances afterwards, a woefully underappreciated problem plaguing lives curiously in many obscure cases. Chemotherapy severely disrupts sleep patterns alongside radiation and psychological pain, badly altering hormonal balances deeply within bodily metabolic functions. Poor sleep quality and insufficient duration have tenuously been linked to adverse effects on key appetite regulators like ghrelin and leptin. Such changes may fuel hankerings for calorie-rich junk food lacking essential micronutrients and exacerbate weight gain, insulin resistance and chronic inflammation, severely hindering cancer prognoses. Recent research underscores the significance of circadian rhythms, intricately regulating human metabolic processes within a complex biological clock oscillating over 24 hours.

Chrononutrition investigates profoundly how the timing of food intake affects metabolic health within novel frameworks marrying dietary habits with circadian rhythms. Eating at night or having erratic meal times strongly correlates with increased oxidative stress and gut microbiota alterations, thereby heightening cancer risk. Time-Restricted Feeding entails eating within a relatively short 10–12 hour window during bustling daytime hours, boosting insulin sensitivity remarkably. TRF has remarkably shown potential for improving sleep quality in breast cancer survivors and reducing fatigue levels substantially in them. Gobbling massive amounts of food before snoozing thoroughly disrupts melatonin secretion and glucose balance, particularly in folks afflicted with metabolic syndrome or desynchronized bodily rhythms. Eating meals earlier in the day possibly enhances metabolic resilience fairly significantly and supports sleep hygiene with some considerable effectiveness.

Cancer care nowadays becomes very holistic when nutritional counselling incorporates sleep patterns and circadian rhythms, rather effectively. Clinicians substantially mitigate inflammation and boost energy balance by tackling complex interplays between nutritional deficits and various sleep disorders, thereby enhancing tolerance of treatments remarkably. Nutrient-dense meals are stressed very early on in the day, and eating schedules curiously align with bursts of frenetic daytime activity. Some patients drastically cut back on stimulant intake and high-sugar foods very sharply in the evening. Cancer survivors benefit enormously from sticking rigorously to consistent sleep schedules, and this greatly improves overall quality of life.

4.4. Stress, Emotional Health, and Eating Behaviours

Psychological stress manifests ubiquitously as a confounding facet of cancer experience, often fraught with turmoil and deep emotional pain. Heightened emotional distress alongside depression is fuelled by changes in body image or physical function, and prognosis uncertainty creeping in slowly. Psychological factors greatly impact appetite regulation and complicate nutrition management during treatment afterwards quite significantly under various circumstances. Stress-induced dysregulation of the hypothalamic-pituitary-adrenal axis spawns elevated cortisol secretion which gets linked rather tenuously to hyperglycemia.

Physiological changes drastically impair metabolic well-being and heighten cancer recurrence risk quite alarmingly alongside numerous comorbid conditions very significantly. Elevated cortisol wreaks havoc on sleep patterns very badly and fatigue sets in rapidly with weight fluctuations stemming from abysmal eating habits. Eating behaviors are influenced heavily by emotional health often manifesting in consumption of extremely high-calorie foods low in essential nutrients during anxious spells or profound sadness. Nausea or depression can trigger highly restrictive eating stemming from severely reduced motivation and a resultant substantial loss of appetite. Disordered eating patterns including bingeing and chronic undereating manifest fairly commonly especially in survivors, struggling mightily to regain some control over their health. Stress and anxiety can provoke nasty gastrointestinal symptoms like bloating and diarrhea or severe abdominal pain reducing food consumption drastically.

Robust psychosocial support frameworks alongside thorough dietary counseling are generally necessitated very much always for effective personalized nutrition . Referral to behavioral health professionals namely psychologists versed in cognitive-behavioral therapy substantially enhances emotional regulation very significantly in most individuals. Flexible meal planning accommodates diverse emotional triggers and peculiar aversions especially during grueling chemo sessions amidst extreme sensory upheaval. Rigid diets often backfire and foster feelings of guilt or deep anxiety in individuals beset by perfectionist tendencies or deeply ingrained disordered eating habits. Emotional well-being gets woven into personalized nutrition frameworks rather effectively fostering compassionately sustainable care models nowadays very remarkably. Cancer survivors need a complex plan involving psychological support and nutrition therapy quite remarkably enhancing life quality and adherence very slowly.

4.5. Cultural and Social Determinants of Nutrition

Culture profoundly shapes beliefs about health and illness while influencing food preferences quite heavily and affecting fasting practices rather noticeably. Personalising cancer nutrition demands sensitivity towards various cultural facets, ensuring nutritionally sound recommendations stay remarkably sustainable and culturally relevant always. Family involvement, caregiver roles, and community resources can significantly hinder or quite effectively reinforce dietary adherence under various specific circumstances. Survivors dwelling amongst multiple generations may crave recipes satisfying therapeutic needs and family members' eccentric palates at the same time. People with restricted culinary skills or minimal access to wholesome ingredients need feasible, budget-friendly meal planning tactics. Individuals possessing rudimentary cooking skills or facing limitations in obtaining nutritious food frequently require down-to-earth strategies for meal organisation and preparation.

4.6. Health Literacy and Behaviour Change Readiness

Precise dietary advice utterly fails without sufficient readiness for behaviour change, and fairly decent health literacy exists among ostensibly keen people. Survivors often get befuddled by conflicting dietary advice swirling around post-treatment misinformation, and dubious wellness claims abound everywhere online daily. Crucial in shaping effective interventions tailored specifically around patients are evaluations of their readiness for change and a basic grasp of nutrition. Personalised goal-setting techniques and visual aids alongside motivational interviewing, spur remarkably enduring changes in lifestyle habits, fostering deep engagement.

Tailoring cancer nutrition plans around lifestyle factors keeps dietary interventions grounded in evidence while remaining very feasible psychologically. Physical activity and genetic factors interact haphazardly with stress and metabolic factors, shaping nutritional needs drastically, with various health outcomes unfolding. Holistic lenses very significantly enhance survivorship care, empowering individuals remarkably in recovery and overall long-term health. Precision oncology advances rapidly nowadays, and synergy between lifestyle factors and personalised nutrition becomes cornerstone of quite integrative cancer care.

5. Nutrigenomics

Nutrigenomics extensively investigates how genetic variations, specifically single nucleotide polymorphisms, influence bodily response somewhat irregularly to various nutrients under certain dietary patterns. Gene function variations profoundly affect nutrient metabolism and detoxification capacity during cancer treatment largely owing partly to stark individual differences. Cancer treatments such as chemo impose substantial physiological strain on various bodily systems and often induce profoundly severe oxidative stress nowadays. Clinicians craft modified nutritional regimens very effectively deciphering a patient's unique nutrigenomic signature thereby encourage treatment efficacy and mitigating nasty adverse reactions. MTHFR gene polymorphisms such as C677T and A1298C significantly impair folate metabolism and DNA methylation in various cancer nutrition studies markedly reducing enzyme activity.

Cell repair gets severely hampered and treatment-related toxicities surge markedly amidst peculiar physiological responses and fluctuating health statuses simultaneously. Patients harbouring specific genetic variants may derive considerable benefit from methylated folate and increased intake of several B vitamins naturally found. Variants in detoxification enzymes GSTM1 GSTT1 and GSTP1 glutathione S-transferases severely impede ability to neutralize reactive oxygen species and chemotherapeutic byproducts rather effectively sometimes. Oxidative balance in individuals can be enhanceed abundantly by consuming selenium and polyphenol-rich foods alongside antioxidants found in cruciferous veggies. Superoxide dismutase 2 very effectively neutralizes superoxide radicals inside cells and mitochondrial enzyme SOD2 is also known by that name. Variant Val16Ala markedly alters enzyme activity with reduced function exacerbating oxidative stress significantly during grueling radiation therapy or intense chemo regimens.

Diets rich in antioxidants may offer fairly targeted protection against various health issues very effectively under certain circumstances or so it seems. Variants in VDR gene profoundly influence cellular response to vitamin D thereby modulating immune system apoptosis and triggering severe inflammation very suddenly. Genotype-tailored vitamin D supplementation according to serum 25(OH)D levels might substantially optimize immune function and mitigate severely nasty inflammatory repercussions very effectively. TNF-α and IL-6 gene polymorphisms significantly sway cytokine production triggering various inflammatory responses nearly simultaneously with profound downstream effects. People carrying variants with high expression may require diets rich in omega-3 fatty acids and polyphenol-rich foods having anti-inflammatory properties.

Cancer nutrition care gets precision tweaks from integrating SNP analysis fairly closely aligning with peculiar genetic makeup of a patient. This strategy holds considerable promise for encourage treatment tolerance very effectively while promoting stability in metabolic processes amidst personalized oncology nutrition. Variants in APOE gene profoundly affect lipid metabolism and may vociferously impact patient responses somewhat differently across various dietary fatty acid regimens. APOE4 carriers may exhibit unusually high inflammation levels and need dietary adjustments featuring drastically less saturated fat yet substantially more omega-3 fatty acids.

5.1. Nutrigenomic Modulation During Cancer Treatment

Nutrigenomics probes gene expression heavily influenced by dietary factors during cancer treatments that go far beyond inherited genetic variations. Chemotherapy and radiation or immunotherapy induces significant alterations in cellular signaling pathways and epigenetic regulation very frequently nowadays. Therapy-induced changes fuel beneficial therapeutic effects and nasty outcomes like cachexia or debilitating fatigue very slowly alongside mucositis. Nutrient-based interventions modulate gene expression patterns very effectively offering a supportive strategy and enhancing treatment efficacy in a remarkably dynamic manner. Turmeric yields curcumin which deeply modulates NF-κB a transcription factor central to regulating pathways of inflammation and cell survival. Curcumin downregulates pro-inflammatory cytokines such as TNF-α and IL-6 very effectively in various preclinical studies and sensitizes tumour cells to chemotherapy rather nicely.

Epigallocatechin gallate significantly influences MAPK and PI3K/Akt signaling pathways in various cancer cells enhancing apoptosis incredibly abundantly found in green tea. EGCG may modulate DNMTs activity quite profoundly thereby affecting gene silencing patterns relevant in various tumour progression contexts significantly. Sulforaphane present in cruciferous veggies activates Nrf2 very effectively; Nrf2 being a master regulator of some antioxidant response elements rather haphazardly. Nrf2 activation quite effectively enhance cellular resilience against radiation-induced oxidative stress and chemotherapeutic onslaughts while simultaneously detoxifying reactive species very rapidly. Omega-3 fatty acids EPA and DHA weirdly influence gene expression via PPAR-γ activation thoroughly promoting anti-inflammatory signaling and modulating immune function very oddly. Preservation of muscle mass and management of cachexia induced by treatment have significant implications arising from this phenomenon essentially.

Vitamin D and resveratrol have been extensively researched for modulating gene expression linked thoroughly to cell cycle regulation and mitochondrial functionality. Clinicians provide highly adaptive support by dynamically tailoring very specific nutritional strategies alongside rapidly unfolding transcriptomic shifts during aggressive cancer therapy with pharmacological interventions. Nutrient bioavailability and precise timing functionally modulate genes significantly without interfering with therapeutic regimen intent down the line. Nutrigenomic insights infused into cancer treatment foster a responsive paradigm encourage anti-tumour efficacy via precision dietary modulation very effectively indeed.

a. Epigenetic Influence

Epigenetics involves heritable changes in gene expression occurring rather frequently nowadays without altering underlying DNA sequence at all. Key epigenetic mechanisms involve DNA methylation and histone modification quite intricately within cells alongside non-coding RNA regulation. Various processes modulate oncogenes and tumour suppressor genes quite variably playing crucial albeit differs in roles in cancer initiation or therapeutic response. Harsh cancer therapies like chemotherapy ravage epigenetic controls thereby surprisingly enough fostering heightened tumour heterogeneity and resistance to treatment. Specific bioactive compounds found in certain foods have been identified as powerful modulators of epigenetic processes affecting gene expression relevant to cancer prevention and cellular regeneration pathways.

Curcumin found in turmeric inhibits histone deacetylases extremely well by condensing chromatin and typically suppressing gene expression effectively. Curcumin hinders HDACs thereby fostering re-expression of silenced tumour suppressor genes while repressing transcription of oncogenes such as c-Myc very effectively. Curcumin influences DNA methyltransferases thereby further enhancing epigenetic regulatory potential significantly inside cells becomes Curcumin profoundly affects DNA methyltransferases and thereby boosts epigenetic regulation very significantly within cellular environments normally. Sulforaphane derived from glucosinolates in cruciferous veggies like kale acts very potently as an epigenetic modulator basically.

Tumour suppressor genes like p21 or PTEN are reactivated thereby as HDAC activity gets inhibited and histone acetylation gets promoted. Sulforaphane very effectively enhance activation of Nrf2 pathway which regulates expression of antioxidant genes via various quirky epigenetic mechanisms and detoxification occurs. Genistein in soy and resveratrol in grapes and various berries similarly affect DNMT activity thereby contributing epigenetically heavily to controlling cancer. Bioavailability stays a limiting factor in clinical translation and effects fluctuate wildly with dose and specific contextual parameters somewhat erratically. Eating whole foods rich in such nutrients very much supports epigenetic stability during cancer treatment with considerable practicality. Clinicians can restore gene expression normally via dietary interventions modulating epigenome and very effectively sensitize tumours to treatment. Epigenetic oncology merges fascinatingly with nutritional science in largely uncharted research territory boasting vast and highly promising therapeutic potential.

b. Inflammation and Immunity

Cancer development gets fueled rapidly by chronic inflammation and stubborn resistance forms rather inexplicably against various treatments in many complex mysterious ways. Tumour microenvironment and cancer therapies such as chemotherapy and radiation alongside immunotherapy induce nasty systemic inflammation heavily contributing to adverse effects. Nutritional strategies offer promising adjuncts by modulating inflammatory pathways deeply via highly specific nutrigenomic influences on expression of various immune-related genes. Nuclear factor kappa B regulates expression of pro-inflammatory cytokines TNF-α and IL-1β frequently in various cell survival pathways downstream. NF-κB gets aberrantly activated fairly often in various tumours and therapeutic stress further upregulates it heavily contributing rather substantially to resistance mechanisms.

Resveratrol a polyphenol abundant in grapes and various berries has been shown alongside other dietary bioactives suppressing NF-κB signaling and encourage immune response quite effectively. Resveratrol very effectively blocks IκB kinase complex thereby inhibiting NF-κB activation and diminishing transcription of various inflammatory mediators subsequently. Resveratrol markedly enhance T-cell functionality and exhibits potential for tumour immune microenvironment improvement thereby heightening responsiveness quite significantly in immunotherapy. Epigallocatechin gallate very significantly downregulates NF-κB and dials back mitogen-activated protein kinase pathways heavily reducing expression of inflammatory cytokines. EGCG vigorously boosts natural killer cell activity and cytotoxic T-cell responses thereby supporting immune surveillance fairly effectively in a somewhat roundabout way.

Eicosapentaenoic acid and docosahexaenoic acid omega-3 fatty acids derived from fatty fish exert effects via numerous mechanisms rather irregularly and they deeply inhibit NF-κB translocation inside cells. They heavily reduce production of pro-inflammatory eicosanoids. Resolvins and protectins are produced at a glacial pace by them. Molecules actively promote resolution of inflammation and may significantly reduce cancer-related cachexia fatigue and treatment-induced injury very effectively nowadays. Modulation of inflammation through dietary changes effectively improves management of symptoms and may enhance efficacy of immunotherapy by downregulating cytokines that are immunosuppressive. Modified nutrition plans incorporating anti-inflammatory nutrients refine cancer care significantly supporting immune resilience and effectively forming key pillar of nutrigenomics informed oncology.

5.2. Personalized Nutrition through Genomic Integration

Nutrigenomics application in oncology nowadays requires melding genetic biochemical and clinical data very thoroughly for tailoring individual nutrition interventions. Precision approach optimizes treatment efficacy remarkably by aligning dietary strategies with a patient's unique genetic makeup and various physiological needs very effectively nowadays. Genetic Screening entails procuring blood or saliva samples painstakingly for scrutinizing quirky single nucleotide polymorphisms linked with shoddy nutrient metabolism and dodgy DNA repair. Panels comprise genes such as MTHFR deeply rooted in folate metabolic pathways and GST family members facilitating glutathione conjugation crucial in certain cancer studies. Biochemical evaluation involves quantifying biomarkers like homocysteine and serum vitamin D alongside folate B12 and antioxidant status very thoroughly for genetic data supplementation.

Cancer type and stage plus various treatment modalities like chemo and radiation therapy precipitate subsequent nutritional challenges in patients quite frequently afterwards. Modified meal plans and supplementation protocols addressing genetic risks identified via testing quietly ensue during subsequent treatment demands. Elevated homocysteine stemming from MTHFR polymorphism may be mitigated greatly by dietary intake of methyl donors found abundantly in eggs and spinach. People with deficient GST enzyme activity may reap huge benefits from munching veggies such as broccoli extremely rich in sulforaphane thereby boosting phase II detox pathways. This integrative approach fosters metabolic resilience and improves clinical outcomes dynamically with biomarker feedback throughout treatment phases somewhat variably. Oncologists and registered dietitians collaborate with genetic counselors ensuring personalized nutrition plans stay rigorously evidence-backed very safely and fairly patient-centric.

6. Individualized Nutritional Interventions for Cancer Prevention and Management

Genetic predispositions coupled with various environmental exposures put certain individuals at significantly elevated risk of cancer necessitating highly tailored dietary interventions. Tailored dietary interventions vigorously tackle peculiar biochemical susceptibilities and enhance innate bodily defenses against cancer development quite naturally over prolonged periods. People with BRCA1/2 or Lynch syndrome mutations might greatly benefit from consuming foods extremely rich in antioxidants and omega-3 fatty acids. Nutritional support can be very specifically tailored for optimal DNA repair in individuals with wonky folate metabolic processes and impaired detoxification. Dietary patterns teeming with phytochemicals and fibre may possibly thwart carcinogenic exposures from tobacco pollutants and lessen chronic inflammation somewhat encourage detoxification and immune function greatly. Modified nutrition plans leveraging genetic data and lifestyle factors that enhance metabolic health can be crafted by healthcare providers simultaneously.

6.1. Genetic Risk Modification

Genetic predispositions sway susceptibility in various cancers markedly within a person's lifetime under specific obscure conditions quite heavily. Mutations in BRCA1 and BRCA2 genes markedly heighten lifetime risk of breast cancer significantly in women harbouring such genetic aberrations. Mutations severely disrupt cellular repair mechanisms rendering cells extremely vulnerable to genomic instability fairly often in many critical biological processes nowadays. Genetic risk stays stubbornly immutable yet dietary tweaks can conceivably slow cancer onset and progression across diverse biological settings rapidly. Evidence indicates BRCA mutation carriers possibly mitigate hormonal dysregulation risks by eating diets rich in omega-3 polyunsaturated fatty acids very effectively. Saturated fats spur estrogen production and pro-inflammatory signaling which may badly exacerbate tumourigenic pathways in genetically predisposed individuals very terribly.

Omega-3 PUFAs occur predominantly in oily fish such as salmon and possess anti-inflammatory properties via eicosanoid synthesis modulation and downregulation of COX-2 enzyme. Vitamins C and E carotenoids and polyphenols found in fruits nuts and veggies can neutralize reactive oxygen species thereby safeguarding DNA. Methylenetetrahydrofolate reductase gene polymorphisms significantly sway cancer risk alongside various genetic variants and utterly alter nutrient metabolism irregularly. MTHFR rather quickly catalyzes conversion of folate into biologically active 5-methyltetrahydrofolate essential for numerous methylation reactions and DNA synthesis. Individuals possessing specific MTHFR variants such as C677T frequently exhibit markedly diminished enzyme activity resulting in erratic folate processing and extremely elevated homocysteine concentrations.

Genome instability and aberrant DNA methylation patterns arise from dysfunction here substantially heightening susceptibility suddenly to breast and colorectal cancer. Personalized nutritional interventions emphasize intake of methylated folate supplements or folate-rich foods like spinach alongside vitamins B6 and B12 very synergistically. Restoring methyl group availability sufficiently and enhancing DNA repair fidelity ultimately reduces risk of carcinogenesis very effectively. Gene-diet interactions are being understood nowadays enabling development of precision nutrition strategies that somewhat effectively modify inherited cancer risk impacts. Genomic integrity gets supported by dietary interventions tailored around individual genetic profiles furnishing a rather proactive cancer prevention strategy nowadays effectively.

6.2. Metabolic and Inflammatory Profiling

Chronic systemic inflammation and metabolic dysregulation increasingly play crucial roles in cancer development and progression rather quietly. Biomarkers like C-reactive protein and pro-inflammatory cytokines such as interleukin-6 indicate systemic inflammation whereas insulin resistance gets evaluated through measures including fasting insulin levels. Elevated levels of those markers often coexist in metabolic syndrome and have been tenuously linked to heightened incidence of various malignancies including colorectal cancer breast tumours and endometrial malignancies. Nutritional strategies customized rather effectively nowadays hold considerable promise for mitigating risk of cancer through metabolic and inflammatory pathways.

Diets heavy in fatty fish rich in omega-3 fatty acids nuts and seeds alongside colorful fruits and veggies very effectively downregulate pro-inflammatory signaling cascades and slash oxidative stress levels significantly. Low-glycemic index diets curtail glucose spikes postprandially and abet improved insulin sensitivity thereby mitigating stimuli fostering neoplastic tumour proliferation vigorously inside human bodies. Mediterranean diet rich in fibre phytochemicals and healthy fats has demonstrated significant efficacy in lowering various inflammatory markers remarkably well nowadays. Such dietary patterns have been observed very frequently nowadays to improve metabolic profiles thereby decreasing cancer risk effectively. Evidence emerging rapidly implicates gut microbiome very deeply in carcinogenesis via roles in immune regulation and metabolism of various dietary constituents.

Dysbiosis namely reduced microbial diversity and imbalance of beneficial versus pathogenic bacteria has been linked fairly significantly to heightened risk of colorectal cancer and fuels systemic inflammation. Customized nutrition strategies nurturing gut flora health can rather effectively enhance cancer prevention efforts these days with quite significant results. Prebiotic fibres found in foods like onions and whole grains very effectively stimulate growth of beneficial bacteria such as Bifidobacterium species selectively. Fermented foods like yogurt and kimchi contain live microorganisms that fairly effectively restore microbial balance and boost mucosal immunity rather significantly.

Interventions remarkably boost production of short-chain fatty acids like butyrate which exhibits anti-inflammatory properties and supports health of epithelial cells very well. Precision dietary regimens formulated under metabolic inflammatory and microbiome profiling guidance effectively mitigate cancer risk by restoring systemic homeostasis and gut balance. Such unconventional approaches underscore increasing paradigm of personalized nutrition in cancer prevention gaining traction nowadays rapidly across various research circles.

6.3. Microbiome-Informed Prevention

Trillions of microorganisms predominantly reside in colon and form intricate ecosystem crucial for host health through various immune function and numerous metabolic processes. Gut microbial composition significantly modulates cancer risk especially in gastrointestinal malignancies such as colorectal cancer with substantial evidence mounting rapidly nowadays. Pathogenic bacteria thrive and gut barrier integrity gets remarkably disrupted in dysbiosis conditions under severely imbalanced microbial diversity. Disruption fosters chronic low-grade inflammation whilst markedly increasing exposure to sundry microbial metabolites harbouring rather ominous carcinogenic potential such as secondary bile acids and various toxins.

Dysbiosis has been tenuously linked through various obscure mechanisms including erratic DNA damage and aberrant cell proliferation with immunosurveillance gone badly awry. Nutritional strategies aimed squarely at gut microbiome restoration emerge increasingly as promising prevention methods with presumably considerable potential. Prebiotic foods bursting with fermentable fibres like inulin and resistant starches found in onions and whole grains feed beneficial gut bacteria readily. Microbes fermenting those fibres produce short-chain fatty acids like butyrate acetate and propionate really quickly deep inside human colon. SCFAs exert anti-inflammatory effects quite effectively by inhibiting nuclear factor kappa B signaling and enhance regulatory T-cell function promoting mucosal tolerance.

Probiotic interventions introduce live beneficial microorganisms via dietary sources like fermented dairy products or kimchi and through formulated supplements sometimes. Probiotics significantly reduce inflammation markers and may attenuate gastrointestinal toxicity related to treatment thereby supporting cancer prevention indirectly. Integrating microbiome-centric dietary regimens remarkably into cancer prevention paradigms nowadays highlights significance of modified systems-biology methodologies rather strikingly. Prebiotic-rich diets and probiotics potentially enhance immune surveillance effectively and diminish chronic inflammation thereby modulating carcinogenic processes in a highly efficacious manner.

6.4. Personalized Nutrition in Cancer Management

Cancer treatment involves surgery and chemotherapy or radiation therapy exerting distinct physiological effects rather vigorously on most patients nowadays. Nutritional requirements fluctuate enormously throughout treatment under influence of factors such as cancer type regimen and patient age baseline status comorbidities. Modified dietary interventions are tailored remarkably well for individuals thereby optimizing symptom management and vastly improving overall treatment efficacy. Rigorous therapy regimens often brutally curtail oral intake and severely hinder absorption of vital nutrients in frail patients undergoing harsh treatment protocols. Chemotherapy and radiation targeting head neck or gastrointestinal tract frequently cause mucositis xerostomia and dysgeusia with nasty nausea and very severe vomiting.

Symptoms severely curtail appetite and impair digestion alongside assimilation of various essential nutrients thereby heightening risk of drastic weight loss or severe deficiencies. Nutrient-dense foods paired rather effectively with texture-modified diets and supplementation carefully tailored to individual tolerances can mitigate such effects very well. Cancer treatment induces drastic metabolic shifts such as hypermetabolism or insulin resistance requiring meticulous macronutrient balancing under conditions of rampant systemic inflammation. Cancer patients with cachexia may benefit significantly from consuming more protein and anti-inflammatory nutrients such as omega-3 fatty acids very effectively. Survivors experiencing treatment-induced insulin resistance or weight gain conversely may need controlled carbohydrate intake with emphasis on low glycemic index foods.

Nutrition plays a rather critical role in supporting immune function and has another vital aspect altogether significantly. Vitamins A C D and E alongside zinc and selenium play crucial roles modulating immune responses possibly requiring optimization based on lab results and genetic predispositions. Polyphenols and probiotics modulate inflammation fairly effectively while gut microbiota get potentially enhanced significantly thereby boosting recovery rather quickly. Implementing personalized nutrition effectively in cancer care nowadays demands collaboration among oncologists, dietitians and various other healthcare providers for ongoing assessment and adaptation. Ongoing tracking of body composition lab results and patient-reported outcomes ensures interventions remain aligned with swiftly changing intricate health needs. Cancer management gets a boost from super personalized nutrition strategies that tackle gnarly eating issues in patients very effectively thereby markedly enhancing survivorship outcomes.

a. Symptom-Driven Customization

Radiation enteritis or bowel resections may require low-fibre or low-residue diets, with gradual reintroduction of fibre based on tolerance. Chemotherapy-induced nausea may necessitate small, bland, energy-dense meals and hydration strategies. Mucositis or dysphagia, common in head and neck cancers, can be managed with texture-modified, nutrient-dense foods and high-protein oral supplements.

b. Immune and Metabolic Support

Cancer treatment intersects intricately with patient's metabolic status and immune function underscoring a crucial role for nutritional interventions specifically targeted in oncology. Robust immune competence and metabolic homeostasis are essentially required for minimizing complications like recalcitrant infections or tissue repair gone awry. Tailored dietary approaches rely heavily on certain nutrients that modulate immunity and tweak metabolic processes effectively for each patient's unique requirements. Glutamine serves as key substrate for rapidly proliferating immune cells and enterocytes during intense physiological stress being conditionally essential. Harsh cancer treatments like chemo deplete glutamine levels drastically often impairing gut health and weakening immune response terribly over time. Glutamine supplementation greatly reduces mucositis severity thereby encourage lymphocyte proliferation and improving patient outcomes by healing intestinal mucosa very quickly.

Vitamin D plays a multifaceted role in regulating immune responses effectively modulating both innate and adaptive immunity with considerable efficacy. Vitamin D rather extensively influences cytokine production and antimicrobial peptide expression beyond its classical roles in bone metabolism. Vitamin D insufficiency afflicts numerous cancer patients fairly often and links strongly with heightened inflammation and generally ghastly prognosis. Vitamin D supplementation calibrated very effectively according norms of serum 25-hydroxyvitamin D and genetic variations within VDR gene optimizes immunomodulatory effects and supports systemic inflammation control. Zinc acts somewhat irregularly as a cofactor for numerous enzymes involved deeply in DNA synthesis and cell division with antioxidant defense mechanisms.

Zinc deficiency severely hampers wound healing and heightens susceptibility of patients to sundry infections throughout treatment owing largely to malabsorption. Tailored zinc replenishment strategies guided by serum zinc concentrations effectively restore impaired immunity and facilitate tissue repair very quickly. Arginine a semi-essential amino acid serves as precursor for nitric oxide synthesis critical for immune cell signaling and fosters tissue regeneration very effectively.

Arginine supplementation enhances immune responses effectively in malnourished patients and supports wound healing rather rapidly after surgical oncology procedures. Cautious deliberation in patients with specific tumour types adept at hijacking arginine metabolic pathways rather effectively is necessitated by its usage. Intricate multifaceted strategies involving various disciplines quietly necessitate modified dietary plans rich in metabolism-boosting nutrients and some immune-supporting compounds. Monitoring various biochemical markers and clinical symptoms regularly facilitates dynamic adjustment of supplementation for great efficacy and safety. Nutritional support tailored to precision boosts cancer care outcomes remarkably by reducing toxicities related to treatment and significantly enhancing bodily resilience.

c. Addressing Sarcopenia and Cachexia

Sarcopenia and cachexia pose stark critical challenges badly in cancer management significantly impacting patients' functional status and overall survival outcomes terribly. Sarcopenia brings about gradual skeletal muscle mass depletion and strength breakdown while cachexia involves severe multifactorial muscle wasting with systemic inflammation. Tailored nutrition strategies remarkably enhance quality of life significantly and boost clinical outcomes under diverse complicated circumstances with great efficacy. Tumour-derived factors fuel muscle protein breakdown and drastically amplify resting energy expenditure thereby altering various metabolic pathways significantly. Profound muscle wasting and precipitous weight loss occur in patients which often defies rectification by conventional caloric supplementation. Nutrition tailored meticulously to individual needs must incorporate interventions targeting preservation of lean body mass extremely slowly.

Cachexia management nutritionally hinges on massive calorie consumption and very high protein diets somewhat countering catabolic losses effectively. Protein intake recommendations fluctuate enormously from 1.2 grams per kilogram body weight daily and adjust according to factors like renal function or metabolic tolerance variably under different treatment phases. Leucine a branched-chain amino acid supplementation plays pivotal role in stimulating muscle protein synthesis via mTOR signaling thereby counteracting rapid muscle tissue degradation. Eicosapentaenoic acid a polyunsaturated omega-3 fatty acid profoundly demonstrates anti-inflammatory properties effectively mitigating cytokine-induced muscle wasting rather oddly. EPA supplementation curbs tumour necrosis factor-alpha levels and catabolic mediators thereby helping attenuate systemic inflammation exacerbating cachexia very significantly. Balancing metabolic homeostasis very effectively aims at encourage appetite remarkably well alongside physical functionality in various dietary plans.

Complex carbs and medium-chain triglycerides provide easily digestible energy supporting caloric needs and minimizing gastrointestinal issues during cancer therapy. Fairly precise assessment of muscle mass changes can be enabled through regular monitoring of body composition via bioelectrical impedance analysis or dual-energy X-ray absorptiometry. Assessments very quickly inform adjustments in protein intake and prevent further muscle loss while imbalances in overall caloric consumption tend to occur. Merging dietary interventions with rigorous exercise protocols and diverse pharmaceutical therapies substantially amplifies muscle anabolism and accelerates functional recuperation afterwards effectively. Ongoing evaluation and modified dietary tweaks underpin a patient-centered multifaceted approach that manages sarcopenia and cachexia vitally in oncology care effectively.

6.5. Post-Treatment and Survivorship Nutrition

Cancer survivorship involves myriad confounding health issues necessitating highly personalized dietary approaches that optimize recovery and mitigate risk of recurrence rather effectively. Survivors often face greatly heightened risk of various comorbidities such as cardiovascular disease osteoporosis and metabolic syndrome after treatment ends abruptly. Risks frequently emerge owing largely to physiological shifts associated with treatment and lifestyle adjustments amidst stubborn underlying inflammation. Personalized nutrition necessitates a rather dynamic multifaceted approach during survivorship integrating various metabolic nutritional microbiome and complex psychosocial factors quite effectively. Weight management plays a crucial role in survivorship nutrition frequently dictated by metabolic markers such as insulin sensitivity and lipid profiles alongside assessments of physical activity. Survivors of hormone-sensitive cancers like breast or prostate cancer frequently experience pronounced weight gain particularly around visceral areas with adverse metabolic outcomes ensuing.

Survivors conversely face undernutrition or significant muscle loss highlighting necessity for tailored energy balance plans with varied macronutrient distributions obviously. Nutrient repletion happens fairly often because various cancer therapies induce severe deficiencies in vitamins or minerals very regularly nowadays. Chemotherapy and radiation very badly impair gastrointestinal absorption or increase losses of vital nutrients like iron and vitamin B12 leading to nasty deficits. Biochemical monitoring done routinely helps correct deficits somewhat and enhances physiological resilience marginally via targeted diet or pharmacologic interventions. Restoration of microbiome assumes vital importance during survivorship owing largely to emerging evidence of gut microbiota's crucial role in modulating host immunity and various metabolic pathways.

Fermented foods like yogurt alongside polyphenol-rich fruits and diverse plant fibres very effectively foster microbial diversity producing short-chain fatty acids. Certain dietary constituents blunt chronic inflammation and significantly enhance intestinal barrier function thereby markedly reducing cancer recurrence and enhancing overall health substantially. Fear of recurrence psychologically wreaks havoc on eating behaviors badly in some folks after a cancer diagnosis and treatment fuels ridiculously restrictive diets. Referrals to specialists or mindfulness-based interventions within nutrition counseling keep dietary plans remarkably sustainable and fairly well balanced overall. Survivorship being wildly dynamic necessitates nutrition counseling adapting quickly through regular reassessments of complex evolving health status and personal lifestyle goals. Survivors gain remarkably effective nutrition strategies from ongoing patient engagement and collaboration with various disciplines fostering long-term health overall.

6.6. Implementation

Highly specialized nutritional interventions require synergy between oncologists and registered dietitians with genetic counselors or various behavioral health specialists sometimes. Nutrigenomic testing alongside metabolic lab panels and dietary intake software can effectively aid highly personalized interventions with body composition assessments. Culturally tailored education and motivational interviewing coupled with goal setting effectively achieves long-term adherence remarkably well over time. Tailored nutritional interventions provide a potent strategy for cancer prevention and effectively manage progression remarkably sometimes with unusual efficacy. Personalized nutrition boosts therapeutic efficacy significantly by merging genetic data with clinical insights and various lifestyle factors quite effectively nowadays. Precision oncology advances rapidly nowadays and nutrition stays vitally integral within cancer care highly personalized across various treatment regimes.

7. The Role of Microbiomes and Epigenetics in Precision Oncology Nutrition

Tumour development stems from intricate interactions between genetic predisposition and environmental factors alongside sundry lifestyle choices that curiously influence cancer progression rather haphazardly. Precision oncology nutrition intricately leverages complexity by tailoring dietary interventions simultaneously for genetic profiles epigenetic regulation and gut microbiome dynamics. Diet profoundly influences cancer risk and therapeutic efficacy gets affected greatly by fields examining various micronutrients and nutrients beyond macronutrients. Trillions of microorganisms inhabiting gastrointestinal tract play a crucial role energetically modulating immune responses and metabolic functions deeply within human body. Dysbiosis aka microbiome composition alterations and diversity changes have been rather starkly linked to heightened risk of carcinogenesis and chemotherapy efficacy impairment.

Polyphenols and prebiotics alongside dietary fibre beneficially shape microbial ecosystems greatly enhancing production of metabolites like short-chain fatty acids supporting mucosal integrity. Personalized dietary regimens focusing on revitalizing gut flora and encourage robustness present potentially efficacious adjunctive cancer interventions alongside standard treatment protocols. Epigenetics nowadays furnishes a mechanistic framework for how various environmental factors and dietary habits influence cancer biology rather quietly these days heavily. Histone acetylation and non-coding RNA activity epigenetically regulate expression of various oncogenes and tumour suppressor genes alongside DNA methylation.

Curcumin and sulforaphane alongside green tea catechins and folate have remarkably shown capacity epigenetically modulating epigenetic marks with considerable efficacy. Diet-driven epigenetic therapies hold promise as modulation rapidly suppresses tumour growth and effectively sensitizes cancer cells for subsequent treatment. Microbiome-derived metabolites intricately amplify regulatory networks by interacting heavily with host epigenome and nutrition influences gene expression variably enough.

Refined biologically informed dietary recommendations emerge from precision nutrition frameworks that incorporate microbiome profiling and epigenetic analyses complementing oncologic treatment regimens very effectively. Personalized interventions can be devised by clarifying molecular interactions between dietary habits microbial communities and gene expression in cancer settings thereby optimizing therapeutic efficacy and boosting long-term survivorship prospects greatly.

7.1. The Microbiome

Gut microbiota orchestrates digestion and nutrient metabolism crucially alongside immune function underpinning sundry cancer development processes quite pertinently in humans normally. Myriad microorganisms constituting microbiome act mysteriously as metabolic interface between host physiological processes and dietary intake somewhat normally. A rather terse utterance was obviously made somewhat brusquely. Gut microbes metabolize dietary fibre and polyphenols into bioactive compounds that rapidly influence various cellular processes deeply inside cells. Fibre fermentation yields butyrate which very effectively promotes anti-inflammatory signaling and epigenetic mods like histone acetylation downstream in cells.

High-fat diets spur production of secondary bile acids that can heavily damage colon cells through oxidative stress and DNA damage thereby contributing significantly to cancer risk. High-fat diets spur formation of secondary bile acids that aggressively promote oxidative stress and DNA damage thereby greatly heightening risk of colon cancer. Dietary inputs and microbial composition somewhat erratically enhance or thwart anti-cancer mechanisms by significantly influencing metabolic byproducts in varying degrees.

a. Microbiota Diversity and Therapy Response

Research nowadays indicates gut microbiota composition profoundly affects cancer therapy effectiveness particularly under specific conditions with immunotherapy approaches being markedly influenced. Certain beneficial taxa including Akkermansia muciniphila and Faecalibacterium prausnitzii correlate remarkably with enhanced efficacy of immune checkpoint inhibitors alongside higher microbial diversity. Antibiotic use and processed diets correlate with diminished treatment tolerance and survival rates largely owing to markedly low gut microbial diversity. Prebiotics alongside probiotics and high-fibre plant-based diets remarkably enhance a microbiome's beneficial role in various cancer therapies quite significantly.

7.2. Epigenetics

Epigenetics involves study of heritable changes in gene expression occurring sans underlying DNA sequence alterations very much everywhere. Genetic tweaks profoundly dictate gene expression status impacting cellular function phenotype in myriad ways beneath seemingly normal surface level appearances. Primary epigenetic mechanisms entail DNA methylation and histone modifications such as acetylation or methylation alongside action of non-coding RNAs heavily influencing cell processes. Malignant transformation unfolds rapidly as epigenetic dysregulation precipitates aberrant oncogene activation or tumour suppressor gene silencing in cancerous cells. Dynamic and reversible epigenetic changes make them unusually appealing targets for certain pharmacological treatments and various dietary interventions. Research endeavors nationwide have recently flagged diet as a potent epigenome modulator across various studies with considerable veracity and intense scrutiny.

Bioactive compounds present in various foods have epigenetically altered genes relevant in cancer biology rather profoundly under certain conditions. Folate and other B vitamins are crucial methyl donors in one-carbon metabolism playing a significant role in DNA methylation processes directly. Nutrient deficiencies can cause global hypomethylation or hypermethylation at specific gene loci thereby affecting genomic stability and cancer risk increases rapidly. Phytochemicals such as curcumin found in turmeric and epigallocatechin gallate from green tea very effectively modulate histone acetylation and methylation states. Compounds inhibit histone deacetylases or activate histone acetyltransferases thereby restoring chromatin structure and reactivating tumour suppressor genes normally silenced. Diet impacts various non-coding RNAs like microRNAs which subsequently play a crucial role in post-transcriptional gene regulation processes.

Altered miRNA expression tweaks pathways that control cell cycles and apoptosis contributing enormously to cancer prevention or rapid tumour progression subsequently. Dietary influences epigenetically impact gene regulation and cancer development quite broadly by linking various environmental exposures crucially. Precision nutrition strategies emerging from understanding complex interactions harness epigenetic modulation quite effectively reducing cancer risk subsequently rather markedly. Dietary epigenetics will likely morph into cornerstone of integrative oncology care rapidly as research advances precipitously in this fairly obscure field.

a. Methyl Donors and DNA Methylation

DNA methylation entails appending a methyl group mostly onto cytosine residues fairly typically within CpG dinucleotides in many instances. This process plays a crucial role in regulation of gene expression and maintenance of genomic stability alongside control of cellular differentiation. Methyl groups utilized in DNA methylation are supplied by metabolites stemming from one-carbon metabolism pathway heavily contingent upon dietary intake of crucial nutrients. Vitamin B9 folate and cobalamin vitamin B12 serve as primary methyl donors along with methionine an essential amino acid and choline in human dietary needs. Folate and vitamin B12 synergize facilitating methyl group transfer through methylation cycle yielding S-adenosylmethionine a universal methyl donor for DNA methyltransferases. Choline and methionine feed into related metabolic pathways that fuel synthesis of SAM thereby somewhat effectively maintaining cellular methylation capacity.

Sufficient intake of methyl donors via dietary sources preserves normal DNA methylation patterns fairly effectively under most circumstances. Low levels severely disrupt methylation balance resulting in global DNA hypomethylation eerily linked to instability of genome and activation of various oncogenes. Hypermethylation of promoter regions in tumour suppressor genes occurs aberrantly thereby silencing their expression and preventing cells from controlling proliferation. Common MTHFR variants greatly impair conversion of folate rather slowly to its active form through one-carbon metabolism pathways. Individuals possessing specific genetic mutations frequently exhibit significantly impaired methylation capacity thus heightening risk of epigenetic dysregulation and increased susceptibility to cancer.

Personalized dietary interventions might utilize methylated folate forms such as 5-methyltetrahydrofolate and vitamin B12 along with other crucial cofactors quite effectively. Modified nutrition plans informed by genetic testing and clinical assessment of nutrient status can restore epigenetic equilibrium supporting DNA repair and ultimately lower cancer risk. Dietary intake of methyl donors profoundly impacts DNA methylation which plays an epigenetically crucial role in regulating genes for cancer therapy. Tailored nutrition plans incorporating genetic susceptibility and eating patterns may yield markedly improved cancer treatment results by modulating epigenetic factors effectively.

b. Histone Modulation by Dietary Compounds

Histone proteins that DNA coils tightly around play a central role regulating gene expression via various drastic changes called histone mods somewhat collectively. Post-translational modifications such as acetylation and phosphorylation alter chromatin structure rather dramatically thereby controlling gene expression very often indeed. Histone acetyltransferases catalyze acetylation while histone deacetylases facilitate deacetylation playing a pivotal role in modulating gene expression deeply related to inflammation and cell growth during cancer progression. Novel research findings have identified multiple bioactive nutrients in foods influencing histone alteration quite effectively serving as potent epigenetic regulators. Sulforaphane a rather recondite phytochemical abounds in cruciferous veggies like broccoli and is studied extensively nowadays by many researchers.

Sulforaphane potently inhibits HDAC thereby promoting hyperacetylation of histones and reactivating tumour suppressor genes silenced in cancer cells quite effectively. Sulforaphane quite effectively inhibits proliferation of cancer cells and induces apoptosis by restoring function of normal genes somewhat. Curcumin very significantly inhibits HDAC activity and modulates histone acetylation rather oddly in turmeric with some epigenetic effects. Curcumin impacts various epigenetic regulators like DNA methyltransferases thereby suppressing oncogenic pathways very significantly and reducing loads of inflammation. Resveratrol profoundly influences histone acetylation by activating sirtuins that regulate cellular stress responses and apoptosis quite vigorously.

Resveratrol modulates histone acetylation in a quite intricate manner thereby exerting profoundly anti-inflammatory effects and pro-apoptotic effects in various murky cellular contexts. Epigallocatechin gallate found majorly in green tea inhibits histone acetyltransferases and histone deacetylases thereby markedly skewing histone acetylation balance. EGCG haphazardly tweaks gene expression patterns related to cell cycle arrest apoptosis and angiogenesis making it rather promising as a potentially efficacious cancer treatment adjuvant. Collectively these dietary compounds modulate histone modifications very effectively influencing gene expression crucial for cancer prevention therapy. Nutriepigenetics integration into precision oncology nutrition strategies remains remarkably an active research area highlighting potential benefits of minimized side effects and reduced resistance.

7.3. Integrating Microbiome and Epigenetic Insights into Nutrition Plans

Personalized cancer prevention support emerges from precision nutrition leveraging microbiome insights and epigenetic markers in myriad unconventional manners pretherapy. Patients may reap huge rewards from diets rich in fermentable fibres and sundry antioxidants that optimize immune function greatly. Epigenetically active compounds and probiotic-rich foods can be added during treatment to boost therapy efficacy and lessen nasty side effects like diarrhea or immune suppression. Post-Treatment Recovery: Targeted use of methylation-supportive nutrients, SCFA-promoting fibres, and anti-inflammatory phytonutrients can aid in epigenetic reprogramming, immune restoration, and recurrence prevention. Targeted use of methylation supportive nutrients and SCFA-promoting fibres alongside anti-inflammatory phytonutrients can aid epigenetic reprogramming and prevent recurrence after treatment.

7.4. Future Directions and Challenges

Merging microbiome and epigenetic science into nutrition has enormous potential, yet several gnarly challenges linger mainly for obtuse reasons apparently. Standardization of testing methods and interpretation across labs remains an issue. Significant variability exists epigenetically and in microbiota among individuals with wildly differing dietary habits very much everywhere apparently. Longitudinal studies are desperately needed now for establishing causality between diet and various epigenetic changes or possibly microbial alterations. Ethical considerations abound greatly in the usage of genomic data and microbiome information quite frequently nowadays. Multi-omics tech advancements and machine learning coupled with systems biology rapidly facilitate design of modified diets based on epigenetic data.

Epigenetics and microbiomes interplay remarkably within human physiology embodying a crucial aspect in evolution of precision oncology nutrition nowadays. Modified approaches can quite effectively improve treatment tolerance and slash cancer risk by tweaking microbial composition via specific dietary regimens. Research in this area grows apace rapidly and microbiome profiling coupled with epigenetic analysis will likely overhaul cancer care eventually in clinical nutrition.

8. Future Directions in Precision Nutrition: Integrating Technology, Genetics, and Personalized Care

Precision nutrition evolves rapidly with genomics advancements and digital health technologies drastically reshaping nutrition science in rather unconventional ways nowadays. Traditional dietary guidelines often falter somewhat in capturing variability in human metabolism and susceptibility to complex diseases like cancer among individuals. Precision nutrition emerges resolutely as a discipline bent on customizing dietary advice according individual's quirky biology and various lifestyle factors quite thoroughly. Cutting-edge tech synergizes with modified care and genetic insights spearheading eerily responsive data-driven transformation that rapidly optimizes human health nowadays.

8.1. The Convergence of Omics Technologies and Nutrition

Precision nutrition relies heavily on systems biology factoring genome transcriptome proteome and metabolome in alongside thorough microbiome understanding of food's deep interaction with human biology. Genomics illuminates genetic polymorphisms affecting nutrient metabolism like certain MTHFR variants that impede folate absorption or FTO variants linked oddly enough to obesity. Various omics layers provide peeks at facets of dietary requirements and diverse human reactions epigenomics explores how diet alters gene expression via mechanisms such as histone acetylation or methylation. Metabolomics measures metabolites to assess real-time nutritional status and metabolic health. Microbiomics evaluates how gut microbial composition and function affect digestion, immunity, and cancer risk. Metabolomics assesses real-time nutritional status and metabolic health by quantifying various metabolites very accurately in human bodies.

8.2. Artificial Intelligence and Digital Tools in Nutritional Personalization

Multi-omics data and clinical information pose significant analytical hurdles nowadays necessitating very sophisticated computational tools fairly frequently. Very personalized dietary recommendations and various outcomes are being predicted nowadays using machine learning algorithms alongside artificial intelligence rather effectively.

a. AI-Powered Diet Planning

AI gets subtly infused into cutting-edge cancer nutrition marking rather transformative strides in modified dietary plans for sufferers of various cancers. AI-powered platforms leveraging multidimensional data convergence comprising dietary logs and physiological data from wearables alongside genomic profiles deliver highly modified nutrition interventions. Machine learning algorithms analyze interactions between genetic predispositions and metabolic status alongside lifestyle factors during various treatment phases very effectively nowadays. Genomic data reveal specific SNPs that influence nutrient metabolism very thoroughly and vehemently affect inflammatory responses alongside various detoxification pathways in humans somewhat mysteriously. Biometric data such as glucose levels and heart rate variability offer insights into patient's physiological state under various dietary regimens quite dynamically.

AI systems devise highly customized meal plans perfectly aligning with therapeutic goals like weight loss and mitigation of nasty side effects very effectively nowadays. Adaptive learning gets incorporated into these platforms and updates recommendations rather continuously based on shifts in biomarkers and patient-reported symptoms. Patients exhibiting markers of insulin resistance and inflammation while undergoing chemo might receive personalized AI-generated dietary regimens emphasizing omega-3 rich food with anti-inflammatory properties. Wearable data indicating dwindling physical activity or erratic sleep patterns enables recalibration of macronutrient ratios supporting homeostasis quite effectively nowadays.

AI-powered diet planning fosters patient engagement remarkably by providing modified shopping lists and actionable evidence-based feedback respecting various cultural nuances. Tailoring interventions dynamically by monitoring outcomes represents significant improvement over static guidelines frequently advocated nationwide by health experts. Multidisciplinary coordination gets enhanceed substantially as evolving platforms integrate deeply with oncology care teams and various electronic health records simultaneously. AI-driven nutrition planning holds immense promise for revolutionizing personalized cancer care and boosts long-term survivorship outcomes amidst gnarly lingering issues.

b. Mobile Health (mHealth) Applications

Mobile health apps represent a rapidly expanding frontier in precision oncology nutrition leveraging smartphones and diverse digital technologies for cancer patients' nutrition plans.mHealth apps integrated with artificial intelligence algorithms deliver adaptive interventions tailored carefully for individual clinical needs quite effectively facilitating comprehensive profiling longitudinally and users track key health metrics including dietary habits symptom severity and physical activity on such platforms. Patients get empowered somewhat mysteriously by dynamic feedback loops and stick fairly closely to highly modified nutrition plans during cancer treatment. A patient undergoing chemo might swiftly receive guidance on food packed with calories and gentle on stomach lining rather quickly. Individuals tracking glucose variability or inflammatory markers reap rewards from AI-driven dietary tweaks stabilizing metabolic function very deeply.

mHealth tools frequently embed behavioral science tenets such as goal setting or social support mechanisms into their architecture nowadays.mHealth platforms facilitate remote monitoring by healthcare providers enabling dietitians and oncologists review patient data and intervene promptly nowadays greatly. Push notifications spur timely hydration or reinforce adherence to specific nutrient targets, thereby encourage holistic care in survivorship. Telehealth integration proves invaluable in managing gnarly cases where dietary tweaks respond with agility to shifting treatment phases or gnarly side effects. MHealth apps deliver personalized nutrition care very effectively despite thorny issues around data privacy and access being unequal among underserved populations. Technological advancements greatly enhance precision nutrition's efficacy in cancer treatment and substantially improve quality of long-term outcomes.

c. Continuous Monitoring Devices

Implantable tech and wearable biosensors are revolutionizing oncology's personalized nutrition nowadays by rapidly spitting out real-time physio data very quickly. Gizmos keenly monitor biomarkers including glucose levels heart rate variability and inflammatory markers thus creating an objective feedback loop between nutrition and bodily response. Physiological states fluctuate rapidly in cancer patients undergoing harsh treatments like chemotherapy impacting metabolic needs greatly and overall well-being suffers terribly. Clinicians and nutritionists keenly observe fluctuations largely through relentless surveillance enabling prompt adjustments in nutritional regimens that substantially enhance treatment tolerance and expedite recovery. Continuous glucose monitors furnish real-time data on blood sugar fluctuations enabling precise dietary carb management thereby preventing hyperglycemia frequently in steroid recipients.

Personalized low-glycemic diets stabilize glucose metabolism radically improving energy and mitigating risk of cancer progression critically. Wearables measuring heart rate variability offer very profound insights into autonomic nervous system functionality and stress levels rather effectively these days systemically. Declines in heart rate variability may presage markedly heightened stress prompting somewhat unorthodox interventions like upping intake of omega-3s or tweaking meal timing drastically. Biosensors emerging rapidly detect cytokines indicating inflammation or biomarkers signifying oxidative stress from sweat and interstitial fluid providing precious biochemical evidence quietly.

Personalized supplementation regimens alongside dietary tweaks mitigating nasty side effects can be informed by such data and tissue repair is fostered vigorously. AI-driven analytics merged quite seamlessly with cutting-edge monitoring tech facilitating rather ingenious predictive modeling that enables quite anticipatory tweaks downstream. Preserving nutritional status and minimizing treatment interruptions directly impact clinical outcomes in oncology with considerable therapeutic value overall. Advancement of user-friendly monitoring devices is promising embedding continuous physiological feedback deeply as cornerstone of precision nutrition in cancer care enhancing survivorship quality markedly.

8.3. Integration with Clinical Practice: The Role of Interdisciplinary Care

Precision nutrition implementation succeeds in oncology largely through deep integration within varied healthcare frameworks that emphasize intensely collaborative care centered on patients. Precision nutrition gets effectively translated into clinical reality via a team-based approach amidst nuances of genomic data interpretation and metabolic variability. Genetic counselors play a pivotal role in deciphering patient's genomic profiles and elucidating significance of various genetic variants related deeply to nutrient metabolism. Their expertise ensures genetic info gets conveyed very accurately thus mitigating risks of misinterpretation and undue anxiety in risk stratification subsequently for personalized dietary advice.

Personalized nutritional regimens are being bridged quite effectively nowadays by clinical dietitians specializing in nutrigenomics with genetic discoveries gaping wide open. Experts meticulously evaluate diverse biochemical indicators and clinical manifestations during treatment phases crafting ultra personalized nutrition plans that accommodate unusual genetic susceptibilities. Their involvement facilitates translation of complex molecular data into actionable guidance tailored around real-world dietary habits with somewhat eccentric specificity for patients. Behavioral health specialists quite effectively provide crucial backing in myriad medical settings addressing various psychosocial aspects of nutritional compliance these days. Cancer treatment side effects and deeply ingrained cultural norms heavily influence dietary changes which can be utterly emotionally exhausting.

Motivational interviewing enhances patients' capacity to stick tenaciously with dietary regimens thereby somewhat improving life quality under certain conditions obviously. Collaboration with bioinformaticians and data scientists enables fairly quick integration of multi-omic data alongside patient-reported outcomes refining precision nutrition algorithms. Precision oncology nutrition will necessitate fostering equitable access to genetic testing and culturally sensitive counseling for patients and healthcare providers persistently. This multidisciplinary model rather quietly leverages rapid technological advances and prioritizes patient autonomy effectively in many clinical settings nowadays. Thus precision nutrition becomes palpably accessible as a facet of comprehensive cancer care rather than some lofty unattainable idealistic notion.

8.4. Personalized Nutrition in Cancer Care and Beyond

Cancer represents a tangled web of precision nutrition possibilities rooted deeply in multifaceted causes and extremely varied patient reactions amidst freakishly heightened metabolic turmoil. Research advances positioned personalized nutrition as crucial oncology care element offering capacity remarkably to tailor dietary regimens supporting treatment efficacy and encourage survivorship prospects effectively. Modulation of immune function through diet potentially substantially augments effectiveness of various immunotherapies in many patients receiving treatment nowadays. Omega-3 fatty acids and polyphenols alongside vitamin D can selectively enhance anti-tumour immunity while mitigating toxicities related to treatment. Immunonutrition approach optimizes patient responsiveness effectively nowadays with novel immunotherapeutic agents in some very rare cases.

Microbiome-directed nutrition very effectively leverages dynamic interplay between gut microbial communities host genetics and various dietary factors these days. Clinicians may markedly improve gastrointestinal tolerance by very specifically tailoring prebiotic fibres probiotics and fermented foods reducing systemic inflammation thereby. Cancer treatment benefits substantially from upkeep of metabolic functionality alongside microbial diversity via a fairly unorthodox holistic therapeutic regimen. Diets rich in methyl donors such as folate and B12 may possibly help restore gene expression in patients with certain epigenetic issues. Nutritional epigenomics represents a fairly intriguing adjunct surprisingly enough to standard cancer therapies at molecular level regulation nowadays. Precision oncology nutrition stands to benefit enormously from real-time nutrient supplementation guided by biomarkers where circulating metabolites inform dietary tweaks dynamically.

Personalized feedback loops can enhance responsiveness rather effectively throughout a care continuum minimizing adverse effects very simultaneously. Principles and technologies underpinning precision nutrition have broad applicability across many chronic diseases involving intricate gene environment interactions. Highly individualized approaches may revolutionize care for neurodegenerative disorders and diabetes mellitus through tailored dietary management and very early intervention. Artificial intelligence alongside interdisciplinary collaboration and multi-omic data integration will be crucial for swiftly translating precision nutrition into routine clinical practice offering new horizons effectively in personalized health management that transcends merely cancer and addresses diverse complex chronic disease nutritional needs.

8.5. Challenges and Ethical Considerations

Precision nutrition's transformative potential faces gnarly hurdles that must be surmounted safely ensuring effective integration into diverse clinical settings equitably. Data privacy and security concerns are paramount fairly significantly nowadays within most global organizations and revolve around sensitive information quite intensely. Precision nutrition heavily relies on gathering sensitive personal data including genomic sequences and microbiome profiles alongside various metabolic biomarkers and lifestyle info. Datasets nowadays demand robust cybersecurity infrastructures very effectively preventing outside breaches and unauthorized access from various malicious sources. Stringent moral guidelines govern consent protocols and data dissemination preserving patient autonomy quietly throughout various often sensitive stages of data utilization.

Globally many communities face significant barriers stemming from risk of health disparities and inequity problematically nowadays in rather complex societal contexts. Steep prices linked with DNA analysis and cutting-edge bioinformatics mainly restrict availability largely to wealthy demographics residing in metropolitan regions. Precision nutrition risks exacerbating existing healthcare inequities nationwide unless subsidized programs and culturally nuanced education are swiftly implemented. Nationwide policy interventions and system-level commitment are desperately needed for effectively bridging divide between inclusivity and affordability. Validation of clinical findings stays a challenge ongoing from fairly esoteric scientific vantage points sometimes rather obscurely. Preliminary studies reveal promising links between genetic variants and nutrient responses but large-scale longitudinal trials are needed for establishing safe efficacy.

Rapid formulation of evidence-based guidelines standardizes nutrigenomic interpretation very quickly and minimizes risk of premature misinformation stemming from faulty application. Precision nutrition's real-world success hinges partly on user engagement and quirky behavioral patterns naturally emerging over quite some time. Tailored nutrition regimens prove efficacious solely when individuals comprehend and practically implement them within their socioeconomic bracket and surroundings normally. Sustaining motivation necessitates psychosocial support alongside culturally sensitive materials for tackling emotional distress and food insecurity effectively with digital tools. Precision nutrition inhabits a rather rarefied frontier of healthcare personalized fairly recently by leaps in genomics and rather sophisticated digital tech. Artificial intelligence tailors nutrition strategies rather precisely in individual biological contexts amidst complex diseases like cancer very dynamically nowadays. Challenges persist in privacy equity validation and engagement yet future trajectory veers decidedly toward adaptive precision-guided nutritional care unfolding gradually alongside each patient's singular odyssey.

9. Conclusion

Nutrition plays a vital role lately in emerging precision medicine paradigms being adopted rapidly within oncology and elsewhere nowadays. Precision nutrition offers a potent strategy quite effectively for cancer prevention and survivorship care grounded in understanding variability in genetics environment. Precision nutrition endeavors surprisingly intricate dietary plans for individuals largely according to idiosyncratic biomarkers and specific medical conditions very precisely nowadays. Clinicians predict patient responses far more accurately nowadays by integrating genomic data epigenetic markers and microbiome composition with specific dietary patterns essentially. Nutrition plans get tailored influencing disease progression significantly and supporting general health or remarkably speeding recovery quite well.

Genetic polymorphisms influencing folate metabolism or vitamin D receptors and detoxification enzymes can drastically alter nutrient requirements and significantly impact efficacy of cancer treatment. Microbiome emerges as malleable intermediary between dietary intake and host reaction markedly influencing drug metabolism and radically reshaping immune homeostasis. Insights like these facilitate development of nutrition plans rooted deeply in biology and are highly adaptable naturally in totally integrative ways. Genetic predispositions intertwine haphazardly with lifestyle factors like stress and sleep quality profoundly influencing cancer biology in myriad unexpected ways.

Oncology precision nutrition requires a nuanced multifaceted approach extremely sensitive to molecular insights and individual psychosocial context alongside keen personal preferences. Patient-centered strategies foster empowerment throughout cancer care continuum remarkably ensuring adherence very effectively and yielding better holistic well-being overall. Precision nutrition teeters on razor-thin margins amidst unfulfilled promise swamped by glaringly obvious data siloing issues and scathing clinical validation shortfalls. Nutrigenomics and bioinformatics advancements are swiftly accelerating personalized nutrition applications nowadays in oncology settings with considerable practical impact.

Precision nutrition represents a seismic shift in cancer treatment by marrying innovative methodologies with modified care fairly effectively nowadays. Healthcare providers can deliver very effective nutrition strategies by leveraging genetic insights alongside various lifestyle factors and leveraging clinical evidence ridiculously well. Nutrition integration within precision oncology remarkably holds great promise redefining cancer care through highly individualized treatment plans with improved outcomes.

References

Ağagündüz D, Cocozza E, Cemali Ö, Bayazıt AD, Nanì MF, Cerqua I, Morgillo F, Saygılı SK, Berni Canani R, Amero P, Capasso R. Understanding the role of the gut microbiome in gastrointestinal cancer: A review. Front Pharmacol. 2023 Jan 24;14:1130562. doi: 10.3389/fphar.2023.1130562. Erratum in: Front Pharmacol. 2025 Jul 30;16:1662597. doi: 10.3389/fphar.2025.1662597. PMID: 36762108; PMCID: PMC9903080.

Al Aboud NM, Tupper C, Jialal I. Genetics, Epigenetic Mechanism. [Updated 2023 Aug 14]. In: StatPearls [Internet]. Treasure Island (FL): StatPearls Publishing; 2025 Jan-. Available from: https://www.ncbi.nlm.nih.gov/books/NBK532999/

Anand P, Kunnumakkara AB, Sundaram C, Harikumar KB, Tharakan ST, Lai OS, Sung B, Aggarwal BB. Cancer is a preventable disease that requires major lifestyle changes. Pharm Res. 2008 Sep;25(9):2097-116. doi: 10.1007/s11095-008-9661-9. Epub 2008 Jul 15. Erratum in: Pharm Res. 2008 Sep;25(9):2200. Kunnumakara, Ajaikumar B [corrected to Kunnumakkara, Ajaikumar B]. PMID: 18626751; PMCID: PMC2515569.

Anderson OS, Sant KE, Dolinoy DC. Nutrition and epigenetics: an interplay of dietary methyl donors, one-carbon metabolism and DNA methylation. J Nutr Biochem. 2012 Aug;23(8):853-9. doi: 10.1016/j.jnutbio.2012.03.003. Epub 2012 Jun 27. PMID: 22749138; PMCID: PMC3405985.

Anjanappa M, Corden M, Green A, Roberts D, Hoskin P, McWilliam A, Choudhury A. Sarcopenia in cancer: Risking more than muscle loss. Tech Innov Patient Support Radiat Oncol. 2020 Nov 9;16:50-57. doi: 10.1016/j.tipsro.2020.10.001. PMID: 33385074; PMCID: PMC7769854.

Antony Dhanapal ACT, Vimaleswaran KS. Vitamin D supplementation and immune-related markers: an update from nutrigenetic and nutrigenomic studies. Br J Nutr. 2022 Oct 28;128(8):1459–69. doi: 10.1017/S0007114522002392. PMCID: PMC9557210.

Ardekani AM, Jabbari S. Nutrigenomics and cancer. Avicenna J Med Biotechnol. 2009 Apr;1(1):9-17. PMID: 23407612; PMCID: PMC3558114.

Baker Rogers J, Syed K, Minteer JF. Cachexia. [Updated 2023 Aug 8]. In: StatPearls [Internet]. Treasure Island (FL): StatPearls Publishing; 2025 Jan-. Available from: https://www.ncbi.nlm.nih.gov/books/NBK470208/

Baskar R, Lee KA, Yeo R, Yeoh KW. Cancer and radiation therapy: current advances and future directions. Int J Med Sci. 2012;9(3):193-9. doi: 10.7150/ijms.3635. Epub 2012 Feb 27. PMID: 22408567; PMCID: PMC3298009.

Calder PC. Omega-3 polyunsaturated fatty acids and inflammatory processes: nutrition or pharmacology? Br J Clin Pharmacol. 2013 Mar;75(3):645-62. doi: 10.1111/j.1365-2125.2012.04374.x. PMID: 22765297; PMCID: PMC3575932.

Chen X, Zhang J, Gao F, Liu N, Du H, Li J, Li Z, Chen R. Exercise therapy: an effective approach to mitigate the risk of cancer metastasis. World J Surg Oncol. 2025 May 16;23(1):192. doi: 10.1186/s12957-025-03846-7. PMID: 40380237; PMCID: PMC12082867.

Coppedè F, Stoccoro A, Tannorella P, Gallo R, Nicolì V, Migliore L. Association of Polymorphisms in Genes Involved in One-Carbon Metabolism with MTHFR Methylation Levels. Int J Mol Sci. 2019 Jul 31;20(15):3754. doi: 10.3390/ijms20153754. PMID: 31370354; PMCID: PMC6696388.

Elsamanoudy AZ, Mohamed Neamat-Allah MA, Hisham Mohammad FA, Hassanien M, Nada HA. The role of nutrition related genes and nutrigenetics in understanding the pathogenesis of cancer. J Microsc Ultrastruct. 2016 Jul-Sep;4(3):115-122. doi: 10.1016/j.jmau.2016.02.002. Epub 2016 Mar 8. PMID: 30023217; PMCID: PMC6014201.

Farhud D, Zarif Yeganeh M, Zarif Yeganeh M. Nutrigenomics and nutrigenetics. Iran J Public Health. 2010;39(4):1-14. Epub 2010 Dec 31. PMID: 23113033; PMCID: PMC3481686.

Fujiwara Y, Kato S, Kurzrock R. Evolution of Precision Oncology, Personalized Medicine, and Molecular Tumor Boards. Surg Oncol Clin N Am. 2024 Apr;33(2):197-216. doi: 10.1016/j.soc.2023.12.004. Epub 2023 Dec 18. PMID: 38401905; PMCID: PMC10894322.

Furman D, Campisi J, Verdin E, Carrera-Bastos P, Targ S, Franceschi C, Ferrucci L, Gilroy DW, Fasano A, Miller GW, Miller AH, Mantovani A, Weyand CM, Barzilai N, Goronzy JJ, Rando TA, Effros RB, Lucia A, Kleinstreuer N, Slavich GM. Chronic inflammation in the etiology of disease across the life span. Nat Med. 2019 Dec;25(12):1822-1832. doi: 10.1038/s41591-019-0675-0. Epub 2019 Dec 5. PMID: 31806905; PMCID: PMC7147972.

Garg S, Sharma N, Bharmjeet, Das A. Unraveling the intricate relationship: Influence of microbiome on the host immune system in carcinogenesis. Cancer Rep (Hoboken). 2023 Nov;6(11):e1892. doi: 10.1002/cnr2.1892. Epub 2023 Sep 14. PMID: 37706437; PMCID: PMC10644337.

Geeleher P, Huang RS. Exploring the Link between the Germline and Somatic Genome in Cancer. Cancer Discov. 2017 Apr;7(4):354-355. doi: 10.1158/2159-8290.CD-17-0192. PMID: 28373166; PMCID: PMC5404740.

Gilani B, Cassagnol M. Biochemistry, Cytochrome P450. [Updated 2023 Apr 24]. In: StatPearls [Internet]. Treasure Island (FL): StatPearls Publishing; 2025 Jan-. Available from: https://www.ncbi.nlm.nih.gov/books/NBK557698/

Greathouse KL, Choudhury A. Precision nutrition and the gut microbiome: Harnessing AI to revolutionize cancer prevention and therapy. Cell Host Microbe. 2025 Jun 11;33(6):766-776. doi: 10.1016/j.chom.2025.05.011. PMID: 40505617.

Haskins CP, Champ CE, Miller R, Vyfhuis MAL. Nutrition in Cancer: Evidence and Equality. Adv Radiat Oncol. 2020 May 24;5(5):817-823. doi: 10.1016/j.adro.2020.05.008. PMID: 33083643; PMCID: PMC7557144.

Hassan FU, Rehman MS, Khan MS, Ali MA, Javed A, Nawaz A, Yang C. Curcumin as an Alternative Epigenetic Modulator: Mechanism of Action and Potential Effects. Front Genet. 2019 Jun 4;10:514. doi: 10.3389/fgene.2019.00514. PMID: 31214247; PMCID: PMC6557992.

Haussler MR, Haussler CA, Whitfield GK, Hsieh JC, Thompson PD, Barthel TK, Bartik L, Egan JB, Wu Y, Kubicek JL, Lowmiller CL, Moffet EW, Forster RE, Jurutka PW. The nuclear vitamin D receptor controls the expression of genes encoding factors which feed the "Fountain of Youth" to mediate healthful aging. J Steroid Biochem Mol Biol. 2010 Jul;121(1-2):88-97. doi: 10.1016/j.jsbmb.2010.03.019. Epub 2010 Mar 20. PMID: 20227497; PMCID: PMC2906618.

Hodges RE, Minich DM. Modulation of Metabolic Detoxification Pathways Using Foods and Food-Derived Components: A Scientific Review with Clinical Application. J Nutr Metab. 2015;2015:760689. doi: 10.1155/2015/760689. Epub 2015 Jun 16. PMID: 26167297; PMCID: PMC4488002.

Kadıoğlu E, Taçoy G, Özçağlı E, Okyay K, Akboğa MK, Çengel A, Şardaş S. The role of oxidative DNA damage and GSTM1, GSTT1, and hOGG1 gene polymorphisms in coronary artery disease risk. Anatol J Cardiol. 2016 Dec;16(12):931-938. doi: 10.14744/AnatolJCardiol.2016.6697. Epub 2016 Apr 26. PMID: 27182613; PMCID: PMC5324912.

Kassem NM, Abdelmegid YA, El-Sayed MK, Sayed RS, Abdel-Aalla MH, Kassem HA. Nutrigenomics and microbiome shaping the future of personalized medicine: a review article. J Genet Eng Biotechnol. 2023 Nov 22;21(1):134. doi: 10.1186/s43141-023-00599-2. PMID: 37993702; PMCID: PMC10665279.

Kiani AK, Bonetti G, Donato K, Kaftalli J, Herbst KL, Stuppia L, Fioretti F, Nodari S, Perrone M, Chiurazzi P, Bellinato F, Gisondi P, Bertelli M. Polymorphisms, diet and nutrigenomics. J Prev Med Hyg. 2022 Oct 17;63(2 Suppl 3):E125-E141. doi: 10.15167/2421-4248/jpmh2022.63.2S3.2754. PMID: 36479483; PMCID: PMC9710387.

Kiani AK, Bonetti G, Donato K, Kaftalli J, Herbst KL, Stuppia L, Fioretti F, Nodari S, Perrone M, Chiurazzi P, Bellinato F, Gisondi P, Bertelli M. Polymorphisms, diet and nutrigenomics. J Prev Med Hyg. 2022 Oct 17;63(2 Suppl 3):E125-E141. doi: 10.15167/2421-4248/jpmh2022.63.2S3.2754. PMID: 36479483; PMCID: PMC9710387.

Krzyszczyk P, Acevedo A, Davidoff EJ, Timmins LM, Marrero-Berrios I, Patel M, White C, Lowe C, Sherba JJ, Hartmanshenn C, O'Neill KM, Balter ML, Fritz ZR, Androulakis IP, Schloss RS, Yarmush ML. The growing role of precision and personalized medicine for cancer treatment. Technology (Singap World Sci). 2018 Sep-Dec;6(3-4):79-100. doi: 10.1142/S2339547818300020. Epub 2019 Jan 11. PMID: 30713991; PMCID: PMC6352312.

L Bishop E, Ismailova A, Dimeloe S, Hewison M, White JH. Vitamin D and Immune Regulation: Antibacterial, Antiviral, Anti-Inflammatory. JBMR Plus. 2020 Sep 15;5(1):e10405. doi: 10.1002/jbm4.10405. PMID: 32904944; PMCID: PMC7461279.

Lagoumintzis G, Afratis NA, Patrinos GP. Editorial: Nutrigenomics and personalized nutrition: advancing basic, clinical, and translational research. Front Nutr. 2024 Jun 14;11:1435475. doi: 10.3389/fnut.2024.1435475. PMID: 38946787; PMCID: PMC11211598.

Lagoumintzis G, Patrinos GP. Triangulating nutrigenomics, metabolomics and microbiomics toward personalized nutrition and healthy living. Hum Genomics. 2023 Dec 8;17(1):109. doi: 10.1186/s40246-023-00561-w. PMID: 38062537; PMCID: PMC10704648.

Liu L, Ancoli-Israel S. Sleep Disturbances in Cancer. Psychiatr Ann. 2008 Sep 1;38(9):627-634. doi: 10.3928/00485713-20080901-01. PMID: 21243092; PMCID: PMC3021374.

Martínez-Garay C, Djouder N. Dietary interventions and precision nutrition in cancer therapy. Trends Mol Med. 2023 Jul;29(7):489-511. doi: 10.1016/j.molmed.2023.04.004. Epub 2023 May 30. PMID: 37263858.

Mazari AMA, Zhang L, Ye ZW, Zhang J, Tew KD, Townsend DM. The Multifaceted Role of Glutathione S-Transferases in Health and Disease. Biomolecules. 2023 Apr 18;13(4):688. doi: 10.3390/biom13040688. PMID: 37189435; PMCID: PMC10136111.

Munteanu C, Schwartz B. The relationship between nutrition and the immune system. Front Nutr. 2022 Dec 8;9:1082500. doi: 10.3389/fnut.2022.1082500. PMID: 36570149; PMCID: PMC9772031.

Pandey H, Tang DWT, Wong SH, Lal D. Gut Microbiota in Colorectal Cancer: Biological Role and Therapeutic Opportunities. Cancers (Basel). 2023 Jan 30;15(3):866. doi: 10.3390/cancers15030866. PMID: 36765824; PMCID: PMC9913759.

Plamada D, Vodnar DC. Polyphenols-Gut Microbiota Interrelationship: A Transition to a New Generation of Prebiotics. Nutrients. 2021 Dec 28;14(1):137. doi: 10.3390/nu14010137. PMID: 35011012; PMCID: PMC8747136.

Prieto I, Montemuiño S, Luna J, de Torres MV, Amaya E. The role of immunonutritional support in cancer treatment: Current evidence. Clin Nutr. 2017 Dec;36(6):1457-1464. doi: 10.1016/j.clnu.2016.11.015. Epub 2016 Nov 24. PMID: 27931879.

Qian L, Zhang F, Yin M, Lei Q. Cancer metabolism and dietary interventions. Cancer Biol Med. 2022 Dec 22;19(2):163–74. doi: 10.20892/j.issn.2095-3941.2021.0461. PMID: 34931768; PMCID: PMC8832959.

Reglero C, Reglero G. Precision Nutrition and Cancer Relapse Prevention: A Systematic Literature Review. Nutrients. 2019 Nov 16;11(11):2799. doi: 10.3390/nu11112799. PMID: 31744117; PMCID: PMC6893579.

Reytor-González C, Simancas-Racines D, Román-Galeano NM, Annunziata G, Galasso M, Zambrano-Villacres R, Verde L, Muscogiuri G, Frias-Toral E, Barrea L. Chrononutrition and Energy Balance: How Meal Timing and Circadian Rhythms Shape Weight Regulation and Metabolic Health. Nutrients. 2025 Jun 27;17(13):2135. doi: 10.3390/nu17132135. PMID: 40647240; PMCID: PMC12252119.

Rituraj, Pal RS, Wahlang J, Pal Y, Chaitanya M, Saxena S. Precision oncology: transforming cancer care through personalized medicine. Med Oncol. 2025 Jun 9;42(7):246. doi: 10.1007/s12032-025-02817-y. PMID: 40488843.

Rivlin N, Brosh R, Oren M, Rotter V. Mutations in the p53 Tumor Suppressor Gene: Important Milestones at the Various Steps of Tumorigenesis. Genes Cancer. 2011 Apr;2(4):466-74. doi: 10.1177/1947601911408889. PMID: 21779514; PMCID: PMC3135636.

Rock CL, Lampe JW, Patterson RE. Nutrition, genetics, and risks of cancer. Annu Rev Public Health. 2000;21:47-64. doi: 10.1146/annurev.publhealth.21.1.47. PMID: 10884945.

Rodriguez-Gonzalez A, Velasco-Durantez V, Martin-Abreu C, Cruz-Castellanos P, Hernandez R, Gil-Raga M, Garcia-Torralba E, Garcia-Garcia T, Jimenez-Fonseca P, Calderon C. Fatigue, Emotional Distress, and Illness Uncertainty in Patients with Metastatic Cancer: Results from the Prospective NEOETIC_SEOM Study. Curr Oncol. 2022 Dec 8;29(12):9722-9732. doi: 10.3390/curroncol29120763. PMID: 36547177; PMCID: PMC9777295.

Rowland I, Gibson G, Heinken A, Scott K, Swann J, Thiele I, Tuohy K. Gut microbiota functions: metabolism of nutrients and other food components. Eur J Nutr. 2018 Feb;57(1):1-24. doi: 10.1007/s00394-017-1445-8. Epub 2017 Apr 9. PMID: 28393285; PMCID: PMC5847071.

Salehi B, Mishra AP, Nigam M, Sener B, Kilic M, Sharifi-Rad M, Fokou PVT, Martins N, Sharifi-Rad J. Resveratrol: A Double-Edged Sword in Health Benefits. Biomedicines. 2018 Sep 9;6(3):91. doi: 10.3390/biomedicines6030091. PMID: 30205595; PMCID: PMC6164842.

Sharma M, Sidhu AK, Samota MK, Gupta M, Koli P, Choudhary M. Post-Translational Modifications in Histones and Their Role in Abiotic Stress Tolerance in Plants. Proteomes. 2023 Nov 22;11(4):38. doi: 10.3390/proteomes11040038. PMID: 38133152; PMCID: PMC10747722.

Singar S, Nagpal R, Arjmandi BH, Akhavan NS. Personalized Nutrition: Tailoring Dietary Recommendations through Genetic Insights. Nutrients. 2024 Aug 13;16(16):2673. doi: 10.3390/nu16162673. PMID: 39203810; PMCID: PMC11357412.

Stefanska B, Karlic H, Varga F, Fabianowska-Majewska K, Haslberger A. Epigenetic mechanisms in anti-cancer actions of bioactive food components--the implications in cancer prevention. Br J Pharmacol. 2012 Sep;167(2):279-97. doi: 10.1111/j.1476-5381.2012.02002.x. PMID: 22536923; PMCID: PMC3481038.

Su X, Jiang X, Meng L, Dong X, Shen Y, Xin Y. Anticancer Activity of Sulforaphane: The Epigenetic Mechanisms and the Nrf2 Signaling Pathway. Oxid Med Cell Longev. 2018 Jun 6;2018:5438179. doi: 10.1155/2018/5438179. PMID: 29977456; PMCID: PMC6011061.

Taylor MK, Sullivan DK, Ellerbeck EF, Gajewski BJ, Gibbs HD. Nutrition literacy predicts adherence to healthy/unhealthy diet patterns in adults with a nutrition-related chronic condition. Public Health Nutr. 2019 Aug;22(12):2157-2169. doi: 10.1017/S1368980019001289. Epub 2019 May 31. PMID: 31146797; PMCID: PMC6827561.

Thompson HJ, Lutsiv T, McGinley JN, Hussan H, Playdon MC. Dietary Oncopharmacognosy as a Crosswalk between Precision Oncology and Precision Nutrition. Nutrients. 2023 May 8;15(9):2219. doi: 10.3390/nu15092219. PMID: 37432381; PMCID: PMC10180692.

Venkatasamy VV, Pericherla S, Manthuruthil S, Mishra S, Hanno R. Effect of Physical activity on Insulin Resistance, Inflammation and Oxidative Stress in Diabetes Mellitus. J Clin Diagn Res. 2013 Aug;7(8):1764-6. doi: 10.7860/JCDR/2013/6518.3306. Epub 2013 Jul 17. PMID: 24086908; PMCID: PMC3782965.

Voltan G, Cannito M, Ferrarese M, Ceccato F, Camozzi V. Vitamin D: An Overview of Gene Regulation, Ranging from Metabolism to Genomic Effects. Genes (Basel). 2023 Aug 25;14(9):1691. doi: 10.3390/genes14091691.

PMID: 37761831; PMCID: PMC10531002.

Wang X, Sun Z, Xue H, An R. Artificial Intelligence Applications to Personalized Dietary Recommendations: A Systematic Review. Healthcare (Basel). 2025 Jun 13;13(12):1417. doi: 10.3390/healthcare13121417. PMID: 40565444; PMCID: PMC12193492.

Zhang P. Influence of Foods and Nutrition on the Gut Microbiome and Implications for Intestinal Health. Int J Mol Sci. 2022 Aug 24;23(17):9588. doi: 10.3390/ijms23179588. PMID: 36076980; PMCID: PMC9455721.

Chapter 14

Dietary Supplements in Cancer: Evidence, Efficacy, and Safety Considerations

Sarfraj Ahmad Siddiqui[1], Ng. Joykumar Singh[2], Lokesh Kumar Mishra[3], and Sheetanshu Gupta[4*]

[1]Department of Biochemistry, King George's Medical University, U.P., India
[2]Department of Food Process Engineering, College of Food Technology, Central Agricultural University (CAU), Imphal, Manipur, India
[3]Department of BPME, College of Agriculture, Central Agricultural University (CAU), Imphal, Manipur, India
[4]Department of Food Safety and Quality Assurance, College of Food Technology, Central Agricultural University (CAU), Imphal, Manipur, India

Abstract

Cancer survivors rely heavily on dietary supplements alongside conventional treatments, hoping for vastly improved outcomes down line in many cases, evidently. Supplements play quite crucial role in cancer patient care and this chapter scrutinizes that role rather thoroughly across diverse scenarios. Evidence surrounding vitamins and antioxidants has been thoroughly reviewed shows surprising results emerging slowly as its impact on cancer prevention is assessed. Efficacy assessment involves scrutinizing preclinical research, observational studies and clinical trials of supplements like omega-3 fatty acids modulating cancer pathways quite vigorously. Chapter highlights challenges translating findings into clinical practice amidst dodgy supplement quality and bioavailability issues plaguing wildly differing dosing regimens overall. This tackles gnarly safety concerns, including dicey interactions between shady supplements and cancer treatments like brutal chemo or edgy immunotherapy, with potentially dire consequences. Healthcare providers must steer patients toward supplements carefully tailored to individual needs and specific cancer types under highly personalized regimens based on evidence.

Keywords: Phytochemicals, Nutraceuticals, Bioavailability, Toxicity, Clinical Efficacy, Pharmacokinetics

DOI: 10.1201/9781042010387-14

1. Introduction

Cancer remains a top killer globally, but survival rates have improved remarkably for many cancer types owing largely to better diagnostic techniques. Rapidly increasing numbers of cancer survivors has sparked interest in optimizing health during and after treatment quite steadily now. Cancer survivors frequently try out weird dietary concoctions as part of some regimen ostensibly geared towards radically enhancing overall wellness and hastening recuperation rapidly afterwards. Cancer care involving dietary supplements necessitates a nuanced grasp of benefits and risks within a backdrop of frequently discordant scientific findings. The efficacy of dietary supplements used in cancer care is grounded in evidence while potential benefits are weighed against safety concerns for patients.

Dietary supplements encompass a vast array of products including vitamins minerals herbal extracts and amino acids, quite irregularly. Stuff like this gets hawked regularly nowadays as utterly fantastic for ramping up immune response and cranking energy production way up. Cancer patients find supplements quite compelling because they seemingly shore up treatment and enhance waning energy amidst nasty deficiencies. Evidence base remains sketchy for many dietary supplements and their effects on cancer outcomes are woefully poorly grasped these days overall. Assessing efficacy of dietary supplements in cancer treatment poses quite a challenge owing largely to wildly varying quality of available evidence. Certain supplements yield tangible benefits in specific cancer types while others may prove utterly useless or even potentially quite deleterious occasionally.

Cancer patients often utilize certain antioxidants such as vitamin C and vitamin E hoping they mitigate oxidative stress caused by harsh treatments. Antioxidants crucially protect cells from oxidative stress yet studies show wildly disparate outcomes regarding their impact on certain cancer therapies. High-dose antioxidants potentially thwart chemotherapy and radiotherapy by mitigating reactive oxygen species crucial for decimating cancerous cells thereby. Antioxidants usage may significantly diminish effectiveness of certain therapies making it imperative rather often to weigh potential benefits against rather significant risks. Omega-3 fatty acids and probiotics garner considerable support nowadays for potentially improving outcomes significantly in cancer patients quite remarkably. Omega-3 fatty acids present in fish oil and some plant oils exert impressively anti-inflammatory effects markedly in various bodily processes.

Probiotics have been thoroughly researched for gut health enhancement and supporting immune function whilst mitigating nasty gastrointestinal side effects from cancer treatments. Probiotics potentially augment gut microbiota thereby mitigating infection risk and encouraging digestive processes throughout therapy a crucial aspect of malnutrition management. Turmeric curcumin and green tea extract have been researched very extensively lately for possibly having anti-cancer properties in various medical studies. Curcumin possesses anti-inflammatory properties and antioxidant effects rather surprisingly, and may enhance cancer prevention via conventional therapies very effectively. Epigallocatechin gallate EGCG and other green tea polyphenols have been associated with anticancer properties, inhibiting tumour growth somewhat and metastasis in certain cancers. Results from various in vitro studies were promising, yet evidence from human clinical trials remains decidedly equivocal and research is still fairly nascent. Rigorous studies must be undertaken thoroughly beforehand endorsing such herbal supplements as wholly viable complementary therapies for treating various cancers effectively.

Efficacy alongside safety of dietary supplements remains very critical very often for numerous reasons, apparently owing to their widespread usage. Supplements are perceived as natural hence very safe but such assumptions can sometimes be glaringly misleading under certain circumstances. Supplements frequently dodge rigorous safety checks that prescription meds face leading to worries about hazardous side effects and sketchy interactions with other medications. Herbal supplements can significantly interfere with chemotherapy drug metabolism thereby increasing risk of toxicity or diminishing efficacy of treatment markedly. St John's Wort frequently interacts with various cancer drugs metabolized by certain cytochrome P450 enzymes being a widely used herbal supplement.

Healthcare providers must stay cognizant of various supplements patients are taking lest adverse interactions with other meds occur quietly. Dietary supplements frequently exhibit very considerable variation in quality apparently. Dietary supplements often fly under radar resulting in worries about contamination or sketchy labeling whereas pharma face tight regs for product purity. Some herbal remedies harbour nasty contaminants such as toxic heavy metals or pesticides posing extra risks for cancer patients already badly ravaged by disease and treatment. Patients should be thoroughly informed about choosing supplements from manufacturers boasting sterling reputations and seek out rigorously tested ones by third-party entities. Healthcare pros gotta step up and shepherd cancer patients through thick of dietary supplement usage more and more these days.

Educating patients thoroughly about potential supplement benefits and risks fosters open discussions daily regarding all supplements being taken for evidence-based recommendations. Recognizing current research limitations and eschewing grandiose assertions about dietary supplement efficacy sans solid clinical trials is crucial very much always. Crucial roles are played by specific supplements in cancer prevention or treatment and further rigorous clinical trials are vital nowadays. Diverse world of dietary supplements gets explored in oncology with evidence supporting their potential benefits and associated safety risks popping up frequently. Cancer patients often utilize various supplements including vitamins minerals and dubious herbal extracts yielding diverse clinical outcomes sporadically. Evidence-based supplement use in patient care will be highlighted alongside crucial considerations regarding supplement-drug interactions and rigorous quality control measures. This chapter endeavours rather sweepingly providing overview of current understanding about dietary supplements in cancer care empowering patients making informed decisions safely.

2. The Role of Dietary Supplements in Cancer Care: An Introduction

Cancer care has lately gained considerable notoriety across various medical research circles for incorporating dietary supplements, rather surprisingly nowadays. People beset by maladies and symptoms of disease often turn towards unconventional nutritional supplements alongside conventional medicinal treatments with great fervour. Supplements comprise a vast array of substances such as vitamins minerals amino acids and very unusual isolated bioactive compounds from sundry obscure botanicals. They frequently rise through ranks supposedly by encourage immune response and diminishing oxidative damage while facilitating detoxification processes relevant mainly to oncological conditions.

Oncology supplements are gaining traction very much everywhere nowadays necessitating a fairly meticulous evidence-based approach in many contemporary medical practices. Some supplements such as omega-3 fatty acids might provide benefits for people suffering from cancer-related cachexia and others harbour substantial peril. High-dose antioxidant supplementation during chemotherapy has sparked worries about shielding malignant cells from oxidative damage right alongside perfectly healthy ones. Supplements interacting with pharmacological agents can alter drug metabolism drastically or ramp up toxicity under fairly specific physiological conditions.

Vitamin C and selenium exhibit antioxidant activity that influences cancer supplement usage alongside zinc and medicinal mushrooms modulating immune responses effectively. Hormonal regulation happens partly via phytoestrogens present abundantly in soy products naturally. Anti-inflammatory effects get attributed largely to curcumin and omega-3s while mitochondrial function gets supported by various cellular repair mechanisms. Dosage bioavailability and synergy with other nutrients heavily influence efficacy fairly critically under certain specific therapeutic conditions or sometimes with various other therapies. Regulation of supplements available commercially varies wildly too and clinical use gets complicated somewhat irregularly by wildly inconsistent oversight.

Dietary supplements should be assessed carefully within diverse patient care contexts tailored from a clinical standpoint for specific individual health needs. Oncologists and registered dietitians along with practitioners of integrative medicine must collaborate to evaluate supplement use appropriateness based on patient's diagnosis and ongoing treatment regimen status heavily influenced by findings from high-quality trials. Patients need clear direction amidst murky info on dietary supplements often tainted by commercial bias and confusing claims. Current dietary supplement use in oncology settings unfolds rapidly here against a frenetic swirl of healthcare practices evolving very quickly nowadays. Supplements are scrutinized rather deeply in cancer prevention contexts and safety considerations surround survivorship treatment generally with regulatory issues looming ominously.

2.1. Rising Use of Supplements among Cancer Patients

Cancer patients have lately turned remarkably to dietary supplements reflecting a broad quirky shift toward patient-driven holistic approaches in oncology. Research across diverse populations indicates that between 30% and 80% of cancer patients use dietary supplements during treatment or survivorship. This wide range reflects various demographic variables cancer type treatment modality cultural influences and disparate healthcare access somewhat unevenly across different populations. Supplement use nowadays stems rather quietly from various deeply personal psychosocial issues and diverse physiological concerns surrounding bodily functions. Patients often turn rather desperately to dietary supplements in effort somewhat alleviating very debilitating side effects like nasty neuropathy or acute nausea.

People heavily rely on dietary supplements owing largely to therapy-induced gut issues or drastically reduced appetite stemming from treatment. Desire fuels immune resilience and radically reduces inflammation thereby fostering a perception that certain supplements offer rather empowering natural means of self-care. Supplement use mostly happens on patients' own initiative very evidently without much input from their respective oncology care providers. Decisions are swayed very frequently nowadays by various online sources or recommendations from family members and alternative healthcare practitioners. Supplements used recklessly without proper monitoring pose considerable risks especially when interacting haphazardly with conventional therapies. High-dose vitamin C or E antioxidants may undermine chemotherapy and radiation therapy efficacy by thwarting pro-oxidative mechanisms very significantly thereby. St John's Wort and similar herbal concoctions drastically revamp metabolism of various chemo agents through induction of cytochrome P450 enzymes thereby affecting efficacy markedly.

Supplements undergo wildly varying quality control measures nowadays and contamination or mislabeling poses significant risks fairly often under certain circumstances. Supplement use must be very safe and weirdly aligned with individual treatment goals through haphazardly integrative communication between healthcare providers or patients evidence-informed very much. Oncology teams nationwide must stay hypervigilant rapidly assessing supplement use and guiding it as part of comprehensive cancer care programs. Education efforts should strongly stress potential benefits and risks fostering informed decision-making quite vigorously and support patients making science-based choices.

2.2. Categories of Supplements Used in Cancer Care

Oncology patients often ingest diverse dietary supplements containing myriad compounds ostensibly boosting nutritional status or alleviating grueling side effects of treatment. Supplements get chunked into various weird functional categories having very distinct biological roles and gnarly therapeutic implications rather broadly. Cancer care nowadays evidently involves very common usage of micronutrient supplements comprising various vitamins and minerals fairly extensively these days. Vitamins A, C, D, E and B-complex alongside minerals like zinc selenium calcium magnesium iron are packed very densely in these essentials. Patients can utilize these during treatment for correcting deficiencies stemming from poor diet malabsorption and greatly heightened metabolic demands quite suddenly.

High-dose antioxidants potentially interfere with oxidative stress-based therapies like chemotherapy and radiotherapy while vitamin D influences immune function significantly alongside zinc for bone health. Serum level monitoring clinically highly recommended under targeted therapeutic regimens, ensures great precision and safe usage extremely effectively always. Extracts from plants like turmeric with curcumin and green tea rich in EGCG are included alongside milk thistle containing silymarin and various adaptogens ginseng. Herbal products frequently exhibit remarkably potent anti-inflammatory properties or yield adaptogenic effects with hepatoprotective benefits and nebulous immunomodulatory activity, meanwhile.

They present significant variability in pharmacokinetics and potential for drug-herb interactions that can drastically alter chemotherapeutic agent metabolism or affect liver enzymes. Branched-chain amino acids and glutamine supplements robustly support tissue repair and muscle mass in patients suffering from mucositis or cachexia. Glutamine has been investigated very extensively for its potential role in mitigating neuropathy and gastrointestinal toxicity caused by chemotherapy, rather haphazardly. Eicosapentaenoic acid and docosahexaenoic acid found in omega-3 fatty acids, are often utilised for their anti-inflammatory effects in cachexia patients supporting weight maintenance quite effectively. Lipids play crucial highly enigmatic roles quietly inside cells in immune regulation and cell membrane structural integrity rather mysteriously.

Growing interest in gut microbiome's role in cancer fuels usage of probiotic supplements haphazardly nowadays alongside prebiotics with increasing recklessness apparently. Risk of infection in severely immunocompromised people must be minimized by carefully considering strain specificity and patient immune status. Supplement classification nowadays lays a fairly solid foundation for oncology nutrition guidance rooted very deeply in systematic evaluation and evidence. Nuanced understanding of therapeutic goals and potential benefits is demanded by safe integration amidst various contraindications within individual treatment contexts very specifically.Dietary supplements in oncology can be broadly categorized into the following groups:

a. Micronutrients

Vitamins A C D and B-complex alongside minerals such as zinc selenium are included fairly often in various dietary supplements very frequently nowadays. Deficiencies frequently surface during cancer treatment largely due to curtailed intake or faulty absorption and skyrocketing metabolic demands so supplementation becomes necessary sometimes. Several nutrients contribute significantly to antioxidant defense mechanisms largely through biochemical processes involving vitamin C. Vitamin D and zinc are crucial for regulating immune responses otherwise they can become severely imbalanced quite rapidly under certain conditions. Folate and B12 facilitate DNA repair and methylation quite remarkably for instance. Lab assessments might reveal whether supplementing with certain nutrients or vitamins is warranted under specific circumstances quite effectively nowadays.

b. Omega-3 Fatty Acids

Fish oil replete with EPA and DHA manifests profoundly anti-inflammatory properties possibly aiding diminution of cancer cachexia and encourage cognitive faculties under specific circumstances greatly enhancing chemotherapy efficacy.

c. Antioxidants

Glutathione alpha-lipoic acid and coenzyme Q10 compounds get heavily hyped for shielding cells rather effectively from oxidative damage very routinely. Their application stays beset by controversy throughout certain chemotherapies and radiation treatments as they might conceivably shield malignant cells and healthy ones at same time.

d. Herbal and Botanical Extracts

Certain herbs like curcumin and astragalus are utilized ostensibly for anti-inflammatory properties or purported anti-cancer effects in various supplements nowadays. Preclinical models suggest some show considerable promise yet clinical evidence varies wildly and risks of serious interactions or contamination loom ominously.

e. Probiotics and Prebiotics

Support for gut microbiome plays some fairly significant role in immunity nutrient synthesis and cancer treatment tolerance. Probiotics may help manage diarrhea or mucositis during radiation therapy or under antibiotic treatment but strain-specific effects necessitate cautious evaluation in immunocompromised patients.

2.3. Potential Benefits of Supplements in Cancer Care

Carefully chosen dietary supplements serve really effectively as valuable adjuncts under clinical supervision in oncology care quite often nowadays. Benefits broadly encompass rectifying deficiencies in essential nutrients and encourage physiological resilience markedly during various treatment regimens essentially. Supplements potentially play therapeutic roles in cancer management heavily based on individual patient needs with validation in diverse treatment settings. Something rather enigmatic exists apparently in some obscure realm. Severe nutrient depletion afflicts cancer patients largely due to malabsorption or catabolic effects of certain tumours and diminished oral intake. Supplementation with vitamin B12 and iron remarkably restores biochemical balance supporting various physiological functions normally within human bodily systems quite effectively.

Replenishing iron and B12 may substantially alleviate fatigue related to anemia while vitamin D plays a crucial role maintaining bone health greatly. Obviously some bizarre text exists here somewhat awkwardly nowadays. Multiple nutrients markedly influence innate immunity and enhance adaptive immune responses vigorously. Glutamine and vitamins C and D alongside zinc or selenium remarkably enhance immune cell proliferation and antioxidant defenses quite effectively. Supplements may mitigate infection risk effectively in patients undergoing harsh chemotherapy treatments or having gravely weakened immune systems naturally over time. C exists rather quietly beneath layers of abstraction. Supplements possibly mitigate harsh therapy side effects very effectively via fiercely anti-inflammatory effects or utterly antioxidant mechanisms.

Glutamine quite effectively mitigates oral mucositis severity in head and neck cancer patients undergoing intense chemoradiation therapy with remarkable outcomes. Omega-3 fatty acids have been rather frequently linked with decreased inflammation and maintenance of lean body mass in cancer cachexia sufferers. Supplements may very significantly boost energy levels and fix deficiencies thereby considerably improving mood and somewhat enhancing cognitive function under obscure surroundings. Melatonin shows potential in improving sleep quality among oncology patients while adaptogenic herbs like ashwagandha are being explored for relieving fatigue somewhat.

Supplements sometimes get woven into supportive care protocols backed by evidence particularly when deficiencies are well documented or certain outcomes show marked efficacy. Unregulated supplement use poses considerable risks frequently for vulnerable individuals lacking proper supervision and medical guidance. Supplementation should be meticulously tailored by qualified healthcare professionals under modified care plans and monitored very closely.

2.4. Risks and Controversies

Cancer patients widely use dietary supplements but murky evidence supporting safety and efficacy fuels heated debate surrounding their role. Incorporating supplements into oncology care must be weighed very carefully against potential harm or meddling with cancer treatment protocols. Things go awry rapidly beneath earth's surface. Quite frequently nowadays concerns surround potential interactions between certain supplements and various anticancer agents with alarming regularity apparently. Herbal compounds and certain nutrients modulate activity of cytochrome P450 enzymes which rapidly metabolize various chemotherapeutic drugs and some targeted therapeutics. St John's wort induces CYP3A4 thereby compromising efficacy of certain chemotherapeutic agents substantially by reducing plasma concentration of these agents potentially.

Grapefruit extract inhibits certain enzymes rapidly leading to toxic accumulation of drug compounds and bizarre phenomena burst forth underneath mundane surfaces. High-dose supplementation can have rather deleterious effects in stark contrast to prevailing notions that more supplementation is better. High doses of specific antioxidants such as beta-carotene consumed by smokers or vitamin E taken during prostate cancer prevention studies may substantially increase cancer risk. Excess iron or fat-soluble vitamins can lead very haphazardly toward toxicity in specific organs highlighting a need for evidence-based dosing very carefully. Cryptic code c appears fairly frequently underneath many sections of text ostensibly serving no discernible illustrative or expository purpose whatsoever.

Patients are opting heavily for unproven regimens around dubious supplements rather than sticking with standard cancer treatments nowadays apparently. Such decisions often get driven by misinformation or deep distrust in conventional western medicine and various strong cultural beliefs prevail. Sadly disease progression may ensue rapidly over time and curative opportunity be irretrievably squandered or prognosis worsened with drastically severe consequences. Healthcare providers must tackle concerns very effectively with empathy and evidence-based guidance every time rather quietly apparently. Dietary supplements often vary wildly in purity or potency unlike heavily regulated pharmaceuticals and lack really stringent oversight. Research has rather alarmingly flagged some products containing heavy metals or biologically active adulterants and undeclared pharmaceuticals in certain cases suddenly.

Inaccurate labeling coupled with batch variability severely undermines reliability of diagnostics in clinical settings under certain unpredictable conditions occasionally. Issues like these underscore need for picking products from manufacturers certified by fairly reputable third-party organisations or bodies occasionally. Some supplements potentially offer therapeutic benefits in oncology care yet their usage necessitates meticulous supervision backed by robust empirical evidence. Oncologist, dietitians and pharmacists must collaborate extensively within fairly integrative cancer treatment frameworks minimizing various risks.

2.5. Clinical Guidance and Shared Decision-Making

Clinicians must nowadays adopt a collaborative evidence-informed approach thoroughly when integrating dietary supplements into cancer care plans very carefully. Crucially assessing nutritional status beforehand and current use of supplements effectively informs formulation of a treatment strategy. Potential benefits and risks of supplement use should be weighed very carefully against each patient's specific treatment regimen and existing comorbid conditions. Clinicians should recommend supplements judiciously only when they have demonstrated safety and shown tangible benefit within a specific therapeutic context. Patients must be vigilantly monitored for symptomatic changes or lab value fluctuations and potential interactions with concurrent therapies.

Education about reputable brand dosing regimens and sobering expectations enables patients make fairly informed decisions under tricky circumstances. Fostering open communication and shared decision-making enables clinicians guide patients safely incorporating supplements into comprehensive cancer treatment plans very effectively nowadays. Dietary supplements may potentially play somewhat supportive roles in various cancer care scenarios but usage must be rooted deeply in scientific evidence tailored for individual patients. Evolving research facilitates judicious integration of targeted supplements into oncology practice offering new resilience avenues alongside conventional medical therapies.

3. Evaluating the Evidence

Oncology evolves rapidly toward patient-centered care and use of dietary supplements surges greatly among cancer patients taking vitamins and botanical extracts. Patients desperately seek such products for nasty treatment side effects or possibly enhancing rather fragile immunity quite extremely nowadays. Thorough examination of scientific literature very much always guides usage appropriately under various circumstances fairly well. Assessing cancer-fighting supplements becomes quite convoluted owing largely to myriad underlying factors existing subtly across diverse regimes and parameters. Supplements embody a motley assortment sprawling haphazardly from solitary vitamins in tablet form to rather intricate botanical concoctions fabricated.

Clinical studies exhibit considerable variability in design dosage and duration alongside patient demographics thereby greatly complicating comparisons across various studies significantly. Sizable disparities emerge between study formulations and ones available consumer largely owing to lack of stringent regulatory oversight subsequently. Vitamin D supplementation holds much promise in encourage bone health and maybe augmenting survival rates largely in patients undergoing hormone therapy for prostate cancer or breast cancer treatments. Meta-analyses indicate somewhat diminished cancer-related mortality rates in individuals having sufficient serum levels mostly across various studied populations generally.

Glutamine has undergone quite thorough scrutiny recently for alleviating mucositis and gut toxicity quite effectively in patients undergoing chemotherapy or radiation treatment with notable improvements orally and nutritionally. Omega-3 fatty acids EPA and DHA profoundly exhibit anti-inflammatory properties potentially helping mitigate cancer-related cachexia or improve quality of life markedly. Conversely other supplements have sparked serious concerns lately among certain groups of people with varied backgrounds. High-dose antioxidants such as vitamin E or selenium have been linked rather inexplicably to heightened cancer risk in some trials involving high-risk populations.

Antioxidant use during chemotherapy and radiation has sparked wariness because oxidative mechanisms remarkably well underlie therapeutic action in such treatments. Most dietary supplements like turmeric and green tea extract are curiously unverified for efficacy due largely to dearth of massive trials. In vitro research and observational studies provide mechanistic insights fairly often but fail to supplant rigorous randomized controlled trials properly conducted. Certain dietary supplements might provide supplementary benefits when employed rather judiciously but others harbor serious health hazards or rest on dubious scientific ground. Meticulous individualized risk-benefit assessment should ideally occur alongside high-quality data analysis within oncology care teams guiding clinical decision-making very carefully.

3.1. Supplements with Evidence of Benefit in Specific Cancer Contexts

Several compounds show significant benefits in targeted evidence-based settings amidst controversy surrounding routine dietary supplement use in cancer patient care. Benefits become strikingly apparent when supplements rectify documented deficiencies or support physiological challenges arising from brutal cancer therapies very quickly afterwards. One entity exists quietly underground. Vitamin D plays a crucial role rather quietly in maintaining calcium homeostasis and regulating cellular differentiation somewhat underappreciatedly. Grim outcomes in breast prostate and various other malignancies correlate strongly with low serum 25(OH)D levels found occasionally in quite rare colorectal cancer. Supplementation may enhance bone mineral density in deficient individuals particularly for patients receiving hormone therapies that heighten fracture risk somewhat mitigating mortality rates according to meta-analyses.

Optimal dosing remains very murky nowadays and researchers are still intensely probing therapeutic thresholds with considerable fervor. Glutamine a conditionally essential amino acid has been evaluated mostly in head and neck cancers for protective effects against chemotherapy induced mucositis. Oral glutamine supplementation quite effectively mitigates mucosal inflammation severity and curtails its duration during catabolic stress in a possibly beneficial manner. Dose escalation manifests clinical benefit variably most efficaciously in patients receiving intense chemotherapy regimens rapidly alongside aggressive treatment protocols.

Certain probiotic strains such as Lactobacillus rhamnosus GG and Bifidobacterium lactis alongside synbiotic formulations show efficacy in reducing antibiotic-associated diarrhea remarkably. Gut barrier function modulation occurs alongside pathogenic microbe suppression and immune signaling support happens simultaneously in a somewhat mysterious manner. Carefully chosen supplements surprisingly offer supportive benefits nowadays in oncology under rigorous monitoring of stringent clinical settings rather effectively. Their application ought to be rooted deeply in singular patient evaluation and treatment objectives with presently available optimum evidence maximizing benefit whilst mitigating hazardous interactions.

Eicosapentaenoic acid and docosahexaenoic acid profoundly exert anti-inflammatory effects very effectively in marine oils by modulating prostaglandin synthesis and cytokine production. Recently compounds have been scrutinized thoroughly within oncology research for possibly mitigating cancer cachexia and preserving lean body mass effectively. Trials indicate chemotherapy response gets somewhat amplified in pancreatic cancers and colorectal ones but conclusive results often remain elusive.

a. Vitamin D

Low vitamin D levels frequently manifest in cancer patients correlating with poorer survival rates especially in breast and prostate malignancies. Vitamin D supplementation rectifies deficiency and has been tenuously linked to improved bone health under certain hormone therapy regimens apparently. Colorectal cancer patients experience diminished recurrence risk with supplementation quite frequently underneath certain conditions. Immune function modulation occurs simultaneously with other processes underneath. Evidence supports supplementation in deficient individuals but high-dose usage outside clinical settings risks peril from hypercalcemia quite suddenly.

b. Omega-3 Fatty Acids (EPA/DHA)

Omega-3 fatty acids profoundly exhibit anti-inflammatory properties and modulate various immune responses effectively in bodily contexts under different conditions. Preserving lean body mass during cachexia and reducing inflammation yields benefits from clinical studies and somewhat improves chemotherapy tolerance. Omega-3s potentially enhance quality of life remarkably in advanced cancer cases and stimulate appetite somewhat irregularly. Omega-3s seem very safe with close monitoring and possibly offer some benefit yet results remain decidedly mixed overall.

3.2. Supplements with Inconclusive or Mixed Evidence

Several dietary supplements display ostensibly fascinating biological plausibility and show substantial preclinical efficacy or yield supportive evidence from relatively small human studies. Very inconsistent results have emerged from large randomized controlled trials studying various compounds thereby limiting their inclusion in cancer treatment protocols. Supplements often dwell in a nebulous realm of dubious effectiveness, warranting rigorous examination and necessitating cautious reserve in therapeutic applications very frequently nowadays. A solitary awkward digit perches quietly on that spot. Vitamin C and Selenium have been researched rather extensively for potentially mitigating nasty reactive oxygen species under harsh chemotherapy regimens. Malignant cells might be shielded from ROS mediated cytotoxicity thereby somewhat diminishing treatment efficacy very significantly under certain circumstances.

High-dose supplementation reckons markedly increased recurrence risk notably in lung cancer patients whereas some research reports drastically reduced treatment side effects like mucositis. Dosage timing and cancer type may rather substantially influence outcomes critically across varied patient populations. Curcumin displays markedly anti-inflammatory properties and surprisingly broad epigenetic regulatory effects in various in vitro settings owing mainly to turmeric's active polyphenol status. Preliminary trials have probed its potential very effectively for enhancing chemotherapy sensitivity and slashing cytokines associated with inflammation rather quickly it seems. Results from clinical trials remain very underwhelming largely owing to lack of standardized formulations and very poor bioavailability.

Larger trials are needed urgently now to confirm therapeutic relevance particularly in cancers like gastrointestinal cancer and very aggressive pancreatic cancer. Epigallocatechin gallate mostly found in green tea extract has shown significant antiproliferative effects and pro-apoptotic activity in various preclinical models. Observational studies hinted very strongly at protective associations in breast cancer and prostate malignancies but interventional data remain rather muddled nowadays. High doses spark concerns about hepatotoxicity thereby complicating clinical adoption rather extensively sometimes.

Bioactive compounds from fungi like Trametes versicolor and Ganoderma lucidum purportedly modulate various immune responses very effectively under certain conditions. Small studies mainly conducted in Asia report markedly improved quality of life and hint at considerable survival benefits quite noticeably. Regional heterogeneity in product standardization hampered adoption in Western clinical practice quite severely due largely to methodological shortcomings recently. Several supplements exhibit ostensibly plausible biological mechanisms and garner preliminary benefit yet their clinical usefulness stays egregiously ambiguous absent stringent validation. Providers of healthcare should exercise extreme caution with these agents until rigorous RCTs establish safety and efficacy under close supervision.

3.3. Supplements with Evidence of Harm or No Benefit

Supplements deemed to be useless or hazardous when taken recklessly without medical supervision and may pose significant risks especially for smokers and asbestos-exposed people. High-dose vitamin E may increase prostate cancer risk; linked to hemorrhagic stroke in some populations. Laetrile (amygdalin) promoted as an alternative therapy, but associated with cyanide toxicity and no proven benefit. High-dose vitamin E supplementation may possibly heighten risk of prostate cancer and has been tenuously linked to hemorrhagic stroke in certain demographic populations.

3.4. Methodological Challenges in Evaluating Supplement Evidence

Research oncology dietary supplement faces huge roadblocks methodologically somewhat problematically limiting reliability of findings and generalizability severely. Challenges significantly obscure data interpretation and muddy clinical decision making processes thereby affecting outcomes very badly in most cases. Cancer patients undergo wildly diverse treatments amidst myriad comorbidities and exhibit various tumour stages in fairly complex clinical settings. Variability creeps in substantially across studies somewhat unpredictably due to differences that obscure effects of various dietary supplements. Immune-modulating compounds behave erratically in chemotherapy patients versus people receiving immunotherapy or radiation making it exceptionally difficult to draw definitive conclusions. Multivitamin preparations and sundry botanical extracts often lack entirely consistent standardization in different studies somewhat inexplicably. Varying chemical makeup and differences in concentration of active ingredients severely hinder comparisons across studies with disparate bioavailability.

Dosage regimens vary substantially across studies rendering determination of therapeutic range or dose response effects rather challenging occasionally. Efficacy of supplements gets assessed in clinical trials that typically last just several months or merely a few brief weeks. Cancer recurrence entails dismal long-term toxicity and survival rates thus necessitating protracted follow-up periods frequently absent in diminutive supplement trials. Obvious short-term gains might not morph into lasting results under clinical scrutiny. Research on dietary supplements under placebo-controlled conditions generally doesn't often feature double-blind study designs fairly uncommonly nowadays. Open-label or single-arm studies abound thereby heightening risk of bias from skewed patient expectations and observer perception and various placebo effects.

Outcomes like mood swings or fatigue are especially susceptible to bias without rigorously assembled control groups in most research studies. Many studies rely on patients' own accounts of dietary habits and supplement intake rather than verifying nutrient levels with blood tests. Observed effects might stem from actual systemic changes or reporting inaccuracies without fairly objective measurement being employed here. Researchers must prioritize standardization in formulation and dosing slowly and extend trial duration aligning with relevant oncology endpoints gradually. Rigorous methodologies alone facilitate fairly reliable identification of genuinely beneficial or possibly detrimental supplements in effectively personalized cancer care. Clinicians must scrutinize existing research meticulously and consider specific treatment milieu of each patient or their nutritional deficiencies very seriously when prescribing supplements.

4. Commonly Used Dietary Supplements in Oncology: Benefits and Risks

Supplementation has grown remarkably prevalent nowadays among cancer patients with estimates suggesting up to 80% of individuals undergoing treatment use it regularly. Supplements wildly diverge across categories like vitamins and minerals but also antioxidants amino acids herbal extracts and very obscure bioactive compounds exist. Motivations of patients vary greatly from alleviating symptoms or boosting immunity and enhancing energy to staving off recurrence requiring nuanced risk-benefit deliberation. Certain supplements potentially offer profoundly marked therapeutic benefits in specific cancer treatment settings quite occasionally underground.

Vitamin D supplements are often touted as crucial for encourage bone density in patients undergoing hormone depleting treatments for breast malignancies or prostate maladies. Glutamine has been shown in some esoteric research studies quite effectively reduce severity of oral mucositis in patients undergoing radical radiation therapy for head and neck cancers. Omega-3 fatty acids EPA and DHA display potent anti-inflammatory effect rather effectively and may counteract cancer cachexia involving severe muscle wasting.

Certain supplements can potentially wreak havoc on bodily functions but others provide zero tangible benefits whatsoever in most cases. High-dose antioxidants such as vitamin E and beta-carotene once hyped as protective agents have been linked somewhat inexplicably to increased cancer mortality in certain demographics especially among lung cancer patients and heavy smokers. Compounds may drastically interfere with pro-oxidant effects of chemotherapy or radiation thereby diminishing treatment efficacy rather markedly in some cases suddenly. St John's Wort and turmeric extract supplements have sparked concern largely owing to their effects on drug metabolism through cytochrome P450 enzyme systems.

Interactions between various factors drastically alter concentrations of certain chemotherapeutic agents leading quite rapidly sometimes to nasty toxicity or therapeutic failure. Herbal products often escape rigorous oversight and harbour contaminants or exhibit wildly varying concentrations of active ingredients very frequently sometimes. Registered dietitians and oncology pharmacists must thoroughly evaluate safety and efficacy before guiding patients on supplement use very carefully nowadays. Supplementation should be grounded basically in documented nutrient deficiencies and various clinical indications alongside specific goals for each patient.

Dietary supplements play a befuddlingly complex role somewhat mysteriously in oncology becomes: Supplements ostensibly integral to certain diets play a befuddlingly complex role rather enigmatically within various oncology disciplines nowadays. Certain supplements effectively fill nutritional voids and enhance immunity whereas others can significantly hinder treatment efficacy or cause considerable harm with improper use. Benefits vary greatly with specific supplement dosage timing and patient's underlying health condition alongside other concurrent medical treatments being administered simultaneously. Clinicians should fervently back modify evidence-based treatment plans that spark open dialogue with patients and deeply embed auxiliary therapeutic regimens. Crucially thorough research and oversight are needed for ensuring safety and efficacy integratively in cancer care with supplement usage nowadays.

5. Efficacy of Vitamins, Minerals, and Herbal Supplements in Cancer Treatment

Growing emphasis on integrative oncology has brought attention sharply into focus on potential role of dietary supplements including various obscure vitamins in cancer treatment lately. Patients gulp down supplements fervently seeking respite from debilitating aftereffects or slightly improved results with success rates that differ enormously. Vitamins and minerals frequently rectify nutritional deficits arising from malnutrition or treatment-induced malabsorption that heightens metabolic demands these days. Vitamin D supplementation tenuously correlates with enhanced bone density in patients undergoing androgen deprivation therapy or receiving aromatase inhibitors irregularly modulating immune responses. Pretty low serum vitamin D levels correlate strongly with dismal outcomes in various cancer types such as breast cancer and colorectal cancer.

Folate and vitamin B12 play crucial role in methylation pathways and DNA synthesis processes very quietly. Deficiencies especially in patients undergoing harsh chemotherapies or possessing MTHFR polymorphisms can severely hamper hematopoiesis and heighten toxicity risk substantially. High-dose supplementation merits very cautious consideration partly owing to potential links with cancer progression in certain subpopulations debatably. Vitamin C and beta-carotene exhibit cytoprotective effects in numerous in vitro experiments yet clinical application stays extremely dubious nowadays. High-dose antioxidant supplementation during chemotherapy or radiation may attenuate oxidative stress necessary for efficacy of treatment thereby diminishing outcomes significantly. Beta-carotene trials among smokers have reported alarmingly high cancer incidence and mortality rates pretty markedly in some rather disturbing findings.

Curcumin and ginseng supplements show potent anti-inflammatory effects suddenly in mice with chronic inflammation induced in various preclinical studies. Sparse human trial data suggest alleviation of symptoms like fatigue nausea or inflammation yet robust evidence backing survival benefits remains woefully scarce. Certain herbal compounds can induce or inhibit various cytochrome P450 enzymes rapidly resulting in significantly altered metabolism of several chemotherapeutic agents quickly. Variability in supplement quality and bioavailability further complicates their clinical application greatly under diverse circumstances apparently. Supplements ought to be prescribed under expert guidance largely based on fairly obvious documented deficiencies backed pretty robustly by clinical evidence. Certain vitamins minerals and herbal products may offer supportive benefits in cancer care with efficacy heavily reliant on specific contexts and circumstances albeit fraught with considerable potential risks. Research nowadays informs evidence-based recommendations quite effectively across various medical fields through rigorous clinical trials and ongoing investigation.

5.1. Vitamins: Supportive, but Context-Dependent

Vitamin D

Vitamin D performs sundry roles rather stealthily in immune modulation and cell differentiation mostly within various bodily tissues and apoptosis. Pretty strongly low vitamin D levels correlate with worse outcomes in breast cancer and prostate cancer and colorectal cancer apparently. Supplementation in deficient individuals may markedly improve survival intervals and reduce bone loss during prolonged endocrine therapy. Randomized controlled trials show mixed results regarding direct anti-tumour effects and some evidence suggests occasional enhancement of immune responsiveness markedly. Vitamin D works best supplementary against deficiency rather than solo as an agent malignantly targeting various types of cancer cells.

Vitamin C

Vitamin C serves as an antioxidant neutralizing free radicals rapidly and may effectively enhance damaged tissue repair somewhat under certain conditions. High-dose intravenous vitamin C has been studied pretty extensively alongside chemotherapy in various early-phase trials showing somewhat surprisingly improved overall quality. Certain studies revealed inflammation reduction pretty nicely underneath specific conditions. Potential pro-oxidant effects may ravage tumour cells selectively and researchers are exploring this avenue further with considerable enthusiasm nowadays. Definitive clinical evidence remains glaringly scarce still nowadays. Oral supplementation could marginally enhance general health but its efficacy in enhancing treatment outcomes solo remains highly dubious.

Vitamin E and Beta-Carotene

Antioxidants have undergone rigorous recent testing for efficacy in cancer prevention and adjunctive therapeutic modalities with quite remarkable success apparently. High-dose vitamin E supplementation substantially heightened prostate cancer risk in SELECT trial participants undergoing rigorous testing and beta-carotene boosted lung cancer incidence alarmingly in smokers. Beta-carotene supplementation markedly elevated lung cancer incidence among heavy smokers in several massive randomized trials focused on prevention efforts.

5.2. Minerals: Targeted Use with Clear Benefits in Deficiency

Zinc

Zinc plays crucial roles in various cellular processes like DNA synthesis and immune regulation alongside antioxidant defense mechanisms that facilitate tissue repair quite effectively. Magnesium acts as a cofactor for numerous enzymes maintaining mucosal integrity remarkably and supporting wound healing pretty effectively in various bodily processes. Zinc supplementation has been researched rather extensively in oncology for alleviating treatment-related side effects mostly in patients receiving intensive chemotherapy regimens or undergoing prolonged radiotherapy. Zinc application is quite clinically relevant in managing dysgeusia a distressing side effect for patients suffering head and neck cancers. Radiation therapy often ravages taste buds and salivary glands thereby impairing zinc-dependent enzymes like gustin or carbonic anhydrase VI crucial for taste perception.

Zinc deficient patients may experience somewhat enhanced taste recovery fairly early on with oral zinc supplementation mostly as zinc gluconate or sulfate. Benefit magnitude seems pretty restricted in patients with fairly adequate zinc levels at baseline ostensibly. Zinc has shown considerable promise in mitigating severity of nasty oral mucositis particularly in patients battling hematologic cancers or getting stem cell transplants. Zinc lozenges or mouthwashes pretty quickly enhance mucosa healing locally by regenerating epithelial tissue and dampen inflammation rapidly therein. Zinc supplementation possibly reduces mucositis duration severely in individuals under high-dose chemoradiotherapy or having pretty low zinc status initially. Excessive zinc intake can cause pretty nasty adverse effects rather quickly including copper deficiency and severely impaired immune function.

Supplementation should be guided by thorough clinical assessment alongside serum zinc levels and dietary intake analysis when such data is readily available. Doses in oncology setting typically range from 25 mg daily up to 50 mg daily but modified regimens are necessitated by patient tolerance and treatment phase specifics. Zinc plays a crucial role biologically in various cancer care applications very specifically nowadays for numerous patients suffering terribly. Targeted zinc supplementation in deficient individuals can markedly improve quality of life during cancer treatment and remarkably facilitate mucosal recovery very effectively afterwards. Biochemical monitoring and sound clinical judgment remain crucial for effective safe use.

Selenium

Selenium plays a critical role quite effectively in human immune systems and thyroid hormone metabolism under normal redox balance conditions. Selenoproteins like glutathione peroxidases and thioredoxin reductases effectively mediate its primary biological functions by quashing reactive oxygen species rather quietly. Selenium has garnered considerable attention for possible adjunctive role in oncology largely owing to its pretty potent antioxidant effects. Selenium supplementation has been rather extensively researched in oncology as a means of reducing toxicity from chemotherapy and radiotherapy quite effectively. Sodium selenite administered orally may mitigate harsh side effects quite effectively in patients receiving intensive chemoradiotherapy for various gastrointestinal malignancies or head and neck cancer. Selenium enhances endogenous antioxidant defenses thereby yielding various benefits ostensibly from this nutrient and modulating inflammatory signaling pathways quite effectively.

Selenium heavily influences immune competence in individuals with low baseline levels particularly under certain conditions quite markedly. Selenium status somewhat effectively enhance antibody responses and appears linked with heightened cytotoxic T lymphocyte activity and natural killer cell functionality. Effects manifest markedly in individuals deficient in selenium and evidence remains scanty for benefit in fairly well-nourished large populations. High-dose selenium supplementation has not yielded consistent cancer prevention benefits despite possessing considerable biological plausibility apparently. Large randomized controlled trials like Selenium and Vitamin E Cancer Prevention Trial failed showing reduction in prostate cancer incidence and raised concerns about potential heightened risk of type 2 diabetes with prolonged high-dose usage.

Indiscriminate supplementation has been met with caution particularly in absence of actual deficiency prompting fairly stringent warnings thereby. Selenium supplementation ought to be judiciously reserved for individuals beset with documented deficiency or suspected malabsorption syndromes amidst cancer therapy. Daily doses over 200 mcg necessitate cautious administration owing largely to risk of selenosis and a pretty narrow therapeutic index. Selenium offers potential adjunctive benefits in cancer care by mitigating treatment related toxicity and encourage immune function very effectively nowadays. Supplementation needs tailoring pretty carefully on individual basis factoring in baseline selenium status and overall risk versus benefit profile obviously.

5.3. Herbal Supplements: Promise with Precaution

Curcumin (Turmeric)

Curcumin a principal polyphenolic compound extracted from Curcuma longa rhizome has been extensively studied for myriad biological properties including profound anti-inflammatory effects. Curcumin has garnered significant attention in oncology circles largely owing to its propensity for modulating molecular pathways heavily implicated in carcinogenesis like NF-κB or COX-2. Curcumin pretty effectively inhibits tumour growth in various cancer models including breast and pancreatic cancer enhancing apoptosis of malignant cells significantly. Curcumin sensitizes cancer cells pretty effectively chemotherapy and radiotherapy thereby potentially amplifying treatment efficacy while mitigating required dosages significantly very often. Curcumin's capacity significantly modulates drug resistance pathways whilst impairing survival of cancer stem cells and reducing inflammatory cytokine production greatly.

Curcumin directly exhibits anticancer activity and potentially mitigates symptoms related to cancer like debilitating fatigue and chronic pain through partly systemic anti-inflammatory effects. Recipients of intensive treatment somewhat surprisingly experience support regarding quality of life under harsh circumstances and functional status improves markedly. Curcumin's clinical application remains stunted largely due to pretty low aqueous solubility and rapid metabolism causing inherently poor bioavailability. Oral curcumin preparations often result in subtherapeutic plasma concentrations spurring creation of fancy delivery systems like nanoparticle carriers and liposomal encapsulation very frequently nowadays. Revised formulations showed greatly enhanced absorption and systemic exposure in various recent pharmacokinetic studies conducted overall with huge success.

Bioavailability-enhanced formulations deployed somewhat quietly in early-phase clinical trials demonstrate potential efficacy in mitigating various tumour-related symptoms and inflammatory markers rather effectively. Robust evidence from sizable randomized controlled trials is still lacking and heterogeneity of curcumin products used in various studies hinders interpretation of results fairly slowly. Curcumin might be deemed potentially viable as adjunctive treatment in oncology under supervision of healthcare professionals particularly for inflammation-driven malignancies. Further rigorous investigation will probably clarify optimal dosing regimens and relevant treatment settings underpinning incorporation into oncology practice backed by empirical research.

Green Tea Extract (EGCG)

Epigallocatechin gallate or EGCG remains biologically active catechin abundant in Camellia sinensis commonly known casually as green tea. Extensive studies on this polyphenol have been fueled by its unusually wide range of biological effects and putative antineoplastic properties largely. EGCG wields potent anticancer effects through sundry cellular routes underlying its efficacy in multifaceted cancer prevention endeavors and various treatment modalities pretty effectively. Oncogene downregulation happens simultaneously with suppression of various signal transduction pathways and inhibition of epidermal growth factor receptor activation alongside HER2/neu. EGCG disrupts DNA methylation or histone acetylation suggesting potential roles epigenetically tweaking tumour suppression rather effectively in various downstream contexts. EGCG triggers apoptosis in malignant cells rather than normal tissue making it a potentially useful adjunct alongside chemotherapy for treating cancer effectively.

EGCG rather effectively inhibits angiogenesis and impairs tumour cell proliferation very significantly in various cancers including breast carcinoma or prostate cancer. Tiny experimental studies done in diverse clinical environments ostensibly boosted chemosensitivity remarkably while observational research purportedly hindered disease advancement irregularly somewhat slowly. Adjunctive EGCG use has been linked with significantly better outcomes in patients having hormone-sensitive breast cancer and largely localized prostate cancer. Beneath its beguilingly benign surface lurk some seriously dicey risks and EGCG's pharmacological profile remains pretty intriguing somewhat dubiously. EGCG appears remarkably well tolerated naturally at physiologic levels attained via drinking copious green tea and seems fairly safe. High-dose EGCG supplements in concentrated extract form have been tied largely to hepatotoxicity probably due mostly to oxidative stress inside hepatocytes. Large amounts of EGCG exceeding 800 mg per day can possibly heighten liver enzyme levels thereby posing a risk of liver damage in susceptible people EFSA says.

Efficacy concerns and potential risks nowadays should significantly temper clinical judgment when using green tea extract in oncology settings variously. EGCG holds potential as complementary therapy in cancers driven by inflammation or sensitive to hormone fluctuations but warrants cautious use in patients with preexisting liver damage. EGCG plausibly confers anticancer benefits requiring scrupulous management of dose and stringent oversight for balancing efficacy with safety.

Mushroom Extracts (e.g., PSK, Reishi)

Extracts from some medicinal mushrooms have garnered considerable attention quickly in integrative oncology largely owing to their immunomodulatory properties and antitumour effects. Triterpenoids from Ganoderma lucidum and protein-bound β-glucan known as Polysaccharide-K extracted from Coriolus versicolor have been widely studied recently. PSK was investigated extensively in Japanese and South Korean clinical trials as adjuvant therapy for gastrointestinal tract cancers mainly gastric and colorectal cancer. PSK significantly boosts natural killer cell activity and stimulates cytokine production including IL-2 and IFN-γ after chemotherapy treatment. Markedly improved disease-free survival emerges in stage II/III colorectal cancer patients undergoing randomized controlled trials with PSK integrated conventional chemotherapeutic regimens mostly in East Asian populations.

Ganoderma lucidum extracts pretty effectively contain bioactive polysaccharides and triterpenes that modulate inflammatory mediators like TNF-α during dendritic cell maturation. Reishi quite effectively inhibits tumour growth and metastasis in cancer hosts while supporting immunologic resilience remarkably well beneath certain conditions. Rather promising initial findings have been reported lately but translation of such results into Western clinical settings remains somewhat hampered still. Trials outside East Asia have been scarce and riddled with dubious methodology or inconsistency in formulation of botanical extracts frequently. Assessing supplements derived from mushrooms poses significant challenges largely due to inconsistent concentrations of bioactive compounds across various product formulations. Variations in gut microbiota makeup and eating habits among diverse populations could heavily impact bioavailability and immune reaction to certain compounds.

PSK and Reishi exhibit fairly favorable safety profiles at therapeutic doses with minimal adverse effects being sporadically reported nonetheless. Caution seems warranted rather curiously in patients receiving pretty intense immunosuppressive therapies or harbouring rather nasty autoimmune conditions posing unforeseen risks. PSK and Reishi extracts show promise in cancer care for encourage immune function during chemotherapy treatments pretty notably and fairly effectively. Further rigorously controlled trials in diverse populations are sorely needed to validate efficacy and inform integration into oncology practice with evidence-based savvy.

Milk Thistle (Silymarin)

Milk thistle Silybum marianum has been used rather traditionally for quite hepatoprotective properties largely owing to active flavonolignan complex silymarin very abundantly. Silibinin and isosilibinin and silychristin and silydianin pretty frequently exhibit antioxidant anti-inflammatory and antifibrotic activities in silymarin mostly. Milk thistle has garnered considerable attention lately for possibly mitigating hepatotoxicity caused by chemotherapy agents like methotrexate and irinotecan recently. Silymarin effectively scavenges reactive oxygen species and boosts glutathione levels somewhat stabilizing hepatocyte cellular membranes thereby limiting injury in liver cells. Silibinin exhibits profoundly suppressive effects on pro-inflammatory cytokines such as TNF-α and IL-1β and extensively attenuates signaling pathways involving TGF-β downstream extensively. Proposed mechanisms suggest theoretical benefits potentially preventing or alleviating hepatic damage during systemic cancer therapy administration quite effectively. Encouraging data emerges from lab settings involving cells and animal yet human clinical evidence stays relatively sparse and pretty murky. Multiple pilot studies and case reports assessed silymarin supplementation pretty thoroughly in cancer patients undergoing chemotherapy with grossly elevated liver enzymes. Tiny sample sizes and lack of blinding severely hinder conclusive findings despite reports of somewhat improved transaminase levels and enhanced subjective well-being.

Silymarin bioavailability differences have greatly complicated standardization efforts in various clinical trials owing largely to poor solubility and extensive first-pass hepatic metabolism. Milk thistle safety data seem pretty favorable on whole. Silymarin tends to be fairly well tolerated by most patients with mild gastrointestinal disturbances happening sporadically or allergic reactions cropping up quite infrequently. Concerns are raised about altered metabolism of co-administered chemotherapeutic agents or medications mainly due to interactions with cytochrome P450 enzymes specifically CYP3A4 and also CYP2C9. Interactions like these aren't particularly well defined and warrant extremely careful watching very closely under a multitude of diverse circumstances.

Milk potentially serves as a remarkably promising supplementary agent in safeguarding liver functionality during cancer treatment particularly in patients with pre-existing liver issues or undergoing highly toxic chemotherapy. Robust randomized controlled trials are desperately needed subsequently in oncology settings and optimal dosing regimens will be determined safely. Its use should be steered by modified risk-benefit appraisal under oncology-savvy healthcare provider supervision until robust data eventually emerge.

5.4. Clinical Considerations and Safety

Meticulous assessment tailored specifically for each oncology patient undergoing vigorous treatment regimens necessitates careful consideration of dietary supplement incorporation. Certain vitamins and minerals alongside herbal compounds may alleviate nasty treatment side effects or rectify underlying deficiencies but scrutinize their use within a patient's overall regimen. Supplementation timing appears pretty critical under most circumstances normally. Antioxidant supplements such as vitamin C or coenzyme Q10 may reduce oxidative stress yet potentially undermine certain chemotherapies relying on reactive oxygen species. Concurrent use during active treatment phases must be approached warily under guidance from emerging evidence in various clinical settings nowadays. Sometimes dosing considerations matter just as much quietly underneath careful medical supervision and in fairly specific circumstances.

Supplements often weirdly display hormesis or a biphasic effect wherein physiological doses yield benefits but supraphysiologic doses induce toxicity fairly often. High doses of selenium have been linked rather alarmingly to increased risk of type 2 diabetes and excessive intake of fat-soluble vitamins A, D, E, K may lead to accumulation and frank toxicity. Drugs and supplements interact in profoundly subtle ways quietly affecting treatment outcomes with significant challenging frequency beneath surface. Rare herbal extracts like St John's wort modulate cytochrome P450 enzymes pretty significantly thereby altering pharmacokinetics of various chemotherapeutic agents. Such interactions potentially lead to somewhat diminished efficacy of interventions therapeutically administered or heightened toxic effects pretty occasionally. Stringent regulations are pretty much lacking throughout various segments of supplement industry and product quality remains somewhat unguaranteed largely.

Dietary supplements often have wildly varying levels of active ingredients and sometimes contain heavy metals or adulterants due partly to spotty manufacturing standards and labeling can be pretty inaccurate. Oncology care should incorporate routine screening for supplement use seamlessly amid numerous complexities surrounding patient health status effectively every time. Oncologists pharmacists and dietitians should collaborate pretty closely reviewing supplement use quite vigorously assessing scientific validity and checking for gnarly side effects. Certain supplements may play a supportive role in managing symptoms or rectifying nutritional deficiencies but direct anticancer efficacy remains woefully unsubstantiated. A judiciously chosen supplement use obviously enhances rather than undermines comprehensive cancer care with evidence-based safety-conscious personalized approach.

6. Safety Considerations: Potential Interactions and Side Effects in Cancer Therapy

Assessing dietary supplement safety among cancer patients receiving active oncology treatment becomes pretty crucial fairly quickly these days nowadays. Certain supplements provide symptomatic relief or rectify micronutrient deficiencies whereas others pose pharmacological interaction risks or cause severely debilitating physiological imbalances. Drug-nutrient interactions pose a primary concern nowadays among many healthcare professionals fairly frequently these days in clinical practice. Herbal supplements and certain nutrients pretty significantly modulate drug metabolism by impacting various cytochrome P450 enzymatic pathways rather thoroughly. Certain compounds drastically alter metabolism of chemotherapeutic agents leading quite often to subtherapeutic levels or markedly heightened toxic side effects suddenly. Such interactions may mercilessly undermine treatment efficacy or markedly escalate severity of adverse effects over time with great ferocity.

High-dose vitamins C and E pose quite an intriguing albeit somewhat inscrutable challenge effectively among various antioxidants nowadays. Assured cancer therapies reliant on oxidative stress like radiation and some chemotherapies may be dissatisfied by them though general health gets somewhat supported. Antioxidants might somewhat capriciously temper cytotoxic effects of treatments across diverse contexts with murky data emerging sporadically from scantily few studies. Toxic effects from supplements themselves must be weighed against potentially hazardous health impacts and various pharmacological interactions quite seriously nowadays. High doses of selenium have been linked anomalously with elevated risk of metabolic disturbances such as insulin resistance and type-2 diabetes. EGCG found in green tea extracts has been tenuously linked to hepatotoxicity mostly in supplement form among folks with preexisting liver issues. Herbal preparations sometimes trigger severely nasty allergic reactions in extremely sensitive people or cause pretty bad gastrointestinal upset. Product quality remains significant concern pretty much everywhere nowadays and regulation stays thorny issue still.

Dietary supplements pretty much evade stringent regulatory scrutiny applied rigorously on actual pharmaceuticals in various nations globally under normal circumstances. Contamination occurs pretty frequently alongside variability in potency and mislabeling happens fairly often too in certain instances. Weird stuff like heavy metals or mystery meds can be lurking in tainted food that people unwittingly chow down on daily. Oncology teams should vigilantly assess supplement usage routinely as part of comprehensive care ensuring patient safety with oversight generally. Oncologists, pharmacists and dietitians must collaborate very closely evaluating potential risks extremely thoroughly under quite current evidence tailoring guidance fairly rigorously nowadays. Ultimately some supplements may offer benefits but safe integration into cancer care demands vigilant monitoring and evidence-based oversight preventing harm.

6.1. Mechanisms of Drug-Supplement Interactions

Cancer patients often ingest myriad dietary supplements comprising vitamins and recondite herbal extracts alongside orthodox therapies with wildly varying efficacy. Certain supplements possibly offer supportive benefits whereas others rather insidiously undermine cancer therapies through sundry largely obscure biochemical mechanisms. Interactions like these often severely compromise treatment efficacy or markedly ramp up toxicity and alter sundry immune responses highlighting necessity for extremely meticulous evaluation. Supplements drastically alter absorption distribution and metabolism profiles of various anticancer drugs very unpredictably in some individuals occasionally. Conversely this situation may eventually result in subtherapeutic drug levels or heightened toxicity over time rather unpredictably. St John's wort induces cytochrome P450 enzymes notably CYP3A4 thereby accelerating metabolism of various chemotherapeutic agents such as irinotecan or imatinib potentially reducing their efficacy.

Grapefruit extract inhibits CYP3A4 and P-glycoprotein transporters thereby markedly boosting bioavailability of certain medications substantially increasing associated toxicity risk. Pharmacodynamic interactions rather subtly alter physiological effects of some drug without significantly changing concentration in most instances. Supplements may amplify action of chemotherapeutic agents pretty significantly or undermine desired therapeutic effects rather badly in certain cases. Ginseng and ginkgo biloba may badly enhance bleeding risk when lumped with anticoagulants or badly impair platelet function thereby messing up certain chemo regimens. Supplements that affect immune function nowadays can significantly hamper treatments involving immunotherapy and immune checkpoint inhibitors rather markedly.

High-dose omega-3 fatty acids or adaptogenic herbs with immunosuppressive properties may significantly blunt mechanisms underlying such novel therapeutic approaches rapidly. Echinacea and astragalus botanicals stimulating immune response may conversely worsen autoimmunity associated toxicities rather badly in some cases unfortunately. Oxidative stress triggers death in tumour cells and various cancer therapies including radiation therapy and alkylating chemotherapies rely heavily on such mechanisms. High-dose antioxidants such as vitamin C or coenzyme Q10 may scavenge reactive oxygen species thereby diminishing efficacy of some therapeutic interventions somewhat slowly.

Antioxidants might considerably mitigate nasty treatment side effects yet their use during cancer therapy remains hotly debated under various murky contexts. Evaluating safety of supplements used in oncology requires grasping underlying mechanisms very critically from various obscure perspectives nowadays. Clinicians must meticulously assess supplement usage on case-by-case basis incorporating current pharmacologic knowledge and relevant clinical guidelines ensuring treatments remain highly efficacious.

6.2. Antioxidants: A Double-Edged Sword

Nowadays cancer patients quite regularly gulp down vitamin C rich antioxidants and beta-carotene supplements along with vitamin E fairly often. Compounds like these are highly prized for neutralizing reactive oxygen species thereby potentially safeguarding normal tissues from damage caused by cancer therapy. Their role in oncology remains beset with controversy largely owing to a delicate balance between shielding healthy cells and preserving treatment efficacy dependent heavily on oxidative stress mechanisms. Cytotoxic effects emerge largely from oxidative stress and free radicals produced by cancer treatments like doxorubicin or radiation therapy and platinum-based compounds. Reactive oxygen species ravage DNA and induce apoptosis rapidly in frenetically dividing tumour cells with utterly catastrophic consequences thereby. High-dose antioxidant supplementation potentially quaches free radicals pretty significantly thereby lessening oxidative stress rather crucial for efficacious treatment outcomes nowadays. Concurrent use of antioxidants during active treatment phases raises concerns largely due to an ominous antagonistic effect unfolding rather problematically.

Antioxidants might undermine chemotherapy's potency or radiation efficacy thereby yielding lower response rates and pretty dismal overall clinical outcomes. Effect varies markedly depending on antioxidant type dosage and timing relative treatment and specific cancer regimen employed simultaneously. Epidemiological studies and interventional research have muddled narrative surrounding antioxidants further in some clinical trials pretty recently. High-dose beta-carotene supplementation significantly increased incidence of lung cancer and mortality amongst heavy smokers under specific pathological conditions apparently. Harm surfaces unexpectedly underscoring necessity of caution when recommending supplements especially in populations beset by pre-existing risk factors and susceptibility.

Clinical guidelines generally advise against routinely using high-dose antioxidant supplements during chemotherapy or radiation unless a deficiency state exists and has been clinically confirmed. Antioxidant support gets prioritized through consumption of veggies and fruits rich in nutrients that work synergistically at various physiological levels. Antioxidants play a vital role in cellular protection and supplementation during cancer therapy remains somewhat thorny issue with various conflicting opinions. Rigorously conducted further research and individualized counseling for patients alongside careful evaluation by healthcare providers mandates potential treatment efficacy blunting.

6.3. Herbal Supplements: Interaction and Contamination Risks

Cancer patients seeking alternative remedies sometimes utilize herbal supplements rapidly alongside conventional treatments deemed fairly safe these days. Supplements pose significant risks related to interactions with certain drugs and shoddy product quality necessitating careful consideration in clinical settings. Numerous herbal compounds markedly affect drug-metabolizing enzymes in particular cytochrome P450 family playing crucial roles in metabolism of various chemotherapeutic agents. St John's Wort and similar herbs powerfully induce CYP3A4 an enzyme that rapidly metabolizes various drugs like irinotecan and paclitaxel in liver cells. St John's Wort induces CYP3A4 accelerating metabolism of these agents resulting in subtherapeutic levels and treatment efficacy gets reduced substantially. Grapefruit extracts and goldenseal Hydrastis canadensis inhibit CYP enzymes badly potentially causing accumulation of chemotherapy drugs to toxic levels and increasing adverse effects very significantly.

P-glycoprotein and other drug transporters are drastically affected by herbal compounds which alter absorption and clearance of chemotherapeutic agents somewhat irregularly. Several herbal supplements modulate immune function weirdly potentially causing gnarly unintended consequences during cancer treatment with dodgy immunotherapies. Echinacea and ginseng contain compounds potentially stimulating immune activity and heavily interfering with checkpoint inhibitors or exacerbating immunity-related adverse events. Conversely other herbs may exert immunosuppressive effects that could dampen efficacy of treatments thereby significantly reducing overall potency of therapeutic interventions. Herbal supplements face pretty lax regulatory oversight in many regions resulting in wildly varying product quality and potency almost everywhere nowadays. Pesticides undeclared pharmaceuticals and heavy metals often contaminate various products posing direct toxicity risks quite frequently in many unfortunate situations.

Batch variability often precipitates wildly inconsistent clinical outcomes and terribly muddles efficacy evaluations under certain obscure circumstances of safety assessment. Adulteration with undeclared substances like corticosteroids or NSAIDs has been reported and may lead quickly to serious nasty reactions or harmful interactions. Risks highlight an urgent need among healthcare providers to get detailed info on supplements and back products from rigorously validated manufacturers. Oncology providers should nowadays routinely quiz patients on usage of herbal supplements and educate them thoroughly on risks ensuring effective coordinated care. Patient safety and treatment outcomes are optimized effectively in complex healthcare scenarios through evidence-based info integration and collaborative decision making.

St. John's Wort

Hypericum perforatum also known as St John's Wort stays pretty popular as a supplement used mainly for somewhat unusual antidepressant effects. It potently induces cytochrome P450 3A4 enzymes and P-glycoprotein transporters which play crucial roles in metabolism of many pharmaceuticals rapidly. Induction accelerates metabolism of various chemotherapeutic agents thereby diminishing plasma concentrations and therapeutic efficacy rather significantly in many cases quite rapidly. St John's Wort pretty remarkably lessens effectiveness of certain pharmaceuticals like irinotecan and imatinib under a variety of fairly diverse conditions. Subtherapeutic drug levels may precipitously lead cancer treatment failure or disease progression and pose substantial risks fairly quickly under certain conditions. Cancer patients gulping St John's Wort without much medical supervision may really mess up their chemotherapy outcomes thereby highlighting necessity of meds review during cancer care.

Green Tea Extract (EGCG)

Epigallocatechin Gallate or EGCG present in green tea extract has garnered rather considerable attention lately exhibiting pretty potent anticancer properties. EGCG may severely inhibit proteasome activity and badly disrupt metabolism of chemotherapeutic drugs via cytochrome P450 enzymes in pretty high doses. Reports of hepatotoxicity linked to green tea extracts in vast amounts have surfaced sparking unease about liver damage in cancer patients suddenly. Meticulous clinical supervision becomes essential when EGCG supplements are taken alongside certain cancer treatments with potentially hazardous interactions.

Turmeric/Curcumin

Turmeric and curcumin exhibit anticancer properties largely via modulation of multiple signaling pathways such as NF-κB or COX-2 pretty effectively. Curcumin inhibits cytochrome P450 enzymes quite badly at high doses thereby potentially altering the metabolism of various chemotherapeutic medications significantly. Curcumin possibly amplifies the effects of anticoagulant medications thereby heightening risk of bleeding issues significantly in certain vulnerable individuals. Curcumin supplements administered alongside cancer treatments demand vigilant monitoring, particularly in patients taking blood thinners or medications metabolized by certain CYP enzymes.

Traditional Medicines

Intricate mixes of botanicals frequently appear in herbal concoctions rooted deeply in obscure ancient medicinal traditions and Indigenous healing modalities. Several products contained heavy metals such as mercury and arsenic alongside undeclared corticosteroids and sundry pharmaceutical adulterants rather alarmingly. Toxic contaminants can greatly heighten risks and foster erratic interactions with cancer treatments potentially undermining the efficacy of such standard therapies. Cancer patients undergoing gruelling treatment regimens should eschew dubious herbal remedies lacking rigorous testing and oversight from medical experts. Sourcing products from reputable manufacturers with rigorous third-party testing pretty much guarantees utmost purity and safety almost every time. Collaboration with integrative medicine specialists provides guidance on safely incorporating traditional remedies, thereby minimizing risks and optimizing supportive care effectively.

6.4. Nutrient Overload and Organ Toxicity

Supplements are used haphazardly in various cancer care settings ostensibly supporting nutrition and somewhat mollifying harsh side effects of treatment regimens. Megadosing with vitamins and minerals often carries significant toxicity risks quietly nowadays owing largely to widespread assumption that more equates better. Excessive micronutrient consumption way beyond normally recommended upper limits precipitates pernicious effects on organ function and disrupts systemic metabolic processes severely. Cancer patients with severely compromised organ systems such as kidneys or liver are particularly vulnerable due to aggressive treatments or disease progression. Excessive doses of vitamin A can trigger hepatotoxicity in severe instances marked by jaundice and hepatic fibrosis with elevated liver enzymes. Vitamin D megadosing precipitates hypercalcemia manifesting insidiously as nausea and vomiting kidney stones or pretty severe impairment of renal function sometimes.

Patients with pre-existing renal issues are extremely vulnerable to nephrotoxic effects caused by excess calcium very frequently nonetheless. Iron supplements often prescribed for cancer patients with anemia can perversely trigger oxidative stress, damaging cellular components and precipitating hemosiderosis, affecting the heart liver endocrine organs severely. Selenium has been linked with heightened risks of type-2 diabetes at supra-physiological doses, possessing antioxidant properties as another obscure trace element. Cancer care complexity muddles safety profiles of nutrient supplements awkwardly in some clinical settings nowadays quite apparently. Anticancer drugs often undergo rapid hepatic metabolism and swift renal excretion so additional nutrient toxicity stress severely exacerbates organ dysfunction, potentially precipitating treatment delays or drastic dose tapering. Supplements in high concentrations can interact heavily with certain hepatic enzymes thereby significantly altering pharmacokinetics and toxicity profiles of various chemotherapeutic agents.

Micronutrient overdose can often cause really severe stomach issues or debilitating nerve damage in many unsuspecting patients suddenly. Supplementation tailored to individuals becomes crucial given lurking risks and unforeseen health hazards highlighted by thorough biochemical assessments and nutritional evaluations. Clinicians should meticulously assess baseline nutrient levels before prescribing supplements and remain vigilant for signs of toxicity throughout therapy. Awareness of upper intake levels and education on proper dosing thresholds alongside counseling against unsupervised megadosing is crucial for safe treatment of cancer patients. Oncologists and dietitians alongside integrative medicine specialists can safely ensure supplementation supports patient health without undermining efficacy of treatment.

Vitamin A and Liver Toxicity

Vitamin A plays a critical role in vision and reproduction while crucially supporting immune function and facilitating subtle cellular processes quietly. Preformed vitamin A namely retinol and retinyl esters exist mainly in animal derived foods and dietary supplements while provitamin A carotenoids like beta-carotene are found mostly in plant sources. Preformed vitamin A consumed excessively especially via dubious supplementary means can lead precipitously to toxicity with liver extremely vulnerable. Liver serves as main storage site for vitamin A accumulating copious amounts remarkably efficiently in hepatic stellate cells almost always. Excessive vitamin A consumption can precipitously lead to dangerously high levels accumulating internally resulting in nasty liver damage suddenly.

Vitamin A toxicity manifests with myriad symptoms ranging from mild nonspecific gripes such as utter fatigue and crippling headaches to severe liver damage including marked hepatomegaly or outright liver failure. Progressive liver damage culminates in cirrhosis and portal hypertension when chronic hypervitaminosis A runs rampant unchecked over prolonged periods. High doses of vitamin A are linked rather seriously with adverse effects besides liver toxicity very frequently and cause serious issues. Prolonged excessive intake may spur bone resorption quite severely and heighten risk of nasty fractures by markedly inhibiting osteoblast activity. Hormone therapy for breast cancer severely undermines bone health posing additional concerns for cancer patients undergoing various grueling treatments. Vitamin A has a pretty dicey rep for wreaking havoc on fetal development rather problematically in certain circumstances apparently.

Women of childbearing age should be pretty careful around vitamin A supplements since excessive intake during pregnancy can severely damage craniofacial development. Supplementation risks underscore importance of strict adherence very carefully always beforehand under guidance from healthcare professionals at recommended dosages. Vitamin A supplementation during cancer care ought be tailored rather gingerly and monitored extremely closely because of such egregious risks. Retinol levels in blood effectively assess vitamin A status and liver function tests detect early ominous signs of toxicity quite alarmingly. Patients should be sternly cautioned against recklessly ingesting high dose vitamin A supplements without proper medical supervision or some sort of oversight. Emphasizing dietary vitamin A sources instead of gulping down massive supplement doses mitigates risk of toxicity while supporting overall nutritional needs fairly adequately. Preformed vitamin A supplements taken excessively pose serious risks like hepatotoxicity bone demineralization and teratogenicity heavily impacting many bodily functions. Incorporating vitamin A safely into oncology nutrition plans requires meticulous assessment and fairly rigorous education with ongoing thorough monitoring.

Selenium and Type 2 Diabetes

Selenium remarkably plays a crucial role in encourage immune function and thyroid hormone metabolism within antioxidant defense systems quite effectively. Selenoproteins such as glutathione peroxidases and thioredoxin reductases rely heavily on it shielding cells from oxidative harm fueling malignant tumour growth rapidly. Selenium intake adequate enough for health maintenance yet both deficient and excessive consumption can sometimes have really nasty detrimental effects on humans. Selenium intake alarmingly correlates with elevated risk of type 2 diabetes mellitus development sporadically under certain conditions somewhat dubiously. Large-scale epidemiological investigations and randomized controlled trials found a U-shaped association between selenium levels and diabetes risk indicating deficiency or excess can be sometimes detrimental. Daily selenium intake exceeding 400 micrograms has been associated with heightened risk of T2DM in some populations quite notably.

Biological mechanisms underlying this phenomenon remain somewhat obscure and may be linked heavily to selenium's impact on various insulin signaling pathways downstream. Selenium's antioxidant properties harbour potential for harm while protecting bodily processes against oxidative stress fairly effectively under certain conditions. Disruption might slowly foster glucose intolerance eventually leading to overt diabetes. Excessive selenium intake triggers selenosis brutally marked by nausea brittle hair loss of nails and nasty peripheral neuropathy symptoms suddenly. Selenosis manifesting chronically may exacerbate severe complications thereby underscoring significance of avoiding overload from habitual excessive selenium ingestion very badly. Selenium supplementation in cancer care must be approached with great vigilance under certain conditions normally with utmost care surrounding such treatments. Selenium possibly enhances antioxidant defenses during treatment and high-dose supplementation recklessly poses severe metabolic risks for diabetes-prone patients notably.

Clinicians must meticulously assess patient's selenium levels at baseline and presence of comorbidities before recommending supplements due largely to heightened metabolic disorder risks in cancer survivors with T2DM. Blood tests nowadays facilitate identification of selenium deficiencies or excesses pretty effectively enabling more tailored nutritional regimens for individuals. Stern warnings ought to be given to patients popping high-dose selenium supplements in absence of clear clinical indications or some documented deficiency. Selenium remains vital for overall health yet excessive daily intake above 400 mcg heightens risk of type 2 diabetes and manifests toxicity symptoms. Meticulous assessment and ongoing monitoring with modified dosing regimens in survivorship nutrition are crucial for safely integrating selenium supplementation into cancer care protocols.

Iron and Oxidative Stress

Iron plays a crucial albeit somewhat obscure role in energy metabolism and is vital for oxygen transport and DNA synthesis. Excess iron wreaks havoc on cells via oxidative stress mostly in cancer care scenarios because too much iron proves pretty toxic. Excessive iron levels catalyze formation of reactive oxygen species via Fenton reaction a notoriously vigorous chemical process producing highly reactive hydroxyl radicals. ROS inflicts severe oxidative damage on lipids proteins and DNA rather frequently under certain conditions with somewhat alarming regularity. DNA damage left unfixed can foster mutations that rather swiftly drive carcinogenesis or significantly boost rapid tumour progression. Iron overload has been implicated rather ominously as risk factor for exacerbating several cancers including liver cancer and notoriously aggressive breast cancer. Repeated blood transfusions or hereditary hemochromatosis and rampant supplementation greatly increase iron overload thereby heightening oxidative stress risk markedly.

Cancer patients undergoing therapies that annihilate red blood cells or suffer malabsorption syndrome often exhibit extremely erratic iron level fluctuations necessitating vigilant monitoring. Iron supplementation should be done judiciously in clinical settings rather than administered hastily without proper diagnosis or serious consideration. Healthcare providers must evaluate serum ferritin and other iron indices very accurately before initiating iron therapy for patients. Supplementation proves beneficial when iron deficiency anemia gets confirmed but excessive iron intake can increase oxidative stress without actual deficiency being present. Daily iron intake ought not to surpass 45 milligrams generally deemed tolerable upper limit for most adults.

Excessive intake beyond a threshold precipitously leads quite nastily to gastrointestinal upset or liver dysfunction and heightened oxidative stress injury. Cancer care decisions regarding iron supplementation must weigh treatment modalities against various cancer types very carefully considering overall patient health. Excess iron may spur oxidative DNA damage fueling tumour progression remarkably in states of iron overload where various biological functions falter badly. Individualized clinical guidance and careful lab evaluation are crucial when pondering iron supplementation in cancer patients precluding severely detrimental pro-oxidant effects that badly compromise treatment efficacy and overall patient safety.

6.5. Immunomodulatory Supplements and Immunotherapy Risks

Immunotherapy advent revolutionized cancer treatment pretty effectively by leveraging body's immune response to target tumour cells for utter destruction rapidly. Modulating immune checkpoints such as PD-1 or CTLA-4 has yielded remarkably high success rates fairly often across diverse cancer types. Robust immune system activation precipitates nasty autoimmune-like effects and various other immune-related adverse events fairly often apparently. Cancer patients on immunotherapy must exercise extreme caution when taking dietary supplements with potentially immunomodulatory properties rather haphazardly. Fungi-derived extracts namely Reishi and Polysaccharide-K gain traction potentially boosting immunity with Ganoderma lucidum being source of such extracts. Bioactive polysaccharides in compounds purportedly stimulate various facets of immune system including T-cells natural killer cells and macrophages quite vigorously.

Mushroom extracts might rev up body's cancer-fighting mechanisms pretty dramatically and supercharge immunotherapy effectiveness thereby encourage innate immunity quite significantly. This immunostimulatory effect might seem rather beneficial down the line yet obviously raises pretty crucial safety concerns subsequently. Immune activity amplification in patients already receiving checkpoint inhibitors may possibly exacerbate severity or probability of irAEs impacting organs such as skin liver lungs or intestines. Immunotherapy's efficacy gets pretty badly undermined by immunosuppressive treatments necessitated sometimes by nasty adverse events in certain tricky situations. Pretty limited evidence presently exists regarding safety and efficacy of immunomodulatory supplements combined with immune checkpoint inhibitors. Data mostly emerge from preclinical studies or small clinical trials featuring heterogeneous patient populations and wildly diverse supplement formulations.

Patients undergoing immunotherapy should divulge each dietary supplement they consume because whacky immune reactions may possibly occur. Healthcare providers nowadays effectively assess risks and benefits while vigilantly monitoring for severe adverse effects pretty regularly with open communication. High-dose vitamins and herbal immunostimulants or probiotics may profoundly disrupt immune balance similarly in some instances alongside other supplements. Prudent clinicians ought to eschew unsupervised use of immunomodulatory supplements during active immunotherapy till fairly robust evidence becomes available. Mushroom extracts and other immunomodulatory supplements offer beneficial effects yet pose risk during therapy with immune checkpoint inhibitors due to overactivation largely. Meticulous assessment of patient health and collaboration with oncologists demands careful patient education for safely integrating various supplements into cancer treatment regimens.

6.6. Quality Control and Regulatory Gaps

Dietary supplements face rather lax regulatory oversight worldwide in many regions but scrutiny varies greatly across this globe. Substantial challenges arise from this regulatory discrepancy particularly in oncology care where patients often surreptitiously take dodgy supplements after treatment. Rigorous quality control lapses spawn serious safety worries making awareness crucial daily for healthcare providers and patients handling efficacy issues. Dietary supplements are viewed as food rather than medicaments in many nations thereby obviating need for rigorous pre-market vetting or safety trials. Manufacturers peddle supplements sans rigorous scientific validation typically demanded by regulatory bodies these days fairly frequently nowadays. Wildly inconsistent potency in ostensibly similar products heightens risk of contamination and mislabeling greatly within significant regulatory void. Presence of noxious agents poses significant threat usually under certain circumstances and with varying degrees of severity every time.

Several studies nowadays document presence of pesticides heavy metals like lead and arsenic mercury or microbial contaminants in various nutritional supplements fairly frequently. Dodgy herbal supplements sold online often harbour clandestine steroids and illicit weight-loss meds alongside other illicit pharmaceutical ingredients surprisingly. Contaminants cause direct toxicity and wreak havoc on cancer therapies rather perilously in some freakishly adverse ways under murky circumstances. Products often contain varying concentrations of active ingredients and dose listed on label may not reflect actual amount delivered accurately sometimes. Dosing decisions become pretty dicey due to such variability and clinicians struggle mightily to give somewhat reliable guidance on treatment outcomes effectively nowadays. Proprietary blends often obscure quantity of individual ingredients thereby further clouding safety assessments under pretty unusual or rare circumstances.

Clinicians and patients should prioritize supplements with rigorous third-party testing or certification mitigating potentially serious inherent health risks somewhat effectively. Organizations like USP and ConsumerLab nowadays rigorously verify supplement quality testing for purity and absence of various contaminants pretty thoroughly. Supplements bearing prestigious seals generally ensure stricter manufacturing protocols and significantly enhanced product dependability overall in most instances naturally. Patients should disclose use of supplements rather candidly with their healthcare providers nowadays. Oncology professionals help navigate safe choices thoroughly amidst cancer treatments and recommend reasonably trustworthy brands with considerable care becomes:

Cancer specialists guide patients through myriad treatment options quite carefully and endorse rather reliable products with utmost vigilance ordinarily under dire circumstances. Cancer care treatment plans that incorporate supplement use should be stringently supervised clinically maximizing benefits while mitigating substantial associated risks. Significant quality control gaps remain starkly alongside glaring regulatory shortcomings while dietary supplements play fairly supportive roles ordinarily in diverse cancer care settings. Verified products must be carefully chosen and awareness heightened for safeguarding patient health while therapeutically optimizing outcomes quite effectively.

6.7. Patient–Provider Communication: A Crucial Safeguard

Cancer patients often withhold info about using supplements largely out of fear that natural remedies are harmless. Clinicians must proactively inquire about supplement usage. Shared decision-making fosters trust and improves safety allowing for early identification of risks. Dietary supplements can be beneficial in cancer care but they also pose risks of interactions with medications and organ toxicity. Clinicians must proactively inquire about usage of various dietary supplements especially those with potentially hazardous interactions with prescribed medications. Shared decision-making fosters trust pretty effectively and enhance safety thereby facilitating detection of lurking hazards fairly early on. Dietary supplements offer supportive benefits in cancer care yet harbor risks of treatment interference and organ toxicity with dubious quality. Pretty thorough grasp of pharmacological interactions evidence-based dosing regimens and often quite open dialogue between patients and various healthcare providers is demanded.

7. Personalized Supplementation: Tailoring Approaches for Individual Cancer Types

Precision oncology advances rapidly and increasingly it's recognized that a one-size-fits-all approach utterly falls woefully short in cancer care nowadays. Cancer types exhibit distinct biological characteristics that necessitate modified nutritional interventions varying remarkably across specific patient populations differently. Tumour traits and genetic predispositions are intricately woven together with patient vitality gut flora and treatment protocols for yielding optimal results. Tumour biology nowadays plays a pivotal role in determining efficacy of various dietary supplements and their safety quite effectively. Cancers sensitive to fluctuations in hormone levels like prostate cancer and breast cancer respond quite variably to phytoestrogens or vitamin D supplements.

Tumours with wildly different metabolic fingerprints or rogue gene mutations may demand highly specific nutrient protocols countering surged oxidative stress pretty effectively. Supplements modulating immune responses might be beneficial in cancers treated with immunotherapies but carefully calibrating timing and type of supplement matters greatly. Cancer treatment modality substantially influences supplemental needs during therapy remarkably and affects patients differently under various conditions. Chemotherapy radiation surgery and targeted therapies impose various physiological stresses altering nutrient requirements differently under odd specific circumstances quite radically sometimes. Patients undergoing chemo often endure malabsorption of vital nutrients or heightened oxidative stress thereby necessitating antioxidants or specific amino acids for repair.

High-dose antioxidants given during radiation therapy may weirdly undermine treatment efficacy by quenching crucial free radicals necessary for eradicating tumour cells. Supplement timing and dosage must be tailored pretty precisely each time in relation to varying treatment schedules individually. Genetic factors profoundly affect metabolism of nutrients variably and bodily response to dietary supplements is altered significantly thereby. Genetic variations such as MTHFR polymorphisms or rare CYP450 variants markedly alter efficacy of various supplements and significantly impact patient responses. Genomic data informs clinical decisions nicely ensuring supplementation dovetails with a patient's peculiar biological makeup rather accurately in most cases. Presence of comorbidities such as diabetes or cardiovascular disease and severe renal impairment drastically alters safety profiles of many dietary supplements.

Excess iron supplementation in patients with hemochromatosis or diabetes may surprisingly exacerbate oxidative damage under some rather unusual circumstances. Profound impacts on nutrient absorption and immune function stem from gut microbiota diversity and overall health suggesting modified interventions involving prebiotics or unusual probiotics. Personalized supplementation in oncology necessitates a rather rigorous multidisciplinary strategy incorporating insights from tumour biology genetics and fluctuating microbiome under various treatment modalities and overall patient health status. Therapeutic synergy gets maximized pretty effectively while risks dwindle and holistic patient care gets a boost in this intricate process. Research evolves rapidly and individualized supplementation protocols will likely become crucial in precision cancer therapy helping patients get vastly better outcomes.

7.1. Breast Cancer: Hormonal Balance and Antioxidant Caution

Breast cancer links intricately with estrogen signaling pathways deeply within cellular mechanisms especially hormone receptor-positive subtypes are affected rather profoundly. Supplementation influencing hormonal balance or oxidative stress and inflammatory processes demands meticulous evaluation very carefully these days with utmost scrutiny. Patients on therapies such as tamoxifen face bone health concerns often, resulting in severe loss of bone density rapidly over time. Breast cancer patients often exhibit vitamin D deficiency which gets linked with poorer overall health outcomes relatively frequently among such individuals. Supplementation plays a dual role supporting skeletal health frequently ravaged during hormone-blocking therapies and potentially modulating myriad cellular processes deeply. Serum 25(OH)D levels should be regularly monitored and supplementation given pretty frequently to maintain ranges typically hovering around 30 ng/mL.

Long-chain omega-3s primarily EPA and DHA present in fish oil exhibit potent anti-inflammatory effects somewhat alleviating fatigue and depression during breast cancer therapy rather effectively. Omega-3 supplementation apparently boosts chemotherapy effectiveness pretty significantly by heavily modulating inflammatory cytokines and altering tumour microenvironment radically. Curcumin a bioactive compound from turmeric profoundly exhibits anti-estrogenic effects and anti-proliferative activity in preclinical breast cancer models influencing NF-κB signaling pathways greatly. Woefully poor bioavailability hampers its clinical use and results from human studies are mostly pretty inconclusive and often downright contradictory. Novel formulations with enhanced bioavailability are being scrutinized pretty thoroughly nowadays for evaluating therapeutic efficacy in diverse clinical settings. Supplements containing soy isoflavones or high-dose flaxseed potentially exert weird estrogen-like effects silently within human bodies daily.

Moderate dietary intake is deemed generally safe yet concentrated supplements might theoretically stimulate estrogen receptors and promote growth pretty readily in hormone-sensitive breast cancer cells. Cautious usage is warranted particularly in patients with ER+ status and strict medical oversight is necessitated under such circumstances. Modified supplementation regimens greatly benefit breast cancer patients by supporting hormonal equilibrium and overall wellbeing while avoiding potentially perturbing supplements. Healthcare providers specializing in nutrition for cancer patients are consulted regularly ensuring safe integration of various dietary supplements fairly effectively nowadays.

7.2. Colorectal Cancer: Micronutrient Restoration and Microbiome Modulation

Colorectal cancer develops in tandem with aberrant gut microbiota composition functioning and chronic inflammation fueled by various dietary factors. Surgical resection and systemic chemotherapy disrupt nutrient absorption and intestinal flora balance severely leading often to various nasty deficiencies. Supporting gut health and optimizing micronutrient status are essential pretty much in comprehensive care for patients who have colorectal cancer. B6 and B12 vitamins alongside folate play crucial roles deeply embedded in one-carbon metabolism and DNA synthesis processes vital for genomic stability. DNA repair and methylation processes rely heavily on such vitamins for proper cellular function and maintenance. Genomic stability gets maintained through highly intricate biochemical processes unusually. B-vitamins play a crucial role pretty much everywhere in myriad complex metabolic pathways unfolding rapidly inside living cells. One-carbon metabolism plays a crucial role in numerous downstream cellular functions rather quietly.

Folate deficiency is fairly common in CRC patients largely owing to aberrant metabolic pathways or malabsorption that gums up DNA repair mechanisms really badly. Supplementation becomes necessary in confirmed deficiency cases but excessive folate intake possibly fosters growth of existing neoplastic cells theoretically warranting caution. Dosing must be tailored rather carefully for each individual patient and monitored extremely vigilantly by healthcare professionals under various circumstances. Probiotics or prebiotics pretty rapidly modulate gut microbiome and significantly enhance barrier function while reducing inflammation in intestines. Grueling chemotherapy regimens frequently precipitate diarrhea and greatly heightened risk of infection due to mucosal damage and ensuing dysbiosis. Preliminary findings indicate a balanced gut microbiota possibly plays a substantial role in mitigating colorectal cancer recurrence and augmenting immunity. Elevated serum vitamin D levels coupled with sufficient calcium intake correlate with reduced CRC recurrence risk in numerous observational studies lately. Vitamin D facilitates immune response quite effectively exerting antiproliferative effects rather aggressively on cells of various colorectal tumour types.

Post-treatment bone health remains worrisome particularly in patients enduring lengthy chemotherapy or beset by lifestyle factors severely limiting sun exposure thus supplementation often becomes necessary. Curcumin's anti-inflammatory and anti-proliferative properties have been researched pretty extensively in a variety of colorectal cancer models with considerable thoroughness. Polyp formation pathways and chronic colon inflammation are suppressed simultaneously in response. Curcumin shows considerable promise as adjunct therapy reducing inflammation substantially and slowing disease progression rather remarkably in various contexts. Colorectal cancer treatment via personalized supplementation should effectively restore essential micronutrients and support gut health by pretty significantly reducing severe inflammation. Collaboration remains utterly critical with oncology specialists and dietitians for ensuring supplements are used safely rather effectively tailored to individual patient needs.

7.3. Prostate Cancer: Antioxidant Balance and Immune Modulation

Prostate cancer often advances quite sluggishly under hormonal influence particularly from androgens. Rather lethargic nature facilitates adoption of peculiar diets geared towards modulating progression of disease and encourages health in patients. Supplementation can be crucial sometimes for prostate cancer patients living quite extended periods with compromised antioxidant status already severely. Pretty much always a careful balance avoids nasty side effects with antioxidant supplementation rather effectively in most cases. Men diagnosed with prostate cancer often have poorer outcomes including faster PSA progression and lower bone density when vitamin D levels are low. Prolonged androgen deprivation therapy substantially accelerates bone loss thereby markedly heightening fracture risk during treatment. Vitamin D supplementation often paired with calcium maintains bone health and may exert antiproliferative effects on prostate tumour cells via cell growth regulation.

Selenium and vitamin E garnered considerable attention as potential chemopreventive agents after early observational studies hinted at profoundly protective anticancer effects. Big scale randomized controlled trials such as Selenium and Vitamin E Cancer Prevention Trial showed utterly no benefit in prostate cancer prevention. High-dose vitamin E supplementation correlated with marginally heightened prostate cancer risk and excessive selenium intake might readily precipitate toxicity under certain circumstances. Nowadays current recommendations basically advise against high dose supplementation of these nutrients outside context of correcting a deficiency. Lycopene a carotenoid predominantly found in tomatoes has garnered considerable attention for potentially lowering prostate-specific antigen levels and thwarting prostate cancer cell proliferation vigorously. It acts as potent antioxidant modulating signaling pathways deeply involved in tumour cell growth erratically rather quietly somewhat.

Lycopene apparently works best when consumed as part of whole foods rather than in high dose isolated supplement form highlighting quirky dietary habits very effectively. Epigallocatechin gallate manifests antioxidant properties and anti-inflammatory effects quite slowly within green tea possibly hindering progression of prostate cancer effectively. Green tea supplementation appears somewhat effective in reducing tumour growth markers and PSA rise significantly in many patients effectively overall. Caution seems warranted owing largely to scattered reports detailing nasty hepatotoxicity incidents linked with reckless use of highly concentrated herbal extracts. Prostate cancer supplementation ought to very carefully focus on rectifying nutritional deficits and supporting skeletal wellness balancing antioxidant consumption with utmost caution. Holistic methods tailored specifically for individual medical needs paired with ongoing treatment offer great potential for markedly enhanced health outcomes effectively.

7.4. Lung Cancer: Antioxidant Risks and Immune-Supportive Interventions

Lung cancer patients often stumble upon a gnarly tangle of oxidative stress inflammation and exposure to sundry carcinogenic substances notably those tied up with tobacco products. Oxidative damage exacts a steep price from lung tissue thereby fostering an environment necessitating judicious supplementation strategies being employed very cautiously under certain conditions. Antioxidants may spur tumour growth in smokers and former smokers especially when taken in very high doses undermining conventional therapies somewhat. Supplementation carefully tailored for immune support and symptom management is essential while avoiding interventions that are potentially risky. Low-dose vitamin C supplementation possibly enhances general antioxidant defenses somewhat during aggressive treatment for lung cancer and enhances immune response. High-dose intravenous vitamin C has garnered considerable research interest as potential adjuvant therapy owing largely to generating hydrogen peroxide inside tumour cells selectively thereby promoting demise of cancer cells.

Intravenous vitamin C remains largely unorthodox as a treatment while this approach still lingers somewhat experimentally in medical practice. Oral supplementation should be given extremely cautiously under very close medical supervision pretty much always. Beta-carotene supplementation has been linked tenuously and somewhat inexplicably with heightened incidence of lung cancer in smokers through dubious large-scale prevention trials. High-dose beta-carotene supplements ought to be shunned in such populations lest they spur carcinogenesis or worsen oxidative stress pretty quickly. Glutamine a conditionally essential amino acid has shown rather considerable promise in somewhat alleviating pretty nasty side effects of various lung cancer therapies. Severity of radiation-induced esophagitis can be somewhat mitigated and chemotherapy-related mucositis greatly alleviated thereby markedly boosting overall patient comfort. Glutamine effectively enhances patients' strength by supporting mucosa repair and modulating immune function thereby fostering treatment adherence remarkably well.

Multimodal treatments for lung cancer severely compromise gut integrity badly and overall gastrointestinal function suffers greatly under chemotherapy radiation and targeted therapies. Probiotic supplementation greatly enhances balance of beneficial gut microbiota and may significantly diminish incidence of nasty infections or diarrhea. Patients receiving aggressive treatments or combo therapies derive substantial benefit especially from such an approach pretty frequently nowadays. Lung cancer supplementation strategies must precariously weigh potential antioxidant benefits against risks of unwittingly abetting neoplastic growth or muddling therapeutic efficacy. Doubtful supplements like beta-carotene potentially spell harm while gut health hangs precariously in the balance and immune support greatly matters. A cautious personalized approach proves essential alongside oncology care team for safely using dietary supplements effectively in treating patients with lung cancer.

7.5. Pancreatic and Gastrointestinal Cancers: Nutritional Repletion and Enzyme Support

Pancreatic cancers and other GI tract malignancies pose peculiar dietary difficulties largely owing severely impaired digestive processes and malabsorption issues suddenly. Tumours afflicting pancreas or stomach swiftly precipitate malabsorption of vital nutrients crucial for sustaining life resulting in drastic weight loss and severe muscle atrophy. Pancreatic resections and bowel surgeries drastically worsen malabsorption in many instances quite obviously for patients undergoing such surgical interventions. Aggressive chemotherapy coupled with radiation may severely impair gut mucosa worsening nutrient uptake badly and cause nasty symptoms like nausea rather frequently. Tailored nutritional supplementation remarkably enhances clinical outcomes in complex scenarios supporting treatment tolerance quite effectively with significant benefits. Pancreatic enzyme supplements play crucial role in treatment of pancreatic cancers and upper GI malignancies through Pancreatic Enzyme Replacement Therapy.

Lipase amylase and protease enzymes remarkably facilitate digestion of fats carbohydrates proteins very well inside human body quite naturally. Pancreatic insufficiency often arises in these patients largely due to tumour obstruction or surgical removal of pancreatic tissue causing steatorrhea and fat-soluble vitamin deficiencies notably A, D, E, K. PERT enhances nutrient absorption remarkably and significantly diminishes various gastrointestinal issues while stabilizing body weight fairly effectively overall in most cases. MCTs get absorbed straight into portal circulation bypassing need for pancreatic lipase whereas long-chain fats undergo extensive processing quite slowly. MCT oil supplementation provides patients with fat malabsorption or steatorrhea a valuable energy source maintaining caloric intake fairly reasonably very well. Malabsorption and chemotherapy-induced depletion often result in deficiencies of water-soluble B-complex vitamins and essential minerals such as magnesium frequently. B vitamins like B12 and thiamine play crucial often murky roles in energy metabolism and contribute somewhat haphazardly to neurological function.

Magnesium vigorously supports nerve health and muscle function while deficiency can significantly exacerbate fatigue or worsen nasty neuropathic symptoms. Targeted supplementation plays a crucial role in preventing disastrous complications while vigilant monitoring supports various metabolic needs quite effectively meanwhile. Cachexia and chronic inflammation often emerge as hallmark complications remarkably in various GI cancers and pancreatic cancer pretty frequently nowadays. Omega-3 fatty acids particularly EPA and DHA exhibit profoundly anti-inflammatory properties and may effectively modulate immune response these days. Omega-3 supplementation proves pretty beneficial in some clinical trials substantially enhancing quality of life by curbing inflammation very effectively. They may enhance heart health significantly in such patients who are often pretty frail and highly vulnerable.

Pancreatic and GI cancer patients require intricate nutritional strategies with varied dietary regimens and supplementary interventions often involving nuanced approaches slowly. Replenishing key vitamins alongside fats such as MCTs and omega-3 fatty acids can collectively result in markedly better overall patient outcomes generally. Interventions must be meticulously tailored into care plans involving specialists like oncologists and dietitians alongside supportive care experts very thoroughly now.

7.6. Hematological Cancers: Immune Support and Antioxidant Balance

Patients face complex treatment regimens involving intensive chemotherapy and targeted agents after being diagnosed with hematological malignancies like aggressive leukemia or nasty lymphoma. Such therapies profoundly suppress bone marrow function leading often enough to neutropenia and anemia and thrombocytopenia in many patients subsequently. Patients face markedly heightened infection risk and thoroughly impaired immune responses as direct result often subsequently in many such cases. Treatment side effects such as mucositis severely impair nutritional status further eroding overall immunity rather quickly in many cases unfortunately. Prudent dietary supplement use supports immune function in vulnerable populations quite effectively while managing treatment-related toxicities but poses risk of adverse effects. Zinc utterly fortifies innate immunity remarkably well while Vitamin C facilitates adaptive immune defenses with astonishing effectiveness.

Zinc plays a crucial albeit somewhat obscure role in T-cell function and antioxidant enzyme activity while vitamin C boosts neutrophil function vigorously becomes: Vitamin C boosts neutrophil function vigorously while zinc plays a crucial role in T-cell function and various antioxidant enzyme activities. Supplementation may enhance immune function and mitigate infection risk especially in patients exhibiting documented deficiencies of certain crucial nutrients. Excessive immune stimulation could possibly exacerbate nasty inflammatory issues or hamper hematologic recovery somewhat during severe neutropenia periods warranting caution. Vitamin D deficiency frequently afflicts hematologic cancer patients largely due to prolonged hospital stays and meager sunlight alongside malabsorption from damaged mucosa. Vitamin D somewhat irregularly modulates immune responses by heavily influencing regulation of T-cells and production of cytokines beyond bone calcium homeostasis. Encourage immune function remarkably with deficiency correction can lead substantially improved outcomes making regular monitoring essential for dosing optimally.

Gut microbiota plays a vital role in development of immune function extensively and helps regulate bodily responses pretty effectively downstream. Probiotic supplementation potentially restores ravaged microbial balance after chemotherapy or antibiotics thereby possibly mitigating nasty gastrointestinal toxicity and various opportunistic infections. Probiotic use carries risk of bacteremia or sepsis in stem cell transplant recipients and other gravely immunocompromised patients rather lamentably. Probiotics should be administered under tight medical supervision preferably in pretty rigorously controlled clinical trials backed by fairly solid evidence. Polysaccharide-K extracts and Ganoderma lucidum exhibit profoundly immunomodulatory properties enhancing natural killer cell activity vigorously boosting cytokine production variably. Early studies on hematologic cancers suggest extracts may enhance immune reconstitution after chemotherapy or marrow transplant potentially reducing infection rates significantly and boosting survival.

Supplements must be administered quite cautiously within care plans involving oncology specialists and experts in integrative medicine owing largely to very erratic product quality. Tailored supplementation exemplifies precision oncology in certain hematological cancers reflecting a broader shift towards interventions shaped by cancer biology uniquely. Genetic polymorphisms drastically modify efficacy and safety of supplement regimens alongside baseline nutritional status and varying microbiome composition. Patients with multiple myeloma undergoing lenalidomide maintenance therapy might greatly benefit from vitamin D supplementation for optimal bone health but necessitate extremely meticulous monitoring of serum zinc levels alongside various antioxidants. Healthcare providers tweak supplement regimens pretty frequently via genetic testing and ongoing monitoring of nutrient levels really effectively. Crafting highly individualized care plans based on evidence necessitates slow collaboration among oncologists and integrative medicine specialists with dietitians and pharmacists. Rigorous evaluation continuously and effective incorporation of dietary supplements into care for hematological cancer depends on careful analysis of risk and benefit.

8. Regulatory and Ethical Challenges in the Use of Supplements in Oncology

Growing demand for dietary supplements amongst cancer sufferers nationwide poses hefty regulatory conundrums and knotty moral dilemmas for healthcare providers. Dietary supplements generally function under somewhat lax oversight whereas conventional pharmaceuticals are subjected normally to fairly rigorous safety and manufacturing scrutiny. Discrepancies spawn erratic product quality and safety issues thereby fueling apprehensions regarding unregulated usage during some pretty aggressive cancer treatment protocols. Numerous nations nowadays regulate dietary supplements as food rather than pharmaceuticals with oversight being woefully shoddy and often resulting in mess. They dodge pre-market approval and clinical trials altogether demonstrating safety rather effectively after landing squarely in consumers hands.

Supplements available contain drastically varying amounts of active ingredients or mysterious contaminants including nasty heavy metals lurking deep within. Labeling frequently turns out glaringly haphazard or downright duplicitous making precise evaluation of actual makeup rather dicey for clinicians. Nationwide dietary supplement usage gets recklessly linked to adverse events that post-market surveillance mechanisms often woefully fail detecting afterwards. Global standards being non uniform severely exacerbates issues surrounding supplements made in dodgy foreign labs and flogged internationally without checks. Products touted for cancer relief often fly under radar of rigorous scrutiny and end up being woefully ineffective or pernicious sometimes. Clinicians often stumble through tricky moral landscapes when patients elect dubious dietary regimens over standard cancer treatments or alongside them. Moral fibre quandaries swirl around patient self-determination pitted against external influence rooted deeply in wildly disparate philosophical standpoints.

Practitioners must rather meticulously balance patients' autonomy in choosing various supplements against duty to deliver efficacious treatment mitigating considerable risk. Oncologists must deftly steer tricky discussions educating patients who opt for some pretty dubious unproven remedies without totally alienating them. Patients often keep quiet about taking supplements mainly because of felt stigma or minimal inquiry from doctors. Crucial data omission endangers safety recklessly due to potentially disastrous drug interactions and supplement combinations with pretty awful side effects sometimes. Providers must foster nonjudgmental surroundings keenly encouraging open dialogue and extremely detailed history-taking with great ethical obligation very vigilantly always. Patients rapidly divert limited financial resources away from conventional therapies toward unproven alternatives that are often pretty pricey these days.

Concerns about equitable access and risk of severe financial toxicity amidst ineffective cancer care are raised pretty significantly these days. Clinicians rather badly flounder without strong evidence or clear guidelines on whether endorsing supplement use or discouraging it is prudent. Such ambiguity potentially precipitates erratic counsel and spawns gnarly moral conundrums surrounding culpability for unfortunate mishaps happening further downstream suddenly. Governments should work toward globally harmonizing ridiculously lax standards while stricter regulatory oversight is urgently needed for dodgy dietary supplements marketed shamelessly. Professional societies must concoct lucid guidelines on supplement usage grounded in rigorous research assisting clinicians counseling cancer patients effectively nowadays. Training clinicians in effective dialogue about supplements fosters trust remarkably among patients and providers and supports shared decision-making quite effectively.

Integrative medicine specialists trained thoroughly provide expert evaluation of various dietary supplements yielding pretty safe and highly individualized treatment recommendations. Regulatory complexities surrounding dietary supplements in oncology necessitate fairly coordinated multifaceted action across various agencies healthcare providers researchers and stakeholders. Supplements can be safely integrated into cancer care pretty thoroughly via open dialogue and rigorous educational oversight generally.

8.1. Regulatory Oversight: Gaps and Inconsistencies

Regulatory frameworks governing dietary supplements differ markedly from those applied for pharmaceutical drugs and this leads substantially concerning product safety. Dietary supplements get regulated as food rather than medicinal products in many nations including United States these days pretty surprisingly enough. Dietary Supplement Health and Education Act of 1994 rather loosely define supplements as products containing various vitamins or certain herbs and minerals. Supplements get marketed freely by manufacturers sans FDA approval provided no explicit disease diagnosis or treatment claims are being made. Significant challenges arise nationwide from various regulatory gaps posing threats particularly for cancer patients and other vulnerable populations obviously. Pre-market evaluation lacks nowadays fairly often in various cases.

Dietary supplements often slip onto market shelves sans rigorous clinical trials proving safety or efficacy unlike most prescription meds sold nowadays. People might unknowingly purchase products flaunting sketchy health perks or harboring fairly heinous poisonous substances rather quietly in stores. Inconsistencies in labeling compound such risks alarmingly further downstream. Ingredient disclosure varies wildly across various products and some labels neglect listing active compounds or spouts outlandish therapeutic claims quite frequently. Inaccurate labeling poses significant risks when consumers or healthcare providers make treatment decisions involving supplement use with conventional medication. Product contamination nowadays remains a pretty major concern obviously. Several investigations recently uncovered anabolic steroids not listed and heavy metals such as lead lurking in various commercial supplements on market shelves.

Contaminants can precipitate dire consequences or greatly hamper efficacy of cancer treatments like chemotherapy and immunotherapy very significantly. Ineffective regulation gets pretty badly hindered by weak enforcement mechanisms ultimately. Regulatory bodies such as FDA frequently lack sufficient capacity to yank non-compliant stuff off global online marketplaces quite rapidly. Regulatory shortcomings pose significant worry particularly for patients undergoing oncology treatments with highly varying degrees of efficacy. Using dietary supplements alongside cancer treatments concurrently may sometimes result in pretty unpredictable deleterious interactions or moderately increased toxicity. Rapidly evolving cancer treatments necessitate urgent implementation of stringent regulatory oversight and transparent labeling practices safeguarding patient health.

8.2. Clinical Ethics: Balancing Autonomy, Safety, and Evidence-Based Care

Ostensibly incorporating dietary supplements into cancer care poses a profoundly knotty and perilously ambiguous moral dilemma with many thorny facets. Clinicians nowadays must pretty carefully navigate tension between respecting patient autonomy and upholding beneficence non-maleficence principles with evidence-based practice. Cancer care spawns vexing issues where patients often opt for unconventional remedies or adjunct therapies regaining agency and alleviating debilitating symptoms pretty quickly. A exists ostensibly. Patient autonomy gets pitched rather vigorously against sundry opposing forces in medical ethics debates these days with marked fervor apparently nowadays. Patient autonomy essentially involves making rather informed decisions about one's health care under a fundamental principle of modern medical ethics nowadays.

Cancer patients frequently snag dietary supplements not just seeking therapeutic benefits but also wresting control of treatment pretty actively. Supplements offer hope or empowerment and culturally rooted healing practices escape acknowledgement by conventional oncology for people with unique needs. Clinicians bear a deeply ingrained professional obligation furnishing patients with relatively safe treatment grounded firmly in copious scientific research and empirical evidence nowadays. Halting usage of potentially pernicious or unproven supplements in contexts confounding cancer treatments plays a significant role. Unqualified support of patient preferences poses serious ethical problems in this context particularly if choices entail grave risks. Nowadays a fairly balanced shared decision-making approach surprisingly lies squarely within most ethical imperatives in various contexts.

Clinicians elucidate current evidence risks and possible interactions with cancer therapies quite clearly in open dialogue fostered by this model between patient and provider. Patients are urged vociferously articulately express deeply seated rather personal core values and long nebulous future aspirations or some quirky preferences. Conversations like these should fairly empower patients with correct information and guide them gently toward reasonably safe and prudent choices. Clinicians must respect informed decisions starkly diverging from standard recommendations provided patients thoroughly grasp complex implications and aren't facing some rather imminent harm. Striking a delicate balance between autonomy and clinical responsibility is essential for promoting patient-centered oncology care and maintaining trust effectively. Cancer patients increasingly need ethical literacy nowadays as usage of dietary supplements rises steadily in this fraught domain. Ongoing education and clear communication alongside interdisciplinary teamwork guarantees ethically sound care medically responsible naturally in most instances.

a. Patient Autonomy vs. Medical Paternalism

Desperate cancer patients sometimes grasp frantically for dubious herbal remedies in a bid for tenuous control over dire circumstances. Outright denial of such an option might feel somewhat paternalistic these days in many rather surprisingly liberal societies anyway. Clinicians must vigilantly ensure patients aren't resorting to dubious remedies and educate them thoroughly on risks of therapeutic efficacy and potential drug interactions. A balanced shared decision making model handles such dicey situations pretty deftly with loads of ethical finesse. Honoring patient choices informed by facts even when drastically deviating from usual treatment protocols stays morally binding pretty much always.

b. Informed Consent

Clinicians ought ethically guide patients toward third-party tested supplements and steer clear of products making dubious claims about therapeutic efficacy. Patients deserve clear info about benefits of supplements and inherent limitations alongside known interactions with prescribed meds pretty frequently nowadays. Concerns about product quality and regulatory status warrant thorough scrutiny and pretty clear disclosure obviously under normal circumstances.

c. Placebo Use and Deceptive Marketing

Supplements peddled very recklessly at desperate cancer victims often originate from dubious assertions leveraging fear or fabulist testimonials of ostensibly miraculous recoveries. Exploitation of vulnerable patients sparks serious ethical qualms and simultaneously fuels worrying erosion of trust in medicine grounded in evidence. Ominous false hope or significant delay looms over unsuspecting individuals awaiting effective treatment rather quietly in dark corners. Healthcare providers must vigorously challenge misinformation while validating patients' desire for exploring unproven integrative options with some legitimacy .

8.3. Research Ethics: Addressing Evidence Gaps Responsibly

Nowadays scarcity of top-notch unprejudiced research greatly hinders formulation of sturdy clinical guidelines for oncology patients using dietary supplements. Efficacy and safety data on supplements widely consumed by cancer patients remains sketchy and frequently at odds with each other. Tackling glaring holes in existing evidence bases spawns thorny issues that demand careful navigation fairly often in somewhat complex situations. Designing rigorous clinical trials for dietary supplements proves exceptionally complex under many circumstances normally owing largely to inherent methodological difficulties. Supplements originate from natural sources with wildly varying compositions pretty erratically dosed and bioavailability fluctuates greatly alongside them. Non-standardized formulations greatly hinder reproducibility of protocols thereby severely undermining reliability of outcomes in various tricky situations mercilessly.

Heterogeneity in patient populations and diverse cancer types along with myriad concurrent therapies rapidly adds layers of complexity to trial design. Supplementing research with industry involvement introduces thorny ethical concerns somewhat problematically across another layer of deliberation. Research into dietary supplements often gets funded by manufacturers thereby raising risk of conflict of interest substantially nowadays obviously. Favorable outcomes get published selectively meanwhile data deemed unfavorable gets suppressed and efficacy claims frequently get exaggerated grossly in various studies. Transparency in funding sources study design and data reporting is essentially always required for maintaining scientific credibility and garnering public trust.

Cancer patients particularly ones with advanced disease or scarce treatment options represent a vulnerable cohort in various clinical research undertakings nowadays. Desire for curative options can make participants vulnerable quite easily to coercion and mistakenly believe trials yield benefits directly for them personally. Ethical research clearly must prioritize informed consent delineating investigational nature of supplement and uncertainties surrounding its potential benefits and myriad associated risks. Research on oncology supplements must adhere quite stringently to high ethical standards and stringent norms scientifically. Sizable samples and control groups operate alongside full transparency in methodology and proper randomization with funding disclosures being pretty thorough.

Researchers should avoid exaggeration regarding preliminary findings particularly in public statements thereby precluding misinformation and fanciful hopes among patients and caregivers rapidly. Rigorously prioritizing ethics and leveraging scientific rigor propels field forward generating credible evidence that informs clinical practice and safeguards patient welfare ultimately.

8.4. Global Disparities in Supplement Regulation and Access

Global dietary supplement regulation differs enormously across regions resulting in vast discrepancies in product quality safety and public health outcomes pretty much everywhere. Stringent regulations govern supplement production and sale in some nations but others allow largely unregulated marketing with scant governmental oversight largely. Divergent regulatory approaches have profoundly far-reaching implications on oncology patients seeking alternative therapies or adjunctive treatments for managing disease effectively nowadays. Supplements are classified as natural health products or complementary medicines in fairly stringently regulated jurisdictions such as Canada or Australia basically. Countries frequently necessitate pre-market clearance alongside rigorous validation of purported health benefits and GMP compliance essentially beforehand very rigorously.

Regions with lax rules permit supplements slipping into market sans thorough vetting thus heightening risk of mislabeling or contamination alarmingly fast. Inconsistencies pretty frequently affect ordinary domestic consumers and foreign buyers purchasing goods online via various platforms these days. Internet opens up global access quite readily enabling circulation of unregulated stuff evading safety checks altogether worldwide with various dodgy supplements available. Consuming such products can have severely detrimental consequences on oncology patients extremely sensitive to treatments and possessing fragile health already. Nationwide deep disparities in economic resources and regulatory infrastructure exacerbate health inequities rather significantly at various times. Hefty prices or lax regulatory oversight can restrict access severely in low and middle-income nations under fairly normal circumstances generally. Wealthier demographics in affluent nations procure high-end verified supplements fuelling debates about global health equity rather vigorously nowadays overseas.

Urgently needed now amidst gnarly, unfolding challenges is greater international harmonization in regulation of dietary supplements rapidly evolving nowadays. Core global standards like ingredient transparency requirements and stringent manufacturing quality controls could improve product safety worldwide pretty rapidly. Global entities like Codex Alimentarius and World Health Organization have established foundational frameworks yet sorely needed concerted efforts remain woefully lacking nowadays globally. Harmonized regulatory environments offer oncology patients clearer guidance and reduce dubious product exposure pretty significantly across various diverse populations.

8.5. The Role of Healthcare Providers and Institutions

Clinicians and cancer centers must take proactive stances through continuing education programs and professional societies must develop some institutional policies. Institutions should empower patients fairly liberally now by fostering open dialogue so they disclose supplement use without much fear. Crucial becomes provision of integrative oncology services staffed by trained practitioners and patient education materials on safe use of supplements. Oncology patients' usage of dietary supplements creates a tangled web of regulatory voids and stubborn clinical enigmas with profoundly unsettling repercussions. Supplements are viewed by patients as a means to empowerment and healing increasingly but significant barrier remains lack of oversight and scientific evidence. Navigating knotty challenges demands diverse hands on deck including regulators and researchers alongside patients establishing transparent practices that safely support patient autonomy.

9. Conclusion

Dietary supplements usage in oncology remains a hotly contested topic nationwide amidst fervent discussion and ferocious disagreement lately still. Cancer survivors view supplements as pretty natural potentially beneficial add-ons alongside conventional therapy for substantially enhancing health outcomes remarkably well. Scientific evidence surrounding efficacy and safety is often shrouded in controversy and ambiguity naturally being highly variable. Thorough evaluation of available evidence surrounding dietary supplement use in cancer care explored potential benefits alongside associated risks quite critically. Certain supplements such as vitamin D shows considerable promise in tempering inflammatory responses pretty effectively while others may cause harm or prove utterly useless.

Efficacy of sundry supplements hinges substantially on dosage alongside individual genetic predispositions during various stages of ongoing cancer therapy. Indiscriminate usage during chemotherapy or radiation can really mess with certain therapeutic mechanisms and exacerbate nasty toxicity pretty badly sometimes. Supplementation within oncology contexts demands an extremely cautious approach remarkably grounded heavily in substantive empirical evidence from various research studies. Clinicians must stay rather current on emerging research and engage patients pretty openly in dialogue about supplement use and various underlying murky motivations. Dietary supplements should be incorporated into cancer care under individual nutritional assessments rather than replacing treatments validated by science. Appealing evidently nowadays challenges related to product quality and regulation persist meanwhile some inconsistency still remains.

Dietary supplements often sidestep stringent pre-market scrutiny unlike pharma drugs resulting in potency variability and contamination concerns fairly frequently nowadays. Patients might ingest dodgy supplements from fly-by-night vendors or recklessly gulp megadoses with nary a peep from their physician. Dietary supplements potentially serve as supportive agents in cancer care but must be used very judiciously with robust scientific backing. Multidisciplinary teams comprising oncologists and researchers along with pharmacists and dieticians should effectively guide safe integration of supplements into patient care nowadays. Future research must clarify mechanisms of action intricately and identify biomarkers vigorously for responsiveness in rigorously designed lengthy clinical trials. Tailored supplementation regimens meticulously devised for individuals can quite effectively mitigate adverse effects and boost overall outcomes pretty significantly.

References

Almatroodi SA, Almatroudi A, Khan AA, Alhumaydhi FA, Alsahli MA, Rahmani AH. Potential Therapeutic Targets of Epigallocatechin Gallate (EGCG), the Most Abundant Catechin in Green Tea, and Its Role in the Therapy of Various Types of Cancer. Molecules. 2020 Jul 9;25(14):3146. doi: 10.3390/molecules25143146. PMID: 32660101; PMCID: PMC7397003.

Almawash S. Revolutionary Cancer Therapy for Personalization and Improved Efficacy: Strategies to Overcome Resistance to Immune Checkpoint Inhibitor Therapy. Cancers (Basel). 2025 Mar 4;17(5):880. doi: 10.3390/cancers17050880. PMID: 40075727; PMCID: PMC11899125.

Chavengkijsakol D, Kongjan J, Suwanwattanakul T, Trakarnsanga B, Areepium N, Siritientong T. Cancer Patients' Behavior and Perception on the Use of Medical Foods and Dietary Supplements During Chemotherapy. Patient Prefer Adherence. 2025 May 9;19:1385-1395. doi: 10.2147/PPA.S514170. PMID: 40370472; PMCID: PMC12075470.

Clusan L, Ferrière F, Flouriot G, Pakdel F. A Basic Review on Estrogen Receptor Signaling Pathways in Breast Cancer. Int J Mol Sci. 2023 Apr 6;24(7):6834. doi: 10.3390/ijms24076834. PMID: 37047814; PMCID: PMC10095386.

de Castro GS, Andrade MF, Pinto FCS, Faiad JZ, Seelaender M. Omega-3 Fatty Acid Supplementation and Its Impact on Systemic Inflammation and Body Weight in Patients With Cancer Cachexia-A Systematic Review and

Meta-Analysis. Front Nutr. 2022 Jan 31;8:797513. doi: 10.3389/fnut.2021.797513. PMID: 35174197; PMCID: PMC8841833.

Didier AJ, Stiene J, Fang L, Watkins D, Dworkin LD, Creeden JF. Antioxidant and Anti-Tumor Effects of Dietary Vitamins A, C, and E. Antioxidants (Basel). 2023 Mar 3;12(3):632. doi: 10.3390/antiox12030632. PMID: 36978880; PMCID: PMC10045152.

Djaoudene, O., Romano, A., Bradai, Y. D., Zebiri, F., Ouchene, A., Yousfi, Y., Amrane-Abider, M., Sahraoui-Remini, Y., & Madani, K. (2023). A Global Overview of Dietary Supplements: Regulation, Market Trends, Usage during the COVID-19 Pandemic, and Health Effects. Nutrients, 15(15), 3320. https://doi.org/10.3390/nu15153320

Esposito T, Pentimalli F, Giordano A, Cortellino S. Vitamins and dietary supplements in cancer treatment: is there a need for increased usage? Expert Rev Anticancer Ther. 2025 Jun;25(6):687-710. doi: 10.1080/14737140.2025.2501077. Epub 2025 May 7. PMID: 40322898.

Gao X, Homayoonfal M. Exploring the anti-cancer potential of Ganoderma lucidum polysaccharides (GLPs) and their versatile role in enhancing drug delivery systems: a multifaceted approach to combat cancer. Cancer Cell Int. 2023 Dec 16;23(1):324. doi: 10.1186/s12935-023-03146-8. Erratum in: Cancer Cell Int. 2024 May 22;24(1):178. doi: 10.1186/s12935-024-03284-7. PMID: 38104078; PMCID: PMC10724890.

Gao Y, Yang H, Zhang X, Ma Y, Wang L. Effectiveness of Glutamine Oral Care in Reducing Oral Mucositis and Improving Oral Health After Neurosurgery: A Randomized Controlled Trial with Microbiome Analysis. Med Sci Monit. 2024 Feb 22;30:e942585. doi: 10.12659/MSM.942585. PMID: 38384124; PMCID: PMC10898191.

Giammarco S, Chiusolo P, Maggi R, Rossi M, Minnella G, Metafuni E, D'Alò F, Sica S. MTHFR polymorphisms and vitamin B12 deficiency: correlation between mthfr polymorphisms and clinical and laboratory findings. Ann Hematol. 2024 Oct;103(10):3973-3977. doi: 10.1007/s00277-024-05937-z. Epub 2024 Aug 28. PMID: 39196375; PMCID: PMC11512882.

Hardy ML. Dietary supplement use in cancer care: help or harm. Hematol Oncol Clin North Am. 2008 Aug;22(4):581-617, vii. doi: 10.1016/j.hoc.2008.04.012. PMID: 18638690.

Harvie M. Nutritional supplements and cancer: potential benefits and proven harms. Am Soc Clin Oncol Educ Book. 2014:e478-86. doi: 10.14694/EdBook_AM.2014.34.e478. PMID: 24857143.

Jabbari P, Yazdanpanah O, Benjamin DJ, Rezazadeh Kalebasty A. Supplement Use and Increased Risks of Cancer: Unveiling the Other Side of the Coin. Cancers (Basel). 2024 Feb 22;16(5):880. doi: 10.3390/cancers16050880. PMID: 38473246; PMCID: PMC10930792.

Jairoun AA, Shahwan M, Zyoud SH. Heavy Metal contamination of Dietary Supplements products available in the UAE markets and the associated risk. Sci Rep. 2020 Nov 2;10(1):18824. doi: 10.1038/s41598-020-76000-w. PMID: 33139833; PMCID: PMC7606431.

Khorashadizadeh S, Abbasifar S, Yousefi M, Fayedeh F, Moodi Ghalibaf A. The Role of Microbiome and Probiotics in Chemo-Radiotherapy-Induced Diarrhea: A Narrative Review of the Current Evidence. Cancer Rep (Hoboken). 2024 Oct;7(10):e70029. doi: 10.1002/cnr2.70029. PMID: 39410854; PMCID: PMC11480522.

Kim YI. Folate: a magic bullet or a double edged sword for colorectal cancer prevention? Gut. 2006 Oct;55(10):1387-9. doi: 10.1136/gut.2006.095463. PMID: 16966698; PMCID: PMC1856406.

Klein EA, Lippman SM, Thompson IM, Goodman PJ, Albanes D, Taylor PR, Coltman C. The selenium and vitamin E cancer prevention trial. World J Urol. 2003 May;21(1):21-7. doi: 10.1007/s00345-002-0314-z. Epub 2003 Mar 8. PMID: 12756490.

Klemow KM, Bartlow A, Crawford J, et al. Medical Attributes of St. John's Wort (Hypericum perforatum) In: Benzie IFF, Wachtel-Galor S, editors. Herbal Medicine: Biomolecular and Clinical Aspects. 2nd edition. Boca Raton (FL): CRC Press/Taylor & Francis; 2011. Chapter 11. Available from: https://www.ncbi.nlm.nih.gov/books/NBK92750/

Knecht K, Kinder D, Stockert A. Biologically-Based Complementary and Alternative Medicine (CAM) Use in Cancer Patients: The Good, the Bad, the Misunderstood. Front Nutr. 2020 Jan 24;6:196. doi: 10.3389/fnut.2019.00196. PMID: 32039227; PMCID: PMC6992534.

Lazard AJ, Nicolla S, Vereen RN, Pendleton S, Charlot M, Tan HJ, DiFranzo D, Pulido M, Dasgupta N. Exposure and Reactions to Cancer Treatment Misinformation and Advice: Survey Study. JMIR Cancer. 2023 Jul 28;9:e43749. doi: 10.2196/43749. PMID: 37505790; PMCID: PMC10422174.

Li S, Fasipe B, Laher I. Potential harms of supplementation with high doses of antioxidants in athletes. J Exerc Sci Fit. 2022 Oct;20(4):269-275. doi: 10.1016/j.jesf.2022.06.001. Epub 2022 Jun 11. PMID: 35812825; PMCID: PMC9241084.

Lin J, Cook NR, Albert C, Zaharris E, Gaziano JM, Van Denburgh M, Buring JE, Manson JE. Vitamins C and E and beta carotene supplementation and cancer risk: a randomized controlled trial. J Natl Cancer Inst. 2009 Jan 7;101(1):14-23. doi: 10.1093/jnci/djn438. Epub 2008 Dec 30. PMID: 19116389; PMCID: PMC2615459.

Luo L, Wang B, Jiang J, Fitzgerald M, Huang Q, Yu Z, Li H, Zhang J, Wei J, Yang C, Zhang H, Dong L, Chen S. Heavy Metal Contaminations in Herbal Medicines: Determination, Comprehensive Risk Assessments, and Solutions. Front Pharmacol. 2021 Jan 14;11:595335. doi: 10.3389/fphar.2020.595335. PMID: 33597875; PMCID: PMC7883644.

Marino P, Pepe G, Basilicata MG, Vestuto V, Marzocco S, Autore G, Procino A, Gomez-Monterrey IM, Manfra M, Campiglia P. Potential Role of Natural Antioxidant Products in Oncological Diseases. Antioxidants (Basel). 2023 Mar 12;12(3):704. doi: 10.3390/antiox12030704. PMID: 36978952; PMCID: PMC10045077.

Mattson MP. Hormesis defined. Ageing Res Rev. 2008 Jan;7(1):1-7. doi: 10.1016/j.arr.2007.08.007. Epub 2007 Dec 5. PMID: 18162444; PMCID: PMC2248601.

Mussa A, Mohd Idris RA, Ahmed N, Ahmad S, Murtadha AH, Tengku Din TADAA, Yean CY, Wan Abdul Rahman WF, Mat Lazim N, Uskoković V, Hajissa K, Mokhtar NF, Mohamud R, Hassan R. High-Dose Vitamin C for Cancer Therapy. Pharmaceuticals (Basel). 2022 Jun 3;15(6):711. doi: 10.3390/ph15060711. PMID: 35745630; PMCID: PMC9231292.

Oczkowski M, Dziendzikowska K, Pasternak-Winiarska A, Włodarek D, Gromadzka-Ostrowska J. Dietary Factors and Prostate Cancer Development, Progression, and Reduction. Nutrients. 2021 Feb 3;13(2):496. doi: 10.3390/nu13020496. PMID: 33546190; PMCID: PMC7913227.

Olson JM, Ameer MA, Goyal A. Vitamin A Toxicity. [Updated 2023 Sep 2]. In: StatPearls [Internet]. Treasure Island (FL): StatPearls Publishing; 2025 Jan-. Available from: https://www.ncbi.nlm.nih.gov/books/NBK532916/

Padayatty SJ, Sun H, Wang Y, Riordan HD, Hewitt SM, Katz A, Wesley RA, Levine M. Vitamin C pharmacokinetics: implications for oral and intravenous use. Ann Intern Med. 2004 Apr 6;140(7):533-7. doi: 10.7326/0003-4819-140-7-200404060-00010. PMID: 15068981.

Peng Y, Ao M, Dong B, Jiang Y, Yu L, Chen Z, Hu C, Xu R. Anti-Inflammatory Effects of Curcumin in the Inflammatory Diseases: Status, Limitations and Countermeasures. Drug Des Devel Ther. 2021 Nov 2;15:4503-4525. doi: 10.2147/DDDT.S327378. PMID: 34754179; PMCID: PMC8572027.

Polyak SJ, Morishima C, Lohmann V, Pal S, Lee DY, Liu Y, Graf TN, Oberlies NH. Identification of hepatoprotective flavonolignans from silymarin. Proc Natl Acad Sci U S A. 2010 Mar 30;107(13):5995-9. doi: 10.1073/pnas.0914009107. Epub 2010 Mar 15. PMID: 20231449; PMCID: PMC2851903.

Prasad AS. Zinc in human health: effect of zinc on immune cells. Mol Med. 2008 May-Jun;14(5-6):353-7. doi: 10.2119/2008-00033.Prasad. PMID: 18385818; PMCID: PMC2277319.

Prasad KN, Cole WC, Kumar B, Che Prasad K. Pros and cons of antioxidant use during radiation therapy. Cancer Treat Rev. 2002 Apr;28(2):79-91. doi: 10.1053/ctrv.2002.0260. PMID: 12297116.

Rombolà L, Scuteri D, Marilisa S, Watanabe C, Morrone LA, Bagetta G, Corasaniti MT. Pharmacokinetic Interactions between Herbal Medicines and Drugs: Their Mechanisms and Clinical Relevance. Life (Basel). 2020 Jul 4;10(7):106. doi: 10.3390/life10070106. PMID: 32635538; PMCID: PMC7400069.

Ronis MJJ, Pedersen KB, Watt J. Adverse Effects of Nutraceuticals and Dietary Supplements. Annu Rev Pharmacol Toxicol. 2018 Jan 6;58:583-601. doi: 10.1146/annurev-pharmtox-010617-052844. Epub 2017 Oct 6. PMID: 28992429; PMCID: PMC6380172.

Sharifi-Rad J, Rayess YE, Rizk AA, Sadaka C, Zgheib R, Zam W, Sestito S, Rapposelli S, Neffe-Skocińska K, Zielińska D, Salehi B, Setzer WN, Dosoky NS, Taheri Y, El Beyrouthy M, Martorell M, Ostrander EA, Suleria HAR, Cho WC, Maroyi A, Martins N. Turmeric and Its Major Compound Curcumin on Health: Bioactive Effects and Safety Profiles for Food, Pharmaceutical, Biotechnological and Medicinal Applications. Front Pharmacol. 2020 Sep 15;11:01021. doi: 10.3389/fphar.2020.01021. PMID: 33041781; PMCID: PMC7522354.

Singh BN, Shankar S, Srivastava RK. Green tea catechin, epigallocatechin-3-gallate (EGCG): mechanisms, perspectives and clinical applications. Biochem Pharmacol. 2011 Dec 15;82(12):1807-21. doi: 10.1016/j.bcp.2011.07.093. Epub 2011 Jul 30. PMID: 21827739; PMCID: PMC4082721.

Singh K, Bhori M, Kasu YA, Bhat G, Marar T. Antioxidants as precision weapons in war against cancer chemotherapy induced toxicity - Exploring the armoury of obscurity. Saudi Pharm J. 2018 Feb;26(2):177-190. doi: 10.1016/j.jsps.2017.12.013. Epub 2017 Dec 19. PMID: 30166914; PMCID: PMC6111235.

Smith EM, Tangpricha V. Vitamin D and anemia: insights into an emerging association. Curr Opin Endocrinol Diabetes Obes. 2015 Dec;22(6):432-8. doi: 10.1097/MED.0000000000000199. PMID: 26414080; PMCID: PMC4659411.

Stefanache A, Lungu II, Butnariu IA, Calin G, Gutu C, Marcu C, Grierosu C, Bogdan Goroftei ER, Duceac LD, Dabija MG, Popa F, Damir D. Understanding How Minerals Contribute to Optimal Immune Function. J Immunol Res. 2023 Nov 1;2023:3355733. doi: 10.1155/2023/3355733. PMID: 37946846; PMCID: PMC10632063.

Steinbrenner H, Duntas LH, Rayman MP. The role of selenium in type-2 diabetes mellitus and its metabolic comorbidities. Redox Biol. 2022 Apr;50:102236. doi: 10.1016/j.redox.2022.102236. Epub 2022 Jan 24. PMID: 35144052; PMCID: PMC8844812.

Sun J, Kato I. Gut microbiota, inflammation and colorectal cancer. Genes Dis. 2016 Jun;3(2):130-143. doi: 10.1016/j.gendis.2016.03.004. Epub 2016 Apr 13. PMID: 28078319; PMCID: PMC5221561.

Talib WH, Ahmed Jum'AH DA, Attallah ZS, Jallad MS, Al Kury LT, Hadi RW, Mahmod AI. Role of vitamins A, C, D, E in cancer prevention and therapy: therapeutic potentials and mechanisms of action. Front Nutr. 2024 Jan 11;10:1281879. doi: 10.3389/fnut.2023.1281879. PMID: 38274206; PMCID: PMC10808607.

Tank M, Franz K, Cereda E, Norman K. Dietary supplement use in ambulatory cancer patients: a survey on prevalence, motivation and attitudes. J Cancer Res Clin Oncol. 2021 Jul;147(7):1917-1925. doi: 10.1007/s00432-021-03594-7. Epub 2021 Apr 6. PMID: 33825025; PMCID: PMC8164602.

Tinggi U. Selenium: its role as antioxidant in human health. Environ Health Prev Med. 2008 Mar;13(2):102-8. doi: 10.1007/s12199-007-0019-4. Epub 2008 Feb 28. PMID: 19568888; PMCID: PMC2698273.

Wang Z, Li L, Wang S, Wei J, Qu L, Pan L, Xu K. The role of the gut microbiota and probiotics associated with microbial metabolisms in cancer prevention and therapy. Front Pharmacol. 2022 Nov 14;13:1025860. doi: 10.3389/fphar.2022.1025860. PMID: 36452234; PMCID: PMC9702994.

Wierzejska RE. Dietary Supplements-For Whom? The Current State of Knowledge about the Health Effects of Selected Supplement Use. Int J Environ Res Public Health. 2021 Aug 24;18(17):8897. doi: 10.3390/ijerph18178897. PMID: 34501487; PMCID: PMC8431076.

Zuvarox T, Goosenberg E, Belletieri C. Malabsorption Syndromes. [Updated 2025 Jul 7]. In: StatPearls [Internet]. Treasure Island (FL): StatPearls Publishing; 2025 Jan-. Available from: https://www.ncbi.nlm.nih.gov/books/NBK553106/

Chapter 15

Translating Science into Practice: Constructing an Anti-Cancer Diet

Praneeth Juvvi[1], Lokesh Kumar Mishra[2], Sheetanshu Gupta[3*], and Sarfraj Ahmad Siddiqui[4]

[1]Department of Food Processing Technology, College of Food Technology-Central Agricultural University, Imphal, Manipur, India
[2]Department of BPME, College of Agriculture, Central Agricultural University (CAU), Imphal, Manipur, India
[3]Department of Food Safety and Quality Assurance, College of Food Technology, Central Agricultural University (CAU), Imphal, Manipur, India
[4]Department of Biochemistry, King George's Medical University, U.P., India

Abstract

Cutting-edge oncology research gets transmuted into actionable meal plans nowadays remarkably well, fostering cancer prophylaxis and encouraging therapeutic efficacy significantly. Supreme wellness and oncogenic hazard mitigation via dietary means are underscored by crucial scientific tenets furnished in a chapter on nutrition regimens. Initially scrutinizing biological mechanisms where diet impacts cancer occurs, including modulation of inflammation and oxidative stress and aberrant cellular metabolism. Bioactive compounds packed in fruits rich with legumes notoriously alter carcinogenesis processes really profoundly every single time in fairly complex manners. Epidemiological studies reveal dietary patterns somewhat akin to the Mediterranean diet or plant-based eating associated with significantly lower overall cancer risk. Antioxidants and fibre remarkably shield human cells from DNA damage and foster detoxification quite effectively inside cells. Modified nutrition factoring genetic, metabolic and environmental intricacies matters profoundly across diverse real-world contexts fraught with hurdles. Cancer patients and clinicians receive very practical, actionable guidelines that remarkably translate cutting-edge science into dietary practices that improve survivorship.

Keywords: Anti-Cancer Diet, Nutrient-Dense Foods, Cancer Prevention, Dietary Guidelines, Macronutrients & Micronutrients, Evidence-Based Nutrition.

DOI: 10.1201/9781042010387-15

1. Introduction

Research into cancer prevention and dietary habits spans decades garnering growing interest amidst mixed results and varying scrutiny levels. Mounting evidence from epidemiological studies and lab research underscores a potentially pivotal role for nutrition in reducing cancer risk and encourage survival outcomes long term. Translating scientific knowledge into practical dietary advice remains a significantly tricky challenge for individuals adopting it daily. Constructing an anti-cancer diet grounded in science involves adopting practical guidelines and somewhat effective management strategies for cancer prevention daily. Cancer erupts quite haphazardly amidst a morass of lifestyle choices and pretty obscure inherited traits under siege from surrounding pollutants.

Genetic cancer predisposition stubbornly remains unchanged, but quirky dietary habits offer chance for radical intervention mercifully through preventive measures. Dietary patterns linked with lower cancer risk have been identified in numerous studies particularly for breast and prostate cancers in certain populations. What precisely demarcates an anticancer dietary regimen and how can people efficaciously implement it amidst their quotidian existence? Grasping biological mechanisms behind certain foods' significant influence on overall cancer risk is crucial for constructing an effective anti-cancer diet rather carefully. Oxidative stress fosters intricate processes such as inflammation and DNA damage within cells alongside dysregulation of various immune responses.

Diet modulates pathways significantly through various nutrients and obscure bioactive compounds mostly found in rather unusual exotic foods. Fruits and veggies pack antioxidants that help mitigate oxidative stress and quell inflammation which fuels cancer growth pretty rapidly. Whole grains and legumes rich in fibre promote healthy microbiota thereby greatly lowering colorectal cancer risk and improving gut health significantly. Fats from fish and flaxseeds possess markedly anti-inflammatory properties and have been shown somewhat effectively to fight various cancers vigorously. Diets high in saturated fats and trans-fats have been linked recently somewhat ominously to increased risk of breast cancer and colon cancer. Plant-based proteins sourced from legumes or soy products fare better than red or processed meats notoriously linked with heightened risks of colorectal cancer.

Phytochemicals profoundly impact bioactive compounds found in various plants having significant implications for effectively preventing cancer in humans naturally everyday. Compounds like flavonoids carotenoids glucosinolates and polyphenols occur pretty much everywhere naturally in such mixtures. Broccoli and kale alongside certain berries contain copious amounts of cancer-fighting compounds and regular consumption has been loosely tied to reduce oncological risks. Curcumin an active turmeric compound has been rather thoroughly studied extensively for anti-inflammatory properties and various anti-cancer effects. Resveratrol present in red wine and grapes alongside green tea catechins induce apoptosis in cancer cells suppressing tumour growth quite significantly.

Creating a potent diet for beating cancer requires examining broad patterns of eating rather than fixating solely on certain nutrients. Evidence galore suggests diets rich in fruits veggies whole grains nuts seeds and legumes greatly reduce risk of getting cancer quite significantly. Diets rich in such food usually flaunt copious antioxidants and fibre pretty much alongside crucial micronutrients that downregulate inflammatory responses pretty effectively. Mediterranean diet rich in plant-based foods and healthy fats has very consistently been linked with reduced risk of numerous chronic ailments.

Grasping which food fosters wellness isn't enough for concocting anticancer cuisine; rationing food and unconventional prep techniques matter greatly too. Eating huge quantities of processed meats or charred food loaded with carcinogens like heterocyclic amines heightens cancer risk pretty significantly. Steaming and boiling offer relatively healthier options while grilling and frying at scorching temperatures ought to be done moderately pretty often. Portion sizes play a crucial role in maintaining a fairly balanced diet with moderately sized servings pretty obviously. Gobbling ostensibly wholesome nosh can rather swiftly precipitate obesity becoming a risk factor for sundry heinous carcinomas including carcinoma of breast. Nowadays constructing an anti-cancer diet requires rigorously prioritizing cancer prevention alongside needs of individuals undergoing treatment for cancer.

Cancer therapies such as chemotherapy and radiation therapy often precipitate nasty side effects like loss of appetite and gastrointestinal distress significantly impacting nutrition. Nutrition optimization happens concurrently with preservation of substantial muscle mass and minimization of heinous side effects from intense treatment during that timeframe. High-protein calorie-dense foods and nutrient supplementation may be required fairly often ensuring patients maintain rather sufficient nutrition. Seeking modified guidance from a registered dietitian proves crucial in devising eating plans that alleviate harsh effects of cancer therapies vigorously.

Whole foods allegedly pack more punch than sum of parts in a pretty vague notion food synergy stresses heavily. Whole foods provide cancer patients a broad spectrum of beneficial compounds necessary for mitigating oxidative stress rather effectively through varied nutritional pathways. Ultimately recognizing essential aspects of anti-cancer diet isn't a panacea but part of broader regimens for holistic cancer prevention naturally. Regular physical activity alongside effective stress management and sufficient sleep lowers cancer risk by avoiding cigarettes and excessive booze consumption habitually. Blending lifestyle habits with anti-cancer diet yields most optimal results in cancer risk reduction and boosts overall health very markedly nowadays.

Nutrients and wholesome foods naturally enhance efficacy of an anti-cancer diet informed by latest groundbreaking scientific research very effectively nowadays. Cancer-fighting key nutrients and dietary patterns will be examined alongside strategies for folding such evidence quietly into everyday life. Evidence-based recommendations can be adopted readily by individuals and healthcare providers effectively optimizing treatment outcomes and diminishing cancer risk substantially. Decoding a vast trove of scientific data meticulously enables cancer prevention through savvy dietary choices and significant lifestyle tweaks for individuals.

2. The Science Behind an Anti-Cancer Diet: Key Mechanisms and Evidence

Growing scientific attention fixates intensely on diet's role in thwarting cancer as mounting evidence links certain nutrients rapidly to carcinogenic pathway modulation. Focusing on whole foods teeming with fibre and phytochemicals supplants singular prescriptions for cancer prevention while heavily curbing refined sugar intake. Cancer development gets significantly influenced by diet through sundry biological pathways and key evidence backs oncology interventions with fervently debated conclusions abound.

2.1. Modulation of Inflammation and Oxidative Stress

Oxidative stress and chronic low-grade inflammation play crucial roles very rapidly in progression of various cancers quite centrally. Both processes cultivate a pro-tumourigenic milieu by spurring frenetic genetic chaos and epigenetic modulations in tandem with unbridled cell division. Evidence showcases diet's pivotal role in modulating biological pathways by exacerbating inflammation or via various antioxidant mechanisms pretty effectively nowadays. Pro-inflammatory dietary patterns typically involve ridiculously high intakes of saturated fats and refined carbohydrates alongside ultra-processed foods and are linked with massively elevated circulating inflammatory biomarkers including interleukin-6 and C-reactive protein. Diets like these spur generation of reactive oxygen species that induce DNA strand breaks and cause protein oxidation fostering mutagenesis. Oxidative stress merged with chronic inflammation spawns microenvironment teeming quite profusely with angiogenesis and sly immune evasion happens quietly thereafter metastasis occurs.

Mediterranean diet furnishes a plethora of bioactive compounds quite effectively thereby exerting protective effects against inflammation rather unusually. Fruits rich in polyphenols and fibre alongside whole grains legumes and nuts are heavily emphasized in this eating model. Vitamins C and E selenium carotenoids and flavonoids scavenge ROS and significantly boost endogenous defenses like glutathione peroxidase remarkably well naturally. Curcumin in turmeric and resveratrol found in grapes remarkably downregulate NF-κB signaling and suppress cyclooxygenase-2 expression showing very potent anti-inflammatory effects. Such diets play protective roles in preventing various cancers effectively nowadays backed by thorough epidemiological and clinical studies. Higher adherence to anti-inflammatory dietary indices strongly correlates with markedly reduced risk of various malignancies, particularly colorectal, breast and prostate cancers.

Diets rich in anti-inflammatory components significantly lower oxidative stress biomarkers and systemic inflammatory markers in prospective cohort studies and randomized controlled trials suggesting mediation of cancer risk reduction through various mechanisms potentially. Modulation of inflammation through dietary changes and mitigation of oxidative stress represents a fairly effective adjunct cancer prevention strategy. Focusing on whole-food heavy diets packed with plants provides an easily available non-surgical method to mitigate biological factors driving cancer growth remarkably well.

2.2. Hormonal Regulation and Endocrine Modulation

Endogenous hormonal activity involving estrogens and androgens influences breast prostate and endometrial cancers significantly through insulin-related pathways. Emerging research suggests diet heavily influences cancer risk and progression through various hormonal mechanisms modulating endocrine function thereby playing a significant role. Estrogen metabolism plays quite a crucial role in hormone-receptor-positive cancers. Insoluble fibre heavily binds estrogens in gastrointestinal tract fostering excretion and fairly quickly boosting elimination of them. This process significantly hampers estrogen reabsorption via enterohepatic circulation resulting in markedly lower systemic levels. Postmenopausal women experience peripheral aromatization mainly in adipose tissue which becomes a primary source of estrogen there subsequently.

Estrogen modulation aside various convoluted pathways involving insulin and insulin-like growth factor 1 IGF-1 are heavily implicated in cancer development rapidly. Diets rich in refined carbs rapidly elevate insulin levels and stimulate hepatic production of IGF-1 a potent mitogen that furthers cellular proliferation vigorously. Elevated IGF-1 levels chronically correlate pretty strongly with heightened risks of various nasty cancers namely breast prostate and very aggressive colorectal cancer. Whole grain diets with legumes and veggies having scant added sugars improve insulin sensitivity and curtail IGF-1 potentially diminishing mitogenic signaling within pre-neoplastic cells. Soy isoflavones like genistein and daidzein are phytoestrogens derived from plants structurally similar apparently to mammalian estradiol. Compounds bind estrogen receptors quite variably exerting estrogenic effects in some tissues but anti-estrogenic effects in others involving different receptor subtypes.

Endogenous hormone levels fluctuate curiously alongside expression of ERβ in a rather intricate manner sometimes. Soy isoflavones pretty vigorously act as estrogen receptor modulators in ER-positive breast cancer competing with endogenous estrogens and somewhat attenuating proliferative effects. Observational studies hint soy has protective effects mainly when consumed quite early in life yet concerns about usage during active cancer treatment linger necessitating guidance extremely tailored closely to individual needs.

High-fibre diets correlate with reduced risk of hormone-related cancers surprisingly whereas plant-based eating patterns yield beneficial outcomes slowly over time. Populations stubbornly clinging to traditional Asian diets rich in phytoestrogens exhibit remarkably pronounced associations with very low intake of processed sugars. Modulation of hormonal pathways through diet offers a promising avenue for preventing and adjunctively managing malignancies related to endocrine function emphasizing nutrition's importance in precision cancer care.

2.3. Gut Microbiome Interactions

Trillions of microorganisms reside in the gut microbiome within gastrointestinal tract and play a pivotal role regulating host metabolism vigorously. Diet profoundly influences microbial composition and activity within various bodily ecosystems like gut flora in a remarkably nuanced manner. Microbial communities profoundly impact cancer development nowadays and influence progression and therapeutic outcomes significantly under various circumstances. Beneficial gut microbes such as Bifidobacterium species and Lactobacillus flourish remarkably with prebiotic dietary components inherent in veggies and whole grains. Microbes ferment dietary fibre rapidly into short-chain fatty acids like butyrate and some acetate with propionate forming in gut.

Butyrate has demonstrated potent anti-inflammatory effects pretty significantly in various murine models and exhibits anti-tumourigenic properties rather effectively elsewhere. It serves as key energy source for colonocytes and promotes epithelial barrier integrity while inhibiting histone deacetylases thereby regulating gene expression suppressing tumour-promoting pathways very effectively. SCFAs modulate immune responses irregularly by influencing T-regulatory cells pretty significantly and reducing production of pro-inflammatory cytokines fairly dramatically. Diets heavily influenced by Western patterns replete with loads of saturated fat and copious red meat correlate with markedly diminished gut microbial diversity. Elevated production of noxious metabolites such as deoxycholic acid occurs in dysbiotic state heavily implicated in colorectal carcinogenesis through DNA damage oxidatively.

Evidence mounts that microbiome plays a huge role variably shaping responses to diverse cancer treatments especially certain immune checkpoint inhibitors pretty significantly nowadays. Distinct microbial patterns correlate with enhanced immunotherapy outcomes while gut dysbiosis intricately links with resistance and treatment related heightened toxicity. Modulation of diet via prebiotics alongside probiotics offers a promisingly efficacious strategy for minimizing nasty side effects pretty effectively overall. Early-phase clinical trials suggest microbiome-targeted interventions like dietary changes and fecal microbiota transplantation remarkably potentiate treatment outcomes by beneficially restoring balance. Pretty thorough large-scale studies must be conducted rigorously establishing causal relationships and formulating standardized dietary guidelines for oncology patients effectively now. Gut microbiome serves as pivotal nexus between dietary patterns and oncogenic processes while manipulation through modified nutritional regimens unlocks novel vistas in oncology therapeutics.

2.4. Regulation of Cell Proliferation and Apoptosis

Tissue homeostasis entails a delicate balance between cell proliferation and apoptosis which often goes awry in various cancers manifesting quite frequently. Bioactive dietary compounds influence critical cellular processes directly with efficacy under various physiological conditions very evidently in many cases. Compounds modulate signaling pathways inside cells fairly effectively and inhibit tumour growth while sensitizing malignant cells quite rapidly to conventional therapies. Broccoli, kale and cauliflower contain glucosinolates hydrolyzed by myrosinase enzymes pretty readily into sulforaphane and various other isothiocyanates. Sulforaphane has demonstrated potent anticancer activity in various preclinical models by triggering mitochondrial-mediated apoptosis and inducing phase II detoxification enzymes. Key regulators like cyclins and cyclin-dependent kinases are modulated thereby suppressing proliferation quite sloppily under some pretty unusual conditions effectively.

Lycopene a carotenoid found predominantly in tomatoes and watermelon has been linked with somewhat surprisingly reduced risk of prostate cancer. Lycopene hinders insulin-like growth factor-1 signaling somewhat in vitro and messes with cell cycle progression suppressing cell proliferation pretty effectively. Antioxidant properties effectively reduce DNA damage in various neoplastic tissue types and oxidative stress gets significantly alleviated. Phytochemicals such as curcumin present in turmeric and resveratrol abundant in grapes berries and peanuts reportedly exhibit significant anticancer properties. These compounds target multiple signaling cascades including NF-κB and Wnt/β-catenin pathways exerting multifaceted effects pretty effectively in various ways. Curcumin hinders pro-inflammatory transcription factors vigorously and promotes activation of caspase leading ultimately to cell death programmed rather abnormally.

Resveratrol has been shown to inhibit angiogenesis and reduce metastatic potential in various cancer cells inducing senescence pretty effectively meanwhile. Preclinical studies yield evidence that early-phase clinical trials validate suggesting certain dietary compounds act as chemosensitizers enhancing efficacy of standard anticancer therapies greatly. Wonky pharmacokinetics and poor bioavailability severely curtail their application in clinical oncology under erratic dosing schedules pretty much everywhere. Bioactives derived from diet offer a promising adjunctive approach regulating cancer cell dynamics somewhat irregularly in various cellular milieus very effectively. Leveraging their efficacy in cancer treatment regimens fully necessitates further probing of formulation methods and synergistic pairings with existing therapies.

2.5. Caloric Intake, Obesity, and Energy Balance

Obesity stays glaringly culpable in development of cancers like postmenopausal breast cancer and colorectal cancer rather quickly underlying several issues. Excess adiposity drastically upsets metabolic homeostasis and hormonal balance thereby fostering quite profoundly a microenvironment extremely conducive to tumourigenesis. Biological mechanisms underlying obesity-cancer link are multifactorial featuring chronic inflammation and insulin resistance with elevated insulin-like growth factor-1 altering sex hormone metabolic pathways. Adipose tissue secretes adipokines like leptin and pro-inflammatory cytokines such as tumour necrosis factor-alpha acting pretty much as an endocrine organ. Molecules promote systemic inflammation pretty much everywhere and enhance oxidative stress rather significantly contributing to immune dysfunction under sundry pathological conditions.

Obesity induces insulin resistance spuriously leading hyperinsulinemia and elevated IGF-1 a growth factor with ostensibly anti-apoptotic mitogenic properties in various cell types. Elevated insulin and IGF-1 levels have been linked aggressively to cancer cell proliferation and survival in various tumour types quite heavily. Postmenopausal women accumulate excess adipose tissue which becomes a key site of aromatization surreptitiously converting androgens into estrogens thereby markedly boosting estrogen levels and stimulating growth of breast cancer tumours. Drastic total energy reduction and certain dietary patterns fostering energy balance have shown promise in mitigating risk of developing various cancers. Nutrient-dense low-glycemic diets facilitate intentional weight loss which significantly lowers insulin levels and various inflammatory biomarkers pretty effectively.

Mortality risk appears significantly lowered among breast and endometrial cancer survivors largely after interventions of such a nature are undertaken. Slowly emerging research substantiates a potential role for intermittent fasting in improving metabolic health and tumour growth reduction occurs gradually in various animal models. Suitable caloric intake and frequent physical activity apparently play a crucial role in preventing cancer and boosting survivorship remarkably. Tackling obesity with subtle dietary adjustments represents a vital aspect of cancer risk reduction strategies and protracted disease management effectively nowadays.

2.6. Dietary Patterns with Anti-Cancer Potential

Dietary patterns offer more meaningful insight into cancer prevention nowadays rather than isolated nutrients or specific foods surprisingly. Interactions between dietary components and genetic individuality intricately suggest holistic nutrition may profoundly impact cancer pathways in surprisingly sustainable ways. A diet rich in fruits vegetables whole grains legumes nuts and olive oil typical of Mediterranean regions has been frequently linked with lower cancer mortality rates. This dietary pattern favorably modulates gut microbiome through anti-inflammatory action and antioxidant defense via multiple mechanisms quite effectively. Meta-analyses and epidemiological studies have extensively linked adherence Mediterranean diet with lowered risk of various cancers including prostate cancer and gastric cancer. Mostly plant-forward omnivorous diets and vegan eating patterns show considerable promise in lowering risks of certain hormone-sensitive cancers and gastrointestinal malignancies.

Diets rich in polyphenols and vitamins tend to be fairly low in saturated fats and heme iron yielding some pretty significant protective benefits subsequently. Fibre intake enhances estrogen excretion and fosters production of short-chain fatty acids by gut microbes whereas polyphenols like flavonoids mitigate oxidative stress greatly. Extremely high fat intake and drastically low carb consumption in a ketogenic diet has sparked interest among oncology researchers studying glioblastoma multiforme lately. Diet exploits Warburg effect by restricting glucose and boosting ketone body production wherein cancer cells hungrily utilizes glycolysis for energy. Preclinical data show considerable promise and small clinical trials indicate potential efficacy but long-term safety necessitates rigorous further investigation very evidently.

An effective anti-cancer diet operates through deeply intertwined mechanisms slowly reducing inflammation extremely inside cells and modulating hormone levels weirdly. Whole foods confer cumulative protective benefits via weirdly synergistic interactions rather than depending on some lone nutrient or cancer-curing food. Precision oncology will rapidly advance with dietary interventions tailored to individual cancer risk and survivorship needs via genomic profiles.

3. Identifying Cancer-Fighting Foods

Cancer biology research evolves rapidly nowadays and dietary choices significantly influence cancer prevention effectively through various intricate mechanisms. Profoundly protective effects against cancer progression stages can be exerted by nutrient-dense whole foods rich in vitamins minerals antioxidants fibre and phytochemicals. Cancer-fighting foods supposedly work through a multitude of convoluted biological pathways and obscure downstream mechanisms very intricately. Many compounds modulating inflammation exist in various substances and inflammation significantly contributes to carcinogenesis in rather complex ways. Others neutralize reactive oxygen species rapidly over time thereby reducing mutation rates and preventing oxidative DNA damage fairly effectively.

Certain compounds augment bodily detox pathways by upregulating hepatic enzymes whereas others foster equilibrium of hormonal fluctuations pivotal in malignancies sensitive to hormonal influences such as breast and prostate cancer. Certain foods sway gut microbiome considerably and foster immune surveillance or thwart processes crucial for tumour survival like metastasis or angiogenesis rapidly. Bioactive compounds such as flavonoids lignans glucosinolates and carotenoids alongside omega-3 fatty acids are behind numerous health benefits remarkably. Thorough examination of foods linked mostly with reduced cancer risk and improved treatment outcomes occur in this chapter for a better grasp.

Preclinical studies alongside epidemiological data and clinical trials remarkably underscore potential roles of active constituents in adjunctive therapy and cancer prevention. Rather exotically foods encompass cruciferous veggies alongside tomatoes and whole grains fatty fish green tea legumes berries various nuts and turmeric. Chapter underscores dietary impact being optimally understood within contexts of overall eating habits lifestyle factors and unique patient requirements. Evidence-based choices complement conventional cancer therapies quite effectively and foster long-term resilience rather than relying on so-called miracle foods. Science-backed nutrition strategies effectively empower patient caregivers and healthcare pros with practical knowledge on crafting a diet protective against cancer.

3.1. Cruciferous Vegetables: Sulforaphane and Detoxification

Cruciferous veggies like cabbage cauliflower and Brussels sprouts are studied alongside broccoli and kale pretty extensively for their cancer-protective properties. Glucosinolates abound in them getting converted fairly rapidly into sulforaphane and indole-3-carbinol during human gut digestion with biological activity. Sulforaphane pretty effectively triggers chemopreventive effects in various cancer models like breast prostate and some pretty rare colorectal ones. It rapidly induces phase II detoxifying enzymes. Apoptosis undergoes significant promotion anomalously within various cancerous cell types. It ordinarily heavily suppresses tumour growth and angiogenesis. Gentle heat applications like steaming help retain beneficial compounds in foods fairly effectively most of time apparently.

3.2. Berries: Antioxidants and Anti-Inflammatory Phytochemicals

Raspberries blackberries and cranberries pack anthocyanins ellagic acid and flavonoids in nutrient-dense packages remarkably bursting with goodness overflowing slowly everywhere. Studies have linked eating berries somewhat rigorously to a reduced risk of various cancers including esophageal breast and colorectal cancer. Antioxidant action pretty effectively counteracts rogue free radicals in bodily systems. Proliferation of cancer cells gets heavily inhibited alongside their invasive tendencies. Chronic inflammation associated with tumourigenesis gets reduced fairly quietly by some mechanism or other greatly over time . Certain research indicates lowered risk of developing cancer quite markedly sometimes. They make quite a savvy decision keeping blood sugar levels in check largely owing to inherently low glycemic load and remarkably stable insulin levels.

3.3. Leafy Greens: Folate and DNA Repair

Arugula mustard greens kale and spinach are consistently recommended nationwide in various dietary patterns that help prevent cancer. Rich sources of folate and vitamin B9 and carotenoids abound with chlorophyll fibre various phytochemicals contributing largely rather significantly to protective effects. Leafy greens exert key anticancer effects mainly through exceptionally high folate content a B vitamin crucial for DNA synthesis and subsequent repair. Folate status sufficiently robust enhances genome integrity by facilitating proper nucleotide synthesis and thwarting uracil misincorporation into DNA thereby triggering fewer chromosomal breaks. Heightened risk of various cancers including notably colorectal and pancreatic cancer correlates strongly with low dietary intake of folate. Folate plays a vital role in cancer prevention and mitigates tumour progression by maintaining genomic stability rather effectively through various biochemical pathways.

Leafy greens furnish chlorophyll a verdant plant pigment harbouring ostensibly significant anticancer properties nestled deep inside sundry bodily systems remarkably. Chlorophyll exerts a possibly chemoprotective effect by binding dietary carcinogens like heterocyclic amines formed during high temperature meat cooking reducing bioavailability and mutagenic potential quite substantially in colon. Leafy greens profoundly affect estrogen metabolism becoming particularly pertinent for cancers sensitive hormonal fluctuations like breast cancer and endometrial cancer occurs frequently nowadays. Arugula and mustard greens being cruciferous leafy greens promote production of protective estrogen metabolites supporting liver detoxification pathways quite effectively facilitating excretion of excess hormones.

Leafy greens abound with dietary fibre that robustly supports gut health and microbiome diversity producing short-chain fatty acids like butyrate having potent anti-inflammatory properties. Regular consumption of diverse leafy greens naturally boosts intake of protective phytochemicals found abundantly in emerald veggies enhancing dietary diversity overall. Vegetables get devoured raw or get steamed eerily into oblivion and are mashed into cancer-fighting smoothies making them super versatile dietary staples. Leafy greens provide surprisingly potent mix of various nutrients and assorted bioactives supporting DNA integrity detoxification processes and hormonal equilibrium remarkably effectively.

3.4. Tomatoes: Lycopene and Hormone Modulation

Tomatoes are crucial fruit eaten extensively in many cancer-protective diets rich in protective nutrients found in Mediterranean dietary patterns. Rich lycopene content has been studied pretty extensively lately for anticancer properties especially in research on prostate cancer. Lycopene exhibits intense antioxidant activity and its protective effects reverberate extensively beyond simply neutralizing rogue free radicals in diverse physiological milieus. Lycopene crucially inhibits signaling of insulin-like growth factor-1 effectively in cancer prevention by thwarting IGF-1 rather remarkably. Elevated IGF-1 levels are associated with heightened risks of various cancers including prostate cancer breast cancer and colorectal cancer quite often. Lycopene downregulates IGF-1 receptor expression significantly, interfering with downstream pathways, such as PI3K/Akt and mTOR suppressing tumour cell proliferation markedly enhancing apoptosis.

Tomatoes may influence sex hormone metabolism rather significantly in hormone-sensitive cancers obviously under certain fluctuations. Lycopene apparently reduces 5-alpha reductase activity thereby hindering conversion of testosterone into dihydrotestosterone a potent form fueling prostate tumour growth significantly. Lycopene possibly tweaks estrogen metabolism by messing with cytochrome P450 enzymes and boosting excretion of nasty estrogen metabolites. Tomatoes harbor a diverse assortment of bioactive compounds including vitamin C beta-carotene flavonoids and chlorogenic acid that pretty effectively enhance antioxidant defenses. Specific enzymes somewhat effectively facilitate neutralization and excretion of carcinogenic compounds during human liver detoxification phase II.

Lycopene bioavailability ramps up quite rapidly upon consumption of cooked tomatoes with olive oil and various health-promoting fatty substances. Heating breaks down plant cell matrix rather effectively thus facilitating absorption of lycopene in intestine pretty quickly. Sauces and pastes made from tomatoes are rich sources of lycopene a compound that protects abundantly in foods like these. Tomatoes ostensibly confer cancer prevention benefits by heavily modulating some hormonal pathways and robustly supporting various bodily detoxification processes in mysterious ways. Consuming cooked tomatoes with unsaturated fats pretty effectively boosts cancer protection in diets backed by considerable evidence.

3.5. Garlic and Allium Vegetables: Sulfur Compounds and Immune Support

Garlic and onions and leeks shallots chives have been used for centuries in traditional folk medicine and modern research increasingly supports their role in cancer prevention. Vegetables contain organosulfur compounds such as allicin and diallyl disulfide responsible for pungent aroma and myriad biological effects. Tumour cells exposed to compounds possessing anticancer properties undergo cell cycle arrest and apoptosis relatively frequently under such conditions. Allicin tweaks multiple signaling pathways deeply involved in cell survival and eradication of cancerous cells happens through p53 cascades subsequently. Compounds vigorously suppress tumour growth in several preclinical cancer models and inhibit angiogenesis simultaneously in various experimental settings effectively.

Allium veggies pretty significantly enhance immune response by egging on activity vigorously of natural killer cells and macrophages and various lymphocytes. Tumour initiation gets thwarted by enhanced immune surveillance especially in primordial carcinogenesis stages serving as rather critical defense mechanism basically. Garlic and allied vegetables remarkably possess capacity for inhibiting various carcinogens effectively within human bodies pretty substantially under certain conditions. Organosulfur compounds markedly suppress activity of some cytochrome P450 enzymes involved in metabolic activation of various procarcinogens and induce phase II detoxification enzymes such as glutathione S-transferases pretty effectively. Dual action significantly enhance bodily capacity for neutralizing carcinogenic substances thereby preventing rapid DNA damage inside cells naturally over time.

Epidemiological studies pretty convincingly back up a protective role of allium veggies in some populations generally. Greater consumption of specific nutrients correlates with diminished cancer risk especially in cohorts consuming largely traditional diets replete with such edibles. Observational and mechanistic evidence strongly underscores potential remarkably despite presently limited data being available from randomized clinical trials. Garlic's bioactivity gets unlocked pretty maximally through various prep methods and its potency varies accordingly with each technique used. Chopping garlic rapidly activates enzyme alliinase that converts alliin into allicin quickly within cells or crushing it does pretty much same thing. Sitting chopped garlic for 5-10 minutes before cooking retains bioactive sulfur compounds that heat degrades pretty quickly and very partially.

Allium veggies furnish broadly sweeping anticancer benefits largely via pro-apoptotic properties and somewhat enigmatic immune enhancement alongside detoxifying machinations. Incorporating them into diet regularly reduces cancer risk somewhat effectively over time with an evidence-informed strategy pretty obviously.

3.6. Whole Grains and Legumes: Fibre and Gut Microbiota Health

Diets rich in whole grains such as oats and brown rice and legumes like lentils and chickpeas often form cancer-protective regimens very effectively. Foods rich in micronutrients such as B vitamins magnesium and various phytochemicals naturally harbor copious amounts of dietary fibre. Beneficial effects manifest largely via interactions with gut microbiota and metabolic regulation occurs alongside haphazard modulation of sundry hormonal pathways. Whole grains and legumes remarkably boost gut microbiota diversity daily through certain primary anticancer mechanisms somewhat effectively. Fermentable fibres and resistant starches in food serve as prebiotics stimulating growth of beneficial bacteria such as Bifidobacterium or Lactobacillus quite effectively underground.

Microbes ferment inside colon producing short-chain fatty acids particularly butyrate and simultaneously forming some acetate and propionate. Butyrate has shown considerable promise amongst SCFAs for exerting remarkably anti-inflammatory effects on colonic epithelial cells very effectively indeed. Butyrate thoroughly enhances gut barrier function and somewhat effectively modulates various immune responses while downregulating inflammatory pathways like NF-κB. It serves as energy source for colonocytes and plays crucial role in maintaining epithelial integrity vital for prevention of colorectal carcinoma development. High-fibre diets quite profoundly impact sundry hormonal processes and metabolic pathways fairly significantly within humans and various other creatures.

Fibre binds bile acids and estrogens quite effectively in gut thereby promoting excretion and subsequently lowering estrogen levels significantly reducing risk of cancers like breast cancer. Fibre-rich foods remarkably enhance insulin sensitivity and mitigate risk of metabolically driven cancers like pancreatic cancer through stable insulin levels. Diets rich in whole grains and legumes strongly correlate with lowered colorectal cancer risk and overall markedly improved metabolic health indicators. Foods like these pretty effectively fuel satiety and lower systemic inflammation thereby reducing risk of cancer and favourably encourage outcomes of treatment. Whole grains and legumes offer synergistic benefits via gut microbiome modulation hormonal regulation and anti-inflammatory signaling in cancer-fighting dietary regimens.

3.7. Fatty Fish and Omega-3-Rich Foods: Inflammation Control

Fatty fish dwelling in frigid waters like salmon harbor copious long-chain omega-3 polyunsaturated fatty acids specifically EPA and DHA abundantly. Essential fats exhibit profoundly anti-inflammatory properties and immunomodulatory effects with potential roles in cancer prevention nowadays as adjunctive therapy extensively. Omega-3 fatty acids exert potent anticancer effects largely by suppressing synthesis of pro-inflammatory eicosanoids specifically prostaglandin E2 from arachidonic acid. EPA competes with arachidonic acid for enzymatic conversion rapidly yielding production of somewhat less inflammatory prostaglandins and leukotrienes of various kinds. Shift in lipid mediator profile curtails chronic inflammation that heavily fuels carcinogenesis through complex biochemical pathways involving various mechanisms.

Omega-3 fatty acids vigorously modulate immune function by enhancing cytotoxic T cell activity and promote resolution of inflammation swiftly through resolvins. Effects may enhance immune surveillance quite vigorously and undermine tumour microenvironment that supports cancer cell survival and subsequent metastasis very effectively. Preclinical models yield emerging evidence suggesting EPA and DHA rather effectively sensitize tumour cells to chemotherapy by altering cell membrane fluidity. Omega-3s reduce tumour proliferation fairly effectively in various cancer types and angiogenesis gets suppressed rather convincingly by them. Omega-3 intake has been tentatively linked inversely to risk of various cancers namely breast and lung cancer in some epidemiological studies albeit with wildly differing results across populations and at different doses. Benefits appear remarkably pronounced when omega-3 intake is balanced against relatively low omega-6 consumption often abnormally high in Western diets.

Flaxseeds chia seeds walnuts and hemp seeds are sources rich in alpha-linolenic acid a precursor crucial for many bodily functions normally. Conversion of ALA into EPA and DHA happens glacially slow in humans so vegetarians or vegans might prudently supplement with algae-based DHA. Foods rich in omega-3 offer robust anti-inflammatory benefits encourage immunological responses that potentially lower cancer risk and amplify therapeutic outcomes significantly.

3.8. Green Tea: Polyphenols and Angiogenesis Inhibition

Green tea Camellia sinensis remains extensively studied for being rich source of polyphenols particularly catechins with highly potent antioxidant properties. Epigallocatechin-3-gallate or EGCG has garnered considerable attention recently owing largely to its anticancer properties in numerous studies. EGCG exerts multifaceted anticancer effects rather haphazardly by modulating cell proliferation apoptosis and metastasis through various cellular processes somewhat irregularly. Tumour angiogenesis inhibition occurs fairly frequently namely formation of new blood vessels supplying nutrients and oxygen for growing tumours. EGCG brutally starves tumours of vascular support by downregulating pro-angiogenic factors like vascular endothelial growth factor and its receptor signaling pathways.

EGCG suppresses matrix metalloproteinases quite vigorously thus impeding tumour invasion and metastasis occurs less frequently in extracellular matrix degradation contexts. It messes with various cancer-promoting signaling routes such as PI3K/Akt and Wnt/β-catenin and NF-κB vital for survival of cancer cells or tumour progression. EGCG's capacity for modulating immune checkpoints like PD-L1 enhances recognition of cancer cells by immune system fairly significantly pretty much. Green tea polyphenols probably assist immunotherapy largely due to somewhat profound immunomodulatory effects gradually unfolding in humans still. Green tea consumption fairly regularly correlates pretty strongly with lowered risks of certain cancer types predominantly in East Asian demographics.

Preclinical models yield consistent findings and enhance biological plausibility supporting a protective role despite evidence from randomized controlled trials being rather scanty. Generally people prefer brewed green tea over high-dose green tea extracts or supplements very importantly for various unclear reasons. High doses of catechin in some formulations recklessly cause liver damage especially when taken alongside other meds without eating food beforehand. Whole tea matrix affords fairly balanced polyphenol intake naturally without undue risk of excessive exposure under normal consumption patterns. Green tea serves as exemplar of dietary phytochemicals vigorously influencing hallmarks of cancer development in a rather natural way. Incorporating it into a nutrient rich diet comprising mostly plants can be fairly safe for effectively reducing overall cancer risk.

3.9. Mushrooms: Immune Regulation and Tumour Suppression

Shiitake mushrooms and reishi have been used extensively in traditional medicine owing profoundly immune-enhancing properties of beta-glucans naturally. Mushroom extracts show considerable promise as adjuvant therapies in gastrointestinal and breast cancers but desperately more human trials are needed. Key benefits include vigorous stimulation of natural killer cells and activation of T-cells effectively. Tumour growth appears markedly suppressed in various preclinical models under intense scrutiny lately. Chemotherapy-related immune response gets significantly enhanced rather dramatically inside tumour tissues after administration of novel therapeutic agents obviously. Whole grains legumes fruits and vegetables along with healthy fats and certain animal-based foods significantly influence prevention of cancer remarkably.

Cancer-fighting foods contribute quite distinctly via phytochemicals and antioxidants alongside various other highly synergistic nutrients obviously in many ways. Focusing on whole foods rather than isolated compounds remarkably boosts effectiveness and fosters safety in most dietary interventions. Ongoing studies nowadays refine understanding of food synergy fairly effectively guiding development of pretty personalized dietary regimens in cancer research.

4. From Bench to Plate: Bridging Research and Real-World Dietary Practices

Recently a plethora of experimental epidemiological and clinical research has shed light on intricate links between cancer biology and dietary habits. Investigations into bioactive nutrients and gut microbiota interactions have established diet quite firmly as crucial component of cancer prevention strategies lately. Rigorous research mostly gained insights slowly and largely aimed at reducing incidence of cancer thereby emerging with evidence-based dietary recommendations. Scientific findings make a pretty rough transition from lab benches into real-world dietary habits around people's plates rather unevenly. Laboratory discoveries frequently occur stealthily beneath sterile conditions using purified compounds or model organisms that crudely simulate human dietary habits.

Clinical trials frequently suffer glaring shortcomings namely woefully short durations and sample sizes remain lamentably small among participants with poor diversity. Implementing research-based nutritional strategies daily in life requires considerable persistence and dedication overcoming several barriers effectively with great effort. Misinformation about diet and cancer persists glaringly amidst stark disparities in food availability and unaffordable healthy eating options for many. Dietary advice must contend vigorously with stubborn deeply ingrained habits and obscure cultural predilections strongly tied to quirky emotional factors surrounding sustenance. Multidisciplinary approaches are vigorously employed nowadays in many fields necessitating bridging sizable gaps between research endeavors and practical applications.

Scientists must work intimately alongside registered dietitians and community leaders nowadays translating findings into fairly actionable guidelines. They must be carefully tailored for diverse populations and pretty sensitive in various local contexts simultaneously. Policymakers quietly play a crucial role in crafting environments through regulations on food labels that foster rather healthy food and agricultural subsidies. Education fosters self-efficacy quite effectively and behavior change happens pretty significantly through empowerment of individuals with health literacy. Daily habits grounded in science remarkably enhance cancer prevention efforts yielding substantial benefits for overall life quality and health. Bench plate pathways unfurl dynamically amidst painstaking iteration within collaborative endeavours rather than along somewhat linear trajectories. Cancer nutrition science succeeds not just through groundbreaking discovery but by being translated into practical equitable eating patterns sustainably for all people.

4.1. The Evidence: Practice Disconnect

Population-level adherence stays remarkably low despite loads of research pretty strongly linking dietary choices with elevated cancer risk nowadays. Multiple factors fuel this chasm partly because scientific findings are often riddled with nuance or contradictory data thus fanning bewilderment among people over soy consumption issues. Promising research findings often get stuck in limbo for years before being reflected in clinical guidelines or public health campaigns. Limited personalization: Many dietary recommendations are generalized, overlooking genetic, cultural, socioeconomic, and behavioral differences that influence food choices. Many dietary recommendations are woefully generalized overlooking crucial differences in genetic makeup cultural background socioeconomic status and deeply ingrained behavioral patterns.

4.2. Translational Nutrition: Turning Mechanisms into Meals

Translational nutrition converts basic research findings into practical edibles via surprisingly tangible food-based recommendations for downright everyday munching. Research on fibre's benefits in modulating gut microbiome spurs recommendations favouring whole grains and legumes pretty strongly nowadays apparently. Gentle steaming of cruciferous veggies retains glucosinolates and studies highlighting sulforaphane's anti-cancer properties in broccoli sprouts prompt some eating adjustments rapidly. Findings on intermittent fasting and caloric restriction mimetics have spurred interest in time-restricted eating protocols tailored for oncology settings. Research on intermittent fasting and caloric restriction mimetics has sparked curiosity about time-restricted eating regimens specifically designed for cancer treatment environments lately.

4.3. Culinary Literacy and Patient Empowerment

Scientific knowledge matters greatly only when it seeps down slowly into lives of people it purports to benefit profoundly. Culinary literacy pretty effectively supports health goals these days in a rather practical and nourishing manner for people generally. Hands-on cooking initiatives paired with nutrition education quite demonstrably boost adherence to diets that help stave off various cancers. Oncology-focused culinary medicine initiatives sprouting at diverse cancer centers furnish survivors with culturally sensitive meal planning guidance rooted in recent nutrition studies. Such programs drastically ramp up consumption of fruits and whole grains while encourage patient confidence making sweeping changes.

4.4. Addressing Social Determinants of Health and Dietary Inequity

Dietary behavior gets shaped heavily by economic factors and various obscure social influences not just knowledge simultaneously under certain conditions. Vulnerable demographics frequently encounter cancer-fighting food like fresh-picked berries or ocean-harvested fish woefully out of reach and obnoxiously pricey. Equitable research translation relies heavily on community-based interventions that utilize local ingredients and traditional cooking methods pretty effectively. Partnerships with food banks and clinics provide nutrient-rich foods at subsidized rates for needy populations. Policy initiatives can drastically cut costs and substantially boost availability of whole foods remarkably across various regions nationwide. Cancer-protective nutrition becomes widely accessible through structural support systems addressing scientific and social hurdles in bridging research and practice.

4.5. The Role of Digital Health and Technology

Technology bridges complex dietary science and modified guidance very effectively nowadays for people with sufficiently keen interest in nutrition nowadays. Nowadays super healthy anti-inflammatory recipes are suggested very frequently by mobile apps obsessively tracking daily nutrient intake. AI-driven platforms recommend meals mainly based on tumour type or genetic markers and gut microbiome profiles. Tele-nutrition services expand access pretty quickly to oncology dietitians mostly in pretty rural areas or ones that are grossly underserved.

4.6. Training and Collaboration across Disciplines

Translating nutrition science into practice effectively requires collaboration across sectors among researcher, clinicians, public health experts and diverse food professionals. Clinicians and dietitians need training in latest evidence on bioactive compounds and cancer metabolism from various experts. Researchers should incorporate behavioral science and implementation frameworks into their work to ensure findings are scalable. Chefs and culinary educators play a vital role in transforming clinical recommendations into appealing and sustainable meals.

Researchers ought to incorporate behavioral science and dodgy implementation frameworks into their work ensuring findings are really quite scalable afterwards. Culinary educators and chefs play a vital role in transforming clinical dietary advice into utterly appealing meals very sustainably. Clinicians require thorough training on bioactive compounds in various dietary patterns extensively and dietitians need training lately on cancer metabolism nowadays. Researchers should pretty deeply infuse behavioral science principles and assorted implementation frameworks into their work ensuring findings scale up effectively somewhat later.

5. Building a Balanced Anti-Cancer Diet: Macronutrient and Micronutrient Considerations

Crafting an anticancer diet involves deliberately weaving in vital nutrients and calibrating them rather meticulously within cells. Pretty frequently nowadays strategic integration of carbohydrates proteins and fats occurs with various bioactive compounds like antioxidants and phytochemicals and vitamins minerals. Carbohydrates should mainly originate from complex sources such as whole grains legumes and vegetables with pretty minimal processing involved typically. Foods rich in fibre considerably enhance diversity of gut microbiome and facilitate excretion of estrogen reducing mechanisms underlying cancer risk significantly.

Limiting carb intake with high glycemic effects potentially alters glucose and insulin thereby mitigating cancer growth via activation of IGF-1 pathway.

Proteins ought to be sourced from fairly diverse plant-based sources such as legumes nuts or soy and occasionally rather lean animal products. Focusing on anti-inflammatory protein sources greatly reduces oxidative stress and enhance tissue repair very effectively during intense therapy sessions. Eating large amounts of red meat and processed meats has been rather strongly linked with heightened risk of colorectal cancer because of heme iron. Fats are quite vital for cell membrane integrity and hormone synthesis while modulating inflammatory pathways rather effectively under various conditions. Omega-3 fatty acids found in fatty fish and flaxseeds may effectively suppress pro-inflammatory eicosanoids and inhibit tumour growth remarkably well. Trans fats and excessive omega-6 fatty acids ought to pretty much be minimized because of their seriously pro-inflammatory effects on bodily functions.

Vitamins A C D E and K selenium zinc magnesium and phytochemicals like polyphenols flavonoids isothiocyanates exert profoundly antioxidant effects naturally with anti-inflammatory properties. Whole foods generally outdo supplements bar certain medically indicated situations where specific compounds interact remarkably well together synergistically. Pretty slowly a diverse eating pattern rich in nutrients tends to be rather sustainable and fairly anti-cancer overall naturally. People can fortify their cancer resilience pretty effectively by aligning food consumption pretty closely with bodily defense systems and backing survivorship initiatives simultaneously.

5.1. Carbohydrates: Quality over Quantity

Carbohydrates serve as vital energy sources but type and processing level significantly impact cancer prevention contexts quite variably.

a. Complex vs. Simple Carbohydrates

Complex carbohydrates found in whole grains, legumes, vegetables, and fruits are rich in dietary fibre, antioxidants, and phytonutrients. Simple sugars and refined carbohydrates (e.g., white bread, pastries, sugar-sweetened beverages) contribute to insulin resistance, chronic inflammation, and elevated levels of insulin-like growth factor-1 (IGF-1), which can stimulate tumour growth. Whole grains legumes vegetables and fruits contain complex carbohydrates richly endowed with dietary fibre various antioxidants and numerous phytonutrients.

b. Glycemic Load and Insulin Response

Anti-cancer diets heavily favor obscure low glycemic index foods reducing ghastly spikes in blood glucose and insulin rather suddenly thereafter. Examples include oats and lentils as well as sweet potatoes and most veggies that aren't loaded naturally with heaps of carbohydrates. Some food drastically minimizes inflammation and helps keep body weight pretty much in check another vital consideration for cancer risk.

5.2. Proteins: Quality, Source, and Timing

Protein serves as vital macronutrient crucial for cellular repair and upkeep of lean body mass in cancer patients undergoing intense therapy slowly. Novel research findings underscore protein quantity quality and consumption timing can profoundly impact cancer risk treatment tolerance survivorship outcomes very markedly. Optimal bodily functions depend heavily on consuming complete proteins rich in essential amino acids for nutrition. Legumes nuts and seeds provide sufficient amino acids unusually when consumed with various whole grains and soy products in eclectic combinations. Soy protein has isoflavones with phytoestrogenic properties exerting protective effects against hormone-sensitive cancers like breast cancer and prostate cancer with varying efficacy across different cancer types.

Protein source variably impacts cancer progression risk somewhat surprisingly across diverse demographics and different populations rather markedly often. Consumption of lots of red meat and processed meat products has been associated with elevated risk of gastric and colorectal cancer largely due to heme iron. Fish poultry and plant-based proteins correlate with lower inflammatory responses and pretty favorable metabolic profiles supporting survivorship mostly in numerous cases. Protein intake timing matters enormously nowadays for cancer sufferers receiving brutal chemo or radiation treatment pretty badly these days. Spreading protein consumption fairly evenly throughout daily meals possibly helps stave off sarcopenia and fuels robust anabolic reactions in body.

Cachexia sufferers benefit greatly from consuming fortified legumes and protein-rich smoothies preserving muscle mass very slowly over time. Protein intake sufficiently supports immune function frequently battered during cancer therapy sessions that drag on interminably with debilitating effects. Cysteine amino acids play crucial roles beneath intestinal barrier integrity in lymphocyte function and antioxidant defense mechanisms significantly. A high-quality predominantly plant-based nutrition strategy should be prioritized drastically during treatment while reliance on processed meats gets slashed pretty rapidly.

a. Plant-Based vs. Animal-Based Proteins

Legumes, soy, nuts, seeds, and whole grains provide high-quality, anti-inflammatory proteins and are linked to lower risks of several cancers. Red and processed meats (e.g., bacon, sausages) are classified as carcinogenic by the World Health Organization, particularly in relation to colorectal cancer. Fish and poultry, when consumed in moderation, can offer lean alternatives, especially those rich in omega-3 fatty acids.

b. Protein Intake during Cancer Therapy

Cancer patients frequently have remarkably elevated protein requirements roughly 1.0 g/kg/day or more especially during intensive medical interventions. Sufficient intake remarkably enhances wound healing and reinforces immune response quite effectively while supporting retention of crucial muscle mass during treatment.

5.3. Fats: Anti-Inflammatory and Essential Sources

Dietary fats play diverse roles quietly in health and disease with nuances especially surfacing within cancer prevention contexts alongside various nuanced management strategies. Fats consumed in excess especially saturated and trans-fats have been linked closely with chronic inflammation and obesity and insulin resistance is exacerbated but other fats play crucial roles in modulation of immune responses. Anti-cancer dietary strategies stress inclusion of protective fats from various unusual sources while diminishing pro-carcinogenic ones down multiple erratic pathways vigorously. Fats saturated with hydrogen atoms lurking predominantly in red meats slathered in fatty sauces high-fat dairy and packaged edibles have been tied pretty strongly to elevated risks of various cancers.

Fats vigorously spur inflammatory pathways like NF-κB and significantly boost expression of pro-inflammatory cytokines in diverse cellular environments. Trans-fats hiding in ultra-processed fare and hydrogenated oils are heinous systemically linked with inflammation and greatly heightened overall cancer risk. Monounsaturated and polyunsaturated fats serve vital yet differing functions playing crucial protective roles inside human bodies fairly differently everyday. MUFAs present abundantly in olive oil and certain nuts are pivotal components of Mediterranean dietary patterns linked frequently to lower cancer rates. Omega-6 and omega-3 fatty acids are both part of PUFAs and balance between these acids greatly matters in various bodily functions.

Omega-3 fatty acids specifically EPA and DHA are found quite abundantly in fatty fish like salmon and have profoundly anti-inflammatory properties. Fats modulate eicosanoid biosynthesis pretty effectively suppressing tumour-promoting prostaglandins while possibly boosting chemotherapy efficacy or enhancing immunotherapy remarkably. Higher omega-3 intake correlates rather strongly with reduced risks of breast and colorectal and possibly lung cancers in numerous observational studies. Fat plays a crucial role in absorption of fat-soluble vitamins A D E and K and maintains cell membrane structure particularly in various immune cells. Fat avoidance completely is not only entirely needless but potentially pretty darn harmful nowadays for many people. Fatty components in anti-cancer diet ought to focus heavily on whole foods rich in copious unsaturated fats like omega-3s with minimal saturated fats. Cellular resilience against cancer-promoting processes gets fostered naturally alongside metabolic health support and inflammation gets controlled rather effectively.

a. Healthy Fats

Monounsaturated fats, found in olive oil, avocados, and nuts, support cardiovascular health and reduce inflammation. Omega-3 fatty acids, primarily from fatty fish (e.g., salmon, sardines) and flaxseeds, can suppress tumour-promoting pathways and support immune function. Short-chain fatty acids (SCFAs) like butyrate, produced by microbial fermentation of fibre, support colon health and reduce carcinogenesis.

b. Unhealthy Fats

High intake of saturated fats (from red meat, butter, cheese) and trans-fats (from processed snacks and margarine) contributes to insulin resistance and inflammation and has been linked to increased cancer risk, especially in breast and prostate cancers.

5.4. Micronutrients

Micronutrients like vitamins and minerals quietly play crucial roles within bodily systems regulating immune responses and maintaining cellular integrity. Nutrients act effectively as cofactors in numerous enzymatic reactions crucial for DNA repair and synthesis normally under various conditions. Micronutrient deficiencies severely impair bodily functions substantially elevating risk of cancer and chronic inflammation pretty drastically over time. Vitamin C acts as potent antioxidant scavenging reactive oxygen species protecting cells from DNA damage caused by oxidation. It enhance collagen synthesis thereby maintaining tissue integrity and stifling invasion by tumour cells effectively meanwhile possibly from within tissues. Vitamin E shields cellular membranes remarkably well from peroxidation of lipids and modulates several immune responses and some inflammatory routes pretty effectively. Vitamin D plays a crucial role deeply in cell cycle regulation and modulates immune responses ambiguously via induction of apoptosis pretty effectively.

Serum 25(OH)D levels appear perilously low in patients diagnosed subsequently with various malignancies including breast cancer and prostate cancer. Folate plays a crucial role rapidly in nucleotide synthesis and DNA methylation occurs within cells during various complex biochemical processes. Folate deficiency triggers uracil misincorporation into DNA thereby inducing strand breaks and genomic instability particularly germane for pancreatic and colon cancers. Selenium and zinc enhance various antioxidant enzyme systems including glutathione peroxidase and superoxide dismutase respectively in fairly complex biochemical pathways normally. Trace elements vitally maintain redox equilibrium and enhance immune function rather effectively under diverse physiological conditions pretty normally. Magnesium plays a crucial role in DNA repair enzymes facilitating cellular energy metabolism pretty effectively alongside genomic stability maintenance.

Deficiency has been linked tenuously over time to rampant inflammation and heightened oxidative stress in various bodily tissues pretty irregularly. Micronutrient imbalances stem partly from inadequate diet and largely from malabsorption during chronic illness or owing to cancer treatment demands. Over-supplementation potentially carries risks especially when interactions between various nutrients aren't taken into account or synthetic forms severely disrupt normal bodily functions. Naturally micronutrient-rich whole foods like veggies fruits legumes nuts and seeds offer optimal status best strategy with whole grains abound. Individualized supplementation becomes necessary pretty frequently under various circumstances during cancer therapy or recovery when clinically indicated. Micronutrients play crucial roles in bodily functions detecting malignant cellular changes and subsequently vigorously repairing and tenaciously defending against them.

a. Key Anti-Cancer Micronutrients

Vitamin D plays roles in immune modulation, cell differentiation, and apoptosis. Vitamin D plays various roles deeply in immune modulation and cell differentiation often alongside apoptosis. Folate is essential for DNA synthesis and methylation. Vitamin D plays multifaceted roles modulating immune responses and regulating cell differentiation alongside apoptosis in various bodily tissues quite effectively always. Vitamin C and E are potent antioxidants protecting cells from oxidative damage and supporting immune surveillance remarkably well.

b. Bioavailability and Food Sources

Micronutrients get absorbed pretty effectively when eaten within whole foods boasting complex nutritional matrices naturally in myriad subtle ways. Lycopene from tomatoes becomes remarkably more bioavailable when simmered in olive oil and curcumin extracted from turmeric gets boosted by piperine abundantly found in black pepper.

5.5. Hydration and Cancer

Hydration plays a vital role rather quietly in cancer prevention yet remains greatly underemphasized in most care settings nowadays. Fluid intake stays vital for upholding cellular homeostasis and metabolic reactions while nutrients get transported via hepatic pathways and toxins get flushed. Grueling chemotherapy and surgery heighten metabolic demands substantially and nasty treatment side effects often cause dehydration in affected individuals. Cancer therapies often trigger ghastly side effects such as protracted vomiting or explosive diarrhea and high fever worsening risk of dehydration severely. Mild dehydration drastically hinders cognitive function and worsens fatigue pretty badly while gastrointestinal motility slows down somewhat leading to quite unpleasant constipation. Dehydration severely impacts kidney function badly in extreme cases potentially heightening nephrotoxicity risk especially in patients receiving cisplatin therapy.

Hydration options like filtered water and unsweetened herbal teas are favored from a nutrition perspective emphasizing disease prevention and bodily support greatly. Pretty decent hydration is offered by these drinks sans nasty glycemic spikes or excess calorie consumption and diuresis fueled by caffeine occurs subsequently. Restricting sugary drinks energy drinks and super caffeinated products rather cleverly helps mitigate inflammation that badly influences cancer growth pretty significantly. Rather obscure herbal infusions provide benefits functionally in some cases with unexpectedly superior results under specific conditions. Green tea has catechins like EGCG exhibiting profoundly antioxidant properties and pretty anti-angiogenic effects in various bodily processes largely. Ginger tea possibly mitigates nausea quite effectively as a distressing side effect stemming from chemotherapy due largely presence of gingerol.

Peppermint and chamomile teas remarkably foster relaxation effectively supporting patient quality of life during lengthy medical treatments. Hydration strategies must be tailored specifically for patients with cardiac issues or renal problems necessitating very strict fluid intake limitations usually. Most adults should drink 2.5 liters of fluid daily unless their healthcare provider directs them otherwise pretty much always. Early intervention relies heavily on closely monitoring symptoms of dehydration like dizziness or unusually dark urine and pretty dry mouth. Strategically implemented adequate hydration remains an essential but woefully overlooked component of mainstream cancer care practice. Fluid intake enormously supports detoxification when paired with nutrient-rich anti-inflammatory diet thereby enhancing outcomes clinically in tissue repair processes.

5.6. The Role of Balanced Dietary Patterns

Emerging evidence strongly backs significance of overall eating habits in mitigating risk of cancer and encourages treatment outcomes fairly substantially. Myriad bioactive compounds fibre fats and proteins interact within a biochemical milieu quite hostile towards cancer development highlighting synergy among various nutrients. Mediterranean diet stays thoroughly studied anti-cancer dietary model globally in various research institutions with frequency and pretty considerable attention nowadays. Nuts and moderate fish intake rich in olive oil and vegetables are accompanied by whole grains and legumes providing diverse polyphenols. Adherence to Mediterranean diet strongly correlates with significantly lower incidence rates and mortality for various cancers including colorectal cancer and breast cancer. Whole-food plant-based diets have been linked with greatly diminished risks of hormone-related cancers and some gastrointestinal malignancies as well pretty frequently.

Diets rich in magnesium and phytochemicals but low in saturated fat promote healthy estrogen metabolism and foster gut microbiota diversity very effectively indeed. Whole plant foods barely processed foster environments rich in antioxidants and reduce chronic disease risk remarkably across entire human lifespan effectively. Time-restricted eating and low-glycemic index diets are garnering considerable attention lately for heavily influencing metabolic pathways linked to cancer. Preliminary data suggest these patterns may rather effectively sensitize tumours for treatment and improve cellular resilience significantly under certain conditions. A balanced anti-cancer diet marries premium macronutrients with diverse micronutrients like vitamins and minerals and sundry polyphenols very naturally.

Whole unprocessed foods are heavily emphasized here whereas pro-inflammatory elements like added sugars and trans-fats get pretty effectively minimized. Dietary effectiveness gets amplified pretty significantly when personalization hinges heavily on age alongside genetic predisposition during distinct treatment phases obviously. Tailoring dietary habits extremely precisely according to individual requirements and fresh research findings makes nutrition an astonishingly potent flexible instrument for cancer prevention across various survivorship stages.

6. Practical Approaches to Implementing an Anti-Cancer Diet in Daily Life

Growing scientific evidence strongly affirms nutrition's crucial role in cancer prevention and treatment support but habitual application of such knowledge remains elusive. Meager budgets severely hinder adoption of health-promoting dietary changes deeply ingrained in cultural eating patterns over time naturally. Emphasis should land squarely on pragmatic strategies that meet people precisely where they are presently dwelling rather than idealistic dietary recommendations. Meal planning acts as bedrock remarkably well for attaining success in multifaceted life aspects with relative ease and considerable effectiveness. Regularly doing prep work for simple meals made from whole foods pretty significantly lessens reliance on heavily processed convenience foods. Batch cooking vastly improves dietary consistency during cancer treatment when fatigue severely limits one's ability to cook suddenly and freezer meals help. Savvy supermarket foraging stays remarkably crucial these days.

Nutrient-rich food options abound at home when meal plans are crafted heavily under influence of currently available whole grains lean proteins fruits and seasonal vegetables. Shopping around grocery store edges where fresh food tends to congregate might steer people clear of sugary salty trash foods loaded with trans-fats. Steaming or roasting preserves nutrient integrity nicely whereas high heat frying and charring generates pretty harmful compounds through nasty chemical reactions. Herbs spices and citrus pretty significantly enhance flavor which reduces sodium dependence and boosts food palatability overall rather nicely. Mindful eating alongside habit tracking remarkably facilitates long-term adherence with considerable success over time when paired with ambitious goal setting. Kin involvement in meal prep reinforces wholesome habits naturally at home and fosters unusually supportive environs around eating with considerable frequency.

Recipes tweaked culturally reflecting venerable local food traditions can remarkably boost meal plans' sustainability in variegated community settings surprisingly. Nationwide equitable anti-cancer dietary strategies depend heavily on addressing stark food insecurity and limited educational access pretty effectively. Nationwide public health initiatives can greatly enhance population-level impact by rapidly expanding access to fresh produce and community gardens with some nutrition education. A multifaceted personalized approach integrating scientific knowledge with culturally sensitive everyday living tips successfully implements an anti-cancer diet effectively nowadays.

6.1. Foundation: Emphasizing Whole, Plant-Based Foods

A diet aimed at fighting cancer essentially revolves around consuming predominantly whole minimally processed foods that originate from various plant sources. Phytochemicals and healthy fats furnished by such foods synergistically reduce inflammation and enhance immune function against remarkable DNA damage effectively. Load up plates daily with vibrantly hued veggies for optimal nutrition and healthy eating habits almost half full obviously. Eat legumes like lentils and beans as protein sources three or four times weekly. Choose whole grains (brown rice, oats, barley, quinoa) over refined grains. Use fruits as natural desserts or snacks to reduce sugar intake. Opt for brown rice and oats and barley or quinoa rather than refined grains whenever possible evidently. Eat fruits as snacks or natural desserts rather quickly reducing overall sugar intake drastically.

6.2. Smart Shopping: Stocking an Anti-Cancer Kitchen

Healthful foods that are readily available predict adherence to diet quite strongly under most circumstances of daily life. Kitchen environments carefully crafted somewhat mitigate decision fatigue and foster healthier eating choices naturally in everyday life. Stick fairly closely around outer perimeter of grocery store where fresh produce whole grains and lean proteins usually abound. Carefully read labels avoiding products laced with added sugars trans-fats and artificial preservatives. Using frozen fruits and vegetables when fresh options are unavailable these retain nutrients and extend shelf life. Keep a well-stocked pantry with spices, legumes, nuts, seeds, and herbal teas. Frozen fruits and veggies are decent alternatives when fresh stuff is not around retaining nutrients pretty well and lasting fairly long.

6.3. Meal Planning and Prepping: Simplifying the Week

Meal planning rather effectively limits frantic resorting to processed junk foods and fosters steady consumption of cancer-protective nutrients. Pretty effective strategies involve meal planning around seasonal produce and core foods known for cancer prevention each week. Batch-cooking staples like whole grains or roasted vegetables, occurs very often in advance for later reheating. Prepare snack boxes with carrot sticks, hummus, fruit, or mixed nuts to avoid vending machine temptations. Rotate "meatless Mondays" or plant-based days, to gradually reduce red and processed meat consumption. Prepare snack boxes with carrot sticks hummus and fruit or a handful of mixed nuts avoiding vending machine temptations altogether daily.

6.4. Cooking Methods: Preserving Nutrients and Flavor

Food preparation methods matter somewhat greatly under various circumstances naturally. Food preparation processes markedly amplify or diminish anti-cancer properties of various ingredients through different cooking techniques quite dramatically. Steamed veggies lightly or deep-fry briskly retaining antioxidants like vitamin C and glucosinolates naturally. Herbs and spices such as turmeric garlic ginger cinnamon can enhance flavor liberally and provide functional benefits. Avoid charring meats or deep frying, which can form carcinogenic compounds like heterocyclic amines (HCAs) and polycyclic aromatic hydrocarbons (PAHs). Choose cold-pressed oils (e.g., olive, flaxseed) and avoid repeated heating of oils. Deep frying and charring meats can produce HCAs and PAHs pretty quickly forming some pretty nasty carcinogenic compounds in the process.

6.5. Behavioral Tools for Sustainable Change

Behavioral change frequently poses a huge hurdle in effectively implementing thorough dietary changes across diverse socioeconomic strata and varied populations nationwide. Psychological tools and sundry environmental factors remarkably enhance motivation quite strongly over time and foster a naturally consistent demeanor. Behavioral techniques entail habit stacking that pairs new behaviors with existing daily routines such as tossing salad into dinner fairly regularly and goal setting involves small measurable objectives like eating three servings of vegetables daily for a week. Mindful eating is best way to reduce overeating and promote appreciation for food quality. Involving family or community in cooking and eating promotes accountability and shared health benefits. Eating mindfully reduces overeating pretty significantly and fosters a deeper appreciation of food quality remarkably well in people almost always.

6.6. Navigating Eating Out and Social Settings

Eating out with careful attention barely sabotages personal healthy eating goals occasionally. Dine out wisely by opting for eateries serving mostly plant-based food or Mediterranean fare with exotic flavors and request extra veggies instead of fries. Limit creamy sauces and deep-fried dishes. Limit rich sauces somewhat and pretty much avoid those deep-fried dishes altogether in favor of much healthier alternatives obviously.

6.7. Addressing Access and Affordability

Many individuals struggle adopting a healthy diet due largely to prohibitive cost and severely limited access across various demographics nationwide. Eating to beat cancer can be pretty cheap and fairly attainable with somewhat deliberate daily meal prep obviously every day. Purchase fresh produce in season as it's typically more affordable and bursting with nutrients. Beans lentils and tofu serve as cheap alternatives to pricey animal-derived proteins. Purchase items in bulk and store staples properly to minimize waste. Support local markets or community-supported agriculture (CSA) programs when possible. Buy stuff in huge quantities and stash staples haphazardly down in basement minimizing unnecessary waste. Beans lentils and tofu are dirt cheap alternatives versus pricey animal proteins which tend to be obscenely expensive usually anyway. Purchase massive amounts of goods and hide necessities haphazardly beneath sink or inside cupboard thereby cutting down on superfluous rubbish substantially.

7. Cultural and Lifestyle Factors in Designing Effective Anti-Cancer Diets

Cancer prevention hinges heavily on evidence-based dietary recommendations but real-world impact gets swayed by varied cultural contexts and lifestyle factors. People's values are reflected very intricately nowadays in cultural traditions and daily life routines deeply embedded with nutrition everywhere. Anti-cancer dietary interventions must nowadays effectively shift focus deeply into lived experiences of diverse human populations beyond nutrient profiles. Cultural norms shape preferences deeply alongside quirky culinary traditions that vigorously influence old cooking methods and warped perceptions of health. Mediterranean-style diets heavily feature olive oil and fish whereas traditional East Asian diets prioritize rice soy and sea vegetables rather frequently nowadays. Leveraging deeply ingrained customs remarkably enhance compliance while cultural identity remains intact largely within societal norms.

Public health messaging should haphazardly tweak cancer-protective principles for local cuisines utilizing familiar flavors and pretty exotic ingredients. Festive rituals profoundly influence eating habits and social norms dictate consumption of delicacies at various times throughout a year. Fasting traditions align rather closely with evidence suggesting significant metabolic benefits accrue from intermittent caloric restriction pretty frequently nowadays. Communal meals and food sharing customs reinforce healthful eating pretty effectively within social support networks every single day basically. Rapid urbanization and hectic work schedules significantly affect dietary feasibility largely due to availability or lack of cooking infrastructure. Nutrient-dense meal solutions and ready-to-eat whole foods are highly recommended for individuals with extremely tight schedules or severely limited kitchen access. Rise of sedentary lifestyles and gobbling down processed food quickly necessitates super targeted tactics that promote sorta mindful munching habits quite vigorously nowadays.

Socioeconomic status heavily influences adoption of anti-cancer diets practically everywhere with education level and food availability playing a crucial role. Interventions must grapple pretty much everywhere with expense and availability of fresh produce alongside requisite nutritional know-how. Culturally tailored cooking classes alongside policy efforts and community-based initiatives effectively foster long-term dietary change by increasing access to healthy options. Incorporating lifestyle factors and cultural subtleties into diet-plans for cancer prevention, boosts remarkably across varied ecological paradigms. Personalized context-aware nutrition empowers individuals extraordinarily within their own communities sustainably and improves adherence in rather meaningful ways.

7.1. The Influence of Cultural Food Practices

Culture plays a profoundly foundational role in shaping mealtime rituals and cooking methods with profoundly varied food preferences deeply. Dietary guidelines ignoring cultural nuances face stiff resistance from various groups despite being grounded in fairly robust scientific evidence.

a. Traditional Diets and Cancer Prevention

Mediterranean diets rich in olive oil and whole grains embodies principles that help thwart cancer growth pretty effectively and regularly. Green tea and fermented foods abundant in Japan and Korea are loaded with polyphenols. Indian diets feature turmeric, ginger, garlic, lentils, and an array of spices with anti-inflammatory properties. Indian diets typically feature ginger and lentils alongside turmeric and various spices possessing ostensibly remarkable anti-inflammatory properties.

b. Cultural Barriers to Change

Meat consumption ostentatiously signifies status or celebration in some cultures with lavish feasts and various ritualistic practices deeply rooted. Drastic cuts in meat consumption are recommended without regard for cultural significance and may ultimately backfire spectacularly in foreign lands. Promoting legumes and exotic mushrooms in traditional Malaysian cuisine can remarkably ease transition in some pretty unusual circumstances naturally.

7.2. Social and Religious Influences on Food Choices

Fasting practices like those observed during Ramadan or Navratri can be reimagined as chances to intermittently fast and potentially prevent cancer quite effectively. Vegetarianism, common in Hindu and Jain traditions, naturally supports plant-based eating when balanced with adequate nutrients like B12 and iron. Communal eating is a key feature in many African, South American, and South Asian societies and can be leveraged to promote collective dietary change. Vegetarianism naturally flourishes in Hindu and Jain traditions when enhanceed with nutrients like B12 and iron pretty adequately.

7.3. Socioeconomic Status and Food Accessibility

Bleak economic prospects and wildly fluctuating food availability severely curtail dietary choices nearly always under very tight unforgiving time constraints. Diets touted as anti-cancer are often deemed prohibitively expensive or super labor-intensive in low-income settings essentially for many folks. Promoting nutrient-rich foods like locally available lentils and seasonal veggies at affordable prices involves equitable implementation strategies and offering community cooking demonstrations. Encouraging use of community gardens, local markets, or food cooperatives is the key to increase access. Promoting community gardens local markets and food cooperatives boosts access quite significantly in various neighborhoods and surrounding areas.

7.4. Lifestyle Factors: Work, Family, and Time Constraints

Prolonged work hours and sluggish lifestyles fueled by a penchant for junk food sabotage efforts to overhaul eating habits severely. Cancer risk rises with behaviors like skipping meals and noshing on highly processed food. Time-saving solutions, such as batch cooking, meal prepping, and using frozen vegetables, make healthy eating more feasible. For busy professionals, portable, nutrient-dense options like homemade smoothies, trail mix, or grain bowls can help maintain dietary goals. Batch cooking and meal prepping with frozen veggies make healthy eating fairly feasible nowadays for busy people. Busy professionals can maintain dietary goals with portable nutrient-dense options like grain bowls or trail mix made at home.

7.5. Personal Beliefs and Misinformation

Patients nowadays get inundated online with a plethora of nutrition info lots of which lacks rigorous scientific backing or seems dodgy. Social media platforms vigorously amplify unsubstantiated claims about efficacy of some detox diets and benefits of so-called miracle foods pretty frequently. Deeply ingrained convictions often starkly contradict evidence-based dietary guidelines thereby fairly significantly undermining public health initiatives and some clinical results. Healthcare professionals wrestle with debunking outlandish myths and respecting stubbornly ingrained folkloric mindsets profoundly influencing personal dietary choices. Effective communication strategies deeply rooted in empathy must be employed pretty skillfully therefore to facilitate successful cultural interactions. A nonjudgmental approach centered on patients fosters recognition of diverse cultural practices surrounding diet without unduly alienating individual persons. Gently correcting egregious errors while affirming pivotal cultural norms, fosters trust and sparks fairly open discussion surprisingly quickly.

Nutrition counseling must prioritize clarity significantly and focus on personalization utmost for broad accessibility amongst diverse population groups. Evidence-based recommendations should morph into pragmatic guidance suited rather neatly for patient lifestyle preferences amidst various sociocultural nuances. Clinicians oughta emphasize overall dietary patterns such as Mediterranean-style food or plant-based chow which has been shown to yield massive benefits in cancer prevention. Patients tend to stick pretty well with nutritional advice when healthcare providers show deep respect and grasp their cultural nuances effectively. Culturally savvy strategies significantly boost effectiveness of dietary interventions fostering long-term change over time in diverse demographics pretty remarkably. Merging scientific insight with cultural nuance quite effectively fosters sound ethical standards and enhanced health results across unusually diverse community groups.

7.6. Designing Personalized, Culturally Competent Diet Plans

Anti-cancer dietary plans emerge effectively from a blend of evidence-based science and nuanced cultural factors under highly individualized circumstances very effectively. Healthcare providers and dietitians must swiftly conduct thorough assessments under various cultural contexts nowadays pretty well understanding food preferences and dietary restrictions. Traditional dishes can be modified with much healthier ingredients using alternative cooking methods. We should recognize emotional connections to food, especially in the context of cancer recovery, where comfort and familiarity are important. We should use attractive relevant cultural examples liberally in nutrition education materials nowadays. Acknowledge emotional ties to food particularly during cancer recuperation when solace and familiarity play rather crucial roles. Traditional dishes get revamped surprisingly effectively over time using altogether healthier ingredients and occasionally alternative cooking methods.

8. Monitoring and Adjusting Anti-Cancer Diets: The Role of Personalized Nutrition

Advancements in nutritional science and oncology have highlighted importance of modified dietary interventions quite frequently nowadays in various cancer care settings. Broad dietary guidelines frequently fail pretty miserably at accounting for drastically different genetic factors and environmental influences on individual disease risk. Precision medicine in oncology now leans heavily on modified nutrition that tailors dietary approaches according to each person's unique biology and contextual factors. Tailored nutrition plans yield considerable advantages nowadays for cancer survivors by optimizing outcomes and mitigating recurrence risk remarkably well. Nutrition planning demands a fairly dynamic responsive approach involving initial assessment and lots of continuous monitoring. Evolving nutritional needs and shifts in physical activity alongside treatment-related side effects must be considered very thoroughly over quite some lengthy period.

Clinicians and nutritionists rely heavily on various tools including biomarkers of nutritional status and genomic profiling alongside patient reported outcomes very frequently nowadays. Such tools quietly facilitate assessment of dietary strategy efficacy and pinpoint need for radical change within normal research environments pretty effectively. Patients undergoing chemotherapy often suffer really severe gastrointestinal symptoms or debilitating taste alterations necessitating temporary dietary adjustments pretty frequently. Cutting-edge technologies for tracking dietary habits are showcased near a novel framework of modified nutrition in cancer treatment and optimum care standards. Integrating real-time data with personalized care plans possibly enhances adherence remarkably yielding better clinical outcomes in numerous cancer patients down the line.

8.1. The Rationale for Personalization in Oncology Nutrition

Cancer manifests variably across disparate tumour types and stages exhibiting diverse molecular signatures and wildly different responses to therapeutic interventions. Biological diversity gets further muddled by individual patient differences such as genetic polymorphisms and epigenetic modifications amidst varied gut microbiota and dietary habits under psychosocial stressors like low socioeconomic standing. Variables exert a rather profound influence on nutritional needs and metabolic responses during disease treatment efficacy of various dietary interventions. Oncology endeavors tackle complexity through modified dietary regimens morphing dynamically alongside patient's nebulous clinical trajectory with rather intricate personalized nutrition. Tailored approaches incorporating biological markers and lifestyle factors zealously facilitate peak bodily function over generic nutrition guidance rather haphazardly. Maximizing nutrient bioavailability and utilization efficiently amid cancer treatment-related disruptions greatly involves primary objectives of personalized nutrition in oncology care.

Therapy frequently triggers nasty side effects such as mucositis or dysgeusia badly compromising nutritional status and utterly torpedoing treatment adherence. Supporting immune function and maintaining metabolic homeostasis effectively anyway are both critical during catabolic stress periods or immunosuppressive therapies. Specific nutrient deficiencies or toxicities stemming from tumour metabolism and drug-nutrient interactions may need correction. Integrative oncology prioritizes patient well-being deeply while elevating quality of life remarkably alongside various psychological aspects and overall physical health. Personalized nutrition evolves quite dynamically over time rather than being a rigid prescription naturally unfolding in a static manner. Dietary plans must be reassessed continually and modified slowly based on treatment phase like surgery or chemotherapy alongside evolving patient tolerances. This adaptive model fosters deep patient engagement within various clinical contexts and ultimately contributes greatly to fairly effective compassionate care for cancer patients.

8.2. Tools and Biomarkers for Monitoring Anti-Cancer Diets

Effective monitoring plays crucial role in assessing impact of anti-cancer dietary interventions, subsequently informing timely evidence-based modifications. Ongoing evaluation enables a quite dynamic responsive approach throughout cancer care from diagnosis through treatment and into survivorship phases fairly effectively. Nutritional status gets revealed through a fairly comprehensive picture emerging from motley biomarkers and patient reported outcomes altogether objectively. Objective assessments crucially facilitate tracking biological outcomes of various nutritional interventions in multiple contexts pretty regularly it seems. Biochemical markers like serum albumin levels and micronutrients including vitamin D iron B12 folate are listed alongside various inflammatory cytokines quietly.

Metabolic therapy protocols entail meticulously tracking various indicators including blood glucose insulin levels lipid profiles and ketone bodies during treatment regimens. Dual-energy X-ray absorptiometry and occasionally CT imaging alongside bioelectrical impedance analysis, track sarcopenia risk with lean body mass and fat mass. Profiling gut microbiome yields insights into microbial diversity heavily interacting with diet components and somewhat modulating systemic inflammation deeply. Subjective evaluations hold equal importance offering context for laboratory findings and highlighting patients' lived experience very deeply inside most clinical settings. Symptom tracking pretty frequently encompasses nausea alongside diarrhea and fatigue as well as rather dramatic taste changes and bouts of vomiting.

Food diaries track caloric intake effectively and assess dietary adherence thoroughly with decent sufficiency evaluations in some rather unusual cases occasionally. EORTC QLQ-C30 and FACT-G instruments assess psychosocial well-being effectively in relation to nutritional care with varying degrees of success somewhat. Healthcare providers can pretty quickly personalize dietary strategies in real time by integrating such tools into routine practice effectively. Feedback loops optimize nutritional status remarkably in oncology settings and enhance overall patient outcomes rather quickly with substantially improved treatment tolerance.

a. Nutritional Status and Body Composition

Assessing nutritional status and evaluating body composition currently serve as foundational elements in effectively monitoring dietary interventions against cancer. Malnutrition and sarcopenia prevail drastically across various cancer types significantly impacting treatment tolerance and overall survival rather quite badly. Ongoing evaluation of nutritional adequacy and body composition essentially tailors interventions thereby improving patient prognosis quite favourably in clinical settings. Anthropometric measurements serve quite effectively as a decent starting point basically for further assessment pretty much everywhere. Body mass index skinfold thickness and waist circumference offer preliminary estimates of body fat distribution lean mass indicating potential metabolic risk fairly accurately nowadays. Simplistic measures often employed for expediency may not wholly capture subtleties of bodily changes particularly in oncology patients experiencing weight flux unlinked to genuine body fat. Sophisticated tools for assessing body composition are used rather often these days to get pretty detailed info on various bodily functions.

Bioelectrical impedance analysis presents a pretty effective non-invasive technique nowadays for estimating body fat mass and total body water fairly accurately. Factors like hydration status and electrolyte imbalances can skew its accuracy yet it remains pretty useful for tracking changes over time. Dual-energy X-ray absorptiometry yields fairly precise quantification regionally and for whole body bone mineral content alongside fat mass and lean tissue measurements. DEXA is deemed gold standard for diagnosing sarcopenia a rather insidious condition marked by progressively dwindling skeletal muscle mass and severely debilitating weakness. DEXA proves useful for spotting cachexia a gnarly metabolic disorder that resists conventional nutrition with stubborn weight loss and muscle wasting rapidly. Incorporating these tools into routine nutritional surveillance enables early identification of at-risk patients and facilitates modified dietary interventions pretty effectively nowadays.

b. Laboratory Markers

Laboratory biomarkers play a pivotal role in monitoring anti-cancer dietary interventions and personalize treatment quite effectively with varying success rates occasionally. They furnish objective insights into micronutrient status and metabolic function while profoundly swaying cancer progression and overall patient well-being in mysterious ways. Cancer patients often exhibit overt deficiencies or subclinical insufficiencies stemming from treatment-induced malabsorption and altered absorption necessitating crucial micronutrient assessments regularly. Nowadays serum levels of vitamin D and B12 alongside folate get evaluated routinely in most medical checkups and zinc and iron levels too. Nutrient deficiencies severely impair immune function and hematopoiesis while badly affecting wound healing and overall neurological health pretty negatively over time. Low vitamin D levels frequently manifest in oncology populations and associate with heightened cancer risk in some pretty nasty malignancies yielding dismal outcomes.

C-reactive protein and interleukin-6 serve as inflammatory markers gauging systemic inflammation which manifests heavily in various cancer-related complications. High CRP or IL-6 levels might indicate necessity of tweaking diet anti-inflammatory by wolfing down omega-3 fatty acids and nutrient dense phyto-rich foods. Tracking markers over time pretty accurately assesses intervention effectiveness meanwhile yielding valuable insights for researchers and practitioners alike very effectively. Fasting glucose levels alongside hemoglobin A1c play crucial roles in managing patients with metabolic syndrome and insulin resistance or frank diabetes. Tight glycemic control may crucially mitigate tumour-promoting effects associated with hyperinsulinemia and excessive glucose levels very effectively in some way. These values effectively guide adjustments in carbohydrate intake and meal timing supporting various therapeutic goals with considerable metabolic balance subsequently. Incorporating lab biomarkers into nutritional assessment frameworks boosts precision of dietary planning and enables early detection of some pretty significant metabolic issues.

c. Dietary Intake and Symptom Logs

Precise evaluation of dietary consumption plays a vital role in assessing adherence to anticancer regimens and informs subsequent adjustments effectively thereafter. Systematic tracking of intake and symptoms gets heavily influenced by quantity of consumed food and treatment-related nasty side effects remarkably. Nowadays food frequency questionnaires and 24-hour dietary recall are used widely evaluating nutrient intake of patients quite thoroughly. FFQs are super useful for gauging habitual dietary intake over very long periods and 24-hour recalls provide detailed snapshots of recent eating habits. Patients can quite readily log meals and portion sizes pretty easily with emerging tech such as mobile apps and digital food diaries nowadays. Such tools significantly boost patient involvement and enable clinicians quite rapidly monitoring dietary adherence in real time.

Symptom generally remain crucial beyond intake for grasping functional barriers impeding adequate nutrition during grueling cancer treatments like prolonged chemotherapy sessions. Nausea and fatigue symptoms drastically affect food choices and nutrient absorption leading to severe malnutrition pretty quickly. Regular symptom tracking enables clinician quite effectively spot trends and make adjustments to food texture or implement supportive strategies like strategic meal timing and potent antiemetics. Melding intake info and symptom data into nutritional monitoring allows fairly thorough evaluation of patient needs from multiple disparate perspectives. Fostering ridiculously precise nutritional care extremely effectively enhances patient quality of life during cancer treatment regimens pretty significantly or so it seems.

8.3. Tailoring Dietary Strategies across the Cancer Journey

Oncology nutritional interventions ought to evolve quickly throughout cancer care as shifting patient needs manifest diversely across various physiological spectrums rather rapidly. Nutritional challenges variably emerge during phases stretching from prevention or diagnosis through active treatment into survivorship afterwards rather slowly. Pretty effectively tailored dietary regimens adapt rapidly according to fluctuating individual needs and support long-term health outcomes remarkably well over time. Minimally processed whole foods bursting with fibre and antioxidants are heavily encouraged during various phases focusing on prevention or risk reduction. Mediterranean fare and plant-based foods loaded diets correlate with diminished cancer risk via inflammation modulation and reduction of oxidative stress naturally.

Nutritional strategies must be tailored rather carefully according to patient condition and tumour type with various comorbidities in subsequent regimens. Emphasis often veers sharply towards effectively encourage immune response while pretty much sustaining bodily vigor and altogether eschewing malnourishment in the process. Patients getting chemotherapy often benefit from eating calorie-dense snacks whereas folks awaiting surgery need nutrient-rich foods for speedy recovery and wound healing. Survivorship phase goals shift decidedly towards recovery and metabolic equilibrium while focusing intently on thwarting subsequent cancer recurrence very gradually afterwards. Nutritional interventions effectively target managing severe long-term treatment effects like debilitating fatigue or osteoporosis and rebuild lean body mass meanwhile encourage emotional well-being generally in patients undergoing rigorous therapy.

Mindful eating habits have grown pretty irregular nowadays and meal prep is often meticulously planned for sustainable lifestyle adjustments frequently. Personalization stays utterly crucial silently throughout each arduous stage always morphs into vital necessity during intensely laborious processes quietly underground. Tailored nutrition must consider deeply personal psychosocial factors alongside functional status and complex medical history and individual quirky cultural preferences. Pretty sustainable dietary recommendations remain realistic within a patient's evolving life through a collaborative patient-centered approach.

a. During Active Treatment

Active cancer treatment phases putting tremendous physiological stress on body encompass chemotherapy radiation surgery and increasingly esoteric immunotherapies of various sorts. Patients frequently endure multifaceted nutrition issues like dysgeusia and nausea alongside mucositis and debilitating fatigue very often. Symptoms severely impair oral intake resulting in stark unintentional weight loss and badly frayed immune function over time pretty badly. Nutritional strategies during this phase must be pretty therapeutic and adaptive enough maintaining nutrition adequacy while enhancing treatment tolerance fairly well. Meals packed with protein and bursting with energy help maintain muscle mass and satiate skyrocketing metabolic needs during intense treatment protocols typically. Frequently eaten small meals are often prescribed instead of large ones which people with gastrointestinal issues or early satiety badly tolerate.

Oral nutrition supplements and nutrient-dense snacks bridge energy and protein gaps pretty effectively in some specific situations usually. Bland food like boiled veggies and soft cereals should be prioritized when nasty gastrointestinal distress or mucositis occurs with mashed spuds rice and bananas. Foods served at room temperature or cold may be tolerated rather better than steaming hot meals served with reckless abandon. Steering clear of acidic or ridiculously fibrous foods rather effectively minimizes irritation and boosts nutrient intake quite remarkably every day. Immunonutrition incorporating nutrients such as omega-3 fatty acids glutamine and arginine has shown pretty effective benefits modulating inflammation in select patients. Bioactive compounds could prove pertinent amidst emerging evidence in surgical oncology for patients sporting unusually high levels of inflammatory markers. Personalization stays remarkably vital rather quietly during some extremely critical phase. Meticulous tracking of symptoms and laboratory results enables real-time adjustments fairly effectively through feedback from patients and weight trends.

b. Post-Treatment and Recovery

Post-treatment recovery signifies a crucial shift from intense cancer treatment regimes toward lengthy survivorship periods slowly afterwards naturally. Nutritional priorities markedly shift from managing symptoms and ensuring caloric adequacy towards fostering metabolic recovery and encourage immune system resilience rapidly. Cancer survivors often struggle with crippling exhaustion and psychological turmoil amidst drastically altered metabolic processes and gut dysfunction alongside sarcopenia. A modified dietary plan carefully tailored around specific individual needs plays quite a pivotal role in enhancing overall wellbeing markedly. Rebuilding lean body mass lost from catabolism during treatment or due to inactivity with concurrently poor nutrition stays a major objective.

Muscle protein synthesis gets a considerable boost from sufficient protein consumption during resistance-based exercise and recovery happens subsequently pretty effectively. Post-treatment diet should heavily emphasize whole-food plant-based nutrition effectively addressing longer-term health goals beyond mere macronutrient repletion slowly. Eating diverse veggies fruits legumes nuts seeds and whole grains rich in phytonutrients and fibre markedly reduces risk of cancer recurrence and comorbidities like cardiovascular disease and type 2 diabetes. Certain foods supply copious antioxidants flavonoids and assorted anti-inflammatory compounds that heavily influence cellular signaling pathways deeply entangled in carcinogenic processes. Cutting back on pro-inflammatory food such as processed meats and refined carbs can enhance anti-inflammatory equilibrium and metabolic well-being quite nicely.

Gut microbiome support becomes crucial pretty quickly in survivorship nutrition plans formulated carefully around individual needs and responses. Chemotherapy and antibiotics frequently disrupt microbial diversity severely within bodily systems and sometimes cause long-term damage to overall health. Eating fermented foods like kimchi with prebiotic fibres found in inulin can reboot gut microbial balance and significantly enhance overall well-being. Nutrient-rich recovery diets tailored to each survivor's needs must be sustainable and aligned with their clinical status and lifestyle preferences supporting well-being naturally long-term.

c. Long-Term Survivorship

Nutritional care evolves fairly slowly during long-term survivorship mainly supporting sustained health and preventing recurrence of cancer or development of chronic comorbidities. Patients moving further away from acute cancer therapy effects slowly experience nutrition focus shifting towards maintenance of overall health. Radical lifestyle overhauls promoting lasting change in dietary habits often necessitate a fairly holistic approach focusing on behavioral modifications quite effectively. Ongoing monitoring assesses metabolic markers such as HbA1c and lipid profiles extremely carefully in survivors highly susceptible to obesity and metabolic syndrome. Screening regularly for depression anxiety and disordered eating influences overall quality of life significantly affecting dietary behaviors rather greatly. Nutritional strategies resonate deeply within personal spheres and get effectively promoted for long-term adherence inside specific cultural milieus normally.

Cultural cuisine preferences in meal plans reinforce identity and amplify eating enjoyment markedly improving overall acceptability pretty significantly over time. Modified traditional food practices thoughtfully align fairly closely with evidence-based health recommendations without sacrificing cultural integrity. Motivational interviewing and other behavioral counseling techniques have proven rather effective nowadays at encourage self-efficacy pretty quickly. Healthcare providers, foster ownership over nutrition decisions effectively by engaging patients in problem-solving activities tailored to individual needs very skillfully. Survivors with evolving needs, benefit effectively from ongoing education through group classes or digital platforms that reinforce key dietary principles. Survivorship care plans enhanceed by dietary advice and peer support groups foster robust community engagement and further enhance considerable accountability remarkably. Successful long-term survivorship nutrition involves deeply embedded dynamic care within a broader framework and plenty of backing psychosocially.

8.4. The Role of Nutrigenomics and Microbiome Insights

Precision medicine evolves rapidly and precision nutrition advances pretty quickly with emerging tools like nutrigenomic analysis offering fresh opportunities suddenly nowadays. Genetic variation profoundly impacts microbial ecosystems which intricately modulate nutrient metabolism disease susceptibility and therapeutic efficacy particularly in contexts centered on cancer prevention. Nutrigenomics examines rather unusually how disparate genetic variations radically impact absorption and utilization of specific nutrients under diverse physiological states. Methylenetetrahydrofolate reductase aka MTHFR gene variants can really bollix folate metabolism thereby hugely ramping up need for bioavailable L-methylfolate forms. APOE gene variations heavily influence lipid metabolism necessitating possibly modified dietary fat intake for mitigating cardiovascular risk or possibly encourage cognitive wellbeing somewhat. By grasping these weird genetic variants clinicians can optimize nutrient delivery and subsequently mitigate nasty metabolic complications and treatment related toxicities.

Gut microbiome profiling nowadays offers remarkably valuable insights into intestinal microbial community composition and function pretty well ordinarily. Disruptions in microbial diversity frequently observed after chemo in cancer patients are linked with metabolic dysfunction and aberrant immune regulation. Strategic deployment of prebiotics and probiotics boosts production of beneficial microbial metabolites such as short-chain fatty acids with anti-inflammatory properties notably butyrate. Modified dietary plans formulated with genetic insights and microbial data now remarkably surpass traditional nutrition guidelines with great efficacy ordinarily. Enhanced patient engagement remarkably boosts promise of this approach for advancing broader precision oncology goals and improving clinical outcomes.

8.5. Multidisciplinary Support for Personalized Monitoring

Personalized nutrition implementation in oncology relies heavily on collaborative models that bring together diverse healthcare professionals with fairly unique expertise. Nutrition-related needs in cancer patients fluctuates erratically necessitating drastic adjustments alongside swiftly progressing treatment and rapidly dwindling bodily functions. Multidisciplinary coordination addresses factors thoroughly via various means in practice normally with considerable effectiveness and a fair degree of thoroughness. Oncology dietitians nowadays play a pretty crucial role assessing dietary intake and fluctuating body composition amidst various debilitating treatment-related symptoms fairly regularly. They develop individualized nutrition plans aligning with patient preferences and clinical goals very meticulously and revise them regularly with great care.

Oncologists and physicians keenly track lab results and treatment efficacy thereby facilitating incorporation of sundry medical data into nutritional choices fairly effectively nowadays. Behavioral psychologists lend crucial support by tackling issues such as disordered eating patterns and anxiety alongside emotional eating problems and depression severely. Their involvement plays a crucial role in encourage motivation and devising effective coping strategies related to body image after cancer treatment. Modified exercise regimes coupled with heavily tweaked nutrition plans attempt boosting muscle mass somewhat slowly and mitigating fatigue very effectively. AI-driven nutrition tracking tools and mobile apps alongside wearable gizmos further enhance personalization pretty effectively in sundry settings. These tools facilitate pretty effective real-time symptom tracking and various behavioral interventions between patients and care teams these days effectively. Personalized nutrition has become a fairly fundamental facet of precision medicine nowadays rather than merely supplemental care for oncology patients. Tailored nutrition strategies leveraging genomic insights and microbiome info can significantly boost treatment tolerance and markedly elevate life quality.

9. Conclusion

Devising sustainable nutrition plans rather effectively nowadays gets fuelled by deepening scientific insight into diet's role within cancer development processes. Nutrients and foods in a comprehensive dietary pattern supporting cellular health boost immune function by modulating metabolism and drastically reducing inflammation. Core principles behind constructing such diets are outlined here drawing heavily from evidence in nutritional science and various meticulous clinical studies. Effective anti-cancer dietary approaches heavily emphasize abundant fruits and whole grains alongside legumes and various vegetables focusing on whole foods. Foods rich in polyphenols supply essential nutrients and bioactive compounds that contribute hugely to DNA protection suppressing tumour pathways greatly. Minimizing exposure happens quite effectively nowadays by eliminating red meats and ultra-processed foods along with excess sugars and nasty trans-fats.

Translating such suggestions into practical reality requires theoretical acumen and pretty deep understanding of individual preferences amidst socioeconomic obstacles. Counseling meticulously tailored around individual patient needs remarkably facilitates sustainable drastic changes in dietary habits over time fairly effectively. Culturally sensitive cookbooks alongside clever meal planning tactics can surprisingly boost long-term adherence pretty well these days with overall significant impact. Dietary interventions alongside clinical oncology care necessitate collaboration quite intensely between healthcare providers nutritionists and several public health practitioners effectively. Cancer risk and treatment response are greatly swayed by dietary patterns while survivorship outcomes teeter on a delicate nutrition fulcrum. Bridging gaps between science and daily food pretty effectively nowadays involves constructing an anticancer diet with surprising regularity and decent odds. Eating nutrient-rich foods and lowering dietary risk factors can foster healthier lives and cancer prevention remarkably quite often.

Ongoing research and policies backing access to healthy food and enlightenment empower patients and practitioners alike wielding such know-how pretty effectively nowadays. Science-based nutrition integrated into daily life naturally serves pretty potently worldwide as a rather potent tool in fight against various cancers.

References

Adams SH, Anthony JC, Carvajal R, Chae L, Khoo CSH, Latulippe ME, Matusheski NV, McClung HL, Rozga M, Schmid CH, Wopereis S, Yan W. Perspective: Guiding Principles for the Implementation of Personalized Nutrition Approaches That Benefit Health and Function. Adv Nutr. 2020 Jan 1;11(1):25-34. doi: 10.1093/advances/nmz086. PMID: 31504115; PMCID: PMC7442375.

Ağagündüz D, Şahin TÖ, Yılmaz B, Ekenci KD, Duyar Özer Ş, Capasso R. Cruciferous Vegetables and Their Bioactive Metabolites: from Prevention to Novel Therapies of Colorectal Cancer. Evid Based Complement Alternat Med. 2022 Apr 11;2022:1534083. doi: 10.1155/2022/1534083. PMID: 35449807; PMCID: PMC9017484.

Al-Shami K, Awadi S, Khamees A, Alsheikh AM, Al-Sharif S, Ala' Bereshy R, Al-Eitan SF, Banikhaled SH, Al-Qudimat AR, Al-Zoubi RM, Al Zoubi MS. Estrogens and the risk of breast cancer: A narrative review of literature. Heliyon. 2023 Sep 17;9(9):e20224. doi: 10.1016/j.heliyon.2023.e20224. PMID: 37809638; PMCID: PMC10559995.

Anand P, Kunnumakkara AB, Sundaram C, Harikumar KB, Tharakan ST, Lai OS, Sung B, Aggarwal BB. Cancer is a preventable disease that requires major lifestyle changes. Pharm Res. 2008 Sep;25(9):2097-116. doi: 10.1007/s11095-008-9661-9. Epub 2008 Jul 15. Erratum in: Pharm Res. 2008 Sep;25(9):2200. Kunnumakara, Ajaikumar B [corrected to Kunnumakkara, Ajaikumar B]. PMID: 18626751; PMCID: PMC2515569.

Arreola R, Quintero-Fabián S, López-Roa RI, Flores-Gutiérrez EO, Reyes-Grajeda JP, Carrera-Quintanar L, Ortuño-Sahagún D. Immunomodulation and anti-inflammatory effects of garlic compounds. J Immunol Res. 2015;2015:401630. doi: 10.1155/2015/401630. Epub 2015 Apr 19. PMID: 25961060; PMCID: PMC4417560.

Barrera S, Demark-Wahnefried W. Nutrition during and after cancer therapy. Oncology (Williston Park). 2009 Feb;23(2 Suppl Nurse Ed):15-21. PMID: 19856583; PMCID: PMC2770876.

Bodur M, Yilmaz B, Ağagündüz D, Ozogul Y. Immunomodulatory Effects of Omega-3 Fatty Acids: Mechanistic Insights and Health Implications. Mol Nutr Food Res. 2025 May;69(10):e202400752. doi: 10.1002/mnfr.202400752. Epub 2025 Mar 30. PMID: 40159804; PMCID: PMC12087734.

Branco, M. G., Mateus, C., Capelas, M. L., Pimenta, N., Santos, T., Mäkitie, A., Ganhão-Arranhado, S., Trabulo, C., & Ravasco, P. (2023). Bioelectrical Impedance Analysis (BIA) for the Assessment of Body Composition in Oncology: A Scoping Review. Nutrients, 15(22), 4792. https://doi.org/10.3390/nu15224792

Bressan V, Stevanin S, Bianchi M, Aleo G, Bagnasco A, Sasso L. The effects of swallowing disorders, dysgeusia, oral mucositis and xerostomia on nutritional status, oral intake and weight loss in head and neck cancer patients: A systematic review. Cancer Treat Rev. 2016 Apr;45:105-19. doi: 10.1016/j.ctrv.2016.03.006. Epub 2016 Mar 14. PMID: 27010487.

Cerletti C, Esposito S, Iacoviello L. Edible Mushrooms and Beta-Glucans: Impact on Human Health. Nutrients. 2021 Jun 25;13(7):2195. doi: 10.3390/nu13072195. PMID: 34202377; PMCID: PMC8308413.

Cole JB, Gabbianelli R. Editorial: Recent advances in nutrigenomics: Making strides towards precision nutrition. Front Genet. 2022 Sep 20;13:997266. doi: 10.3389/fgene.2022.997266. PMID: 36204315; PMCID: PMC9531153.

Colella M, Charitos IA, Ballini A, Cafiero C, Topi S, Palmirotta R, Santacroce L. Microbiota revolution: How gut microbes regulate our lives. World J Gastroenterol. 2023 Jul 28;29(28):4368-4383. doi: 10.3748/wjg.v29.i28.4368. PMID: 37576701; PMCID: PMC10415973.

Corr PG, Hudson W, Kalita N. Cancer Care and Nutrition Counseling: The Role of the Oncologist in Patient Learning and Behavior Change. Glob Adv Integr Med Health. 2024 Sep 13;13:27536130241285029. doi: 10.1177/27536130241285029. PMID: 39280090; PMCID: PMC11402076.

Deka A, Vita JA. Tea and cardiovascular disease. Pharmacol Res. 2011 Aug;64(2):136-45. doi: 10.1016/j.phrs.2011.03.009. Epub 2011 Apr 6. PMID: 21477653; PMCID: PMC3123419.

Deledda A, Annunziata G, Tenore GC, Palmas V, Manzin A, Velluzzi F. Diet-Derived Antioxidants and Their Role in Inflammation, Obesity and Gut Microbiota Modulation. Antioxidants (Basel). 2021 Apr 29;10(5):708. doi: 10.3390/antiox10050708. PMID: 33946864; PMCID: PMC8146040.

Ding Z, Zhou L, Zhou Y, Jin K, Wu R, Gui Y. Nutritional status and body composition of patients with head and neck cancer treated with perioperative evidence-based nutritional management. J Clin Biochem Nutr. 2024 Jul;75(1):71-77. doi: 10.3164/jcbn.24-35. Epub 2024 May 21. PMID: 39070536; PMCID: PMC11273269.

Donaldson MS. Nutrition and cancer: a review of the evidence for an anti-cancer diet. Nutr J. 2004 Oct 20;3:19. doi: 10.1186/1475-2891-3-19. PMID: 15496224; PMCID: PMC526387.

Ducrot P, Méjean C, Aroumougame V, Ibanez G, Allès B, Kesse-Guyot E, Hercberg S, Péneau S. Meal planning is associated with food variety, diet quality and body weight status in a large sample of French adults. Int J Behav Nutr Phys Act. 2017 Feb 2;14(1):12. doi: 10.1186/s12966-017-0461-7. PMID: 28153017; PMCID: PMC5288891.

Facchin S, Bertin L, Bonazzi E, Lorenzon G, De Barba C, Barberio B, Zingone F, Maniero D, Scarpa M, Ruffolo C, Angriman I, Savarino EV. Short-Chain Fatty Acids and Human Health: From Metabolic Pathways to Current Therapeutic Implications. Life (Basel). 2024 Apr 26;14(5):559. doi: 10.3390/life14050559. PMID: 38792581; PMCID: PMC11122327.

Franco GA, Interdonato L, Cordaro M, Cuzzocrea S, Di Paola R. Bioactive Compounds of the Mediterranean Diet as Nutritional Support to Fight Neurodegenerative Disease. Int J Mol Sci. 2023 Apr 15;24(8):7318. doi: 10.3390/ijms24087318. PMID: 37108480; PMCID: PMC10139089.

Fu J, Zheng Y, Gao Y, Xu W. Dietary Fiber Intake and Gut Microbiota in Human Health. Microorganisms. 2022 Dec 18;10(12):2507. doi: 10.3390/microorganisms10122507. PMID: 36557760; PMCID: PMC9787832.

Ghaseminejad-Raeini A, Ghaderi A, Sharafi A, Nematollahi-Sani B, Moossavi M, Derakhshani A, Sarab GA. Immunomodulatory actions of vitamin D in various immune-related disorders: a comprehensive review. Front Immunol. 2023 Jul 14;14:950465. doi: 10.3389/fimmu.2023.950465. PMID: 37520529; PMCID: PMC10379649.

Golovinskaia O, Wang CK. Review of Functional and Pharmacological Activities of Berries. Molecules. 2021 Jun 25;26(13):3904. doi: 10.3390/molecules26133904. PMID: 34202412; PMCID: PMC8271923.

Hamelers IH, Steenbergh PH. Interactions between estrogen and insulin-like growth factor signaling pathways in human breast tumor cells. Endocr Relat Cancer. 2003 Jun;10(2):331-45. doi: 10.1677/erc.0.0100331. PMID: 12790794.

Hertzler SR, Lieblein-Boff JC, Weiler M, Allgeier C. Plant Proteins: Assessing Their Nutritional Quality and Effects on Health and Physical Function. Nutrients. 2020 Nov 30;12(12):3704. doi: 10.3390/nu12123704. PMID: 33266120; PMCID: PMC7760812.

Hiatt RA, Clayton MF, Collins KK, Gold HT, Laiyemo AO, Truesdale KP, Ritzwoller DP. The Pathways to Prevention program: nutrition as prevention for improved cancer outcomes. J Natl Cancer Inst. 2023 Aug 8;115(8):886-895. doi: 10.1093/jnci/djad079. PMID: 37212639; PMCID: PMC10407697.

Hodges RE, Minich DM. Modulation of Metabolic Detoxification Pathways Using Foods and Food-Derived Components: A Scientific Review with Clinical Application. J Nutr Metab. 2015;2015:760689. doi: 10.1155/2015/760689. Epub 2015 Jun 16. PMID: 26167297; PMCID: PMC4488002.

Hossain MS, Wazed MA, Asha S, Amin MR, Shimul IM. Dietary Phytochemicals in Health and Disease: Mechanisms, Clinical Evidence, and Applications-A Comprehensive Review. Food Sci Nutr. 2025 Mar 19;13(3):e70101. doi: 10.1002/fsn3.70101. PMID: 40115248; PMCID: PMC11922683.

Hwa YL, Kull MR. The why and how of maintaining hydration during cancer therapy. Curr Opin Support Palliat Care. 2020 Dec;14(4):324-332. doi: 10.1097/SPC.0000000000000526. PMID: 33009008.

Jeong M, Collins N. Nutritional modulation of antitumor immunity. Curr Opin Immunol. 2024 Apr;87:102422. doi: 10.1016/j.coi.2024.102422. Epub 2024 May 9. PMID: 38728931; PMCID: PMC11288377.

Kapała A, Szlendak M, Motacka E. The Anti-Cancer Activity of Lycopene: A Systematic Review of Human and Animal Studies. Nutrients. 2022 Dec 3;14(23):5152. doi: 10.3390/nu14235152. PMID: 36501182; PMCID: PMC9741066.

Karthikayan A, Sureshkumar S, Kadambari D, Vijayakumar C. Low serum 25-hydroxy vitamin D levels are associated with aggressive breast cancer variants and poor prognostic factors in patients with breast carcinoma. Arch Endocrinol Metab. 2018 Aug;62(4):452-459. doi: 10.20945/2359-3997000000062. PMID: 30304110; PMCID: PMC10118730.

Kerschbaum E, Nüssler V. Cancer Prevention with Nutrition and Lifestyle. Visc Med. 2019 Aug;35(4):204-209. doi: 10.1159/000501776. Epub 2019 Jul 23. PMID: 31602380; PMCID: PMC6738231.

Kiousi DE, Kouroutzidou AZ, Neanidis K, Karavanis E, Matthaios D, Pappa A, Galanis A. The Role of the Gut Microbiome in Cancer Immunotherapy: Current Knowledge and Future Directions. Cancers (Basel). 2023 Mar 31;15(7):2101. doi: 10.3390/cancers15072101. PMID: 37046762; PMCID: PMC10093606.

Klek S, Laviano A, Chrostek H, Cardenas D. Nutrition in Oncology: Overcoming Challenges to Optimize the Patient Journey from Prehabilitation to Rehabilitation. Oncol Ther. 2025 Sep;13(3):577-593. doi: 10.1007/s40487-025-00358-y. Epub 2025 Jul 11. PMID: 40643833; PMCID: PMC12378855.

Krupa KN, Fritz K, Parmar M. Omega-3 Fatty Acids. [Updated 2024 Feb 28]. In: StatPearls [Internet]. Treasure Island (FL): StatPearls Publishing; 2025 Jan-. Available from: https://www.ncbi.nlm.nih.gov/books/NBK564314/

Lampe JW. Diet and Cancer Prevention Research: From Mechanism to Implementation. J Cancer Prev. 2020 Jun 30;25(2):65-69. doi: 10.15430/JCP.2020.25.2.65. PMID: 32647647; PMCID: PMC7337006.

Loman BR, Luo M, Baggs GE, Mitchell DC, Nelson JL, Ziegler TR, Deutz NE, Matarese LE; NOURISH Study Group. Specialized High-Protein Oral Nutrition Supplement Improves Home Nutrient Intake of Malnourished Older Adults Without Decreasing Usual Food Intake. JPEN J Parenter Enteral Nutr. 2019 Aug;43(6):794-802. doi: 10.1002/jpen.1467. Epub 2018 Nov 22. PMID: 30565718; PMCID: PMC6924274.

Messina MJ, Wood CE. Soy isoflavones, estrogen therapy, and breast cancer risk: analysis and commentary. Nutr J. 2008 Jun 3;7:17. doi: 10.1186/1475-2891-7-17. PMID: 18522734; PMCID: PMC2443803.

Milliron BJ, Packel L, Dychtwald D, Klobodu C, Pontiggia L, Ogbogu O, Barksdale B, Deutsch J. When Eating Becomes Torturous: Understanding Nutrition-Related Cancer Treatment Side Effects among Individuals with Cancer and Their Caregivers. Nutrients. 2022 Jan 14;14(2):356. doi: 10.3390/nu14020356. PMID: 35057538; PMCID: PMC8781744.

Mirmiran P, Bahadoran Z, Gaeini Z. Common Limitations and Challenges of Dietary Clinical Trials for Translation into Clinical Practices. Int J Endocrinol Metab. 2021 May 1;19(3):e108170. doi: 10.5812/ijem.108170. PMID: 34567133; PMCID: PMC8453651.

Mittelman SD. The Role of Diet in Cancer Prevention and Chemotherapy Efficacy. Annu Rev Nutr. 2020 Sep 23;40:273-297. doi: 10.1146/annurev-nutr-013120-041149. Epub 2020 Jun 16. PMID: 32543948; PMCID: PMC8546934.

Narimatsu H, Yaguchi YT. The Role of Diet and Nutrition in Cancer: Prevention, Treatment, and Survival. Nutrients. 2022 Aug 14;14(16):3329. doi: 10.3390/nu14163329. PMID: 36014835; PMCID: PMC9414571.

Ottaiano A, Ianniello M, Santorsola M, Ruggiero R, Sirica R, Sabbatino F, Perri F, Cascella M, Di Marzo M, Berretta M, Caraglia M, Nasti G, Savarese G. From Chaos to Opportunity: Decoding Cancer Heterogeneity for Enhanced Treatment Strategies. Biology (Basel). 2023 Aug 29;12(9):1183. doi: 10.3390/biology12091183. PMID: 37759584; PMCID: PMC10525472.

Paradisi G, Smith L, Burtner C, Leaming R, Garvey WT, Hook G, Johnson A, Cronin J, Steinberg HO, Baron AD. Dual energy X-ray absorptiometry assessment of fat mass distribution and its association with the insulin resistance syndrome. Diabetes Care. 1999 Aug;22(8):1310-7. doi: 10.2337/diacare.22.8.1310. PMID: 10480776.

Passaro A, Al Bakir M, Hamilton EG, Diehn M, André F, Roy-Chowdhuri S, Mountzios G, Wistuba II, Swanton C, Peters S. Cancer biomarkers: Emerging trends and clinical implications for personalized treatment. Cell. 2024 Mar 28;187(7):1617-1635. doi: 10.1016/j.cell.2024.02.041. PMID: 38552610; PMCID: PMC7616034.

Pavlicek R, Cradock KA. Behaviour change techniques, intervention features and usability of diet apps. Prev Med Rep. 2025 May 2;54:103085. doi: 10.1016/j.pmedr.2025.103085. Erratum in: Prev Med Rep. 2025 May 30;55:103121. doi: 10.1016/j.pmedr.2025.103121. PMID: 40458474; PMCID: PMC12127858.

Pendergast FJ, Ridgers ND, Worsley A, McNaughton SA. Evaluation of a smartphone food diary application using objectively measured energy expenditure. Int J Behav Nutr Phys Act. 2017 Mar 14;14(1):30. doi: 10.1186/s12966-017-0488-9. PMID: 28288657; PMCID: PMC5348892.

Picó C, Serra F, Rodríguez AM, Keijer J, Palou A. Biomarkers of Nutrition and Health: New Tools for New Approaches. Nutrients. 2019 May 16;11(5):1092. doi: 10.3390/nu11051092. PMID: 31100942; PMCID: PMC6567133.

Reuter S, Gupta SC, Chaturvedi MM, Aggarwal BB. Oxidative stress, inflammation, and cancer: how are they linked? Free Radic Biol Med. 2010 Dec 1;49(11):1603-16. doi: 10.1016/j.freeradbiomed.2010.09.006. Epub 2010 Sep 16. PMID: 20840865; PMCID: PMC2990475.

Shakhshir MH, Salameh HT, Amer R, Zyoud SH. An evaluation of nutritional impact symptoms and their association with reduced dietary intake in patients with solid tumors at tertiary care hospitals: a multicenter, cross-sectional study from palestine. BMC Cancer. 2024 Apr 25;24(1):524. doi: 10.1186/s12885-024-12289-4. PMID: 38664802; PMCID: PMC11046763.

Singh BN, Shankar S, Srivastava RK. Green tea catechin, epigallocatechin-3-gallate (EGCG): mechanisms, perspectives and clinical applications. Biochem Pharmacol. 2011 Dec 15;82(12):1807-21. doi: 10.1016/j.bcp.2011.07.093. Epub 2011 Jul 30. PMID: 21827739; PMCID: PMC4082721.

Song B, Wang W, Tang X, Goh RMW, Thuya WL, Ho PCL, Chen L, Wang L. Inhibitory Potential of Resveratrol in Cancer Metastasis: From Biology to Therapy. Cancers (Basel). 2023 May 14;15(10):2758. doi: 10.3390/cancers15102758. PMID: 37345095; PMCID: PMC10216034.

Story EN, Kopec RE, Schwartz SJ, Harris GK. An update on the health effects of tomato lycopene. Annu Rev Food Sci Technol. 2010;1:189-210. doi: 10.1146/annurev.food.102308.124120. PMID: 22129335; PMCID: PMC3850026.

Thomsen M, Kersten C, Sorbye H, Skovlund E, Glimelius B, Pfeiffer P, Johansen JS, Kure EH, Ikdahl T, Tveit KM, Christoffersen T, Guren TK. Interleukin-6 and C-reactive protein as prognostic biomarkers in metastatic colorectal cancer. Oncotarget. 2016 Nov 15;7(46):75013-75022. doi: 10.18632/oncotarget.12601. PMID: 27738330; PMCID: PMC5342719.

Trabelsi K, Ammar A, Boujelbane MA, Puce L, Garbarino S, Scoditti E, Boukhris O, Khanfir S, Clark CCT, Glenn JM, Alhaj OA, Jahrami H, Chtourou H, Bragazzi NL. Religious fasting and its impacts on individual, public, and planetary health: Fasting as a "religious health asset" for a healthier, more equitable, and sustainable society. Front Nutr. 2022 Nov 24;9:1036496. doi: 10.3389/fnut.2022.1036496. PMID: 36505246; PMCID: PMC9729557.

Vliet SV, Beals JW, Martinez IG, Skinner SK, Burd NA. Achieving Optimal Post-Exercise Muscle Protein Remodeling in Physically Active Adults through Whole Food Consumption. Nutrients. 2018 Feb 16;10(2):224. doi: 10.3390/nu10020224. PMID: 29462924; PMCID: PMC5852800.

Wan L, Tan HL, Thomas-Ahner JM, Pearl DK, Erdman JW Jr, Moran NE, Clinton SK. Dietary tomato and lycopene impact androgen signaling- and carcinogenesis-related gene expression during early TRAMP prostate carcinogenesis. Cancer Prev Res (Phila). 2014 Dec;7(12):1228-39. doi: 10.1158/1940-6207.CAPR-14-0182. Epub 2014 Oct 14. PMID: 25315431; PMCID: PMC4259248.

Yin R, Kuo HC, Hudlikar R, Sargsyan D, Li S, Wang L, Wu R, Kong AN. Gut microbiota, dietary phytochemicals and benefits to human health. Curr Pharmacol Rep. 2019;5:332-344. doi: 10.1007/s40495-019-00196-3. Epub 2019 Aug 19. PMID: 33224717; PMCID: PMC7678755.

Zanetti M, Gortan Cappellari G, Barazzoni R, Sanson G. The Impact of Protein Supplementation Targeted at Improving Muscle Mass on Strength in Cancer Patients: A Scoping Review. Nutrients. 2020 Jul 16;12(7):2099. doi: 10.3390/nu12072099. PMID: 32708527; PMCID: PMC7400018.

Zhang AMY, Wellberg EA, Kopp JL, Johnson JD. Hyperinsulinemia in Obesity, Inflammation, and Cancer. Diabetes Metab J. 2021 May;45(3):285-311. doi: 10.4093/dmj.2020.0250. Epub 2021 Mar 29. Erratum in: Diabetes Metab J. 2021 Jul;45(4):622. doi: 10.4093/dmj.2021.0131. PMID: 33775061; PMCID: PMC8164941.

Chapter 16

Emerging Paradigms: Future Directions in Nutritional Oncology Research

Sarfraj Ahmad Siddiqui[1], Praneeth Juvvi[2*], Sheetanshu Gupta[3], and Ng. Joykumar Singh[4]

[1]Department of Biochemistry, King George's Medical University, U.P., India
[2]Department of Food Processing Technology, College of Food Technology-Central Agricultural University, Imphal, Manipur, India
[3]Department of Food Safety and Quality Assurance, College of Food Technology, Central Agricultural University (CAU), Imphal, Manipur, India
[4]Department of Food Process Engineering, College of Food Technology, Central Agricultural University (CAU), Imphal, Manipur, India

Abstract

Nutritional oncology evolves rapidly, driven by increasing insight into the diet's profound impact on cancer biology and cancer prevention outcomes vary greatly nowadays. Pioneering breakthroughs redefine cancer treatments via novel nutrition regimens rapidly under newly emerging frameworks, and inventive strategies are being implemented. Research on molecular mechanisms linking diet and tumour progression yields novel insights into epigenetics and metabolic reprogramming of the gut microbiome rapidly. Genetic microbiome profiling and metabolic analysis optimize treatment efficacy nowadays by tailoring dietary recommendations with great precision, very frequently. Novel dietary regimens such as intermittent fasting and ketogenic diets, alongside nutraceuticals, are explored deeply for synergising with traditional cancer treatments and significantly lowering recurrence rates. Examining bioinformatics advances alongside systems biology enables sophisticated diet-cancer interaction models incorporating rather recondite precision medicine techniques. Forthcoming clinical trials heavily emphasise validating the dietary intervention survivorship impact after cancer diagnosis. New therapeutic avenues emerge rapidly in nutritional oncology as gaps in knowledge are identified and current trends synthesized revealing exciting possibilities.

Keywords: Nutritional Genomics, Microbiome, Personalized Nutrition, Cancer Metabolism, Epigenetics, Artificial Intelligence

DOI: 10.1201/9781042010387-16

1. Introduction

Nutritional oncology lately has garnered significant attention by probing deeply complex interplays between dietary habits and diverse cancer forms. Recognition of nutrition's role in cancer prevention and treatment evolves swiftly, while understanding of cancer biology undergoes rapid mutation. Novel findings progressively unveil a deep influence of nutritional elements on cancer cell behavior and therapeutic results in patients with diverse malignancies. Novel paradigms and cutting-edge technologies are revolutionising cancer care at a pivotal moment for the rapidly evolving field of nutritional oncology. Tremendous growth has lately manifested in nutritional oncology research with emerging trends poised to revolutionise increasing fields fairly rapidly now. Studies on cancer and nutrition have mostly focused on prevention through diet, identifying certain foods and nutrients that could potentially lower risk.

Studies nowadays yield valuable insights yet often merely correlate diet with cancer risk substantially under various extremely complicated circumstances. A significant shift has occurred recently exploring interactions between dietary components and various cellular processes that influence cancer initiation and progression quite starkly. Mechanistic approaches are radically altering nutritional oncology nowadays by offering highly modified targeted therapeutic strategies rather than fairly generic dietary advice. Nutrigenomics and nutrigenetics integration significantly impacts cancer risk and treatment outcomes amidst emerging nutritional oncology paradigms fairly nowadays. Scientists gain profoundly deeper insight into how genetic quirks heavily influence individual responses to varied dietary regimens with next-generation sequencing tech advancements rapidly nowadays.

Specific genetic variations related to processing omega-3 fatty acids and folate metabolism greatly impact efficacy of dietary cancer prevention measures. Precision nutrition involves tailoring dietary recommendations rather specifically according to a person's genetic makeup and various cancer risk factors very rapidly. Tailored strategies rather quietly amplify cancer treatment efficacy and significantly enhance patient outcomes over an extended period naturally. Emerging focus in nutritional oncology highlights gut microbiome's enigmatic influence on cancer progression alongside efficacy of assorted treatment modalities remarkably. Trillions of microbes inhabit human gut microbiome fairly effectively regulating metabolism and immune function nowadays with crucial roles. Evidence mounts rapidly that microbiome profoundly influences drug metabolism tumour progression and broadly impacts immune surveillance in complex physiological contexts.

Prebiotics found in whole grains and probiotics present in fermented foods greatly support a healthy microbiome and potentially enhance cancer treatment outcomes remarkably. Dietary tweaks drastically reshape microbiome hence potentially influence cancer progression in a super promising research direction for nutritional oncology. Cancer cells display wildly aberrant metabolic routes representing a fascinating frontier in oncology connected to dietary habits fairly recently. Cancer cells exhibit drastically altered metabolism characterized by reliance on glycolysis despite abundant oxygen and heightened demand for nutrients fueling rapid proliferation. Cancer hallmark involves peculiar metabolic shift presenting uniquely ripe opportunity suddenly for novel interventions via diet.

Researchers investigate how cancer cell metabolism reacts quite effectively to dietary tactics such as severe caloric restriction or ketogenic diet inclusion. Emerging evidence indicates profoundly altering diet can markedly impede tumour growth and sensitize cancer cells extremely to chemotherapy meanwhile inhibiting metabolism. Rapidly evolving this field could yield novel cancer therapies quite effectively by integrating dietary strategies into care alongside traditional treatment modalities.

Epigenetics has emerged rather centrally in cancer research as study of gene expression changes without DNA sequence alteration underlying them. Bioactive compounds and vitamins alongside minerals present in food have been shown influencing epigenetic modifications such as histone mods and DNA methylation heavily. Dietary interventions might possibly tweak genes fueling cancer progression quietly thereby reversing aberrant epigenetic changes linked with various forms of cancer underground. Phytonutrients present rather abundantly in cruciferous veggies berries and green tea may effectively prevent or reverse epigenetic changes leading cancer. Future research in nutritional oncology will heavily rely on well-designed trials that effectively evaluate various dietary interventions during cancer treatment rigorously.

Nutritional assessments in clinical trials allow researchers grasp pretty effectively how diet interacts with cancer therapies such as dodgy chemotherapy. Evaluating cancer survivors quite thoroughly remains crucial for overall quality of life and prevention of recurrence after dietary interventions. Nutritional interventions are gaining recognition rapidly as vital parts of cancer care, and soon needs for evidence-based guidelines will become critically imperative. Nutritional oncology lately is embracing concept of food systems and their quite significant role in public health maintenance rather slowly. Societal and environmental factors such as socioeconomic status and dubious food production practices heavily influence cancer risk nowadays apparently everywhere. Restructuring food systems at population level for cancer prevention and investigating broader factors shaping dietary patterns is crucial nowadays quite evidently.

Nationwide cancer risk reduction efforts will significantly benefit from boosting availability of nutrient-dense foods in underserved areas and tackling food access disparities effectively. Diverse perspectives from genomics and microbiome research alongside epigenetics will be crucial for grasping diet's potential in cancer treatment fully nowadays. Nutritional oncology research hurtles into an extremely exhilarating phase where science of food metabolism genetics and cancer converge creating rather modified cancer therapies effectively. Emerging paradigms in nutritional oncology will be probed deeply offering fresh perspectives on future research trajectories that promise revolutionizing cancer comprehension and forging innovative evidence-backed stratagems for cancer prophylaxis treatment and survivorship endeavors.

2. Advances in Nutritional Genomics

Nutritional genomics emerges quite intricately as transformative science fusing nutrition and molecular biology with fascinating complexity slowly unfolding in obscure ways. Genetic variations influence nutrient metabolism rather profoundly and specific dietary components tweak gene expression remarkably under certain peculiar physiological conditions. Significant insights gained in oncology reveal cancer risk progression hinges on genome exposome interplay involving dietary habits and epigenetic factors deeply. Nutritional recommendations have long relied heavily on broad guidelines geared towards population level needs rather than specifics of individual cases. Substantial variability in nutrient requirements and metabolic responses amongst individuals with differing disease susceptibility rates is often quietly overlooked by this approach. Polymorphisms in genes such as MTHFR and FTO rather profoundly affect individual metabolic handling of folate and energy variably.

Oncology variations might badly affect cancer risk and alter treatment toxicity profiles thereby undermining overall survivorship outcomes in a quite significant manner. Nutritional genomics applied in cancer care offers promising pathways toward rather personalized dietary regimens aligning subtly with individual's peculiar genetic profile and tumour biology. Patients harbouring MTHFR polymorphisms potentially benefit from highly bioavailable folate forms whereas individuals with pro-inflammatory genotypes respond remarkably well to omega-3 fatty acid rich diets. Genomic insights remarkably inform nutritional support composition during treatment and remarkably aid recovery afterwards with substantial effectiveness subsequently. Nutritional genomics foundational principles and cutting-edge research on gene-diet interactions relevant to cancer development are examined alongside practical applications in clinical nutrition settings vigorously. Precision oncology evolves rapidly and stands poised redefining diet's role enabling biologically tailored interventions that enhance cancer survivorship care treatment efficacy greatly.

2.1. Understanding Nutritional Genomics

Nutritional genomics evolves rapidly as it seeks grasping individual genetic makeup's interaction with diet profoundly influencing health outcomes and disease risk. Nutrigenetics and nutrigenomics offer modified insights into tailored nutrition plans mainly for cancer prevention in rather complex biological contexts. Nutrigenetics probes deeply into how quirky single nucleotide polymorphisms drastically affect individual responses to certain nutrients in vastly different ways. Polymorphisms can tweak enzyme activity rather dramatically thereby skewing metabolic pathways linked oxidative stress and carcinogen metabolism very subtly inside cells. Variants in MTHFR gene pretty badly impair folate metabolism and DNA methylation thereby potentially elevating cancer risk whereas GST polymorphisms significantly reduce detoxification capacity of some nasty carcinogens. Clinicians nowadays tailor nutrient intake very precisely according largely to individual genetic predispositions and varying metabolic requirements.

Nutrigenomics delves deeply into epigenetic modifications of gene expression via DNA methylation and histone acetylation by nutrients and bioactive compounds. Reversible epigenetic changes occur under specific dietary conditions offering potential targets for nutritional intervention in cell cycle regulatory pathways deeply implicated in cancer. Sulforaphane and curcumin pretty significantly alter gene expression through various epigenetic mechanisms involving modifications evidently in different cellular contexts. Nutrigenetics and nutrigenomics furnish foundational knowledge for grasping variability in individual responses somewhat differently to specific dietary interventions pretty much always. Researchers illuminate diverse reactions extensively to standardize dietary regimens and highlight modulating carcinogenic processes rather effectively at molecular level.

2.2. Genetic Variants and Cancer-Related Nutritional Needs

Scientists currently pinpoint particular genetic variants that modulate metabolic processes and heavily influence cancer risk through whole genome sequencing and extensive epigenomic analysis. Nutritional interventions informed by gene insights potentially mitigate risk and enhance outcomes effectively with considerable therapeutic benefits downstream . Methylenetetrahydrofolate reductase gene facilitates DNA methylation pretty effectively in one-carbon metabolism playing a somewhat crucial albeit obscure role. Genetic variations such as C677T and A1298C drastically impair MTHFR enzyme function leading to substantially raised homocysteine levels and hypomethylation of sundry oncogenes. Individuals possessing such genetic variants might benefit enormously from eating folate rich foods naturally like leafy greens rather than taking synthetic folic acid supplements. GSTM1 and GSTT1 encode enzymes crucial for xenobiotic metabolism in glutathione S-transferase family normally vital for various detoxification processes.

Homozygous gene deletions severely impair detoxification capacity and neutralization of oxidative stress occurs poorly under such hapless circumstances rather slowly. Folks sporting certain genetic quirks may reap huge benefits from chomping down cruciferous veggies such as broccoli packed with isothiocyanates that crank up alternative detox routes. Apolipoprotein E polymorphisms specifically ε2, ε3 and ε4 alleles significantly sway lipid metabolism inflammation and oxidative stress in cancers driven hormonally. People carrying APOE ε4 allele may show heightened susceptibility to saturated fat intake ratcheting up prostate or breast cancer risk substantially. Dietary recommendations sometimes prioritize consumption of mono and polyunsaturated fats over saturated ones quite heavily in specific cases apparently. Clinicians proactively pinpoint metabolic vulnerabilities and devise highly individualized dietary plans dovetailing effectively with oncologic risks and varied therapeutic outcomes.

2.3. Epigenetics:

Epigenetic regulation plays a pivotal albeit subtle role in carcinogenesis by influencing gene expression without messing with underlying DNA sequence. DNA methylation histone modification and non-coding RNA expression are dynamic reversible processes offering sundry targets for dietary interventions rather interestingly apparently. Emerging evidence underscores that certain bioactive dietary compounds profoundly influence epigenome thereby altering expression of various oncogenes and tumour suppressor genes heavily involved in carcinogenesis. Sulforaphane a naturally occurring isothiocyanate found in cruciferous veggies like broccoli gets studied pretty thoroughly by various researchers nowadays. Sulforaphane pretty effectively inhibits histone deacetylases thereby boosting histone acetylation and ramping up transcription of tumour suppressor genes like Nrf2 and p21.

Epigenetic changes drastically promote apoptosis in various cancer models and reduce cell proliferation rates significantly overall in most cases. Curcumin's principal polyphenol modulates DNA methyltransferases and HDACs thereby reactivating epigenetically silenced tumour suppressor genes such as p53 or PTEN in turmeric. Curcumin profoundly alters histone acetylation patterns remarkably and influences signaling pathways such as NF-κB which are pivotal in inflammation-driven cancers. Polyphenols like epigallocatechin-3-gallate in green tea and resveratrol in grapes exert epigenetic effects alongside anthocyanins quite frequently. Cell cycle apoptosis and immune response are affected quite profoundly downstream by regulation of MicroRNA expression via these compounds.

EGCG suppresses oncogenic miR-21 pretty effectively while upregulating tumour-suppressive miRNAs thereby fairly significantly enhancing anti-cancer response in a major way. Diet acts as an epigenetic reprogramming tool modulating gene expression fairly complementary to conventional therapies supporting these findings collectively. Epigenome-targeting nutritional strategies may drastically slash cancer risk and sensitize tumours for treatment, thereby encourage diet's value as non-invasive precision modality.

2.4. Nutritional Genomics in Cancer Therapy and Survivorship

Nutritional genomics integration into cancer care goes far beyond prevention offering unusually significant promise during active treatment phases and survives long term. Clinicians can decipher complex gene-nutrient interactions pretty effectively thereby encourage therapeutic efficacy and mitigating adverse effects with remarkable specificity. Nutrient metabolism and efficacy of certain drugs are affected by genetic variability during cancer treatment with diverse dietary compounds in patients. Genetic variations in certain enzymes notably CYP450 family members heavily influence tolerance of chemotherapeutic agents like methotrexate during drug metabolism processes. Tailoring nutritional interventions remarkably boosts patient outcomes and drastically cuts toxicity associated with distinct genomic profiles.

Gene-diet interactions involving inflammatory cytokines such as IL-6 or TNF-α might facilitate selection of anti-inflammatory nutrients modulating systemic inflammation effectively during therapy. Nutrition goals markedly shift toward promoting metabolic recovery and managing comorbid conditions like obesity and cardiovascular disease during post-treatment survivorship. Genomic data guides peculiar dietary habits pretty well based on individual susceptibility to malnutrition or risk for dyslipidemia pretty unusually. People with polymorphisms affecting lipid metabolism like APOE4 may benefit from tweaking fat quality but those with GST variants might need higher nutrient doses supporting detoxification pathways.

Epigenetic memory forged during cancer therapy profoundly influences gene expression long after treatment ostensibly terminates quite abruptly afterwards. Diets rich in methyl donors polyphenols and omega-3 fatty acids very effectively restore gene expression and maintain anti-inflammatory cellular states. Nutritional genomics provides a somewhat potent framework quite remarkably for tailoring dietary interventions across various cancer stages boosting therapy efficacy.

a. During Treatment

Active cancer treatment such as chemo or radiotherapy often entails profound metabolic stress and severe systemic inflammation with drastically altered nutrient demands frequently. Nutritional management must adapt rapidly during this phase responding keenly to physiological shifts and unique genetic quirks influencing treatment efficacy very differently now. Dihydropyrimidine dehydrogenase or DPYD metabolizes fluoropyrimidines such as capecitabine and 5-fluorouracil pretty significantly in gene-nutrient interactions. Individuals possessing specific DPYD variants often exhibit severely reduced enzyme function resulting in accumulation of toxic byproducts and heinous adverse reactions such as mucositis or neurotoxicity. Nutritional interventions may necessitate fairly radical adjustments in oral intake for patients coping with nasty side effects ensuring they stay hydrated with soft-textured nutrient-dense foods.

Genetic variation in taste perception genes such as TAS2R38 which encodes bitter taste receptors can sway food preferences drastically during cancer treatment. Veggies like broccoli and Brussels sprouts normally packed with beneficial phytochemicals are bitterly avoided by extremely sensitive patients for their health. Dietitians utilize knowledge of sensory-related genotypes quite effectively to select nutrient-rich food alternatives and promote adherence readily. Treatment-induced symptoms such as anorexia interact very badly with underlying nutrigenetic issues affecting appetite regulation pretty negatively messing with nutrient absorption mechanisms.

Genetic variations in IL-1β and TNF-α gene potentially amplify pro-inflammatory conditions warranting consumption of foods rich in omega-3 fatty acids. Ultimately healthcare providers tailor nutrition strategies quite effectively during treatment incorporating genomic insights that mitigate really nasty adverse effects. Highly personalized dietary support is required essentially during this vulnerable phase to preserve patient quality of life and optimize treatment outcomes.

b. Post-Treatment and Long-Term Survivorship

Patients enter a precarious phase after wrapping up aggressive cancer treatment and focus on protracted recuperation staving off recurrence very slowly. Latent frailties surface pretty frequently during this stage in individuals harbouring specific genetic predispositions and facing risk of severe metabolic derangement. Survivors harboring peculiar genetic polymorphisms linked to metabolic regulation like FTO gene or TCF7L2 face considerably heightened risk of insulin resistance and obesity negatively influencing cancer recurrence. Tailor-made anti-inflammatory meal plans prove vital in peculiar cases with beneficial effects emerging slowly over time rather unusually. Phytonutrient-rich diets remarkably lower inflammatory biomarkers such as C-reactive protein alongside omega-3 fatty acids and low-glycemic index carbs. Such diets mitigate chronic low-grade inflammation thereby supporting cellular homeostasis extensively and encourage immune surveillance quite effectively across various physiological conditions.

Targeted nutritional supplementation might be necessary based on genetic assessments and biochemical evaluations to optimize nutrient status or address severe deficiencies quickly. Individuals possessing specific vitamin D receptor gene variants frequently exhibit aberrant processing necessitating supplementation via highly bioavailable formulations on occasion. Omega-3 fatty acid supplementation might greatly benefit individuals harbouring specific FADS gene variants severely impeding endogenous fatty acid conversion processes naturally. Clinicians modify interventions effectively over time by tracking serum 25(OH)D levels and various inflammatory markers with fairly good precision usually. Modified precision-based strategies remarkably equip survivors with effective tools for managing long-term health over protracted periods of time quite effectively. Nutritional genomics substantially enhance survivorship yielding rather effective science-driven nutrition strategies against cancer recurrence and various comorbid conditions often simultaneously.

2.5. The Role of Multi-Omics and Technology

Multi-omics tech encompassing genomics transcriptomics metabolomics proteomics and microbiomics has revolutionized understanding of diet interactions with cancer biology at a systems level. Integrative approaches yield novel insights into molecular mechanisms underlying individual responses to dietary interventions enabling precision oncology nutrition research rather quietly nowadays. Metabolomics facilitates discovery of distinctive metabolic fingerprints linked with dietary consumption and tumour metabolic processes fairly easily these days. Researchers detect disruptions in key metabolic pathways such as glycolysis by scrutinizing small-molecule metabolites present in blood samples quite thoroughly. Optimizing fat intake versus carbohydrate consumption fine-tunes dietary macronutrient ratios in patients with wonky glucose or lipid profiles somewhat effectively.

Microbiome profiling amplifies personalization by starkly revealing gut microbial communities often profound influence on nutrient metabolism alongside sheer inflammation. Dysbiosis or reduced microbial diversity has been tenuously linked to pretty dismal cancer outcomes and markedly impaired efficacy of various therapies. Targeted prebiotic interventions and probiotic treatments can significantly improve metabolic function and reduce pro-tumourigenic signals by modulating gut microbiome effectively. New developments are happening fast making real-time adaptive nutrition management fairly feasible these days with emerging tech advancements underway rapidly. Wearable sensors track bodily functions pretty deeply now monitoring physiological responses like heart rate variability or glucose levels with uncanny accuracy. AI-powered dietary tracking apps rapidly adjust plans in response to biological markers and quirky symptom patterns exhibited by patient behavior. Multi-omics and digital tools meld together rather intricately forming a foundation for systems biology approach in cancer nutrition care. Cancer nutrition gets pretty tailored with this model that caters dynamically evolving interventions reflecting a patient's current biological profile and current clinical situation quite effectively.

2.6. Ethical, Practical, and Accessibility Considerations

Nutritional genomics holds vast potential in oncology yet navigating thorny ethical economic and tricky educational conundrums very carefully necessitates broad clinical uptake. Major concerns swirl around hefty expenditure and somewhat poky accessibility these days awkwardly in many places. Genetic testing and multi-omics analysis stays prohibitively costly nowadays for many patients hailing from rural or ridiculously under-resourced settings. Innovations of this sort risk amplifying existing inequities in healthcare provision absent subsidized schemes or swift assimilation into national public health frameworks. Various ethical considerations surrounding genomic data privacy are paramount especially nowadays. Robust safeguards must be firmly in place protecting patient confidentiality as clinicians daily amass sensitive genetic data and scrutinize it. Vital guidelines surrounding data ownership and transparency of usage uphold trust and lofty ethics pretty well in shaky clinical settings normally.

Patients and healthcare providers still face a pretty formidable challenge regarding health literacy pretty much everywhere nowadays. Translating genetic data into actionable nutrition guidance necessitates esoteric expertise often sorely lacking across diverse healthcare cohorts in various understaffed clinical settings. Misinterpretation of genomic data could precipitously lead to anxiety or drastic dietary changes unnecessarily at times somewhat inexplicably. Genomics-informed nutrition counseling now requires interdisciplinary education and training that underscores its crucial importance in present times markedly.

Nationwide efforts should simultaneously focus on democratizing genomic tools through development of low-cost testing and multilingual educational materials. AI-based decision support systems and digital health tech can rapidly spit out salivating dietary blueprints and bridge yawning knowledge chasms effectively nowadays. Nutritional genomics spearheads radical change in cancer treatment morphing populous static dietary guidelines into modified therapeutic regimens informed by genes suddenly. Illuminating complex nutrient-genome dynamics enables precision nutrition tailored rather intricately with each patient's remarkably distinct biological configuration. Nutritional genomics will profoundly shape cancer prevention and treatment as access barriers crumble now and comprehension slowly gains considerable traction.

3. The Role of the Microbiome in Cancer Prevention and Treatment

Human microbiome has emerged remarkably fast as crucial arbiter of overall health quietly exerting a profound sway over immune function and genetic expression. Evidence mounting rapidly suggests microbiome acts as modulator of cancer risk and determinant of therapeutic efficacy garnering significant attention in oncology lately. Interactions between host microorganisms and dietary factors bidirectionally influence carcinogenesis and body's response to radiotherapy and other therapies somewhat variably. Tumour development gets triggered pretty rapidly by alterations in microbial diversity through chronic inflammation and genotoxic metabolite production. Microbiome diversity fosters protective metabolic pathways and mediates potent anti-tumour effects while encourage mucosal immunity very effectively underneath epithelial layers.

3.1. Microbiome Overview

Trillions of microorganisms including bacteria fungi and archaea thrive very remarkably within human gut alongside protozoa and various kinds of viruses. Microbial ecosystems co-evolved stupendously with various hosts over a long period and now play quite an ostensibly crucial role in human bodily functions. Microbiome functions rather like another bodily system carrying out diverse biochemical processes vital for maintaining overall health and preventing sundry maladies. Fermentation of recalcitrant dietary fibres occurs pretty rapidly within gut regions yielding short-chain fatty acids like butyrate and acetate mostly. SCFAs energetically fuel colonocytes and enhance mucosal barrier function while exerting profoundly anti-inflammatory effects via regulatory T cell modulation.

Microbiome synthesizes essential vitamins like K and B-group fairly readily and produces neurotransmitters such as serotonin systemically across various bodily systems. A diverse microbiota fosters maturation of immune system particularly early in life and maintains integrity of epithelial barrier preventing translocation of pathogens. Detoxification of heterocyclic amines and polycyclic aromatic hydrocarbons happens simultaneously with biotransformation of carcinogens present in daily consumed food. Pro-inflammatory signaling pathways get suppressed thereby reducing oxidative stress quite significantly and subsequently fostering a decrease in cellular damage overall. Reduced microbial diversity coupled with rampant pathobiont overgrowth can spark chronic inflammation and severely compromise intestinal barrier functionality suddenly. Dysbiosis fosters genotoxic metabolite production pretty readily and significantly exacerbates cellular damage over fairly long periods. Dietary probiotic and prebiotic interventions remarkably advance cancer prevention and therapy by restoring balance and function of microbes quite effectively.

3.2. Microbiome and Cancer Prevention

Increasing data troves nowadays underscore pivotal roles gut microbiota plays in thwarting various cancers pretty effectively beneath surface level. Commensal microbes help maintain cellular homeostasis through a plethora of epigenetic mechanisms and counteract carcinogenic processes rather effectively in various tissues. Malignant cells undergo apoptosis quite effectively when gut microbiota ferments dietary fibres into short-chain fatty acids specifically butyrate inducing robust cellular changes. SCFAs also diminish inflammation locally and systemically a well established driver of tumour genesis occurs subsequently in neoplastic progression environments. Microbiome plays a rather crucial role mostly within bodily environments and gets deeply involved in immune system regulation simultaneously.

Bifidobacterium and *Lactobacillus* taxa pretty effectively stimulate regulatory T cells thereby promoting anti-inflammatory responses while suppressing pro-inflammatory cytokines like TNF-α. Immune balance remarkably reduces chronic inflammation underlying various cancers including colorectal and gastric cancer pretty significantly every single day. A healthy microbiome reinforces tight junction proteins deeply within intestinal epithelium thus thwarting microbial translocation and subsequently preventing endotoxemia. This barrier function pretty effectively shields host from microbial components like lipopolysaccharide under certain conditions acting as tumour-promoting agents. Microbial enzymes pretty effectively facilitate biotransformation and detoxification of xenobiotics and carcinogens that originate from ingested food in various cases.

Gut bacteria break down nasty stuff like heterocyclic amines and polycyclic aromatic hydrocarbons lurking in charred meats thereby greatly reducing genotoxic potential. Microbiota harbouring β-glucuronidase activity deconjugates estrogens thereby modulating systemic hormone levels significantly in aggressive breast cancer. Myriad microbial genes crucial for estrogen metabolism in a balanced estrobolome may significantly help modulate risk of various cancers rather quietly. Several mechanisms link the gut microbiota to cancer prevention:

a. Detoxification and Protection against Carcinogens

Gut microbiota crucially prevents cancer by detoxifying dietary carcinogens and systemically mitigating their profoundly genotoxic effects quite effectively. Lactobacillus and Bifidobacterium bacterial genera largely mediate protective effects through enzymatic actions and binding capabilities that neutralize nasty compounds pretty effectively. Carcinogens such as heterocyclic amines form readily during extremely high-temperature cooking, causing DNA adducts that initiate mutagenic reactions subsequently. Aflatoxins produced by certain Aspergillus species lurking in spoiled grains and nuts are pretty potent hepatocarcinogens almost everywhere basically. Lactobacillus rhamnosus strains and Bifidobacterium longum have markedly bound mutagens rather tightly onto cell walls thereby largely reducing bioavailability and subsequent absorption in gastrointestinal tracts quite effectively.

Gut bacteria enzymatically break down carcinogens into rather less toxic metabolites while facilitating physical binding in sundry obscure biochemical processes. Certain probiotic strains produce glutathione-S-transferase and other detoxifying enzymes that facilitate excretion of reactive intermediates pretty effectively meanwhile. Others facilitate metabolism of nitrates and nitrites thereby lowering formation of potentially carcinogenic N-nitroso compounds deep within gut flora heavily. Microbes maintain redox balance pretty indirectly thereby mitigating oxidative stress induced by various carcinogenic substances and encourage immune surveillance quite effectively. Production of short-chain fatty acids gets boosted thereby enhancing integrity of mucosal barrier and stimulating anti-inflammatory pathways that protect host tissues effectively from DNA damage. A diverse gut microbiome crucially diminishes cancer risk effectively stemming from varied dietary exposures and myriad environmental toxins. Prebiotics and probiotics alongside dietary interventions could effectively nurture beneficial microbes offering promise for prevention of certain cancers meanwhile very effectively.

b. SCFA Production and Anti-Proliferative Effects

Gut microbiota ferments dietary fibre into short-chain fatty acids like butyrate and acetate pretty quickly thereby exerting significant anti-cancer effects. Butyrate has been researched rather extensively for its anti-inflammatory properties and epigenetic effects particularly in contexts involving colorectal cancer. Butyrate serves as primary energy source for colonocytes and plays a crucial albeit oft-underappreciated role in maintaining intestinal barrier integrity remarkably effectively. Butyrate exhibits profoundly anti-carcinogenic effects well beyond its foundational functions apparently in various contexts. Pro-apoptotic signaling cascades activation promotes apoptosis of dysplastic cells via caspase pathways sparing normal cells in the process meanwhile. Butyrate exhibits selective cytotoxicity rendering it rather uniquely promising as a metabolite for thwarting cancer development potentially in various cellular milieus.

Butyrate pretty effectively inhibits histone deacetylase thereby epigenetically influencing gene expression through various somewhat obscure modulation mechanisms. HDAC inhibition results in accumulation of acetylated histones that promote expression of tumour suppressor genes and genes involved heavily in cell cycle arrest. Butyrate pretty effectively halts proliferation of potentially malignant cells and reduces tumour progression by enhancing transcription of genes like p21. Butyrate and other SCFAs modulate immune responses with weird effectiveness in tumour microenvironments quite significantly and rather effectively apparently. Production of pro-inflammatory cytokines like IL-6 and TNF-α gets suppressed and differentiation of regulatory T cells gets heavily promoted thereby contributing to an anti-inflammatory milieu somewhat less conducive for tumourigenesis. Gut microbiota produces SCFA at varying rates and this capacity significantly influences risk of colorectal cancer elsewhere within bodily tissues. Diets heavy with soluble fibres sourced from legumes whole grain stuff fruits and veggies can foster growth of beneficial SCFA-producing gut bacteria and offer a rather potent non-invasive cancer prevention route.

c. Immune Surveillance and Inflammatory Regulation

Gut microbiome crucially shapes immune homeostasis vital for cancer prevention and effectively surveilling neoplastic cells always with utmost precision. Commensal microbes modulate immune responses through continuous interaction with host immune system ensuring a delicate balance between tolerance of harmless antigens and vigorous defense against pathogens lurking everywhere. Diverse microbiota profoundly promotes development of regulatory T cells and antigen-presenting cells including rather unusual kinds of dendritic cells. Crucial immune cells maintain unusually rigorous surveillance and fairly effectively thwart aberrant cells escaping from most immunosurveillance mechanisms. Butyrate and propionate greatly enhance Treg differentiation and IL-10 production thereby fostering deep immune tolerance against various chronic inflammatory conditions.

Dysbiosis conversely sparks immune dysregulation and low-grade systemic inflammation thereby fostering quite effectively a pro-tumourigenic microenvironment. Heightened pro-inflammatory cytokine production correlates with certain microbial profiles under various conditions including interleukin-6 and tumour necrosis factor-alpha apparently. Cytokines foster angiogenesis and tumour cell proliferation while inhibiting apoptosis particularly within inflammation-driven malignancies like liver cancer and pancreatic cancer. Commensal bacteria profoundly modulate expression of sundry pattern recognition receptors like Toll-like receptors on disparate immune cell populations heavily downstream. Dysbiosis often triggers aberrant activation rapidly leading to chronic inflammation and nasty oncogenic processes whereas proper microbial stimulation fosters balanced signaling pretty well. Microbiome exerts significant influence over immunomodulation and thereby noticeably enhances host's ability for spotting cancer cells pretty early. Prebiotics and fecal microbiota transplantation show rather considerable promise for fairly effectively encourage cancer defense mechanisms mediated largely by immune system.

3.3. Microbiome and Cancer Treatment Response

Emerging research reveals gut microbiome plays quite a crucial albeit oft underappreciated role in modulating efficacy or toxicity of various cancer therapies. Gut microbiota composition crucially impacts therapeutic efficacy significantly in precision oncology by encourage or undermining treatment responses fairly often nowadays. Microbiota profoundly affects metabolic processes of various drugs and modulates host immune responses somewhat erratically during many chemotherapy treatments. Bacterial species harbour enzymes that swiftly reactivate chemotherapeutic agents within gastrointestinal tracts altering drug bioavailability and side effects pretty drastically. Dysbiosis conversely hampers metabolic processes of certain pharmaceuticals and boosts toxicity of mucosa thereby fostering nasty complications like severe mucositis or systemic inflammation. *Blautia* and *Faecalibacterium* prausnitzii depletion has been associated with rather severe intestinal damage during diverse treatments involving anti-inflammatory activity.

Radiotherapy disrupts intestinal barrier function rather profoundly via modulation of microbiome thereby exacerbating toxicity induced by radiation or tumour radiosensitivity somewhat unpredictably. Surprisingly diverse microbiota protects against radiation-induced gastrointestinal damage heavily by modulating pathways associated with oxidative stress and enhancing mucosa repair. Microbiome unusually influence on cancer immunotherapy efficacy notably enhance immune checkpoint inhibitors like anti-PD-1 therapy remarkably in various clinical contexts. Elevated levels of salutary microbes like Akkermansia muciniphila markedly enhance responsiveness in patients undergoing immunotherapy treatment fairly often with great success apparently. Bacteria enhance anti-tumour immunity rather effectively through enhanced antigen presentation and cytokine production and pretty significant T-cell infiltration occurs subsequently. Antibiotic use preceding immunotherapy correlates with dismal outcomes probably owing to severely disrupted microbial flora in patients undergoing treatment. Microbiota-targeted interventions like prebiotics and fecal microbiota transplantation are facilitated quietly by grasping complex interactions between microbiome and therapy.

a. Modulation of Immunotherapy Response

Cancer therapy has been revolutionized pretty significantly nowadays by efficacy of immune checkpoint inhibitors targeting programmed cell death protein 1. Response rates remain erratically inconsistent and many patients derive scant benefit from treatment nowadays altogether in most such cases. Novel breakthroughs have incriminated gut microbiota as crucial factor in immunotherapy efficacy offering modified treatment modalities very suddenly now. Certain gut microbial taxa correlate remarkably with favorable outcomes in patients receiving anti-PD-1 therapy alongside treatment with anti-CTLA-4 antibodies. Akkermansia muciniphila enhances anti-PD-1 therapy efficacy remarkably by recruiting dendritic cells vigorously and activating $CD4^+$ T-helper cells deeply in tumour microenvironments. Faecalibacterium prausnitzii produces butyrate and anti-inflammatory metabolites thereby contributing heavily to immune homeostasis and anti-tumour immunity with improved ICI responsiveness correlating strongly with its abundance.

Immunotherapy treatments have lately been complicated by antibiotic-induced dysbiosis which has weirdly surfaced as rather ominous prognostic factor. Broad-spectrum antibiotics administered before or during ICI treatment disrupt gut microbiota linking it to reduced diversity and impaired T-cell priming and decreasing production of immunostimulatory metabolites like short-chain fatty acids. Microbial depletion severely hampers maturation of antigen-presenting cells and weakens cytotoxic T-cell infiltration thereby really dampening immune response against tumour cells. Findings highlight microbiome's crucial role remarkably well nowadays as modulator of host immunity and potential biomarker predicting various immunotherapy responses effectively. Novel approaches incorporating dietary regimens probiotics or fecal microbiota transplants squeeze gut microbiota thereby rather effectively optimizing immunotherapy outcomes somewhat silently. Ongoing clinical trials are exploring microbiota-targeted adjuncts alongside ICIs signaling a promising frontier in cancer immunotherapy informed by microbiome research.

b. Chemotherapy and Microbiome Crosstalk

Complex bidirectional interactions between gut microbiome and various chemotherapeutic agents heavily influence efficacy and toxicity of cancer treatment surprisingly. Microbial modulation influences immune responses somewhat erratically alongside drug metabolism amidst systemic inflammation driven crosstalk thus positioning microbiome as crucial entity in optimizing chemotherapeutic regimens effectively. Cyclophosphamide and similar chemotherapeutics require a gut microbiome immunologically pretty active for working effectively against various tumour types really well. Cyclophosphamide induces translocation of Gram-positive bacteria such as Enterococcus hirae from gut into secondary lymphoid organs vigorously stimulating differentiation of Th17 cells and memory T cells thereby encourage anti-tumour immune responses.

Antibiotics or germ-free conditions severely disrupt microbial translocation resulting in markedly diminished therapeutic efficacy thereby underscoring microbiota's crucial role in modulating potent immune responses effectively. Gut microbiota can sometimes detrimentally affect chemotherapy efficacy through fairly unpredictable biotransformation into rather toxic or curiously inactive compounds. Microbial β-glucuronidase enzymes readily deconjugate irinotecan metabolites in colon sometimes leading to mucosal injury and severe diarrhea occurs fairly frequently. Microbiome-targeted inhibitors of bacterial β-glucuronidase have shown considerable promise in pretty effectively reducing fairly nasty side effects. Modulation of intestinal permeability by microbes profoundly influences chemotherapy side effects like mucositis and nausea downstream quite frequently. Chemotherapy-induced dysbiosis precipitates drastic loss of beneficial commensals such as *Bifidobacterium* alongside unchecked proliferation of various highly pathogenic microbial species. Such changes exacerbate toxicity markedly and may interfere substantially with absorption of certain drugs subsequently distributed systemically throughout bodily tissues. Novel therapeutic interventions emerge rapidly nowadays upon thoroughly grasping intricacies of chemo-microbiome axis dynamics in a very detailed manner. Preclinical models indicate probiotics or fecal microbiota transplantation can rather effectively ameliorate nasty side effects and restore efficacy. Personalized microbiome profiling may guide chemotherapy regimens effectively by predicting patient-specific risks and optimizing therapeutic outcomes in various ways.

c. Radiation-Induced Gut Damage

Radiotherapy blasted at abdominal areas frequently spawns nasty gastrointestinal toxicity and sometimes mucositis down the line with diarrhea being another upshot. Evidence points increasingly towards gut microbiota orchestrating a crucial role in modulating host response to radiation thereby influencing tissue injury and repair subsequently. Radiation directly ravages epithelial cells and spawns inflammatory responses somewhat indirectly within intestinal mucosa resulting in gut barrier disruption and microbial composition shifts a phenomenon often dubbed radiation-induced dysbiosis. Dysbiosis manifests with pronounced depletion of beneficial commensals such as Lactobacillus and an overabundance of opportunistic pathogens like Enterobacteriaceae occurs simultaneously.

Microbial imbalance severely exacerbates intestinal permeability and pro-inflammatory cytokine production such as IL-1β badly compounding mucosal injury with oxidative stress. Research on humans and animals has revealed that modulating gut microbiota before undergoing radiation therapy can remarkably alter treatment outcomes significantly. Probiotic supplementation with unusual strains such as Lactobacillus rhamnosus GG has been shown pretty effectively and rather deeply to attenuate radiation-induced mucositis.

Enhanced tight junction integrity mediates these effects alongside upregulation of anti-inflammatory cytokines like IL-10 and restores butyrate generating SCFA-producing bacteria. Non-digestible fibres namely prebiotics rather effectively boost production of SCFA and stimulate growth of beneficial microbes quite substantially. Synbiotics comprising prebiotics and probiotics alongside fecal microbiota transplantation emerge as novel therapeutic approaches restoring homeostasis in severely affected radiation enteropathy patients. Microbiome modulation shows considerable promise in effectively mitigating radiotherapy-induced gastrointestinal toxicity across diverse clinical contexts pretty successfully. Microbiota-preserving strategies incorporated into radiation oncology protocols might significantly boost comfort and ameliorate quality of life for long-term cancer survivors remarkably.

3.4. Microbiome-Targeted Interventions in Oncology

Emerging evidence on microbiome's role in cancer development has sparked creation of innovative therapies targeting gut flora quite effectively for improved cancer treatment outcomes. Efficacy of treatment gets enhanced thoroughly here with employed strategies reducing toxic effects of therapy supporting overall patient well-being significantly. Probiotics teeming with live beneficial microbes somewhat anomalously restore balance and pretty effectively modulate assorted immune responses within mucosal tissue barriers effectively. *Lactobacillus rhamnosus* GG and *Saccharomyces boulardii* strains can markedly lessen severity of diarrhea induced by radiation therapy remarkably well. Probiotics markedly boost local and systemic immunity beneath epithelial layers potentially greatly enhancing anti-tumour surveillance. Prebiotics such as inulin and fructooligosaccharides fuel SCFA-producing bacteria remarkably well deep within diverse gut microbiota ecosystems every day. Fermentation yields butyrate and other SCFAs with anti-inflammatory properties that deeply support colonocyte health while suppressing tumour-promoting pathways variably.

Synbiotic formulations comprising probiotic elements alongside prebiotics are being rather thoroughly investigated nowadays for yielding synergistic benefits in oncology settings. FMT entails transferring fecal matter from a healthy donor into a patient's gut thereby repopulating it quickly with myriad diverse microbiota. FMT initially emerged for treating recurrent *Clostridioides difficile* infection and now gets explored heavily in various oncology research settings worldwide. FMT from immunotherapy responders boosts checkpoint inhibitor efficacy in non-responding melanoma patients by introducing microbial taxa such as Akkermansia muciniphila effectively. Tumour microenvironment gets deeply infused with T-cell infiltration and immune activation by these taxa so efficacy enhancement occurs remarkably. Diet modulates gut microbiota powerfully alongside various factors that irregularly influence overall health and microbial equilibrium within human bodily systems.

Diets rich in polyphenols and whole grains with high fibre content coupled with fermented foods remarkably support anti-inflammatory microbial species these days. Precision nutrition interventions emerge erratically as adjunctive strategies modulating gut microbiome profiles in various cancer patients with somewhat altered microbial composition. Postbiotics comprising unusual bioactive compounds like butyrate and secondary bile acids produced by certain microbes are now being explored very vigorously. These metabolites directly influence gene expression and significantly modulate several immune checkpoints whilst enhancing repair of epithelial tissues pretty substantially. Postbiotics offer advantages in safety and peculiar stability thus rendering them fiendishly attractive candidates for potential integration into assorted cancer care support regimens.

Broad-spectrum antibiotics usage in cancer treatment strongly correlates with severely disrupted gut flora and subsequently significantly diminished efficacy in various immunotherapy settings. Implementing rigorous antibiotic stewardship programs preserves microbial integrity pretty effectively by drastically curtailing unnecessary exposure to antimicrobials for patients. Microbiome-targeted approaches signify a drastic shift rapidly in oncology treatment toward highly personalized cancer care by effectively altering microbial ecosystems. Research advances will gradually reveal complex interactions between tumour cells and microbes thoroughly paving way for precision oncology treatments informed by rich microbiome data. Recognizing the microbiome's influence on cancer outcomes has led to several intervention strategies:

a. Probiotics and Prebiotics

Supplementation with specific probiotic strains like *Lactobacillus rhamnosus* GG and *Saccharomyces boulardii* has shown considerable potential in modulating immune responses rather effectively. Probiotics often mitigate diarrhea and mucositis alongside systemic inflammation associated with chemotherapy and radiotherapy pretty frequently these days. Prebiotics like inulin and fructooligosaccharides serve as fermentable fibres nourishing beneficial microbes fairly selectively within normally occurring gut environments. Fermentation by them fosters production of short-chain fatty acids especially butyrate which possesses remarkably anti-inflammatory properties and pro-apoptotic characteristics. Enhanced SCFA production rather effectively fosters improved epithelial health and suppresses inflammation that promotes tumours maintaining homeostasis quite steadily. Synbiotics involving combined probiotics and prebiotics usage are being pretty vigorously investigated nowadays for potentially highly synergistic effects in various cancer therapies.

b. Dietary Modulation

Dietary composition profoundly shapes gut microbiome thereby modulating cancer risk and significantly influencing various treatment outcomes under diverse clinical settings. A fibre-rich plant-based diet teeming with whole grains legumes and fruits enhance microbial diversity and ramps up production of short-chain fatty acids like butyrate having potent anti-inflammatory effects. Phytochemicals and polyphenols in diverse plant-based foods such as flavonoids and lignans profoundly impact microbial metabolic processes and significantly enhance immune response thereby contributing favorably to tumour microenvironment conditions. Diets loaded with processed meats saturated fats and weird food additives like emulsifiers trigger gut permeability and nasty chronic inflammation. Carcinogenesis may be vigorously facilitated by such conditions and treatment response severely impaired quite dramatically over long periods. Modulating diet strategically provides a rather non-invasive and quietly cost-effective method for enhancing therapeutic efficacy and microbiome health effectively.

c. Fecal Microbiota Transplantation (FMT)

Fecal microbiota transplantation entails transferring gut microbiota from a healthy donor into recipients thereby somewhat restoring microbial equilibrium irregularly. FMT traditionally treats recurrent Clostridioides difficile infections but oncology researchers are now pretty heavily exploring its potential. Preclinical studies imply FMT potentially boosts responses to immune checkpoint inhibitors in patients with malignancies stubbornly entrenched notably in melanoma. Donor-derived microbiota modulates systemic immunity deeply inside tumours and restores favorable microbial metabolites quite effectively supporting antitumour immunity. FMT shows considerable promise in rapidly alleviating chemotherapy-induced gastrointestinal toxicity by re-establishing gut barrier integrity and microbial diversity somewhat effectively. FMT in oncology remains largely experimental facing gnarly hurdles like lack of standardization in dodgy donor screening and freaky safety concerns. Novel microbiome restoration methods are being assessed quite vigorously in various cancer care settings for personalized treatment efficacy and overall safety.

d. Microbiome-Based Biomarkers

Gut microbiota composition and function offer tantalizing glimpses into cancer therapy responses fraught with recurrence risk and excruciatingly severe adverse effects. Recently metagenomics and metabolomics advances enabled oncology researchers to non-invasively identify specific microbial taxa functioning as biomarkers alongside certain metabolites. Elevated Akkermansia muciniphila and Faecalibacterium prausnitzii at baseline often correspond with successful immunotherapy outcomes but presence of pro-inflammatory microbes may foretell poor tolerance or grievous immune-related complications during treatment. Microbial metabolite profiles eerily mirroring host microbe interactions relevant slowly to tumour progression include short-chain fatty acids and various tryptophan catabolites.

Microbiome-based biomarkers confer numerous benefits clinically by markedly enhancing treatment efficacy prediction thereby optimizing therapy regimens substantially at initial stages. Survivors' recurrence risk can be effectively monitored over time using these biomarkers. Microbial signature analysis enables targeted interventions such as administering probiotics and drastically altering a patient's usual diet quite effectively. Microbial biomarkers need rigorous validation in diverse sizable cohorts before being harnessed for cancer treatment strategies. Sequencing methods and data interpretation standardization remains critical for translating microbiome diagnostics from research labs into routine clinical settings effectively.

3.5. Challenges and Future Directions

Microbiome research in oncology holds promise yet substantial hurdles remain before full implementation clinically occurs eventually in many research settings. Differences between individuals in microbial composition and functional capability greatly hampers attempt to devise a notion of healthy microbiome applicable universally. Genetics alongside geography influence variability markedly with medication use and various lifestyle factors under certain dietary conditions quite unpredictably. Fecal microbiota transplantation and other microbiome-targeted interventions remain under intense scrutiny especially in cancer patients with severely compromised immune systems. Modified therapeutic interventions and validated diagnostic tools are demanded alongside standardized protocols for data interpretation and microbial profiling by successful clinical implementation.

Metagenomics and systems biology advancements remarkably revamp real-time microbiome mapping capabilities nowadays with rather high precision. Novel analytical platforms facilitate profoundly intricate characterization of host-microbe interplay offering modified insights into tumour biology influenced by microbes heavily. Microbiome poised ahead becomes cornerstone of precision oncology quite lately with growing importance beneath surface. Its influence pervades cancer dynamics rather thoroughly from reduction of risk modulating immune responses and pretty significantly enhancing efficacy of various therapies. Microbiome informed strategies will probably become standard in integrative cancer care as understanding of science gets progressively deeper. Various microbial aspects are encompassed within modifiable dimensions of cancer prevention strategies effectively nowadays.

Microbiome-modulating therapies are frequently customized rather haphazardly for chemotherapy response optimization or immunotherapy yielding wildly varying efficacy rates sometimes. Personalized dietary regimens and probiotic supplements are utilized maintaining equilibrium of microbial flora in gut. Microbial biomarkers guide treatment choices effectively and monitor recurrence risk stratification pretty accurately in many cancer patients nowadays. Microbiome research surprisingly powerful could revolutionize treatment of cancer significantly. Integrating this complex ecosystem into oncology remarkably holds transformative potential for advancing personalized medicine and greatly improving patient outcomes.

4. Integrating Artificial Intelligence and Big Data in Nutritional Oncology Research

Artificial intelligence and big data analytics are now rapidly transforming nutritional oncology by facilitating profoundly nuanced understandings of complex diet-oncogenesis interplays quickly. Cancer manifests as a complex multifaceted disorder heavily swayed by myriad genetic and epigenetic factors alongside immunological perturbations and environmental stressors. Nutrition intricately modulates various cancer hallmarks but conventional research methodologies falter in capturing interindividual variability amidst dynamic dietary patterns over time. Sophisticated analytical tools are now required due to an abundance of complex data emerging alongside genomics and real-time dietary tracking tech. Artificial intelligence and big data play a transformative role rather profoundly here in some obscure manner very effectively.

Machine learning algorithms dig up obscure patterns deeply within data and predict treatment responses quite effectively in previously unseen ways. Technologies facilitate integration of diverse datasets including electronic health records omics profiles and wearable sensor data alongside sporadic dietary logs into strangely comprehensive models. AI-enabled predictive modeling substantially enhances modified dietary regimen design for clinicians based on tumour characteristics and patient's lifestyle factors largely. Emerging AI applications and big data slowly seep into nutritional oncology for risk stratification and precision diet recommendations mostly nowadays. Rapidly emerging federated learning mechanisms and unsupervised clustering alongside natural language processing drive progress, underneath various underlying technologies. Critical challenges surrounding data privacy equity and algorithm bias are tackled vigorously alongside clinical validation and sundry thorny ethical concerns about data quality. Ridiculously accessible AI tools and big data are redefining precision nutrition in oncology making it predictively super personalized nowadays effectively.

4.1. The Promise of Big Data in Nutritional Oncology

Nutritional oncology infused with big data has dynamically opened unprecedented avenues for grasping intricate diet interactions and cancer treatment responses. Big data entails not only a sheer volume of info but also velocity and variety and weirdly high accuracy of datasets gleaned rapidly from sundry obscure sources. Genomics and epigenomics data alongside patient-reported outcomes and wearable sensor info heavily influence cancer nutrition research these days very significantly. Somewhat unorthodox analytical techniques applied effectively nowadays unearth subtle patterns and obscure associations by aggregating diverse datasets. Correlating prolonged eating habits with tumour characteristics and patient outcomes may yield fresh nutritional indicators for evaluating cancer risk remarkably well. Metabolomic profiles merged with dietary data expose weird metabolic footprints of dietary influences slowly shaping tumour behavior or therapy resistance somewhat.

Big data analytics enable stratification of patient populations based on variability in individual dietary responses thereby paving way for super personalized dietary regimens subsequently. Big data analysis longitudinally empowers researchers quite effectively assessing cumulative diet effects on cancer incidence and survivorship across hugely diverse populations. Big data holds considerable promise nowadays in oncology by pretty effectively supporting evidence-based precision nutrition approaches grounded thoroughly in research. Modified nutritional regimens are crafted by researchers using advanced statistical modeling and systems biology tools heavily informed by genetic profiles and various lifestyle factors. Big data will become a cornerstone of translational research and clinical innovation in nutritional oncology as analyzing such massive datasets evolves rapidly nowadays.

4.2. Role of Artificial Intelligence in Data Interpretation and Prediction

Artificial intelligence plays a pivotal role rapidly in deciphering big data complexity via machine learning and deep learning techniques in nutritional oncology. Sophisticated computational techniques quietly uncover non-linear trends and predictive cues within complex datasets far beyond scope of traditional statistical analysis. Machine learning algorithms excel remarkably well at ferreting out intricate links between dietary factors and various kinds of cancer outcomes typically nowadays. Supervised learning models get trained pretty thoroughly on patient data predicting treatment responses deeply rooted in dietary habits and some genetic predispositions. Unsupervised learning such as clustering facilitates discovery of patient subgroups exhibiting disparate metabolic responses or nutritional requirements thereby informing highly tailored dietary interventions pretty effectively.

Neural networks and other deep learning techniques prove especially valuable nowadays in analyzing high-throughput data like gene expression profiles effectively. Models directly process raw data unearthing aberrant hierarchical representations that facilitate classification of cancer subtypes or prognostication based on specific dietary habits. Nowadays natural language processing quite effectively extracts relevant dietary info and clinical data from sources like electronic health records. NLP automates extraction and categorization of dietary habits fairly effectively nowadays in nutritional oncology with real-world evidence integration. Predictive modeling embodies an eerily potent AI application yielding remarkably transformative insights fairly well across swaths of diverse industries these days. AI models effectively predict cancer risk progression by merging molecular features with diet-related data and various other clinical characteristics. Nowadays they can pretty effectively forecast adverse treatment responses or nutritional deficiencies enabling proactive management of patients rather than reactive ones. AI-driven tools furnish highly personalized dietary advice effectively in clinical settings and optimize treatment synergy drastically. Data-driven dynamic systems remarkably improve cancer care outcomes and quality of life fairly nowadays holding considerable promise. AI technologies will eventually serve as indispensable tools in translating vast nutritional oncology big data into pretty actionable precision medicine strategies.

a. Diet-Cancer Associations

AI algorithms rapidly discern subtle relationships between diet and cancer outcomes by integrating huge datasets multidimensionally nowadays with considerable accuracy. Machine learning approaches manage non-linear interactions effectively uncovering associations hidden from conventional statistical analyses fairly easily with surprising frequency. ML models such as gradient boosting and support vector machines have detected dietary patterns correlating with cancer risk and prognosis pretty effectively. Models incorporate variables such as genetic predisposition and socioeconomic status alongside age and nutritional intake remarkably improving prediction accuracy.

High dietary fibre intake correlates with significantly reduced risk of colorectal cancer in AI-driven analyses of diverse cohort data surprisingly. Breast cancer sufferers have yielded somewhat favorable outcomes on diets low in glycemic load bursting with omega-3 fatty acids curiously enough. AI models have unearthed dietary patterns sparking inflammation marked by copious consumption of processed meats and sweetened beverages associated with elevated cancer incidence rates. AI enables modified risk profiling assessing impact of specific dietary components rather remarkably in context of individual's unique genetic and microbiome profiles. Precision nutrition strategies in oncology gain support nowadays from this development replacing broad outdated public health guidelines quite effectively. AI tools facilitate assessment of temporal dietary patterns allowing researchers to track long-term exposures influencing cancer development slowly over quite extended periods. A longitudinal perspective yields critical insight into periods of vulnerability and opportunity for somewhat effective dietary interventions being implemented subsequently. AI subtly reshapes understanding of diet-cancer relationships through revealing interactions between various nutrients and convoluted cancer biology mechanisms very quietly. Insights paving way effectively for highly individualized evidence-based dietary recommendations squarely aimed at cancer prevention and long-term survivorship care.

b. Personalized Dietary Recommendations

Modified dietary plans tailored rather cleverly to a patient's peculiar biological makeup might be forthcoming thanks largely to artificial intelligence in nutritional oncology. AI systems quite effectively analyze genomics data and lifestyle factors to predict how certain diets impact cancer pathways and treatment outcomes. Fairly sophisticated models analyze gene-nutrient interactions in various metabolic states effectively nowadays using machine learning quite intricately. Algorithms identify gene-diet interactions quite precisely in specific cancer patients where certain foods starkly alter tumour-promoting genes. Clinicians craft modified interventions pretty effectively now informed by molecular cancer subtype and vulnerabilities alongside a patient's immune status. AI systems can pretty crudely incorporate microbiome profiles alongside genetic data accounting for individual variations in obscure microbial metabolic pathways. Dietary recommendations enhancing beneficial microbes such as SCFA-producing bacteria can be strategically crafted for effectively supporting cancer prevention therapy. AI-driven platforms crudely model how regimens like ketogenic diets or Mediterranean eating habits affect tumour metabolism and systemic inflammation in cancer patients. These tools predict potential adverse effects or nutrient-drug interactions thereby minimizing toxicity related to treatment and improving tolerability vastly often. AI-driven digital health tools swiftly recalibrate suggestions responding haphazardly and irregularly to fluctuations in patient condition or symptom severity in real time.

Chemotherapy patients might get daily dietary tweaks suddenly based on gut microbiota shifts or rising inflammatory markers over several days perhaps. AI makes oncology nutrition remarkably scalable pretty clinically actionable these days with great precision. Biologically informed personalized dietary roadmaps updated dynamically are poised utterly to become ridiculously indispensable in delivery of cancer care centered on patients.

c. Predictive Models for Treatment Response

Machine learning utterly transforms predictive ability rapidly by integrating genomic information with various metabolic factors and nutritional data. Emerging predictive models evaluate impact of dietary habits on efficacy and patient tolerance of various cancer treatments including immunotherapy and radiation. Recent studies have trained ML algorithms on datasets encompassing pre-treatment nutritional biomarkers such as serum albumin or body mass index with gut microbiota composition. Variables influencing drug metabolism subsequently impact treatment efficacy greatly through various murky immune modulation pathways altering toxicity profiles radically. Malnourished patients or those beset by systemic inflammation typically fare quite badly with chemotherapy and suffer rather higher complication rates now eerily predictable by machine learning models.

Predictive models stratifying patients likely responding well now incorporate dietary factors and microbiome-derived metabolites such as short-chain fatty acids and bile acid profiles. AI systems help tailor nutritional interventions enhancing responsiveness quite effectively or mitigating resistance remarkably during therapy sessions occasionally. Predictive analytics are being integrated into somewhat antiquated clinical decision-support systems with fanfare nowadays rather quietly in real-time. Such platforms perpetually scrutinize patient info like nutrient intake fluctuations or metabolic markers and revamp dietary recommendations with great rapidity nowadays. Clinicians dynamically tailor nutrition plans during cancer treatment thereby markedly boosting efficacy while mitigating super nasty side effects like mucositis. AI-guided predictive tools will likely become crucial in precision oncology as models get more robust and are validated clinically so nutrition becomes modifiable determinant of treatment success rather than just passive component of cancer care.

4.3. Integrating Multi-Omics and AI for Precision Nutrition

Artificial intelligence applications in nutritional oncology profoundly integrate genomics transcriptomics proteomics metabolomics and microbiomics data into clinically relevant insights rather unified. Highly individualized nutrition strategies emerge from a comprehensive systems biology approach that fosters deeper understanding of complex interactions between dietary components and cancer biology. Gene variants and expression patterns interact heavily with dietary factors influencing cancer susceptibility via genomic data and various transcriptomic profiles. AI algorithms pinpoint SNPs heavily linked with aberrant folate metabolism or polyunsaturated fatty acid processing that quietly affect numerous DNA repair pathways. Modified dietary regimens informed by genetic predispositions help suppress tumours and mitigate oncogenic risk thereby promoting wellness in patients rapidly. Proteomics alongside metabolomics offers a dynamic albeit somewhat blurred snapshot of cellular activity beneath varied metabolic responses during diverse dietary interventions.

Machine learning tools swiftly discern proteomic signatures indicative of oxidative stress or inflammation and correlate those with diverse cancer outcomes very effectively nowadays. Metabolomic profiling particularly of lipid mediators and amino acid derivatives uncovers biomarkers responsive heavily to dietary changes influencing drug metabolism. Microbiomic data vividly enrich pictures by mapping modulation of nutrient availability through various gut microbial populations and altering immune signaling mechanisms. AI models effectively uncover highly predictive microbial signatures of responses to fibre-rich diets and resistance against dietary carcinogens oftentimes successfully. Manipulating microbiome-driven nutrient metabolic processes quite slowly introduces a fresh nuanced dimension of personalization in oncology nutritional therapy nowadays effectively. AI-driven platforms intricately build molecular profiles by deeply integrating omics datasets and subsequently rendering modified dietary advice for individual patients precisely. Precision nutrition plans are designed rather complementarily with conventional cancer treatments and they optimize immune resilience somewhat longterm with minimized toxicity. Food becomes biologically active intervention tailored meticulously by patient's unique genetic blueprint with considerable influence from molecular signature obviously nowadays. As multi-omics tech becomes ridiculously accessible and AI algorithms get pretty darn sophisticated integration of these tools promises redefining oncology nutritional care standards with evidence-based interventions precisely.

4.4. Digital Health and Real-Time Monitoring

Artificial intelligence merges with digital health tech revolutionizing oncology landscapes by facilitating real-time monitoring of dietary habits and physiological responses quite effectively. Wearable devices and mobile health apps quietly facilitate capture of high-resolution real-world data outside most traditional clinical settings nowadays. Cutting-edge tech yields granular Intel on daily nutrient consumption and physical activity alongside sleep hydration gut function and crucial patient-reported outcomes in oncology nutrition research. Machine learning algorithms somewhat effectively synthesize various data into intelligence that supports adaptive nutritional care dynamically these days pretty successfully. AI-enhanced gizmos tracking dietary habits pretty heavily nowadays assess food quality via image recognition and barcode scanning with minimal user fuss.

Automatically these tools detect dietary trends and flag nutritional risks like deficiencies or sugars intake excessive in meal plans daily. Intelligent systems swiftly adjust nutritional recommendations in real time according to a patient's treatment phase or emerging side effects suddenly. A patient undergoing chemotherapy might receive unusual meal recommendations and keep energy reserves fairly stable despite stomach woes being partially mitigated. Patients undergoing immunotherapy might receive alerts about maintaining hydration and boosting protein intake in response to fluctuating body weight and various biomarker levels. Real-time interventions greatly enhance patient adherence and tolerance of treatment which are crucial factors determining therapeutic success quite significantly overall. Clinicians gain leverage from automatically generated dashboards and predictive analytics that flag impending nutritional decline or treatment-related complications pretty timely. Digital platforms empower patients pretty actively in health management and foster deeply collaborative care environments remarkably effectively with great overall effectiveness. Digital tools foster accountability and self-monitoring pretty effectively thereby supporting behavioral changes crucial in interventions promoting sustainable nutrition practices normally. Emerging tech holds considerable promise nowadays for scalable precision-driven nutrition strategies within oncology care. Digital health tools evolve into perspicacious partners in cancer prevention therapy optimization and survivorship care when paired rather elaborately with artificial intelligence.

4.5. Challenges and Ethical Considerations

Merging artificial intelligence with big data in nutritional oncology spawns thorny conundrums and holds transformative potential for rather vexing scientific and deeply knotty ethical issues. Inconsistencies plague data sources significantly and data quality standardization efforts remain a primary hurdle nationwide every day pretty much. App-based logs and self-reported food frequency questionnaires often yield inaccuracies owing largely to variability in methods of collecting dietary data. Incompatibilities between various electronic health record formats and disparate genomic sequencing platforms significantly impede data interoperability, limiting reproducibility of AI models across diverse clinical environments. Deep learning AI systems mystifyingly deliver eerily accurate predictions yet shrouded in obscurity sans transparent reasoning or lucid explanatory mechanisms.

Unexplained recommendation generation erodes trust in clinical nutrition badly when provider accountability and patient understanding are compromised significantly. Using evidence-based practice with clinician intuition in an interpretable manner to develop AI models nowadays necessitates pretty considerable effort. Sensitive data usage raises significant ethical concerns nowadays regarding ownership and confidentiality of genetic profiles and microbiome sequences fairly often. Robust data governance frameworks must be established squarely upholding patient autonomy in data-driven care and ensuring compliance with legal standards like GDPR. AI tools risk magnifying cancer care disparities if trained largely on data from affluent urban areas or predominantly majority populations. Model development should crucially incorporate measures for inclusivity and deployment processes must prioritize accessibility effectively for underrepresented communities. Affordability alongside digital literacy and access to health technologies must be heavily prioritized for broadly democratizing AI-driven nutritional oncology benefits.

Tackling intricate problems necessitates wildly diverse cooperation between oncologists and nutrition experts data wranglers bioethicists and various health officials. Pretty equitable implementation strategies must be developed slowly alongside standardized protocols and transparent algorithms with secure robust data infrastructures. Artificial intelligence and big data remain poised to revolutionize nutritional oncology by enabling deep personalization with rather unusually predictive risk assessment dynamically.

5. Innovative Dietary Interventions

Nutritional oncology undergoes a somewhat swift paradigmatic shift towards modified therapeutics that leverage biologically nuanced understandings rather than broad sweeping dietary proscriptions. Convergence of two trends fuels transformation with expanding use of funky foods offering health benefits way beyond basic nutritional value and emergence of genomics-guided personalized nutrition rooted deeply in microbiome science. Phytochemical-rich plant products and probiotic formulations alongside fortified staples have garnered interest owing largely to potential modulation of oxidative stress within immune function central to cancer development. Bioactive compounds intricately interact with various cellular pathways and epigenetic mechanisms offering non-toxic complementary approaches supporting cancer prevention rather effectively alongside therapeutic efficacy.

Personalized nutrition surge empowers clinicians tailoring dietary interventions pretty effectively nowadays based on individual genetic makeup and gut microbiota composition. Precision approaches remarkably enable dietary strategies effectively aligned with each patient's unique biology in a surprisingly sustainable manner. Sophisticated tools including AI-driven diet modeling and nutrigenomic assays help translate complex data into modified guidance effectively these days. Innovations hold promise remarkably well throughout cancer continuum by reducing risk in people susceptible and enhancing resilience during arduous treatment. Personalized nutrition approaches and functional ones may enhance therapy adherence remarkably while reducing recurrence risk by tackling behavioral factors modifiable effectively.

5.1. Functional Foods

Functional foods quietly bestow myriad health benefits far beyond basic nutrition serving as dietary components replete with subtle advantageous properties. They play increasing roles naturally thwarting disease or mitigating its devastating effects within various cancer contexts especially through dietary fortification. Bioactive compounds in such foods heavily interact with various molecular pathways deeply involved in carcinogenesis and systemic inflammation. Phytochemicals teeming with polyphenols and flavonoids exhibit strikingly anti-inflammatory effects and possess potent antioxidant properties quite naturally in various organisms. Quite remarkably various signaling pathways are modulated and angiogenesis suppressed in numerous studies on diverse fruits and vegetables by these compounds. Live beneficial microbes like Lactobacillus and Bifidobacterium often referred to as probiotics profoundly enhance gut health and curb systemic inflammation.

Prebiotics such as inulin act as substrates for beneficial microbes in gut flora thereby substantially increasing production of short-chain fatty acids encourage health in colon. EPA and DHA present in fatty fish and flaxseeds heavily modulate inflammatory responses while profoundly influencing membrane fluidity and regulating gene expressions. Incorporation into cell membranes pretty significantly alters eicosanoid synthesis and enhanced anti-tumour immunity with dramatic effect in many instances. Fibres enhance gut health markedly enhancing microbial diversity and production of SCFAs such as butyrate exhibiting potent anti-inflammatory properties in colorectal tissue. Products fortified remarkably with vitamin D and selenium or iron can correct deficiencies linked heavily to cancer risk and its insidious progression. Vitamin D-fortified dairy products may enhance immune surveillance pretty significantly and reduce tumour proliferation fairly effectively in humans overall nowadays.

Functional foods in oncology are viewed pretty significantly as therapeutic adjuncts influencing critical processes such as epigenetic modifications and oxidative stress alleviation. Integration into dietary strategies enables a non-invasive low-risk approach centred on patients that rather effectively complements conventional treatments these days. Research advances will make identification of bioactive compounds central quite rapidly in evidence-based dietary recommendations for cancer care nationwide. Incorporating such foods strategically rather substantially enhances treatment efficacy and improves outcomes effectively across various cancer types long term.

a. Anti-inflammatory and Antioxidant Effects

Functional foods exert cancer-protective effects pretty effectively via a central mechanism that modulates inflammation and oxidative stress rather thoroughly. Oxidative stress triggers DNA damage and aberrant cell signaling whilst chronic inflammation fosters a deeply pro-tumourigenic microenvironment. Curcumin a principal polyphenol found deeply embedded in turmeric has garnered extensive research attention for its capacity inhibiting nuclear factor-kappa B quite effectively. Curcumin effectively mops up highly reactive oxygen species protecting cellular components from oxidative damage in a somewhat sloppy manner meanwhile. Resveratrol a stilbene found in grapes berries and red wine downregulates various inflammatory mediators like cyclooxygenase-2 and inducible nitric oxide synthase markedly. It enhances activity of endogenous antioxidant enzymes like superoxide dismutase and catalase thereby counteracting oxidative DNA damage quite effectively downstream.

EGCG or epigallocatechin gallate present abundantly in green tea reduces oxidative stress effectively by quenching free radicals and upregulating Nrf2 pathway. EGCG thwarts inflammatory pathways such as MAPK and STAT3 thereby substantially augmenting chemopreventive potential under diverse cellular contexts rather mysteriously. Compounds paired with conventional therapies exhibit synergistic effects potentially boosting treatment response markedly and minimizing toxicity quite effectively. Modulating cellular redox remarkably highlights therapeutic relevance across various cancer stages from prevention in high-risk individuals during treatment afterwards. Efficacy of such compounds hinges precariously on bioavailability and metabolic milieu necessitating copious research into varied formulations and obscure delivery methods. Incorporating them into functional food-based interventions appears rather promisingly as a strategy against oxidative and inflammatory carcinogenic mechanisms pretty effectively.

b. Modulation of Cell Signaling Pathways

Bioactive compounds present in various functional foods heavily impact cancer cell behavior by profoundly influencing cell signaling pathways and modulating gene expression. Dietary components profoundly perturb transcriptional regulation and epigenetic mods governing proliferation apoptosis and angiogenesis inside cells somewhat irregularly. Sulforaphane occurs naturally and seems rather abundant pretty frequently in cruciferous veggies like broccoli sprouts. Sulforaphane inhibits histone deacetylase activity pretty effectively thereby altering chromatin structure and reactivating silenced tumour suppressor genes in various cancer cells. Sulforaphane emerges as fairly selective epigenetic modulator inducing apoptosis readily in various malignant cells but sparing mostly normal bodily tissue.

Nrf2 pathway gets activated swiftly leading tortuously to heightened expression of various detoxifying enzymes and a slew of antioxidant proteins rather gradually. Simultaneously disrupting redox homeostasis thoroughly shields healthy cells and sensitizes cancer cells extremely well for chemotherapy or radiation treatment. Genistein a soy isoflavone profoundly modulates estrogen receptor signaling and heavily downregulates various oncogenes interfering with tyrosine kinase activity quite extensively. Quercetin a flavonoid abundant in apples and onions disrupts PI3K/Akt and MAPK pathways thereby markedly dampening cell proliferation and inducing apoptosis subsequently. Apigenin sourced from parsley or chamomile heavily influences Wnt/β-catenin signaling and STAT3 pathways thereby markedly stifling tumour growth and further metastasis.

Compounds exhibit anticancer properties directly and reprogram tumour surroundings fairly often suppressing inflammatory responses while restoring somewhat normal immune responses in patients. Epigenetic modulation occur frequently thereby drastically altering DNA methylation or histone modification and significantly heightening cancer risk with minimal genetic alteration present. Molecularly active foods infused into cancer treatment regimens robustly support holistic modalities wherein dietary tactics target key oncogenic pathways. Further investigation remains crucial for development of evidence-based dietary therapies underlying their clinical applications and bioavailability.

c. Gut Microbiota Interactions

Evidence nowadays highlights crucial interplay between functional foods and gut microbiota in effectively modulating various cancer outcomes. Fermentable fibres and prebiotics alongside probiotics in functional foods variably influence systemic inflammation and alter gut microbiome composition profoundly. Prebiotics like inulin and fructooligosaccharides serve as fermentable substrates for beneficial gut bacteria such as Bifidobacterium and some Lactobacillus strains naturally. Fermentation yields short-chain fatty acids like butyrate and propionate exerting profoundly anti-inflammatory effects very effectively on immune systems. Butyrate quite effectively promotes apoptosis in colorectal cancer cells and inhibits proliferation. Strengthening intestinal barrier integrity reduces systemic endotoxemia and chronic inflammation somewhat slowly over time in most individuals naturally.

Gene expression gets regulated via rather obscure epigenetic mechanisms such as peculiar histone acetylation processes occurring inside cells. Probiotics containing certain Lactobacillus strains and Bifidobacterium species rather significantly modulate immune responses and contribute greatly to microbial equilibrium. Probiotic supplementation boosts chemotherapy efficacy and immunotherapy remarkably by largely preserving gut integrity during treatment. Emerging evidence suggests microbiome pretty significantly influences metabolic pathways of various drugs thereby altering bioavailability of some anticancer agents substantially. Probiotics pretty significantly mitigate nasty gastrointestinal side effects such as mucositis thereby improving treatment tolerance quite substantially. Probiotic use effectively suppresses regulatory T cell mediated immune evasion and cytotoxic T cell responses skyrocket while dendritic cell activity gets heavily modulated.

Certain microbial taxa are tenuously linked often enough to improved outcomes with various immune checkpoint inhibitors underscoring microbiome's pivotal role in immunotherapy response effectively. Fermented food like kefir and kimchi alongside fibre-rich nosh substantially enhance beneficial microbes thereby modulating microbiota interactions effectively reducing carcinogenic metabolites while promoting protective pathways. Aiding cancer therapy pretty effectively via dietary means represents a fairly low-risk non-invasive strategy for prevention efforts alongside other treatments. Personalized oncology benefits remarkably from microbiome-informed dietary strategies that potentially amplify therapeutic efficacy and enhance long-term survivorship very effectively.

5.2. Personalized Nutrition: Tailoring Diet to the Individual

Modified dietary regimens informed by distinct genetic makeup and lifestyle factors embody a revolutionary shift in oncology through personalized nutrition. Personalized nutrition optimizes health outcomes effectively by factoring genetics epigenetics microbiome composition metabolic biomarkers and varied environmental exposures into equation. A seems pretty ambiguous ostensibly. Genetic variations such as single nucleotide polymorphisms sway nutrient metabolism pretty significantly alongside inflammatory responses and detoxification pathways concurrently. People with MTHFR gene variations often display wonky folate processing necessitating tweaked folate intake for sustaining DNA methylation processes and genetic repair. Genetic variants such as GSTT1 and SOD2 heavily influence protective antioxidant effects against carcinogenesis by regulating oxidative stress pretty significantly. Epigenetic tweaks such as DNA methylation or histone modification keenly respond to dietary factors and crucially influence gene expression underlying tumourigenesis.

Polyphenols and micronutrients like choline and selenium and folate heavily influence epigenetic mechanisms thereby modulating cancer susceptibility significantly and tumour progression. Diet profoundly impacts health through gut microbiome which varies greatly in composition and mediates responses differently under multifarious dietary regimens. Modified dietary regimens emerge from microbiome profiling thereby enhancing beneficial microbial activity like SCFA production and quashing noxious metabolites implicated in colorectal cancer. Emerging AI assisted platforms now integrate microbiome data with dietary inputs generating real-time personalized nutrition strategies pretty effectively in oncology care. A lowercase letter appears third somewhat mysteriously in alphabet. Personalized nutrition reckons with metabolic profiles including blood glucose levels alongside inflammatory markers and various deficiencies in essential nutrients quite frequently nowadays. Indicators help adjust macronutrient balance naturally for patients undergoing therapy and prevent nasty conditions like cachexia or stubborn insulin resistance.

Energy balance support boosts somewhat immune competence during recovery periods. Lifestyle factors including physical activity and stress heavily influence cancer outcomes as they interact irregularly with dietary patterns obviously beneath surface tensions. Wearables and AI-driven analytics facilitate tracking diet and physiological responses remarkably in myriad obscure ways quite continuously nowadays. Keen feedback mechanisms and highly adaptive meal planning strategies in these tools remarkably improve adherence very slowly over time. Detecting risk signals fairly early on ordinarily proves crucial but they generally do it quite well under normal circumstances. Patient empowerment blossoms rather naturally with such innovative tools in dietary care. Personalized nutrition embodies a vital shift in dietary science profoundly impacting cancer care nowadays rather than being just another fleeting trend. Tailoring nutritional regimens extremely carefully around each person's singular genetic makeup ushers in precision nutrition as cornerstone of oncology that enhances survivorship significantly.

a. Genetic and Epigenetic Profiling

Personalized oncology nutrition relies heavily on genetic and epigenetic profiling yielding keen insights into individual's genomic makeup altering nutrient metabolic pathways substantially. Clinicians can pretty effectively tailor dietary interventions by leveraging nutrigenomics and sometimes nutrigenetics for a patient's unique genetic makeup. Genetic variations like single nucleotide polymorphisms inside nutrient uptake or elimination genes can very dramatically change bodily reactions against certain food constituents. MTHFR or Methylenetetrahydrofolate Reductase entails folks carrying mutations like C677T or A1298C variants that badly impair folate metabolism. People with specific health issues may greatly benefit from extra methylated folate supplements such as L-methylfolate supporting crucial cancer prevention and DNA methylation processes. CYP1A2 gene modulates metabolism of xenobiotics and various compounds like caffeine or certain polycyclic aromatic hydrocarbons fairly effectively nowadays.

Fast metabolizers tend pretty well tolerate caffeine whereas slow metabolizers may face heightened risks upon exposure to various dietary carcinogens especially in hormone-influenced cancers like prostate cancer. Deletions in GSTT1 and GSTM1 genes may severely hamper bodily detoxification of various carcinogens prompting necessity for significantly augmented antioxidant intake or completely avoiding pro-oxidant foods. Dietary components subtly tweak epigenetic mechanisms such as DNA methylation or histone modification thereby altering gene expression quietly without mutating DNA sequence. Bioactive nutrients exhibiting epigenetic activity mostly comprise folate and vitamin B12 donating methyl groups heavily regulating DNA methylation influencing tumour suppressor genes.

Sulforaphane present in cruciferous veggies pretty vigorously inhibits histone deacetylases and promotes apoptosis in various kinds of cancer cells. Genistein and curcumin irregularly modulate miRNA expression very deeply impacting cellular processes like inflammation and proliferation somewhat variably. Modified diets informed by such insights can harness epigenetic modulation or offset genetic predispositions supporting cancer prevention vigorously with therapeutic backing.

b. Metabolic and Microbiome Assessments

Modified nutrition strategies slowly emerge vital in thwarting cancer onset when metabolic profiling converges with gut microbiome analysis for cancer care regimens. Assessments provide pretty dynamic snapshots of an individual's physiological status thereby facilitating rather modified dietetic interventions for metabolic function and immune modulation effectively. Metabolic assessments involve evaluation of crucial blood biomarkers in an individual's profile that signify risk or progression of cancer pretty accurately. Elevated triglyceride levels or abnormal cholesterol signal metabolic dysregulation linked with chronic inflammation and heightened risk of various cancers including breast prostate and colorectal cancer. Elevated fasting glucose or insulin resistance fuels hyperinsulinemia boosting insulin-like growth factor-1 activity thereby enhancing tumour growth across diverse cancer types vigorously.

Biomarkers like C-reactive protein help assess systemic inflammation effectively guiding dietary plans rich in omega-3 fatty acids usually. Personalized nutrition plans informed by specific biomarkers could involve adopting very low-carb regimens or radically anti-inflammatory eating protocols yielding surprisingly robust health benefits. Gut microbiome modulates immune function intricately within systemic inflammation deeply entwined with carcinogenic processes and nutrient metabolism occurs simultaneously. Shotgun metagenomics and 16S rRNA sequencing furnish insights into microbial diversity pretty haphazardly these days with somewhat varying degrees of success.

Microbial diversity depletion often correlates pretty strongly with chronic inflammation and generally poor cancer outcomes in people harbouring metabolic disorders. Folks wrestling with gut dysbiosis may derive considerable benefits from regularly consuming fermented food or popping probiotics and prebiotics supplements pretty frequently. Certain microbial communities produce beneficial metabolites such as short-chain fatty acids possessing anti-inflammatory and anti-proliferative properties very naturally. Others may harbour potentially carcinogenic proclivities thereby necessitating meticulously modulated nutritional interventions through diverse biochemical routes very carefully.

Gut microbiome significantly influences efficacy or toxicity of certain treatments particularly some immunotherapies under various complex physiological conditions pretty markedly. Dietary tweaks can significantly revamp microbiome composition and potentially boost tolerance remarkably enhancing overall success of treatment very effectively. Merging metabolic data with microbial insights facilitates a holistic nutrition approach enhancing therapeutic efficacy remarkably in individuals having distinct physiological makeup.

c. Lifestyle and Behavioral Considerations

Personalized nutrition works best when deeply psychosocial individual nuances and lifestyle behavioral aspects are incorporated beyond mere biological data. Dietary interventions become scientifically sound rather practical extremely sustainable deeply patient-centered by recognizing peculiar daily routines and individual preferences effectively. Exercise has a profoundly beneficial impact on metabolic function and also diminishes inflammation while encourage immune responses crucial for cancer prevention overall. Tweaking macronutrient intake and calories based on activity levels supports optimal body composition and maintaining muscle mass during treatment effectively. Active individuals undergoing chemotherapy may require rather higher protein intake very quickly preserving lean tissue and promoting swift repair.

Nutrient-rich foods effectively combat fatigue related to treatment in patients struggling with anorexia who lead sedentary lifestyles pretty frequently. Swift recovery and enhanced treatment tolerance are key considerations for modified nutrition plans formulated meticulously around individual patient needs. Nutrient-rich foods extremely high in energy are usually deemed very desirable and highly recommended by virtually all nutrition experts nowadays. Chronic stress ravages eating habits terribly and grossly disrupts gut health severely compromising immune function in the process very badly. Personalized interventions assess stress-related eating patterns alongside cortisol-associated metabolic shifts rather quietly including emotional eating and appetite suppression effectively.

Mood microbiota and diet interactions get factored in very slowly beneath surface layers of gut biome complexity and nutrient uptake. Dietary strategies often get paired with mindfulness-based eating or behavioral counseling in such instances very frequently nowadays. Ashwagandha and similar adaptogenic foods support emotional resilience remarkably and physiological balance remains intact through such dietary approaches effectively. Pharmacological treatments often radically alter appetite and change taste digestion nutrient absorption in suddenly very unpredictable ways. Personalized diets should be aligned with individual meds mainly for mitigating nasty side effects like mucositis thereby encourage therapeutic efficacy pretty significantly. Patients using corticosteroids might require drastic sodium restriction or extra blood sugar management measures subsequently. Folks undergoing immunotherapy occasionally reap huge benefits from nutrition that supports a healthy microbiome quite remarkably sometimes.

Personalization should deeply respect individual's quirky cultural identity and deeply rooted ethical values including religious dietary laws and peculiar flavor preferences. Familiar foods patients enjoy immensely enhance therapeutic alliance between patient and practitioner remarkably improving psychological comfort in a most satisfying manner. Ultimately successful personalized nutrition melds scientific precision with deep behavioral insight ensuring recommendations stay deeply aligned with individual lived quirky experience. This holistic strategy galvanizes individuals into assuming active roles in personal care while fostering surprisingly sustainable dietary shifts throughout arduous cancer treatment.

5.3. Bridging Functional Foods and Personalization

Functional foods converge with personalized nutrition in a transformative shift within cancer care dietary strategies pretty interestingly nowadays. Practitioners can match specific bioactive compounds rather precisely to individual metabolic genetic profiles and microbiome characteristics with targeted dietary components. Clinicians enhance therapeutic potential of diet very uniquely for each patient's specific physiological and pathological oncology state. Functional foods furnish myriad bioactive compounds ostensibly possessing anti-inflammatory antioxidant properties and potentially immunomodulatory effects alongside some markedly anti-carcinogenic benefits. Carefully chosen compounds produce specific effects that match a patient's clinical characteristics benefiting mostly those having high inflammatory markers or metabolic issues. Omega-3 fatty acids sourced from fatty fish or flaxseed benefit people exhibiting cachexia rather quietly alleviating related severe symptoms.

Fatty acids modulate cytokine production effectively reducing inflammation that fuels tumour growth and possibly enhancing tolerance of harsh chemotherapy regimens substantially. Blueberries and blackberries rich in polyphenols contain ellagic acid and flavonoids that modulate estrogen receptor pathways quite heavily in various cellular contexts. Foods potentially serve as natural adjuncts reducing cancer risk in individuals harbouring BRCA1/2 mutations or other hormone sensitive cancer susceptibilities naturally. Patients battling gut dysbiosis after intense chemotherapy treatments greatly benefit from fermented foods containing live probiotics like pungent kimchi or savory miso. Specific nutrients remarkably enhance gut barrier function and foster resilience during treatment over fairly protracted periods of time normally.

Tailoring functional food interventions very significantly boosts biological relevance and enhances effectiveness remarkably well in quite a few patients. Modified dietary regimens get incorporated into daily life mostly when they align nicely with personal food preferences and specific health goals. Dosing frequency can be tweaked significantly matching individual metabolic capacity and quirky absorption kinetics thereby boosting outcomes markedly under varying physiological conditions. This integrative model bridges gap between nutritional science and clinical application ensuring functional foods wield precision quite effectively in oncology care. Future evidence-based personalized nutrition therapy in oncology gets exemplified by aligning dietary bioactives with molecular diagnostics very effectively and patient-specific variables.

5.4. Technology as a Catalyst for Innovation

Technological advancement fuels successful implementation of personalized oncology nutrition thereby bridging gaps between theoretical science and real-world application quite murkily. Nowadays technology rapidly morphs nutrition into highly individualized therapy via large-scale data aggregation and super personalized feedback loops. Wearable devices and mobile health apps have drastically altered capture of nutritional data remarkably in recent times rather quickly. Tools facilitate dietary intake tracking via image recognition or barcode scanning and voice logging while monitoring physical activity simultaneously and sleep patterns overnight. Patients report treatment side effects and emotional well-being rather haphazardly in real time now and then pretty regularly. Clinicians tweak interventions rapidly under evolving conditions and feedback keeps patients fairly engaged in nutritional care somewhat effectively. AI and machine learning intricately converge quite rapidly with predictive analytics in ferreting out genomic data yielding modified dietary advice.

Algorithms unearth diet-gene interactions and nutrient-response patterns within vast datasets with remarkable quickness and surprising frequency nowadays. Nutritional status and a patient's dietary history rather thoroughly predict treatment responses or adverse events based on somewhat obscure correlations. Tumour biology's intricate metabolic pathways and immune responses are simulated under drastically different dietary regimens with considerable complexity. Models evolve swiftly enhancing precision and adaptability of nutrition plans uniquely tailored for each patient's distinct biology and specific treatment regimen. Mobile apps serve as portals for personalized nutrition delivering modified meal plans rooted deeply in genetic predispositions rather slowly nowadays. Platforms offer modified educational content for specific cancer types and phases of treatment with remarkable precision during therapy.

Goal tracking remarkably improves long-term adherence in patients with peculiar needs and behavioral coaching does so pretty effectively too apparently. These platforms simplify access to expert guidance considerably and foster patient autonomy effectively over time reducing various implementation barriers. Intelligent data analysis and digital delivery systems operate in real time transforming personalized nutrition into precise oncology care strategy effectively nowadays. Sophisticated tools will pretty significantly redefine cancer prevention outcomes as they become ridiculously accessible and pretty effective in various ways.

5.5. Clinical Applications and Evidence

Functional personalized nutrition merged into oncology care has transitioned rapidly from esoteric exploration into somewhat practical implementation rather lately nowadays. Nutritional interventions lately demonstrated significantly remarkable outcomes in cancer management alongside survivorship and various supportive care measures effectively. Mediterranean diet consists largely of monounsaturated fats from olive oil fibre-rich legumes whole grains and fruits veggies rich in omega-3 fatty acids from fish. A specific dietary pattern has been associated with improved metabolic health and reduced systemic inflammation and better outcomes in breast cancer survivors. Large-scale epidemiological studies and several randomized trials suggest adherence strongly correlates with substantially reduced cancer recurrence and significantly improved overall survival rates. Copious fat consumption fosters ketosis while severely curtailing carbohydrate intake in ketogenic diets being probed as oncology research metabolic therapy options.

Ketogenic interventions may exploit altered metabolic dependencies of tumour cells rather heavily particularly in glioblastoma and some extremely aggressive malignancies. Fasting-mimicking diets simulate metabolic effects of fasting pretty effectively without necessitating super strict caloric restriction for quite long periods. FMDs pretty significantly heighten cancer cells' susceptibility thus boosting chemotherapy efficacy while sparing non-malignant cells from somewhat collateral damage. Interventions may modulate immune response quite effectively promoting autophagy thereby adding unusual therapeutic benefit in significant layers down the line. Novel dietary approaches are being assessed for safety and effectiveness in varied cancer patient populations through utterly critical longitudinal cohort studies. Nutrigenomics and metabolic profiling advances are evolving rapidly and poised to deliver precision nutrition strategies complementing conventional cancer treatments pretty quickly nowadays. Personalized dietary interventions may remarkably enhance survivorship in oncology and improve overall quality of life significantly with notable efficacy.

6. Targeting Cancer Metabolism: Emerging Nutritional Strategies for Therapy

Cancer understood increasingly not solely as result of genetic mutations but also as disease riddled deeply with obscure metabolic dysregulation. Tumour cells undergo odd metabolic shifts allowing super rapid proliferation alongside stubborn therapy resistance and stealthy immune evasion downregulating apoptosis. Aberrant lipid synthesis and heightened glutamine uptake alongside elevated aerobic glycolysis rates known as Warburg effect frequently transpire in reprogrammed metabolism. Frenzied cancer cells proliferating at alarming rates necessitate customized adjustments satisfying hectic bioenergetic requirements and spawning insidious metabolic soft spots awaiting exploitation. Novel research suggests targeted nutritional interventions disrupt cancer-specific metabolic pathways thereby remarkably encourage therapeutic efficacy and mitigating off-target toxicity rather effectively. Ketogenic regimens drastically curtail glucose availability a vital fuel for tumours and instead elevate ketone bodies quite substantially in the process.

Metabolic pressure may thwart tumour expansion fairly effectively while maintaining viability of cells pretty well in nearby healthy tissue. Fasting and fasting-mimicking diets represent another rather promising approach being explored deeply in various research circles surrounding nutrition pretty intensely nowadays. Therapeutic regimens instigate drastic metabolic flux potentially rendering malignant cells vulnerable to chemotherapy or radiotherapy amidst uneven stress tolerance mechanisms. Fasting pretty significantly spurs autophagy and tweaks immune responses encourage anti-cancer effects under various unusual conditions rather effectively. Scientists investigate peculiar nutrient-centric strategies such as stifling glutamine in tumours glutamine-addicted and sabotaging serine and methionine metabolic pathways in malignancies hooked on one-carbon metabolic processes.

Metabolomics advances and tumour-specific metabolic profiling inform these approaches rapidly alongside increasing transcriptomics research nowadays with increasing frequency. Nutritional strategies are gradually shifting towards potential therapeutic modalities from supportive care as cancer metabolism becomes increasingly understood more profoundly. Dietary modulation remarkably serves as a strategic tool disrupting tumour bioenergetics and complements conventional oncologic treatments within a precision medicine framework effectively.

6.1. Cancer Metabolism

Tumour cells rapidly undergo extensive reprogramming metabolically enabling heightened energy demands for biosynthesis and redox balance maintenance quite effectively. Metabolic flexibility has emerged as cancer's hallmark lately providing a fertile foundation for novel interventions deeply rooted in nutritional strategies. Cancer cells predominantly harness glycolysis for energy production even with oxygen availability being quite ample exhibiting a pronounced Warburg effect. Excessive lactate production fosters biomass synthesis and promotes an acidic tumour microenvironment that facilitates invasion and enhance immune evasion. Malignancies often display glutamine addiction and anomalous glucose metabolism rapidly in various cancerous cells with pretty high frequency.

Glutamine fuels tricarboxylic acid cycle and nucleotide synthesis through glutathione production thereby maintaining redox homeostasis quite effectively. Tumour growth gets severely hampered upon glutamine deprivation or disruption of a metabolic pathway and cells become highly sensitized to chemotherapy. A hallmark involves drastically altered lipid metabolism exhibiting rampant de novo lipogenesis alongside greatly enhanced fatty acid oxidation simultaneously in cells. Phospholipids are supplied by these processes for synthesizing membranes and energy substrates are needed rapidly for cellular proliferation or metastasis and also signaling molecules. Tumour survival somewhat benefits from metabolic adaptations harbouring peculiar vulnerabilities susceptible to targeted nutritional strategizing in a rather peculiar manner.

Manipulating intake of specific nutrients and metabolic substrates can rather remarkably impair tumour growth selectively while sparing normal cells quite effectively. Such strategies offer complementary avenues alongside traditional oncologic therapies potentially enhancing efficacy pretty significantly and mitigating treatment-associated toxicity rather effectively. Cancer metabolism presents a vital target for devising dietary interventions grounded in oncology's metabolic underpinnings effectively in practice.

6.2. Ketogenic Diets and Glycolysis Inhibition

Ketogenic diet involves drastically cutting carbohydrate consumption and ramping up fat intake to target cancer metabolism rather extensively these days. Ketogenic diet drastically slashes carbohydrate availability forcing body drastically to switch primary energy source from glucose and utilizing ketone bodies produced deeply in liver. Therapeutic potential lurks within this metabolic shift particularly via glycolysis inhibition on which numerous tumour cells heavily rely for survival. Ketogenic dietary intervention rationale stems from Warburg effect where cancer cells voraciously utilize glucose via aerobic glycolysis rapidly biosynthesizing and generating energy in presence of oxygen abundantly. Severely restricting glucose can quite effectively starve tumour cells thereby significantly impairing their proliferative capacity in a rather dramatic fashion normally.

Cancer cells oftentimes strangely display a markedly impaired ability harnessing ketone bodies owing mostly to mitochondria gone haywire or sparse crucial enzyme expression. Normal cells adapt readily to ketone metabolism thereby creating a therapeutic window sparing healthy tissue and targeting malignant cells very selectively. Ketogenic diets impeded tumour growth significantly in glioblastoma models and remarkably in various prostate cancer models under certain experimental conditions. KDs may enhance chemotherapy efficacy and radiation therapy heavily via altering tumour microenvironment reducing insulin levels and modulating systemic inflammatory responses profoundly. Ketogenic diets remain under intense scrutiny nowadays in cancer therapy obviously still. Further research seems necessary now for determining long-term safety and patient adherence across various cancer types basically. Ketogenic diet potentially serves as game-changing adjunct in standard cancer care by uniquely exploiting glycolysis in vulnerable cancer cells effectively.

a. Mechanism of Action

Ketogenic diet's therapeutic potential in oncology stems largely from its capacity to vigorously disadvantage cancer cells by manipulating metabolism quite selectively. Drastically cutting dietary carbs plunges body into nutritional ketosis where it heavily relies on fat-derived ketones for energy instead of glucose. Several antitumour effects arise rather quietly from this metabolic shift upending crucial pathways many cancers depend on effectively. Glucose levels in circulation plummets rapidly reducing substrate availability for glycolysis, a metabolic pathway preferred by most tumour cells largely owing to Warburg effect. Reduction in insulin and insulin-like growth factor 1 levels further suppresses anabolic signaling pathways like PI3K/Akt/mTOR often upregulated in various cancers fueling tumour growth vigorously.

Ketogenic state yields copious ketone bodies namely β-hydroxybutyrate and acetoacetate remarkably in greatly elevated amounts quite often. Normal cells such as neurons readily adapt to utilizing ketones via mitochondrial oxidative phosphorylation while many cancer cells remain metabolically inflexible. Such discrepancy renders cells pretty metabolically stressed subsequently making them far more vulnerable to various treatments.

Ketogenic diet fosters a metabolic milieu favoring oxidative phosphorylation in healthy tissues whilst precipitating energy crises and oxidative stress rapidly in glycolysis-reliant cancer cells. Tumours subjected to ketogenic conditions often exhibit altered redox states and mitochondrial dysfunction which markedly heightens susceptibility to chemotherapy or oxidative insult. Tumour cell proliferation gets hindered collectively by these mechanisms and conventional therapies become markedly more selective and effective under certain conditions. Further research endeavors elucidate molecular mechanisms underlying effects and pinpoint specific patient cohorts likely benefiting greatly from ketogenic dietary regimens in various oncology settings nowadays.

b. Clinical Applications

Interest in ketogenic diets remarkably grew as therapeutic adjuncts in oncology lately driven by promising preclinical research findings surprisingly. Ketogenic dietary interventions effectively suppress tumour progression in cancers with high glycolytic activity such as glioblastoma multiforme and some prostate cancers. KDs inhibit tumour growth effectively and markedly prolong survival while enhancing efficacy of various chemotherapeutic agents or radiotherapy pretty significantly. Glioblastoma persists as a wickedly aggressive glucose-dependent brain tumour having sparse treatment options and a pretty dismal prognosis usually. Preliminary human trials indicate KDs are feasible for certain GBM patients and potentially enhance metabolic parameters significantly stabilizing disease somewhat. Ongoing research investigates whether ketogenic interventions might synergize rather effectively with standard therapies by subtly altering tumour microenvironments.

Ongoing clinical trials are probing KDs' broader utility across various cancer types evaluating tumour responses and metabolic shifts quite vigorously. Ketogenic diets in oncology ought be approached extremely cautiously and selected meticulously for rather specific rare cases despite increasing enthusiasm. Malnourished individuals exhibiting severe muscle atrophy alongside advanced pathology may struggle mightily with metabolic pressures of a very low-carb high-fat regimen. People with underlying metabolic issues or those exhibiting liver dysfunction and kidney problems may subsequently display extremely adverse reactions quite frequently downstream. Multidisciplinary teams comprising oncologists and metabolic specialists must conduct thorough assessments pretty regularly and monitor patients for safe execution. Ketogenic diets show promising adjunctive potential in metabolically active tumours but clinical application must be grounded in evidence-based protocols under close monitoring.

6.3. Fasting and Fasting-Mimicking Diets (FMDs)

Fasting and fasting-mimicking diets have emerged rather surprisingly as promising interventions garnering considerable attention in oncology quite effectively targeting cancer cells. Certain dietary strategies remarkably effectively exploit vulnerabilities of tumour cells under specific physiological conditions while safeguarding normal tissues very subtly. Intermittent fasting entails irregular bouts of fasting and refeeding that can last from a few hours to several days sometimes. Fasting-mimicking diets are deliberately crafted regimens remarkably low in calories and protein and carbohydrates mirroring the physiological effects of prolonged water-only fasting quite precisely. FMDs are decidedly more feasible for implementation and remarkably more enduring making them quite suitable for clinical use effectively. Fasting triggers catabolic metabolism shifting away from anabolic processes, thereby lowering glucose insulin and insulin-like growth factor 1 levels in circulation quite drastically.

Cancer cells strangely falter here owing largely to utter reliance on steady nutrient and growth factor supplies in their surroundings. Normal cells enter a protective state termed differential stress resistance on other hand characterized by energy conservation under fairly specific conditions. Fasting or FMDs substantially boost chemotherapy efficacy and radiotherapy results while slowing tumour growth and lessening many treatment-related side effects. Healthy cells exhibit enhanced DNA damage repair and autophagy gets ramped up subsequently while immune responses undergo subtle modulation thereafter. Fasting may sensitize tumours rather substantially to oxidative stress and diminish various cellular resistance mechanisms effectively under certain conditions simultaneously. Early-phase clinical trials yield promising results demonstrating markedly enhanced patient well-being overall and reduced hematological toxicity from chemotherapy. Fasting-based interventions should be somewhat individually tailored especially in patients with advanced cancer malnutrition or considerable metabolic derangement obviously. Fasting and FMDs emerge as novel non-pharmacological approaches effectively integrated with standard cancer treatments yielding pretty decent clinical gains.

a. Cellular Mechanisms

Fasting and fasting-mimicking diets spark rather dramatic metabolic shifts disadvantageous to tumour cells yet sparing normal tissues pretty selectively. Multiple convoluted cellular processes mediate these effects quietly beneath surface. Fasting yields dramatic reductions in circulating glucose and insulin-like growth factor 1 levels quickly alongside insulin apparently. Pivotal anabolic hormones IGF-1 and insulin activate various growth-promoting pathways like PI3K/Akt/mTOR axis often upregulated highly in malignant cells. Fasting curtails such signals thereby fostering an environment restrictive to growth that gravely hinders tumour cell survival and proliferation. Glucose availability reduction directly stunts glycolytic flux thereby disrupting primary energy source severely for many fast growing malignant tumour cells.

Cells under severe nutrient stress surprisingly activate various protective mechanisms like autophagy a quirky recycling system for ridding damaged cell parts. Fasting triggers adaptive cellular response somewhat encourage resilience of healthy cells against oxidative stress and DNA damage from chemotherapy or radiation therapy. Fasting exerts a pretty effective protective effect on various non-malignant tissues largely due to differential stress resistance phenomenon manifesting therein. Fasting simultaneously ramps up oxidative stress and greatly impairs antioxidant defenses in cancer cells rendering them vulnerable to various therapeutic insults. Metabolic stress intensifies markedly under specific conditions and certain cytotoxic agents can quite selectively precipitate tumour cell death precipitously. Fasting mechanisms underscore potential as a metabolic adjuvant boosting efficacy of conventional therapies significantly while reducing collateral damage pretty substantially. Fasting interventions offer quite a potent system-wide strategy for treating cancer grounded rather deeply in resilience at cellular level.

b. Therapeutic Synergy

Fasting and fasting-mimicking diets can significantly boost efficacy of conventional cancer treatments remarkably while improving tolerability pretty substantially. Cancerous cells and non-cancerous ones exhibit disparate metabolic responses under nutrient deprivation quite effectively harnessed to reduce toxicity rather remarkably. FMDs or short-term fasting administered with chemotherapy have been shown remarkably well to shield healthy tissues from quite severe cytotoxic insult. Fasting remarkably shifts normal cells into quiescent stress-resistant states by reducing insulin and IGF-1 signaling perhaps surprisingly quite effectively. Cancer cells stay highly proliferative and metabolically inflexible under fasting-induced metabolic stress rendering them susceptible to DNA damage and apoptosis by chemotherapeutic agents.

Patients undergoing chemotherapy while fasting reportedly experience fewer side effects like fatigue and nausea without any reduced efficacy therapeutically. Benefits manifest strikingly in hormone-sensitive tumours and solid malignancies like breast cancer or prostate cancer with well characterized metabolic dependencies. FMDs remarkably enhance anti-tumour responses mediated by immune systems and modulate tumour microenvironments significantly favoring responsiveness to various treatments pretty effectively. Fasting-based interventions wield multifaceted effects that robustly endorse their deployment as potent adjuvants alongside chemotherapy or potentially with targeted agents and radiotherapy. Sizable trials defining optimal protocols for carefully selected patients under disparate conditions ultimately necessitate broader clinical adoption and validation of safety parameters. Crucially individualized assessment remains vital for vulnerable populations like elderly folks or people suffering badly from various nasty metabolic issues.

6.4. Amino Acid Restriction Strategies

Nutritional oncology now entails drastically limiting certain amino acids rather cleverly to capitalize on cancer cells' rather peculiar metabolic vulnerabilities. Tumours often bizarrely depend on certain amino acids making them highly vulnerable to severe dietary regime changes rather drastically. Methionine glutamine and serine are highly studied targets playing crucial epigenetic roles in tumour cell proliferation and various redox processes. Methionine a vital sulfur-containing amino acid plays a crucial role in synthesizing S-adenosylmethionine which donates primary methyl groups during DNA methylation. Cancer cells frequently display defective methionine recycling through methionine salvage pathway rendering them unusually vulnerable to abrupt severe methionine depletion.

Preclinical studies reveal that restricting dietary methionine thwarts tumour growth and boosts chemotherapy efficacy by disrupting methylation processes somewhat effectively. Glutamine, a non-essential amino acid, enhances multiple anabolic pathways and redox homeostasis in various kinds of cancer cells. Pancreatic adenocarcinoma and triple-negative breast cancer exhibit pronounced reliance on glutamine for survival and they proliferate rapidly. Tumour growth stalled remarkably under targeted glutamine intake reduction coupled with glutaminase inhibitors and cells became unusually sensitive to treatment. Carefully managed modest dietary restriction may enhance therapeutic responses because entirely eliminating glutamine is not feasible owing largely to its crucial role in immune function. Serine another non-essential amino acid plays a somewhat obscure role in one-carbon metabolism and synthesizes nucleotides with fairly remarkable efficiency. Dietary serine and glycine restriction pretty effectively shows anti-tumour effects in some models when paired with inhibitors of folate metabolism. Nutritional status and tumour metabolic profiling inform controlled dietary modulation a potentially supportive yet relatively safe strategy in cancer therapy. Modified amino acid restriction regimens enhance targeted treatments quite effectively while maintaining overall nutritional adequacy fairly intact.

6.5. Lipid Metabolism and Dietary Fat Manipulation

Tumour cells rely heavily on glucose and amino acids displaying markedly altered lipid metabolic processes that sustain extremely rapid proliferation mechanisms. Rampant fatty acid uptake alongside upregulated β-oxidation and de novo lipogenesis, demonstrate cancer types with diverse metabolic landscapes. Lipid metabolism emerges as a tantalizing target for dietary manipulation furnishing crucial substrates rampantly for energy production and biosynthesis of cellular membranes. Modifying fat intake pretty effectively disrupts lipid dependencies of cancer cells rather non-invasively these days through altering composition and quantity. Eicosapentaenoic acid and docosahexaenoic acid found in omega-3 polyunsaturated fatty acids have exhibited remarkably potent anti-inflammatory effects in numerous cancer models very recently. Fatty acids insidiously infiltrate cellular membranes, knocking arachidonic acid out of kilter and utterly disrupting lipid raft domains crucial for tumour cell signalling.

Omega-3 PUFAs profoundly disrupt key proliferative pathways such as PI3K/Akt and NF-κB in cancer cells while heavily promoting oxidative stress. High intake of saturated fats fosters pro-tumourigenic microenvironments especially in hormone sensitive malignancies like breast cancer and prostate cancer aggressively. Reducing saturated fat intake possibly hinders lipid substrates fueling oncogenic signaling and hormone production thus slowing disease progression somewhat gradually. Dietary fat composition fairly significantly modulates tumour microenvironment crucially in many complex ways. Omega-3 fatty acids substantially enhance immune cell infiltration and rather effectively foster anti-tumour macrophage polarization thereby somewhat diminishing angiogenesis which may amplify responsiveness to diverse immunotherapies. Lipid-rich environments rather quietly support peculiar immunosuppressive phenotypes and effectively promote highly metastatic behavior under some very specific conditions. Altering fat intake quite collectively represents rather promising adjunctive strategy in certain cancer therapies. Precisely tailored interventions may modulate tumour biology effectively and enhance intake of beneficial fatty acids significantly in oncology personalized for each patient.

6.6. Integrative and Personalized Approaches

Nutritional strategies tailored metabolically for oncology require highly personalized approach factoring complex interactions between tumour-specific metabolic needs patient genetic makeup and treatment protocols under diverse overall nutritional conditions. Cancer metabolism fluctuates erratically across various tumour types and a universal dietary regimen basically falls flat in most cases. Multi-omics tech advances pretty effectively enable in-depth characterization nowadays of tumour metabolic landscape through transcriptomics proteomics and metabolomics. Such tools can occasionally pinpoint specific nutrient dependencies and metabolic bottlenecks pretty effectively for exploitation in highly tailored dietary regimens. Tumours riddled with glutamine addiction or methionine dependence or festooned with supercharged glycolytic flux can be thwarted via modified dietary tweaks or supplemental wizardry.

Biomarker monitoring in real time enables fairly dynamic adjustment of dietary interventions throughout a treatment course with pretty good effectiveness. Monitoring boosts safety fairly effectively by facilitating early detection of nasty complications or malnutrition and intolerance to treatment quite swiftly now. Integration with digital nutrition platforms like wearable biosensors and app-based meal tracking empowers patients pretty actively in their nutritional care and further supports personalized implementation. Nutritional interventions embody a potent stratagem in oncologists' arsenal albeit grossly underutilized ultimately by cancer specialists very effectively nowadays. Strategically applied interventions markedly enhance efficacy of conventional therapies and significantly improve long-term outcomes now under certain conditions effectively. Clinicians can tap into precision nutrition's vast therapeutic potential for cancer care by leveraging evidence-based dietary regimens extremely effectively nowadays. Translational research and rigorous clinical trials will be utterly essential in oncology practice for validating outcomes and establishing stringent safety parameters eventually.

7. Exploring Epigenetic Modifications

Recently epigenetics involving heritable gene expression changes has profoundly reshaped cancer development understanding without altering underlying DNA sequence. Epigenetic modifications such as DNA methylation or histone post-translational modifications play a pivotal role controlling gene activity pretty effectively downstream. Epigenetic changes dynamically shift and reverse rendering them attractive targets for therapy unlike genetic mutations that often stubbornly persist permanently. Nutrition emerges as a potent modifiable influencer among various environmental factors heavily influencing epigenetic regulation via complex pathways in multiple ways. Nutrients and bioactive dietary components serve as substrates for cellular metabolism and directly modulate epigenetic machinery fairly effectively downstream. Folate and vitamins B6 and B12 play crucial roles in one-carbon metabolism providing methyl groups necessary for various DNA methylation processes.

Epigallocatechin gallate found in green tea alongside curcumin markedly influence histone acetylation with polyphenols having been shown to do so previously. Sulforaphane and other isothiocyanates found pretty abundantly in cruciferous veggies rather significantly affect expression of tumour suppressive microRNAs. Aberrant epigenetic regulation often silences tumour suppressor genes quite pertinently in oncology amidst nutrient-epigenome interactions that are fairly significant really. Oncogenic pathways get activated thereby facilitating cancer progression alarmingly fast. Dietary interventions may possibly restore normal epigenetic patterns quite effectively and cancer prevention efforts thereby gain considerable momentum. Oncology's nutritional epigenetics burgeons rapidly examining how certain dietary elements deeply modulate epigenetic configurations in rather complex cellular processes. Modified nutrition may complement molecular therapies and thwart carcinogenesis by elucidating mechanistic links between diet and gene regulation quite effectively one day.

7.1. Epigenetic Mechanisms and their Role in Cancer

Epigenetic regulation entails heritable gene expression changes that are reversible and occur fairly often sans underlying DNA sequence modification nowadays. Modifications orchestrate development normally and cellular differentiation proceeds via radical restructuring of chromatin for purposes of gene expression essentially. Malignant transformation and progression in cancer frequently stem from disruption of epigenetic control which often precedes or vigorously interacts with genetic mutations. Three primary epigenetic mechanisms regulate it pretty intricately. DNA methylation entails addition of a methyl group covalently at cytosine residues' 5' position within CpG dinucleotides often clustered in promoter-associated islands.

DNA methylation maintains genomic stability pretty effectively in healthy cells and silences various repetitive elements under normal physiological conditions.

Tumour suppressor genes in cancer get transcriptionally silenced pretty quietly due to promoter hypermethylation and cell proliferation runs amok. Global hypomethylation occurs frequently in tumour genomes and promotes chromosomal instability and oncogene activation often spuriously in various cancer types. Histone proteins undergo diverse post-translational modifications like methylation and phosphorylation ubiquitination alongside acetylation that radically alter gene expression and chromatin structure. Histone acetyltransferases catalyze acetylation reactions typically correlating with gene activation whereas histone deacetylases conversely promote deacetylation mostly linked with repression. Aberrant histone modifications in cancer cells precipitously silence tumour suppressor genes and concurrently activate various pro-tumourigenic signaling pathways rapidly.

Non-coding RNAs encompass microRNAs and long non-coding RNAs that regulate gene expression quietly at various cellular levels post-transcriptionally. Dysregulation of ncRNAs manifests aberrantly in various cancers and influences numerous pathways related obscurely to cell cycle control and metastasis very deeply. Epigenetic alterations play a crucial role in almost all cancer hallmarks and offer novel mechanistic insights alongside fresh therapeutic opportunities simultaneously. Their reversible nature renders them pretty attractive targets simultaneously for dietary modulation and quite effective pharmacological interventions.

7.2. Diet as an Epigenetic Modulator

Growing evidence starkly highlights nutrition's potent role as a malleable epigenetic regulator right from embryogenesis through human existence till natural senescence occurs. Dietary components serve as energy sources and act as epigenetic modulators influencing gene expression through histone modification heavily modifying cellular processes. Nutriepigenomic interactions yield profoundly significant consequences somewhat irregularly for cancer prevention and progression or response under therapeutic interventions. Diet profoundly influences epigenetics by furnishing methyl donors and cofactors necessary for one-carbon metabolism generating S-adenosylmethionine a universal methyl donor for DNA methylation. Folate vitamin B12 and other nutrients like choline and betaine play crucial roles in a complex biochemical pathway deeply.

Methylation patterns in cells get drastically altered by nutrient deficiencies potentially leading to aberrant gene expression heavily involved in oncogenic processes. Bioactive dietary compounds directly influence epigenetic enzyme activity markedly under various physiological conditions. Sulforaphane present quite abundantly in cruciferous vegetables pretty effectively inhibits histone deacetylases promoting expression of tumour suppressor genes rather remarkably. Epigallocatechin gallate mostly found in green tea may inhibit DNA methyltransferases and effectively modulate expression of various miRNA. Resveratrol found in red grapes and various berries interacts heavily with SIRT1 and histone acetylation pathways regulating gene expression pretty slowly. Interactions are context-dependent phenomena heavily swayed by genetic makeup and microbiome and age and sundry obscure environmental factors. Dietary epigenetic effects persist remarkably beyond exposure and get transmitted eerily across multiple generations highlighting potential long-term catastrophic health impact. Nutritional interventions aimed squarely at epigenetic plasticity offer cancer prevention and pretty personalized therapy down a rather promising road. Formulating cancer treatments now relies pretty heavily on grasping subtle connections between epigenome and diet pretty obscurely these days.

a. Methyl Donors and Cofactors

Methyl groups are donated liberally in DNA methylation processes via a crucial biochemical network that fuels epigenomic changes heavily. Generation of S-adenosylmethionine SAM plays a crucial role in this pathway serving as universal methyl donor for myriad methyltransferase reactions. Folate vitamin B12 and choline act pretty much as crucial cofactors or methyl donors alongside methionine in various methylation-related biological processes. Folate acts as one-carbon unit carrier in tetrahydrofolate derivatives facilitating methionine synthesis via remethylation of homocysteine pretty efficiently. Vitamin B12 acts rather obscurely as coenzyme for methionine synthase a crucial enzyme during remethylation step. Choline donates methyl groups somewhat mysteriously for SAM synthesis through betaine a metabolite entirely outside folate pathways.

Methionine directly serves as precursor for SAM production being an essential amino acid. Methyl group transfer efficiency gets severely hampered amidst gross nutrient deficiency or utterly skewed nutritional profiles fostering gnarly epigenetic chaos. Disruptions in cancer cause global DNA hypomethylation promoting genomic instability while hypermethylation silences tumour suppressor gene promoters facilitating oncogenesis effectively. Heightened risks of various malignancies including colorectal cancer and pancreatic tumours are associated frequently with low levels of folate or B12. Synthetic folic acid intake excessively may potentially spur progression of pre-existing neoplasms highlighting importance of striking optimal delicate balance.

Modulating methyl donors through dietary changes targets one-carbon metabolism which represents a promising epigenetic strategy for cancer therapy. Research must ferret out subtle interactions between timing of dosage and genetic context rendering some nutrients surprisingly beneficial or remarkably pernicious.

b. Histone Modification Modulators

Epigenetic regulators modulating chromatin structure rely heavily on histone modifications such as phosphorylation and ubiquitination very profoundly. Modifications mostly occur on amino-terminal tails of histone proteins and are dynamically regulated by various enzymes like histone acetyltransferases or histone deacetylases and histone methyltransferases. Evidence demonstrates convincingly certain nutrients influence enzyme activity thereby exerting potent epigenetic effects and anticancer properties rather remarkably inside human cells. Sulforaphane a naturally occurring isothiocyanate abounds in cruciferous veggies like broccoli and modulates histones quite effectively in dietary contexts. Sulforaphane strongly inhibits HDAC enzymes which repress gene expression by heavily promoting chromatin condensation in a quite complex manner.

Sulforaphane pretty frequently reactivates epigenetically silenced tumour suppressor genes like p21 and Bax by inhibiting HDAC activity in various cancer cell lines. Butyrate a short-chain fatty acid produced vigorously by gut microbiota during dietary fibre fermentation holds considerable significance apparently. Butyrate exhibits HDAC inhibitory properties particularly relevant in colorectal cancer contexts where it heavily accumulates in colonic lumen gradually over time. It fosters differentiation and apoptosis mainly in cancerous cells while exerting fairly minimal effects mostly on normal epithelial cells. Curcumin present in turmeric and epigallocatechin gallate or EGCG sourced from green tea seemingly modulate histone acetylation and methylation at same time.

Polyphenolic compounds extensively reprogram cancer epigenome by inhibiting HDACs and HATs while modulating activity of HMTs and various HDMs. They quite strikingly exhibit antioxidant properties and display anti-inflammatory effects thereby significantly amplifying overall therapeutic potential in various applications. Nutritional epigenetics shows promise in cancer prevention efforts effectively modulating gene expression linked with malignancy through various bioactive compounds.

c. MicroRNA Modulation

MicroRNAs are short non-coding RNAs about twenty two nucleotides long binding post-transcriptionally to complementary sequences on target messenger RNAs. Dysregulation of specific miRNAs heavily implicates initiation and progression of various cancers with distinct profiles often serving as oncomiRs nowadays. Bioactive dietary compounds have emerged as potent modulators of miRNA expression thereby influencing cancer-related pathways significantly in recent times. Resveratrol a rather reclusive polyphenolic compound dwells mainly in red grape skin and certain berries or peanuts ostensibly. Resveratrol modulates multiple miRNAs effectively in various key oncogenic processes irregularly and deeply within cellular pathways sometimes. Upregulation occurs pretty aggressively for tumour-suppressive miRNAs like miR-34a targeting genes involved in proliferation and anti-apoptotic signaling pathways.

Resveratrol significantly contributes to anti-proliferative effects and pro-apoptotic outcomes during epithelial-mesenchymal transition by modulating pathways like p53 activation and NF-κB inhibition. Genistein remarkably regulates miRNA networks in hormone-responsive cancers especially in breast cancer cells and also quite abundantly in prostate cancer cells. Genistein alters expression of miRNAs like miR-155 and miR-221 and miR-222 intricately involved in estrogen receptor signaling pathways heavily modulating cell cycle progression. Genistein pretty effectively restores ER expression in ER-negative breast cancer cells by subtly tweaking specific miRNAs and suppressing tumour growth rapidly. Diet-derived compounds act as potent epigenetic regulators of miRNA expression offering novel noninvasive cancer therapy and prevention strategies fairly effectively nowadays. Studies on nutrient-miRNA interplay hold much promise for devising highly tailored dietary regimens aimed squarely at cancer sufferers harbouring distinct miRNA signatures.

7.3. Timing and Duration of Exposure

Nutritional exposure timing plays a crucial role in shaping epigenome significantly during fetal development and somewhat surprisingly early adulthood periods. Epigenetic windows of vulnerability signify periods like infancy or adolescence when epigenome stays highly plastic and extremely responsive to various dietary inputs. Epigenome gets heavily shaped by various environmental cues during formative childhood years quite significantly under normal circumstances apparently. Such windows pivotally determine long-term epigenetic changes many years after initial exposure occurs under certain conditions apparently. Major developmental stages display rather differing levels of epigenetic plasticity under fairly normal circumstances usually. Certain developmental stages are extremely vulnerable to external influences like nutrition and lifestyle under specific conditions quite frequently.

Nutritional interventions during sensitive developmental windows profoundly impact gene expression inducing long-lasting effects on overall susceptibility to various diseases. Maternal nutrition during pregnancy affords quite persuasive evidence strangely. Methyl-donating nutrients such as folate and vitamin B12 if inadequately ingested during gestation can trigger quite persistent epigenetic alterations in a developing fetus. Epigenetic alterations may silence tumour suppressor genes or crank up dodgy oncogenes thereby heightening malignancy likelihood pretty substantially later on. Maternal diet potentially programs protective gene expression profiles significantly reducing cancer susceptibility through complex biological pathways and various other mechanisms. Emerging research underscores adolescence and early adulthood as pivotal stages owing largely to swift cellular changes and profound hormonal upheaval. During puberty mammary tissues undergo drastic epigenetic remodeling heavily influenced by diet which modulates lifetime risk of cancers like breast and prostate cancer. Research findings underscore significance of adopting lifespan approach in nutritional epigenetics where diverse dietary patterns profoundly impact health outcomes and cancer risk over lengthy periods. Formulating age-specific preventive nutrition strategies that foster epigenetic robustness against cancerous processes relies heavily on grasping diet-epigenome interplay dynamics over prolonged periods roughly.

7.4. Epigenetic Diets and Cancer Prevention

Epigenetic diets frequently comprise foods extremely rich in bioactive compounds deliberately targeting epigenetic mechanisms like DNA methylation and histone modification. Epigenetic diets heavily modulate gene expression pathways implicated in carcinogenesis and bypass traditional macronutrient balancing with rather weird specificity entirely. Sulforaphane-rich cruciferous veggies play a pivotal role in epigenetic modification by quite effectively reactivating dormant tumour suppressor genes. Grapes bursting with polyphenol and berries furnish resveratrol which modulates microRNAs heavily in various inflammatory pathways exerting profoundly anti-cancer effects. Epigallocatechin-3-gallate pretty effectively inhibits DNA methyltransferases in green tea thus restoring gene function in cancer-prone cells remarkably. Genistein and other soy isoflavones markedly alter expression of estrogen receptors and show substantial epigenetic activity in various hormone-sensitive cancers.

High-fibre foods including whole grains and legumes robustly support microbial fermentation in gut producing butyrate fairly effectively as a potent HDAC inhibitor downstream. Substantially enhancing anti-inflammatory properties occurs when nuclear receptors are modulated and histone acetylation is altered in an omega-3 rich dietary regimen found in fatty fish. Dietary elements rather quietly enhance genomic stability and foster apoptosis mostly in premalignant cells or dysplastic ones very effectively. Epigenetic diets possibly reduce cancer risk significantly and enhance therapeutic outcomes by modulating tumour microenvironment irregularly altering immune response somewhat. New evidence pretty strongly supports nutritional regimens epigenetically active as a remarkably low-risk strategy to thwart cancer and enhance overall healthspan.

7.5. Clinical and Therapeutic Implications

Nutritional epigenetics insights are being leveraged slowly into innovative clinical strategies with considerable promise for remarkably improving human health outcomes. Rapid breakthroughs in cutting-edge epigenomic tech and omics integration platforms are hastening shift from preclinical stages toward actual clinical usage quickly. Bioactive dietary components reversing aberrant epigenetic modifications that silence tumour suppressor genes or activate various oncogenes emerge via chemoprevention. Sulforaphane and EGCG potentially restore gene expression in premalignant tissues quite effectively offering a pretty non-toxic dietary approach for cancer risk reduction. Epigenetically active diets may serve quite effectively as adjuncts in diverse therapeutic contexts rather significantly enhancing tumour sensitivity towards chemotherapy. Nutrients reprogram epigenome via modulation of DNA methylation or histone acetylation lowering treatment resistance and often ameliorate toxicity in cancers.

Novel research findings substantially back employing epigenetic indicators such as DNA methylation patterns and histone alteration profiles for tailoring highly modified nutritional regimens. Biomarkers may facilitate identification of individuals most likely benefiting from epigenetic modulation and enable real-time monitoring of response effectively. Precision oncology incorporating highly personalized epigenetic nutrition nowadays holds remarkably substantial potential in various fairly influential medical research arenas. Clinicians can remarkably boost therapeutic efficacy by tailoring dietary strategies according to an individual's unique epigenomic landscape and improve long-term outcomes pretty significantly. Widely adopting such approaches requires robust clinical trials and stringent protocols validating efficacy and ensuring utmost safety beforehand in most cases.

7.6. Challenges and Future Directions

Merging epigenetics with nutrition nowadays remarkably sparks a paradigm shift in comprehending etiology prevention and cancer treatment profoundly. Epigenetic modifications like DNA methylation or histone alterations get profoundly influenced irregularly by diet in a somewhat very dynamic reversible manner. Malleability positions nutrition as central modulator of gene expression and tumour behavior rather than just some supportive cancer care component. Various bioactive compounds and nutrients like methyl donors and histone deacetylase inhibitors showed epigenetic activity in several in vitro models fairly effectively. Tumour suppressor genes long silenced can be reactivated somewhat by compounds modulating signaling pathways and boosting conventional therapies' efficacy influencing cancer susceptibility variably throughout life. Nutritional exposures profoundly shape cancer risk during critical epigenetic windows identified in early development and adolescence with lifelong importance.

Nutritional epigenetics has immense potential yet faces rather formidable challenges ahead with considerable uncertainty surrounding its future development slowly. Genetic background and nutrient metabolism variability modulate epigenetic effects of diet significantly and pretty heavily complicating efforts at generalization. Scarcity of large-scale longitudinal human trials and dearth of standardized epigenetic biomarkers severely hobble immediate translation into clinical practice. Amalgamating epigenomic insights with various omics technologies including genomics and metabolomics forges sturdy predictive models of diet's impact on oncogenic pathways effectively. Epigenetic profiling remarkably guides evolution of precision nutrition holding considerable promise downstream for remarkably personalized cancer prevention therapy. Tailor-made nutrition plans based on singular metabolic profiles and molecular traits might lessen reliance on meds and enhance long-term health outcomes exceedingly well.

Food becomes a super potent tool recalibrating epigenetic expression rather than just being sustenance and thwarting malignant cellular transformation dead in its tracks. Nutritional epigenetics offers rather compelling framework that bridges molecular oncology with lifestyle medicine facets pretty effectively nowadays. Rapidly accumulating scientific evidence nowadays underscores pivotal roles of epigenetic-based dietary strategies in future cancer care pretty effectively.

8. Collaboration across Disciplines

Cancer treatment complexity requires deeply interdisciplinary collaboration often remarkably well integrated into shifting paradigms under various circumstances nowadays. Merging oncology with nutritional insights and cutting-edge emerging tech yields profoundly transformative cancer care models spanning prevention and palliative interventions effectively. Oncologists, dietitians and molecular biologists collaborate intimately to deciphering tumour biology amid various systemic metabolic factors starkly influencing disease progression pathways. Nutrition stands potent as a largely modifiable determinant in cancer risk management across various populations quite effectively worldwide now. Modified treatment regimens for individuals with vastly different needs require real-time metabolic data and intricate molecular profiling pretty much always nowadays. Wearable gadgets and AI-driven diet analysis software facilitate dynamically personalized interventions across various mobile platforms with remarkable flexibility nowadays.

Clinicians and data scientists collaborate pretty seamlessly alongside nutritionists ensuring oncology interventions are backed by solid evidence and very actionable. Fresh insights into tumour metabolism emerge rapidly from advancements in genomics and epigenomics offering opportunities for tailoring nutrition strategies cleverly now. High-level personalization becomes feasible through synergy of diverse teams where clinical expertise intersects with computational modeling and nutritional science suddenly. Collaboration has become utterly imperative in our rapidly evolving ecosystem rather than being merely some optional nicety nowadays. Precision oncology demands a seismic overhaul of cancer care through deeply embedding nutrition alongside state-of-the-art tech into a fiercely personalized framework. Collaborative frameworks substantially enhance treatment efficacy and obliterate debilitating side effects by actively empowering patients in their own healthcare regimen. Cancer care will heavily bank on partnerships across disciplines for garnering peak results through tech-enabled nutritionally dense science-backed approaches down line.

8.1. The Evolving Role of Nutrition in Oncology

Nutrition has emerged somewhat weirdly as a critical determinant of clinical outcomes in oncology shedding its ancillary role pretty entirely now. Emerging evidence nowadays vividly underscores nutritional status impact on initiation of cancer progression and survivorship outcomes rather markedly. Malnutrition obesity sarcopenia systemic inflammation and insulin resistance are modifiable through diet and now widely regarded as key prognostic factors influencing therapeutic efficacy overall survival and quality of life very heavily. Registered dietitians and clinical nutrition specialists frequently collaborate with oncologists and palliative care providers in oncology teams nowadays in various settings. Responsibilities span cancer care continuum entailing early identification of nutritional risk through validated screening tools and formulation of highly modified dietary plans. Surgery patients and those getting treatments like chemo or radiation frequently endure side effects such as mucositis and really debilitating fatigue.

Targeted nutrition strategies are employed pretty effectively nowadays modulating immune function and attenuating inflammation in various esoteric clinical settings. Nutrition plays a pivotal role in reducing recurrence risk and managing comorbidities during survivorship thereby improving functional outcomes very greatly. Maximizing potential of nutrition in oncology nowadays necessitates rapid integration with rather emerging disciplines across various healthcare domains effectively. Rapid advancements in genomics and metabolomics are uncovering sizable differences in individual responses necessitating pretty modified nutrition plans rather quickly nowadays. Mobile apps and wearables facilitate rather robust tracking of eating habits and pretty decent patient involvement in a fairly continuous manner. Oncology care veers sharply toward holistic patient-centered models suddenly and nutrition emerges as a vital therapeutic modality necessitating extensive collaboration across disciplines.

8.2. Integrating Technological Innovation into Nutritional Oncology

Digital tech converges haphazardly with nutritional science quietly reshaping oncology care landscapes eerily from behind largely unnoticed by many observers. Technology emerges nowadays as crucial enabler of data-driven nutritional interventions markedly improving outcomes and fostering collaboration pretty effectively across various disciplines. Advanced bioinformatics melds rather effectively with real-time dietary tracking optimizing efficacy of nutritional support across cancer care continuum pretty significantly. Mobile health apps and digital platforms empower patients remarkably well now tracking physical activity weight changes and symptoms rather accurately. Patient engagement and self-management are facilitated by these tools which generate copious data streams remotely for clinicians effectively monitoring nutritional status.

Digital feedback loops pretty quickly facilitate adjustments in dietary plans thereby mitigating malnutrition dehydration and nasty complications associated with various treatments. Wearable devices equipped with biosensors extensively monitor physiological parameters sporadically offering obscure insights into various fluctuating metabolic demands nowadays. Dietary data insights synergize with this nowadays facilitating much targeted nutrition interventions relatively effectively with considerable precision and some flair. Machine learning algorithms and artificial intelligence are being utilized heavily on massive datasets like electronic health records and copious molecular profiles predicting nutritional risks. Secure video conferencing and cloud-based platforms enable tele-nutrition services surmounting geographical hurdles nationwide very slowly with expanding access.

Clinical decision support systems are being developed very effectively nowadays under guidance of updated clinical guidelines and modified risk profiles. Technology evolves swiftly nowadays and integration into nutritional oncology promises markedly enhanced care coordination and enhanceed patient adherence very effectively. Key areas of integration include:

a. Wearables and Mobile Health Platforms

Digital tools effectively facilitate real-time monitoring of dietary intake and physical activity alongside various treatment-related symptoms and sleep patterns. Clinicians harness mobile apps and wearable sensors pretty effectively monitoring patient adherence dynamically adjusting nutritional plans based on physiological feedback.

b. Telehealth and Remote Nutrition Counseling

Telemedicine platforms facilitate virtual consultations between patients and care teams heavily reducing access barriers in notably underserved rural areas. Such platforms facilitate seamless care continuity and allow swift adaptation to fluctuating nutritional requirements with relative ease amidst diverse situations.

c. Artificial Intelligence and Big Data

Machine learning algorithms scrutinize copious genomic data alongside treatment outcomes and dietary logs very meticulously uncovering modified nutritional regimens often quietly. Therapeutic efficacy gets predictably enhanceed by these somewhat obscure tools which facilitate decision making and pinpoint modifiable dietary factors yielding vastly improved prognostic outcomes.

8.3. The Microbiome: A New Nexus of Collaboration

Recently gut microbiome has emerged as a critical interface between nutrition and cancer biology necessitating wildly transdisciplinary collaboration in oncology. Commensal microbes are deemed active players in host metabolism regulation and systemic inflammation suppression exhibiting wildly varying degrees of somewhat therapeutic efficacy. Microbiome modulates immune responses and influences bioavailability of certain drugs while metabolizing diverse dietary components thereby acting as pivotal cancer determinant. Turbocharged mapping of individual microbial ecosystems via recent advances in high-throughput sequencing and metagenomics reveals dysbiosis strongly linked to tumourigenesis.

Oncologists and bioinformaticians propel key initiatives forward energetically alongside microbiologists with expertise in nutrition science research. Microbiome-based diagnostics emerging slowly stratify patients crudely by response to immunotherapy or various chemotherapy regimens quite effectively nowadays. Probiotic therapies are being studied intensely these days for potentially rectifying microbial dysbiosis and encourage mucosal immune function pretty significantly. Fermented edibles and fibre-rich food are being scrutinized pretty thoroughly nowadays potentially flipping gut microbial activity towards markedly anti-carcinogenic pathways. Robust platforms integrating diverse datasets including metagenomic and genomic data alongside advanced computational tools decipher complex interactions between host and microbe under various dietary regimens. Microbiome inhabits a nebulous frontier nowadays where cutting-edge tech converges pretty interestingly with oncology and nutritional science. Unlocking microbiome informed dietary strategies' full potential in cancer care relies heavily on effectively forging synergy across various disparate domains.

8.4. Genomics and Precision Nutrition

Genomic science converges rather haphazardly with nutritional oncology heralding a novel era of precision medicine wherein dietary interventions get carefully tailored somewhat bizarrely around an individual's genetic makeup. Genetic variability and epigenetic differences profoundly impact metabolism of nutrients and responsiveness quite significantly in various cancer patients undergoing nutritional therapies. Genomic profiling enables identification of single-nucleotide polymorphisms in genes such as MTHFR, that heavily affect folate metabolism and FTO awkwardly regulates lipid metabolism. Somatic mutations reprogram cellular metabolism in tumours creating vulnerabilities like glutamine addiction which can be exploited rather effectively via specific nutrition interventions.

Epigenetic modifications such as DNA methylation or histone acetylation respond haphazardly to certain dietary compounds like methyl donors and various polyphenols. Genomic information's clinical utility precariously hinges on collaboration between nutrigenomic researchers and molecular oncologists with computational biologists in various clinical nutrition fields. Modified nutrition plans aligned eerily with genotype and tumour phenotype are developed during remarkably painstaking therapy sessions for each patient specifically. Algorithm-driven systems swiftly assimilate genomic info with dietary data providing evidence-backed suggestions fairly accurately in real time these days.

Mobile apps play a significant supporting role as digital dashboards and wearables track patient biomarkers and tweak dietary regimens very accordingly. This approach enhances therapeutic precision remarkably by situating nutritional interventions within genomic contexts and it fosters patient engagement very effectively. Genomic-informed nutrition plays a vital role nowadays in personalized oncology care effectively mitigating toxicity and various metabolic issues.

8.5. Building Collaborative Care Models

Multidisciplinary care models have become fairly imperative lately in various medical circles as cancer diagnosis complexity grows steadily nationwide. Silos of traditional approaches are getting supplanted by novel frameworks uniting diverse clinical expertise with sterling research acumen for patient-centered oncology care. Cancer outcomes depend heavily on gnarled factors like metabolic mayhem and tricky environmental stressors rather than solely on fancy pharmacological treatments. Multidisciplinary cancer centers spearhead radical transformation by implementing tumour boards and integrative care teams with specialists from various fields. Modified nutritional interventions are devised very carefully nowadays by registered dietitians for individual metabolic needs and highly personalized treatment regimens. Psychologists quite effectively alleviate emotional turmoil associated with cancer diagnoses and foggy cognitive states in many cases remarkably well.

Exercise physiologists devise rigorous exercise protocols that mitigate exhaustion and preserve considerable muscular bulk remarkably well in most individuals. Pharmacists adeptly manage polypharmacy and scrutinize nutrient-drug interactions extremely thoroughly in most cases with great precision daily. Bioinformaticians and data analysts frequently decipher complex patient data in real time informing clinical decisions somewhat irregularly nowadays. Tech-savvy healthcare gurus enable remote patient tracking largely through modified digital tools that considerably enhance user involvement nowadays. This integrative model boosts care coordination significantly and fosters shared decision-making thereby ensuring patient voice stays pretty central. Rapid exchange and testing of cross-disciplinary insights within same infrastructure enables swift translation of research into clinical practice effectively.

Collaborative models facilitate integration of nutrition science into clinical mainstream quite crucially elevating its role from supportive care to cornerstone of oncology highly personalized. Evidence accumulates rapidly on interplay between diet metabolism genomics and treatment response necessitating collaborative models for delivering next-gen precision oncology very essentially nowadays.

8.6. Challenges and Opportunities

Oncology nutrition and tech integration holds transformative potential in cancer care with significant benefits nowadays quite obviously in diverse settings. Navigating multifaceted obstacles deeply inherent across various fields necessitates collaboration pretty effectively with multiple disciplines involved simultaneously. Differing terminologies and priorities among clinicians nutritionists data scientists and technologists spawn various glaringly obvious communication barriers right upfront in various instances. Disparities like these can hinder swift decision-making pretty badly and slow down translation of innovations into practice over considerable periods. Data fragmentation and interoperability issues stubbornly present significant obstacles meanwhile posing thorny problems down line for various stakeholders. Healthcare systems often function in isolated silos with EHRs and research databases largely failing alongside various quirky digital health platforms.

Inadequate integration gravely impedes synthesizing diverse data forms such as clinical genomic nutritional and behavioral data into profoundly insightful actionable information. Training gaps awkwardly hinder efficacy of collaborative efforts rather significantly. Healthcare pros often go woefully undertrained in wildly diverse fields such as oncology and nutritional science within swiftly shifting digital health spheres. Specialists extremely adept at traversing complex intersections of multiple fields are in glaring shortage nowadays within murky waters very effectively. Bureaucratic slowness stymies adoption of unconventional therapies and novel data sharing methods within ossified institutional frameworks rather quietly. Strategic investments in areas such as holistic education initiatives foster a skilled workforce proficient in cancer care extremely effectively these days. Sorely needed over there are super fancy data platforms and wonky EHRs that facilitate analytics across multiple modes with shared digital infrastructure.

Cross-sector partnerships spur innovation among stakeholders including shady biotech firms academic institutions and healthcare systems or somewhat obscure digital health companies. Systems-level thinking will pretty thoroughly shape oncology's future by embracing highly complex facets of disease and interconnected biological behavioral aspects. Cancer care can be radically reconfigured by deeply embedding nutrition within highly collaborative frameworks and thoroughly disrupting ossified siloed thinking patterns utterly. Nutrition becomes foundational rather than ancillary in this model a pillar of cancer therapy validated through scientific rigour and enabled by emerging technologies.

9. Conclusion

Evolving nutritional oncology landscape reflects growing recognition of profound diet influence on cancer biology and treatment response quite remarkably nowadays. Scientific inquiry deepens very effectively revealing nutrition plays a crucial role in cancer prevention and therapy within systems-based approaches. Cutting-edge trends are shaping future of this field rapidly from super personalized dietary interventions and microbiome strategies to integration of fancy omics technologies. Precision nutrition will be cornerstone of future research endeavors unfolding rapidly and fueling significant clinical breakthroughs down the line eventually.

Genomics and epigenetics advances enable development of modified dietary plans according to a patient's molecular makeup and disease subtype slowly. Tailored interventions hold promise of vastly improving treatment outcomes remarkably well in cancer patient's longterm while minimizing toxicity quite effectively. Gut microbiome has emerged quite rapidly as a crucial mediator of cancer progression under numerous dietary conditions somewhat mercurially. Future cancer research probably focuses on manipulating microbiome via diet prebiotics or probiotics slowly modulating various immune responses in cancer. Pretty darn crucial technological innovations facilitate real-time monitoring of dietary intake alongside tracking patient adherence and metabolic responses effectively. Artificial intelligence infused mobile health apps and wearable devices will markedly boost data accuracy in nutritional oncology research empowering patients greatly nowadays.

Emerging paradigms bring vexing challenges quite suddenly with them and spawn fresh turmoil under surprisingly hazy circumstances. Interactions between nutrients and genes and microbiome vary hugely between individuals necessitating ridiculously long high-quality clinical trials undertaken collaboratively across many disciplines. Bridging gaps between basic science and clinical research public health policy will be essential for fully tapping enormous untapped potential of oncology nutrition. Nutritional oncology's future hinges pretty effectively on deeply insightful biology revelations merging with spot-on personalized care and some fancy tech wizardry. Researchers devise highly effective patient-centered strategies nowadays by harnessing nutrition as a potent tool in cancer treatment and recovery. Further hefty investment catapults scientific understanding forward rapidly nationwide yielding tangible gains in health outcomes eventually with marked frequency.

References

Aghajanpour M, Nazer MR, Obeidavi Z, Akbari M, Ezati P, Kor NM. Functional foods and their role in cancer prevention and health promotion: a comprehensive review. Am J Cancer Res. 2017 Apr 1;7(4):740-769. PMID: 28469951; PMCID: PMC5411786.

Al Aboud NM, Tupper C, Jialal I. Genetics, Epigenetic Mechanism. [Updated 2023 Aug 14]. In: StatPearls [Internet]. Treasure Island (FL): StatPearls Publishing; 2025 Jan-. Available from: https://www.ncbi.nlm.nih.gov/books/NBK532999/

Alsaedi S, Ogasawara M, Alarawi M, Gao X, Gojobori T. AI-powered precision medicine: utilizing genetic risk factor optimization to revolutionize healthcare. NAR Genom Bioinform. 2025 May 5;7(2):lqaf038. doi: 10.1093/nargab/lqaf038. PMID: 40330081; PMCID: PMC12051108.

Bai X, Fermandez E, Gould G, Strong R. Homozygous Deletion of Glutathione Peroxidase 1 and Aldehyde Dehydrogenase 1a1 Genes Is Not Associated with Schizophrenia-Like Behavior in Mice. J Biochem Pharmacol Res. 2013 Dec 1;1(4):228-235. PMID: 24494173; PMCID: PMC3909525.

Barker AD, Lee JSH. Translating "Big Data" in Oncology for Clinical Benefit: Progress or Paralysis. Cancer Res. 2022 Jun 6;82(11):2072-2075. doi: 10.1158/0008-5472.CAN-22-0100. PMID: 35416976; PMCID: PMC9306452.

Bhinder B, Gilvary C, Madhukar NS, Elemento O. Artificial Intelligence in Cancer Research and Precision Medicine. Cancer Discov. 2021 Apr;11(4):900-915. doi: 10.1158/2159-8290.CD-21-0090. PMID: 33811123; PMCID: PMC8034385.

Birla M, Rajan, Roy PG, Gupta I, Malik PS. Integrating Artificial Intelligence-Driven Wearable Technology in Oncology Decision-Making: A Narrative Review. Oncology. 2025;103(1):69-82. doi: 10.1159/000540494. Epub 2024 Jul 25. PMID: 39072365; PMCID: PMC11731833.

Blaževitš O, Di Tano M, Longo VD. Fasting and fasting mimicking diets in cancer prevention and therapy. Trends Cancer. 2023 Mar;9(3):212-222. doi: 10.1016/j.trecan.2022.12.006. Epub 2023 Jan 14. PMID: 36646607.

Bouyahya A, Mechchate H, Oumeslakht L, Zeouk I, Aboulaghras S, Balahbib A, Zengin G, Kamal MA, Gallo M, Montesano D, El Omari N. The Role of Epigenetic Modifications in Human Cancers and the Use of Natural Compounds as Epidrugs: Mechanistic Pathways and Pharmacodynamic Actions. Biomolecules. 2022 Feb 25;12(3):367. doi: 10.3390/biom12030367. PMID: 35327559; PMCID: PMC8945214.

Bouyahya A, Omari NE, El Hachlafi N, Jemly ME, Hakkour M, Balahbib A, El Menyiy N, Bakrim S, Naceiri Mrabti H, Khouchlaa A, Mahomoodally MF, Catauro M, Montesano D, Zengin G. Chemical Compounds of Berry-

Derived Polyphenols and Their Effects on Gut Microbiota, Inflammation, and Cancer. Molecules. 2022 May 20;27(10):3286. doi: 10.3390/molecules27103286. PMID: 35630763; PMCID: PMC9146061.

Buono R, Longo VD. Starvation, Stress Resistance, and Cancer. Trends Endocrinol Metab. 2018 Apr;29(4):271-280. doi: 10.1016/j.tem.2018.01.008. Epub 2018 Feb 17. PMID: 29463451; PMCID: PMC7477630.

Calancie L, Keyserling TC, Taillie LS, Robasky K, Patterson C, Ammerman AS, Schisler JC. TAS2R38 Predisposition to Bitter Taste Associated with Differential Changes in Vegetable Intake in Response to a Community-Based Dietary Intervention. G3 (Bethesda). 2018 May 31;8(6):2107-2119. doi: 10.1534/g3.118.300547. PMID: 29686110; PMCID: PMC5982837.

Cha RR, Sonu I. Fecal microbiota transplantation: present and future. Clin Endosc. 2025 May;58(3):352-359. doi: 10.5946/ce.2024.270. Epub 2025 Mar 25. PMID: 40468650; PMCID: PMC12138360.

Davani-Davari D, Negahdaripour M, Karimzadeh I, Seifan M, Mohkam M, Masoumi SJ, Berenjian A, Ghasemi Y. Prebiotics: Definition, Types, Sources, Mechanisms, and Clinical Applications. Foods. 2019 Mar 9;8(3):92. doi: 10.3390/foods8030092. PMID: 30857316; PMCID: PMC6463098.

David A, Lev-Ari S. Targeting the Gut Microbiome to Improve Immunotherapy Outcomes: A Review. Integr Cancer Ther. 2024 Jan-Dec;23:15347354241269870. doi: 10.1177/15347354241269870. PMID: 39223798; PMCID: PMC11369881.

Do LK, Lee HM, Ha YS, Lee CH, Kim J. Amino acids in cancer: Understanding metabolic plasticity and divergence for better therapeutic approaches. Cell Rep. 2025 Apr 22;44(4):115529. doi: 10.1016/j.celrep.2025.115529. Epub 2025 Apr 6. PMID: 40193251; PMCID: PMC12038367.

Dumitru IG, Todor SB, Ichim C, Helgiu C, Helgiu A. A Literature Review on the Impact of the Gut Microbiome on Cancer Treatment Efficacy, Disease Evolution and Toxicity: The Implications for Hematological Malignancies. J Clin Med. 2025 Apr 25;14(9):2982. doi: 10.3390/jcm14092982. PMID: 40364013; PMCID: PMC12072304.

Dutta D, Lim SH. Bidirectional interaction between intestinal microbiome and cancer: opportunities for therapeutic interventions. Biomark Res. 2020 Aug 12;8:31. doi: 10.1186/s40364-020-00211-6. PMID: 32817793; PMCID: PMC7424681.

Essa MM, Bishir M, Bhat A, Chidambaram SB, Al-Balushi B, Hamdan H, Govindarajan N, Freidland RP, Qoronfleh MW. Functional foods and their impact on health. J Food Sci Technol. 2023 Mar;60(3):820-834. doi: 10.1007/s13197-021-05193-3. Epub 2021 Jul 8. PMID: 36908338; PMCID: PMC9998796.

Farhud D, Zarif Yeganeh M, Zarif Yeganeh M. Nutrigenomics and nutrigenetics. Iran J Public Health. 2010;39(4):1-14. Epub 2010 Dec 31. PMID: 23113033; PMCID: PMC3481686.

Fenton JI, Hord NG, Ghosh S, Gurzell EA. Immunomodulation by dietary long chain omega-3 fatty acids and the potential for adverse health outcomes. Prostaglandins Leukot Essent Fatty Acids. 2013 Nov-Dec;89(6):379-90. doi: 10.1016/j.plefa.2013.09.011. Epub 2013 Sep 30. PMID: 24183073; PMCID: PMC3912985.

Fernandes MR, Aggarwal P, Costa RGF, Cole AM, Trinchieri G. Targeting the gut microbiota for cancer therapy. Nat Rev Cancer. 2022 Dec;22(12):703-722. doi: 10.1038/s41568-022-00513-x. Epub 2022 Oct 17. PMID: 36253536.

Gao J, Cahill CM, Huang X, Roffman JL, Lamon-Fava S, Fava M, Mischoulon D, Rogers JT. S-Adenosyl Methionine and Transmethylation Pathways in Neuropsychiatric Diseases Throughout Life. Neurotherapeutics. 2018 Jan;15(1):156-175. doi: 10.1007/s13311-017-0593-0. PMID: 29340929; PMCID: PMC5794704.

Gerber M, Corpet D. Energy balance and cancers. Eur J Cancer Prev. 1999 Apr;8(2):77-89. doi: 10.1097/00008469-199904000-00002. PMID: 10335454; PMCID: PMC2565800.

Golob N, Oblak T, Čavka L, Kušar M, Šeruga B. Aggressive anticancer treatment in the last 2 weeks of life. ESMO Open. 2024 Mar;9(3):102937. doi: 10.1016/j.esmoop.2024.102937. Epub 2024 Mar 11. PMID: 38471241; PMCID: PMC10944113.

Greathouse KL, Wyatt M, Johnson AJ, Toy EP, Khan JM, Dunn K, Clegg DJ, Reddy S. Diet-microbiome interactions in cancer treatment: Opportunities and challenges for precision nutrition in cancer. Neoplasia. 2022 Jul;29:100800. doi: 10.1016/j.neo.2022.100800. Epub 2022 Apr 29. PMID: 35500546; PMCID: PMC9065883.

Gregg JR, Lopez DS, Reichard C, Zheng J, Wu W, Ye Y, Chapin B, Kim J, Daniel CR, Davis J. Coffee, Caffeine Metabolism Genotype and Disease Progression in Patients with Localized Prostate Cancer Managed with Active Surveillance. J Urol. 2019 Feb;201(2):308-314. doi: 10.1016/j.juro.2018.08.048. PMID: 30179617; PMCID: PMC9798525.

Gu M, Ren B, Fang Y, Ren J, Liu X, Wang X, Zhou F, Xiao R, Luo X, You L, Zhao Y. Epigenetic regulation in cancer. MedComm (2020). 2024 Feb 19;5(2):e495. doi: 10.1002/mco2.495. PMID: 38374872; PMCID: PMC10876210.

Gyamfi J, Kim J, Choi J. Cancer as a Metabolic Disorder. Int J Mol Sci. 2022 Jan 21;23(3):1155. doi: 10.3390/ijms23031155. PMID: 35163079; PMCID: PMC8835572.

Handy DE, Castro R, Loscalzo J. Epigenetic modifications: basic mechanisms and role in cardiovascular disease. Circulation. 2011 May 17;123(19):2145-56. doi: 10.1161/CIRCULATIONAHA.110.956839. PMID: 21576679; PMCID: PMC3107542.

Hardy TM, Tollefsbol TO. Epigenetic diet: impact on the epigenome and cancer. Epigenomics. 2011 Aug;3(4):503-18. doi: 10.2217/epi.11.71. PMID: 22022340; PMCID: PMC3197720.

Hiatt RA, Clayton MF, Collins KK, Gold HT, Laiyemo AO, Truesdale KP, Ritzwoller DP. The Pathways to Prevention program: nutrition as prevention for improved cancer outcomes. J Natl Cancer Inst. 2023 Aug 8;115(8):886-895. doi: 10.1093/jnci/djad079. PMID: 37212639; PMCID: PMC10407697.

Jain N, Nagaich U, Pandey M, Chellappan DK, Dua K. Predictive genomic tools in disease stratification and targeted prevention: a recent update in personalized therapy advancements. EPMA J. 2022 Nov 12;13(4):561-580. doi: 10.1007/s13167-022-00304-2. PMID: 36505888; PMCID: PMC9727029.

Jain S, Jain PK, Puranik AK. Digital Health Technology & Cancer Care: Conceptual Framework Leading Comprehensive Fruitfulness. J Healthc Leadersh. 2024 Dec 8;16:525-535. doi: 10.2147/JHL.S486263. PMID: 39679178; PMCID: PMC11645248.

Kaphingst KA, Blanchard M, Milam L, Pokharel M, Elrick A, Goodman MS. Relationships Between Health Literacy and Genomics-Related Knowledge, Self-Efficacy, Perceived Importance, and Communication in a Medically Underserved Population. J Health Commun. 2016;21 Suppl 1(Suppl 1):58-68. doi: 10.1080/10810730.2016.1144661. PMID: 27043759; PMCID: PMC5546792.

Khan A, Barapatre AR, Babar N, Doshi J, Ghaly M, Patel KG, Nawaz S, Hasana U, Khatri SP, Pathange S, Pesaru AR, Puvvada CS, Billoo M, Jamil U. Genomic medicine and personalized treatment: a narrative review. Ann Med Surg (Lond). 2025 Feb 13;87(3):1406-1414. doi: 10.1097/MS9.0000000000002965. PMID: 40213198; PMCID: PMC11981433.

Konstantinidi M, Koutelidakis AE. Functional Foods and Bioactive Compounds: A Review of Its Possible Role on Weight Management and Obesity's Metabolic Consequences. Medicines (Basel). 2019 Sep 9;6(3):94. doi: 10.3390/medicines6030094. PMID: 31505825; PMCID: PMC6789755.

Kunzmann AT, Coleman HG, Huang WY, Kitahara CM, Cantwell MM, Berndt SI. Dietary fiber intake and risk of colorectal cancer and incident and recurrent adenoma in the Prostate, Lung, Colorectal, and Ovarian Cancer Screening Trial. Am J Clin Nutr. 2015 Oct;102(4):881-90. doi: 10.3945/ajcn.115.113282. Epub 2015 Aug 12. PMID: 26269366; PMCID: PMC4588743.

Lee HS. Impact of Maternal Diet on the Epigenome during In Utero Life and the Developmental Programming of Diseases in Childhood and Adulthood. Nutrients. 2015 Nov 17;7(11):9492-507. doi: 10.3390/nu7115467. PMID: 26593940; PMCID: PMC4663595.

Leonard JM, Toro DD. Defining the Microbiome Components (Bacteria, Viruses, Fungi) and Microbiome Geodiversity. Surg Infect (Larchmt). 2023 Apr;24(3):208-212. doi: 10.1089/sur.2023.014. PMID: 37010972; PMCID: PMC10061322.

Li L, Yang Z, Yi Y, Song Y, Zhang W. Gut microbiota and radiation-induced injury: mechanistic insights and microbial therapies. Gut Microbes. 2025 Dec;17(1):2528429. doi: 10.1080/19490976.2025.2528429. Epub 2025 Jul 6. PMID: 40618373; PMCID: PMC12233896.

Li T, Copeland C, Le A. Glutamine Metabolism in Cancer. 2021 May 21. In: Le A, editor. The Heterogeneity of Cancer Metabolism [Internet]. 2nd edition. Cham (CH): Springer; 2021. Available from: https://www.ncbi.nlm.nih.gov/books/NBK573682/ doi: 10.1007/978-3-030-65768-0_2

Li Z, Zhang H. Reprogramming of glucose, fatty acid and amino acid metabolism for cancer progression. Cell Mol Life Sci. 2016 Jan;73(2):377-92. doi: 10.1007/s00018-015-2070-4. Epub 2015 Oct 23. PMID: 26499846; PMCID: PMC11108301.

Ling H, Fabbri M, Calin GA. MicroRNAs and other non-coding RNAs as targets for anticancer drug development. Nat Rev Drug Discov. 2013 Nov;12(11):847-65. doi: 10.1038/nrd4140. PMID: 24172333; PMCID: PMC4548803.

López-Gómez L, Alcorta A, Abalo R. Probiotics and Probiotic-like Agents against Chemotherapy-Induced Intestinal Mucositis: A Narrative Review. J Pers Med. 2023 Oct 12;13(10):1487. doi: 10.3390/jpm13101487. PMID: 37888098; PMCID: PMC10607965.

Martin SE, Kraft CS, Ziegler TR, Millson EC, Rishishwar L, Martin GS. The Role of Diet on the Gut Microbiome, Mood and Happiness. medRxiv [Preprint]. 2023 Mar 21:2023.03.18.23287442. doi: 10.1101/2023.03.18.23287442. PMID: 36993403; PMCID: PMC10055576.

Marzola E, Nasser JA, Hashim SA, Shih PA, Kaye WH. Nutritional rehabilitation in anorexia nervosa: review of the literature and implications for treatment. BMC Psychiatry. 2013 Nov 7;13:290. doi: 10.1186/1471-244X-13-290. PMID: 24200367; PMCID: PMC3829207.

Masood W, Annamaraju P, Khan Suheb MZ, et al. Ketogenic Diet. [Updated 2023 Jun 16]. In: StatPearls [Internet]. Treasure Island (FL): StatPearls Publishing; 2025 Jan-. Available from: https://www.ncbi.nlm.nih.gov/books/NBK499830/

Matson V, Chervin CS, Gajewski TF. Cancer and the Microbiome-Influence of the Commensal Microbiota on Cancer, Immune Responses, and Immunotherapy. Gastroenterology. 2021 Jan;160(2):600-613. doi: 10.1053/j.gastro.2020.11.041. Epub 2020 Nov 28. PMID: 33253684; PMCID: PMC8409239.

Meeran SM, Ahmed A, Tollefsbol TO. Epigenetic targets of bioactive dietary components for cancer prevention and therapy. Clin Epigenetics. 2010 Dec 1;1(3-4):101-116. doi: 10.1007/s13148-010-0011-5. PMID: 21258631; PMCID: PMC3024548.

Molla G, Bitew M. Revolutionizing Personalized Medicine: Synergy with Multi-Omics Data Generation, Main Hurdles, and Future Perspectives. Biomedicines. 2024 Nov 30;12(12):2750. doi: 10.3390/biomedicines12122750. PMID: 39767657; PMCID: PMC11673561.

Nagy S, Petrosky SN, Demory Beckler M, Kesselman MM. The Impact of Modern Dietary Practices on Cancer Risk and Progression: A Systematic Review. Cureus. 2023 Oct 7;15(10):e46639. doi: 10.7759/cureus.46639. PMID: 37937022; PMCID: PMC10627144.

Nencioni A, Caffa I, Cortellino S, Longo VD. Fasting and cancer: molecular mechanisms and clinical application. Nat Rev Cancer. 2018 Nov;18(11):707-719. doi: 10.1038/s41568-018-0061-0. PMID: 30327499; PMCID: PMC6938162.

Nicastro HL, Trujillo EB, Milner JA. Nutrigenomics and Cancer Prevention. Curr Nutr Rep. 2012 Mar 1;1(1):37-43. doi: 10.1007/s13668-011-0007-6. PMID: 24910810; PMCID: PMC4047824.

Ozaki Y, Broughton P, Abdollahi H, Valafar H, Blenda AV. Integrating Omics Data and AI for Cancer Diagnosis and

Prognosis. Cancers (Basel). 2024 Jul 3;16(13):2448. doi: 10.3390/cancers16132448. PMID: 39001510; PMCID: PMC11240413.

Padin AC, Hébert JR, Woody A, Wilson SJ, Shivappa N, Belury MA, Malarkey WB, Sheridan JF, Kiecolt-Glaser JK. A proinflammatory diet is associated with inflammatory gene expression among healthy, non-obese adults: Can social ties protect against the risks? Brain Behav Immun. 2019 Nov;82:36-44. doi: 10.1016/j.bbi.2019.07.031. Epub 2019 Jul 26. PMID: 31356923; PMCID: PMC6800628.

Park JH, Yoo Y, Park YJ. Epigenetics: Linking Nutrition to Molecular Mechanisms in Aging. Prev Nutr Food Sci. 2017 Jun;22(2):81-89. doi: 10.3746/pnf.2017.22.2.81. Epub 2017 Jun 30. PMID: 28702424; PMCID: PMC5503416.

Pérez Guerra N. The Impact of Probiotics, Prebiotics, and Functional Foods on Human Health. Nutrients. 2025 Apr 30;17(9):1529. doi: 10.3390/nu17091529. PMID: 40362839; PMCID: PMC12073198.

Peterson SN, Bradley LM, Ronai ZA. The gut microbiome: an unexpected player in cancer immunity. Curr Opin Neurobiol. 2020 Jun;62:48-52. doi: 10.1016/j.conb.2019.09.016. Epub 2019 Dec 6. PMID: 31816571; PMCID: PMC7274858.

Phan LM, Yeung SC, Lee MH. Cancer metabolic reprogramming: importance, main features, and potentials for precise targeted anti-cancer therapies. Cancer Biol Med. 2014 Mar;11(1):1-19. doi: 10.7497/j.issn.2095-3941.2014.01.001. PMID: 24738035; PMCID: PMC3969803.

Qian L, Zhang F, Yin M, Lei Q. Cancer metabolism and dietary interventions. Cancer Biol Med. 2022 Dec 22;19(2):163–74. doi: 10.20892/j.issn.2095-3941.2021.0461. PMID: 34931768; PMCID: PMC8832959.

Rahman A, Debnath T, Kundu D, Khan MSI, Aishi AA, Sazzad S, Sayduzzaman M, Band SS. Machine learning and deep learning-based approach in smart healthcare: Recent advances, applications, challenges and opportunities. AIMS Public Health. 2024 Jan 5;11(1):58-109. doi: 10.3934/publichealth.2024004. PMID: 38617415; PMCID: PMC11007421.

Ratti M, Lampis A, Ghidini M, Salati M, Mirchev MB, Valeri N, Hahne JC. MicroRNAs (miRNAs) and Long Non-Coding RNAs (lncRNAs) as New Tools for Cancer Therapy: First Steps from Bench to Bedside. Target Oncol. 2020 Jun;15(3):261-278. doi: 10.1007/s11523-020-00717-x. PMID: 32451752; PMCID: PMC7283209.

Reuter S, Gupta SC, Park B, Goel A, Aggarwal BB. Epigenetic changes induced by curcumin and other natural compounds. Genes Nutr. 2011 May;6(2):93-108. doi: 10.1007/s12263-011-0222-1. Epub 2011 Apr 24. PMID: 21516481; PMCID: PMC3092901.

Sebastian AM, Peter D. Artificial Intelligence in Cancer Research: Trends, Challenges and Future Directions. Life (Basel). 2022 Nov 28;12(12):1991. doi: 10.3390/life12121991. PMID: 36556356; PMCID: PMC9786074.

Sedley L. Advances in Nutritional Epigenetics-A Fresh Perspective for an Old Idea. Lessons Learned, Limitations, and Future Directions. Epigenet Insights. 2020 Dec 18;13:2516865720981924. doi: 10.1177/2516865720981924. PMID: 33415317; PMCID: PMC7750768.

Shams M, Abdallah S, Alsadoun L, Hamid YH, Gasim R, Hassan A. Oncological Horizons: The Synergy of Medical and Surgical Innovations in Cancer Treatment. Cureus. 2023 Nov 22;15(11):e49249. doi: 10.7759/cureus.49249. PMID: 38143618; PMCID: PMC10743204.

Shankar S, Kumar D, Srivastava RK. Epigenetic modifications by dietary phytochemicals: implications for personalized nutrition. Pharmacol Ther. 2013 Apr;138(1):1-17. doi: 10.1016/j.pharmthera.2012.11.002. Epub 2012 Nov 16. PMID: 23159372; PMCID: PMC4153856.

Sharma P, Dwivedi S. Nutrigenomics and Nutrigenetics: New Insight in Disease Prevention and Cure. Indian J Clin Biochem. 2017 Oct;32(4):371-373. doi: 10.1007/s12291-017-0699-5. Epub 2017 Sep 22. PMID: 29062169; PMCID: PMC5634986.

Silbermann M, Pitsillides B, Al-Alfi N, Omran S, Al-Jabri K, Elshamy K, Ghrayeb I, Livneh J, Daher M, Charalambous H, Jafferri A, Fink R, El-Shamy M. Multidisciplinary care team for cancer patients and its implementation in several Middle Eastern countries. Ann Oncol. 2013 Oct;24 Suppl 7(Suppl 7):vii41-47. doi: 10.1093/annonc/mdt265. PMID: 24001762; PMCID: PMC3767159.

Singar S, Nagpal R, Arjmandi BH, Akhavan NS. Personalized Nutrition: Tailoring Dietary Recommendations through Genetic Insights. Nutrients. 2024 Aug 13;16(16):2673. doi: 10.3390/nu16162673. PMID: 39203810; PMCID: PMC11357412.

Son MY, Cho HS. Anticancer Effects of Gut Microbiota-Derived Short-Chain Fatty Acids in Cancers. J Microbiol Biotechnol. 2023 Jul 28;33(7):849-856. doi: 10.4014/jmb.2301.01031. Epub 2023 Mar 30. PMID: 37100764; PMCID: PMC10394342.

Su LJ, Mahabir S, Ellison GL, McGuinn LA, Reid BC. Epigenetic Contributions to the Relationship between Cancer and Dietary Intake of Nutrients, Bioactive Food Components, and Environmental Toxicants. Front Genet. 2012 Jan 9;2:91. doi: 10.3389/fgene.2011.00091. PMID: 22303385; PMCID: PMC3266615.

Supic G, Jagodic M, Magic Z. Epigenetics: a new link between nutrition and cancer. Nutr Cancer. 2013;65(6):781-92. doi: 10.1080/01635581.2013.805794. PMID: 23909721.

Talib WH, Mahmod AI, Kamal A, Rashid HM, Alashqar AMD, Khater S, Jamal D, Waly M. Ketogenic Diet in Cancer Prevention and Therapy: Molecular Targets and Therapeutic Opportunities. Curr Issues Mol Biol. 2021 Jul 3;43(2):558-589. doi: 10.3390/cimb43020042. PMID: 34287243; PMCID: PMC8928964.

Tan PY, Moore JB, Bai L, Tang G, Gong YY. In the context of the triple burden of malnutrition: A systematic review of gene-diet interactions and nutritional status. Crit Rev Food Sci Nutr. 2024;64(11):3235-3263. doi: 10.1080/10408398.2022.2131727. Epub 2022 Oct 12. PMID: 36222100; PMCID: PMC11000749.

Tan-Shalaby J. Ketogenic Diets and Cancer: Emerging Evidence. Fed Pract. 2017 Feb;34(Suppl 1):37S-42S. PMID: 30766299; PMCID: PMC6375425.

Thapa D, Kumar V, Naik B, Kumar V, Gupta AK, Mohanta YK, Mishra B, Rustagi S. Harnessing probiotic foods: managing cancer through gut health. Food Sci Biotechnol. 2024 Jun 28;33(9):2141-2160. doi: 10.1007/s10068-024-01638-5. PMID: 39130664; PMCID: PMC11315834.

Wang H, Bian S, Yang CS. Green tea polyphenol EGCG suppresses lung cancer cell growth through upregulating miR-210 expression caused by stabilizing HIF-1α. Carcinogenesis. 2011 Dec;32(12):1881-9. doi: 10.1093/carcin/bgr218. Epub 2011 Sep 28. PMID: 21965273; PMCID: PMC3220612.

Wang X, Sun Z, Xue H, An R. Artificial Intelligence Applications to Personalized Dietary Recommendations: A Systematic Review. Healthcare (Basel). 2025 Jun 13;13(12):1417. doi: 10.3390/healthcare13121417. PMID: 40565444; PMCID: PMC12193492.

Wang X, Zeng H, Li L, Fang Z, Xu L, Shi W, Li J, Qian J, Tan X, Li J, Qian Y, Xie L. Personalized nutrition intervention improves nutritional status and quality of life of colorectal cancer survivors in the community: A randomized controlled trial. Nutrition. 2022 Nov-Dec;103-104:111835. doi: 10.1016/j.nut.2022.111835. Epub 2022 Aug 28. PMID: 36183482.

Wang Z, Li L, Wang S, Wei J, Qu L, Pan L, Xu K. The role of the gut microbiota and probiotics associated with microbial metabolisms in cancer prevention and therapy. Front Pharmacol. 2022 Nov 14;13:1025860. doi: 10.3389/fphar.2022.1025860. PMID: 36452234; PMCID: PMC9702994.

Wei W, Sun W, Yu S, Yang Y, Ai L. Butyrate production from high-fiber diet protects against lymphoma tumor. Leuk Lymphoma. 2016 Oct;57(10):2401-8. doi: 10.3109/10428194.2016.1144879. Epub 2016 Feb 17. PMID: 26885564.

Woo V, Alenghat T. Epigenetic regulation by gut microbiota. Gut Microbes. 2022 Jan-Dec;14(1):2022407. doi: 10.1080/19490976.2021.2022407. PMID: 35000562; PMCID: PMC8744890.

Xia H, Wang L, Wang H. Current research trends, hotspots, and frontiers of medical nutrition therapy on cancer: a bibliometric analysis. Front Oncol. 2023 May 5;13:1170198. doi: 10.3389/fonc.2023.1170198. PMID: 37213299; PMCID: PMC10196469.

Xu Y, Gao Z, Liu J, Yang Q, Xu S. Role of gut microbiome in suppression of cancers. Gut Microbes. 2025 Dec;17(1):2495183. doi: 10.1080/19490976.2025.2495183. Epub 2025 Apr 20. PMID: 40254597; PMCID: PMC12013426.

Yang SY, Han SM, Lee JY, Kim KS, Lee JE, Lee DW. Advancing Gut Microbiome Research: The Shift from Metagenomics to Multi-Omics and Future Perspectives. J Microbiol Biotechnol. 2025 Mar 26;35:e2412001. doi: 10.4014/jmb.2412.12001. PMID: 40223273; PMCID: PMC12010094.

Zamani MR, Šácha P. Immune checkpoint inhibitors in cancer therapy: what lies beyond monoclonal antibodies? Med Oncol. 2025 Jun 19;42(7):273. doi: 10.1007/s12032-025-02822-1. PMID: 40536609; PMCID: PMC12178997.

Zhang G, Liu X, Zeng Y. Advancements in oncology nursing: Embracing technology-driven innovations. Asia Pac J Oncol Nurs. 2024 Feb 8;11(3):100399. doi: 10.1016/j.apjon.2024.100399. PMID: 38465238; PMCID: PMC10920149.

Zhang J, Lacroix C, Wortmann E, Ruscheweyh HJ, Sunagawa S, Sturla SJ, Schwab C. Gut microbial beta-glucuronidase and glycerol/diol dehydratase activity contribute to dietary heterocyclic amine biotransformation. BMC Microbiol. 2019 May 16;19(1):99. doi: 10.1186/s12866-019-1483-x. PMID: 31096909; PMCID: PMC6524314.

Zhang M, Zhang Q, Huang S, Lu Y, Peng M. Impact of ketogenic diets on cancer patient outcomes: a systematic review and meta-analysis. Front Nutr. 2025 Jul 18;12:1535921. doi: 10.3389/fnut.2025.1535921. PMID: 40756563; PMCID: PMC12313497.

Zhao LY, Mei JX, Yu G, Lei L, Zhang WH, Liu K, Chen XL, Kołat D, Yang K, Hu JK. Role of the gut microbiota in anticancer therapy: from molecular mechanisms to clinical applications. Signal Transduct Target Ther. 2023 May 13;8(1):201. doi: 10.1038/s41392-023-01406-7. PMID: 37179402; PMCID: PMC10183032.

For Product Safety Concerns and Information please contact our EU representative GPSR@taylorandfrancis.com
Taylor & Francis Verlag GmbH, Kaufingerstraße 24, 80331 München, Germany

www.ingramcontent.com/pod-product-compliance
Ingram Content Group UK Ltd.
Pitfield, Milton Keynes, MK11 3LW, UK
UKHW052224190926
475702UK00007B/1186

* 9 7 8 1 0 4 1 3 7 1 6 4 9 *